online and in-print Internet
directories in medicine

ENDOCRINOLOGY & METABOLISM

MARCH 2001 — FEBRUARY 2002

AN INTERNET RESOURCE GUIDE

CONSULTING EDITOR
Paul W. Ladenson, M.D.

*John Eager Howard Professor
of Endocrinology and Metabolism*

*Director, Division of Endocrinology and Metabolism
Johns Hopkins University School of Medicine*

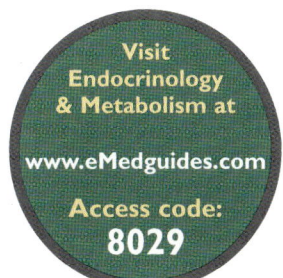

eMedguides.com, Inc., Princeton, New Jersey

© 2001 eMedguides.com, Inc.
eMedguides.com, Inc.
Princeton, NJ 08543

All rights reserved. No part of this book may be reproduced in any form by any electronic or mechanical means (including photocopying, recording, or information storage and retrieval) without permission in writing from the publisher.

For electronic browsing of this book, see
http://www.eMedguides.com/endocrinology

The publisher offers discounts on the eMedguides series of books. For more information, contact:

Sales Department
eMedguides.com, Inc.
P.O. Box 2331
Princeton, NJ 08543
tel   800-230-1481
fax   609-520-2023
e-mail sales@eMedguides.com
web   http://www.eMedguides.com/books

This book is set in Avenir, Gill Sans, and Sabon typefaces and was printed and bound in the United States of America.

10 9 8 7 6 5 4 3 2 1

ISBN 0-9700525-1-0

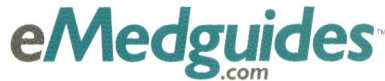

ENDOCRINOLOGY & METABOLISM
AN INTERNET RESOURCE GUIDE

Daniel R. Goldenson
Publisher

Paul W. Ladenson, M.D.
*Consulting Editor,
Director,
Division of Endocrinology and Metabolism,
Johns Hopkins University School of Medicine*

Karen M. Albert, MLS
*Consulting Medical Librarian,
Director of Library Services,
Fox Chase Cancer Center*

Alysa M. Wilson
Editor-in-Chief

Adam T. Bromwich
Managing Editor

Sue Bannon
Designer

eMEDGUIDES.COM

Raymond C. Egan
Chairman of the Board

Daniel R. Goldenson
President

Adam T. Bromwich
Chief Operating Officer

Raymond Egan, Jr.
Marketing Director

P.O. Box 2331
Princeton, NJ 08543-2331
Book orders 800.230.1481
Facsimile   609.520.2023
E-mail   endocrinology@eMedguides.com
Web   http://www.eMedguides.com/endocrinology

2001 ANNUAL EDITION

Anesthesiology & Pain Management
Arthritis & Rheumatology
Cardiology
Dental Medicine
Dermatology
Diet & Nutrition
Emergency Medicine
Endocrinology & Metabolism
Family Medicine
Gastroenterology
General Surgery
Infectious Diseases & Immunology
Internal Medicine
Neurology & Neuroscience
Obstetrics & Gynecology
Oncology & Hematology
Ophthalmology
Orthopedics & Sports Medicine
Otolaryngology
Pathology & Laboratory Medicine
Pediatrics
Physical Medicine & Rehabilitation
Plastic Surgery
Psychiatry
Radiology
Respiratory & Pulmonary Medicine
Urology & Nephrology
Veterinary Medicine

Disclaimer

eMedguides.com, Inc., hereafter referred to as the "publisher," has developed this book for informational purposes only, and not as a source of medical advice. The publisher does not guarantee the accuracy, adequacy, timeliness, or completeness of any information in this book and is not responsible for any errors or omissions or any consequences arising from the use of the information contained in this book. The material provided is general in nature and is in summary form. The content of this book is not intended in any way to be a substitute for professional medical advice. One should always seek the advice of a physician or other qualified healthcare provider. Further, one should never disregard medical advice or delay in seeking it because of information found through an Internet Web site included in this book. The use of the eMedguides.com, Inc. book is at the reader's own risk.

All information contained in this book is subject to change. Mention of a specific product, company, organization, Web site URL address, treatment, therapy, or any other topic does not imply a recommendation or endorsement by the publisher.

Non-liability

The publisher does not assume any liability for the contents of this book or the contents of any material provided at the Internet sites, companies, and organizations reviewed in this book. Moreover, the publisher assumes no liability or responsibility for damage or injury to persons or property arising from the publication and use of this book; the use of those products, services, information, ideas, or instructions contained in the material provided at the third-party Internet Web sites, companies, and organizations listed in this book; or any loss of profit or commercial damage including but not limited to special, incidental, consequential, or any other damages in connection with or arising out of the publication and use of this book. Use of third-party Web sites is subject to the Terms and Conditions of use for such sites.

Copyright Protection

Information available over the Internet and other online locations may be subject to copyright and other rights owned by third parties. Online availability of text and images does not imply that they may be reused without the permission of rights holders. Care should be taken to ensure that all necessary rights are cleared prior to reusing material distributed over the Internet and other online locations.

Trademark Protection

The words in this book for which we have reason to believe trademark, service mark, or other proprietary rights may exist have been designated as such by use of initial capitalization. However, no attempt has been made to designate as trademarks or service marks all personal computer words or terms in which proprietary rights might exist. The inclusion, exclusion, or definition of a word or term is not intended to affect, or to express any judgment on, the validity or legal status of any proprietary right that may be claimed in that word or term.

VISIT US ON THE INTERNET

Instant access to all of our selected Web sites at http://www.eMedguides.com

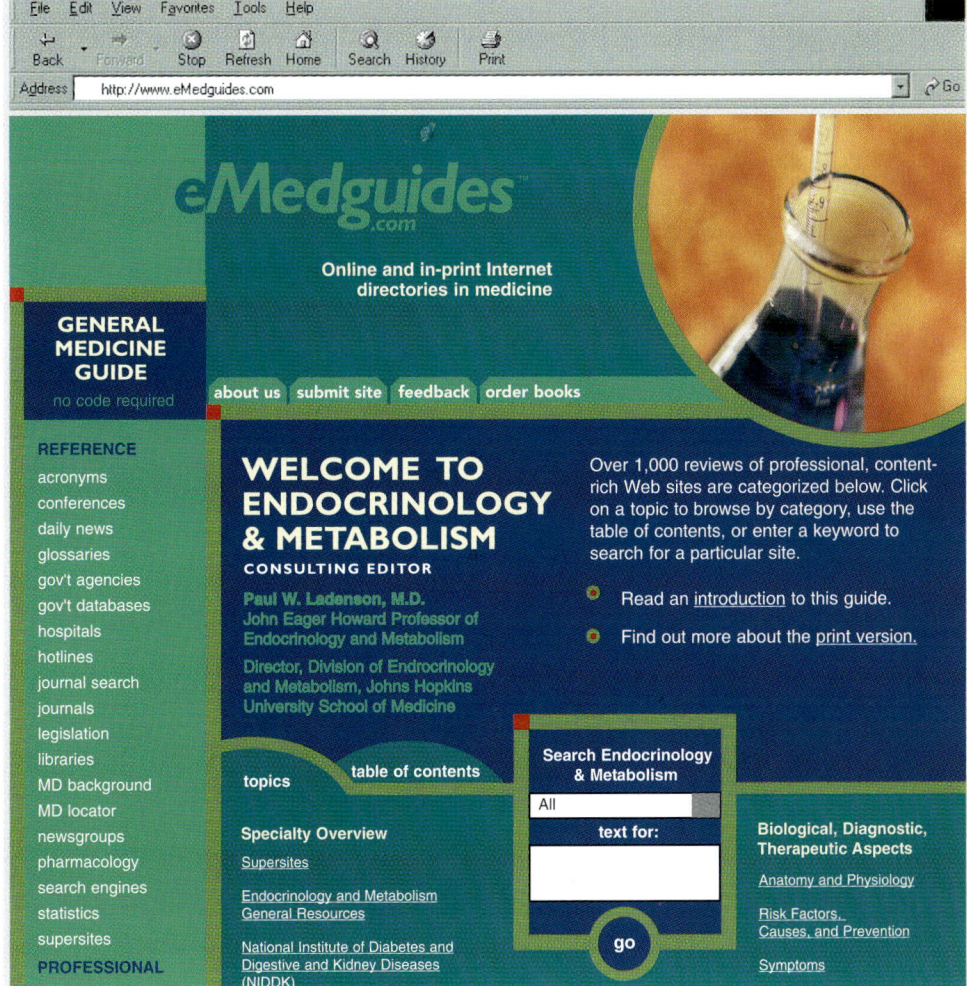

Each print edition is online, *in its entirety*, so you can browse with your mouse, never typing in a single Web address. Simply visit http://www.eMedguides.com, click the appropriate specialty, enter your access code (printed in a circle on the title page), and you are presented with every site, listed by topic. Browse through the book online, or enter a keyword term to search the entire specialty.

Visit us often—we are continually adding new sites to each specialty database!

- Surf straight to selected Web sites in the medical topic of your choice.

- Read the latest medical headlines in *your* specialty.

- Check out the latest issue of up to 100 journals in your field.

- Use over 50 medical search engines to research information in any field.

Summary Table of Contents

INTRODUCTION 3
  Ratings and Site Selection 5
  Getting Online 6

PART ONE ENDOCRINOLOGY & METABOLISM WEB RESOURCES

2. Quick Reference 13
3. Journals, Articles, and Latest Books 21
4. Continuing Medical Education (CME) 49
5. Overview Sites 55

PART TWO BIOLOGICAL, DIAGNOSTIC, AND THERAPEUTIC RESOURCES

6. Anatomy and Physiology 67
7. Diagnostics and Monitoring 87
8. Therapeutic Procedures and Surgery 123
9. Pharmacology 141
10. Pathology and Case Studies 167
11. Clinical Practice & Guidelines ..171

PART THREE TOPICAL RESOURCES AND ORGANIZATIONS

12. Public Health and Policy Topics 177
13. Subspecialty Topics 199
14. Other Topical Resources 209
15. Organizations and Institutions ..215

PART FOUR DISORDERS OF ENDOCRINOLOGY & METABOLISM

16. General Resources 261
17. Neuroendocrine System 263
18. Thyroid Gland 273
19. Adrenal Glands 291
10. Gastrointestinal Tract 301
21. Female Endocrinology 307
22. Male Endocrinology 315
23. Development and Sexual Differentiation 327
24. Bone and Mineral Metabolism ..335
25. Vitamin and Trace Mineral Deficiencies 351
26. Fluid, Electrolyte, and Acid-Base Metabolism 353
27. Diabetes Mellitus 359
28. Energy Metabolism 373
29. Lipoprotein and Cholesterol Metabolism 377
30. Metabolism, Inborn Errors 385
31. Paraendocrine and Neoplastic Syndromes 411
32. Polyendocrine Disorders 415
33. Systemic Diseases: Endocrine Manifestations 417
34. Rare Disorders 421

PART FIVE GENERAL MEDICAL WEB RESOURCES

35. Reference Information and News Sources 425
36. Professional Topics and Clinical Practice 475
37. Student Resources 499
38. Patient Education & Planning ..505

39. Web Site and Topical Index 531

Table of Contents

FOREWORD **1**

1. INTRODUCTION **3**

1.1 Welcome to eMedguides 3
*How to Benefit
  Most from this Book* 4
*The Benefits of Both
  Print and Online Editions* 5
Accessing the Online Edition ... 5
1.2 Ratings and Site Selection 5
Site Selection Criteria 5
Ratings Guide 6
Abbreviations 6
1.3 Getting Online 6

**PART ONE   ENDOCRINOLOGY
            & METABOLISM
            WEB RESOURCES**

2. QUICK REFERENCE **13**

2.1 Endocrinology
    Disease Profiles 13
2.2 Endocrinology Glossaries 14
2.3 Topical Search Tools 15
2.4 Endocrinology News 16
2.5 Conferences................ 17
2.6 Statistics 17
2.7 Clinical Studies and Trials 18
2.8 Approved and Developmental
    Therapeutic Agents 19

**3. JOURNALS, ARTICLES,
    AND LATEST BOOKS** **21**

3.1 Abstract, Citation,
    and Full-text Search Tools 21

3.2 Journals on the Internet...... 22
*Selected Articles
  and Commentaries* 22
Individual Journal Web Sites .. 22
3.3 Books on Endocrinology
    Published in 1999/2000 39

**4. CONTINUING MEDICAL
    EDUCATION (CME)** **49**

5. OVERVIEW SITES **55**

5.1 Supersites 55
5.2 General Resources 57
5.3 National Institute of
    Diabetes and Digestive and
    Kidney Diseases (NIDDK).... 58
NIDDK Web Site Features 58
Intramural Research 60
Extramural Research 60
Health Education Programs... 61
5.4 Other Government
    Agencies and Programs 62

**PART TWO   BIOLOGICAL,
            DIAGNOSTIC,
            AND THERAPEUTIC
            RESOURCES**

**6. ANATOMY
    AND PHYSIOLOGY** **67**

6.1 General Principles 67
6.2 Hormones................. 69
Biochemical Categories 69
Endocrine Rhythms 70
*Feedback Control
  in Endocrine Systems*....... 70

Over 5 Million Prescriptions Dispensed*

Impressive Glycemic Control That Lasts

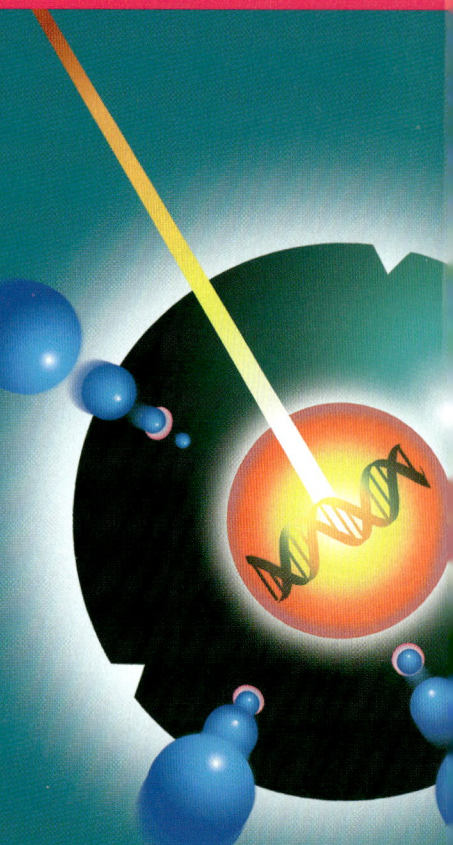

▶ **Provides long-lasting control versus glyburide**

▶ **Enhances efficacy in combination with sulfonylureas or metformin**

▶ **Substantial reductions as monotherapy**

▶ **Important clinical considerations**

- **Liver monitoring:** Recommended at baseline, every 2 months for the first 12 months, and periodically thereafter. *Avandia* should not be initiated in patients with clinical evidence of active liver disease or ALT >2.5X the upper limit of normal

- **Fluid retention:** Since thiazolidinediones can cause fluid retention, which can exacerbate congestive heart failure, patients at risk (particularly those on insulin) should be watched for signs/symptoms of heart failure†

- **Hypoglycemia:** Patients receiving *Avandia* in combination with a sulfonylurea may be at risk, and a reduction in the sulfonylurea dose may be necessary

- **Anemia:** In clinical trials, the frequency was greater with the combination of *Avandia* plus metformin (7.1%) compared to metformin alone (2.2%). Lower pretreatment hemoglobin/hematocrit levels may have contributed to this higher reporting rate

* Scott-Levin SPA, August 2000.
† *Avandia* is not indicated for use in combination with insulin.

Please see Appendix A at the end of this book for complete prescribing information.

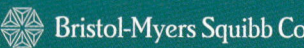
SmithKline Beecham Pharmaceuticals
Philadelphia, PA 19101

Bristol-Myers Squibb Company

Avandia is a registered trademark of SmithKline Beecham.
AV7636   © SmithKline Beecham, 2000

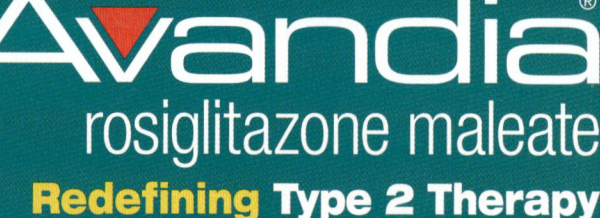
Avandia®
rosiglitazone maleate
Redefining Type 2 Therapy

	Mechanisms of Action 71
	Synthesis,
	Storage, and Release 71
6.3	Neuroendocrine System. 72
	General Resources 72
	Hypothalamic-Pituitary
	Hormones and Function 73
	Pineal Gland
	and Melatonin Physiology . . . 77
6.4	Thyroid Gland. 77
6.5	Adrenal Glands 78
6.6	Kidney. 79
6.7	Gastrointestinal Tract 79
6.8	Reproductive Organs 80
	Ovaries and
	Female Reproductive Tract . . 80
	Testes 80
6.9	Bone and
	Mineral Metabolism 81
	Bone Physiology 81
	Calcium, Vitamin D,
	and Parathyroid Hormone . . . 81
	Parathyroid Gland A
	natomy and Physiology 82
6.10	Energy Metabolism 82
	Cellular Metabolism:
	General 82
	Cellular Metabolism:
	Carbohydrate 83
	Cellular Metabolism: Lipid . . . 83
	Cellular Metabolism: Protein. . 84
	Cholesterol and
	Lipoprotein Metabolism 84
	Metabolic Regulation 84
	Pancreatic Anatomy
	and Physiology 85

7.	**DIAGNOSTICS AND MONITORING. 87**
7.1	General Endocrinology Tests . . 87
	General Resources 87

	Genetic Tests. 88
	Overview of Dynamic
	Tests in Endocrinology 90
7.2	Hypothalamic-
	Pituitary Testing 91
	General Resources 91
	Antidiuretic
	Hormone Testing 92
	Follicle-
	Stimulating Hormone 92
	Growth Hormone 92
	Prolactin 93
	Imaging. 93
	Inferior Petrosal
	Sinus Sampling 93
	Stimulation Testing 94
	Suppression Testing. 95
7.3	Thyroid Gland. 96
	General Resources 96
	Imaging. 97
	Immunoassays. 98
	Thyroid Biopsy 99
	Thyroid Function Tests 100
7.4	Adrenal Glands 100
	ACTH Stimulation Test. . . . 100
	Dexamethasone
	Suppression Testing. 101
	Hormones 101
	Hypertension
	Evaluation, Adrenal. 102
	Imaging. 103
	Urine Free Cortisol 104
7.5	Kidney. 104
	Blood Urea Nitrogen 104
	Creatinine 105
	Imaging. 105
7.6	Gastrointestinal Tract 106
	Imaging. 106
	Tests 107
7.7	Reproductive Glands 108
	Gonadal Hormone Tests 108
	Imaging. 109

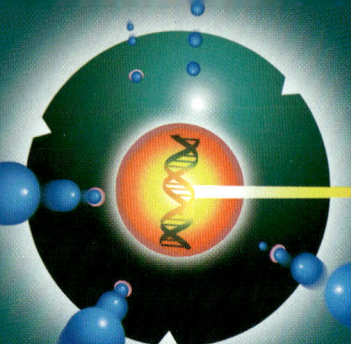

Compared to metformin or sulfonylureas...

AVANDIA® Works Differently

▶ **The primary effect of AVANDIA® is to improve insulin sensitivity in peripheral tissues**[1-4]

Avandia	Metformin	Insulin Secretagogues
Skeletal Muscle/Adipose Tissue	**Liver**	**Pancreas**
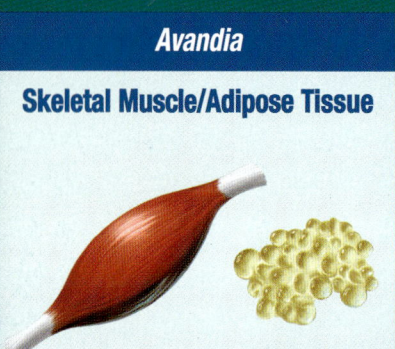	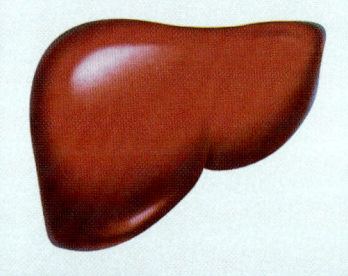	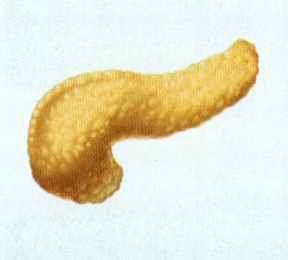
↑ Insulin Sensitivity/ Peripheral Glucose Uptake	↓ Glucose Production	↑ Insulin Secretion
Primary effect: Thiazolidinediones[5] Secondary effect: Metformin	Primary effect: Metformin Secondary effect: Thiazolidinediones	Primary effect: Sulfonylureas, Meglitinides

▶ **AVANDIA® exhibits powerful insulin-sensitizing effects**[2]

- Thiazolidinediones (TZDs) work primarily by increasing the rate of glucose disposal in **peripheral tissues** whereas metformin acts primarily by decreasing glucose production **in the liver**[3,4]*

* Both studies discuss the TZD, troglitazone, which is no longer available in the US.

References:
1. Jabbour SA, Goldstein BJ. Improving disease management with new treatments for type 2 diabetes mellitus. *Clin Geriatr.* 2000;8:44-56.
2. *Avandia* [package insert]. Philadelphia, Pa: SmithKline Beecham Pharmaceuticals; 2000.
3. Inzucchi SE, Maggs DG, Spollet GR, et al. Efficacy and metabolic effects of metformin and troglitazone in type II diabetes mellitus. *N Engl J Med.* 1998;338:867-871.
4. Yu JG, Kruszynska YT, Mulford MI, Olefsky JM. A comparison of troglitazone and metformin on insulin requirements in euglycemic intensively insulin-treated type 2 diabetic patients. *Diabetes.* 1999;48:2414-2421.
5. Data on file, SmithKline Beecham Pharmaceuticals, 2000.
6. Scott-Levin data, September 2000.

And Provides Convenient Once-daily Dosing

▶ **Low incidence of hypoglycemia as monotherapy**

▶ **Low occurrence of GI upset as monotherapy**

▶ **Simple and convenient once daily**
- 4 mg qd—the most commonly prescribed dose[6]
- May be dosed bid for convenience with concomitant dosing schedules

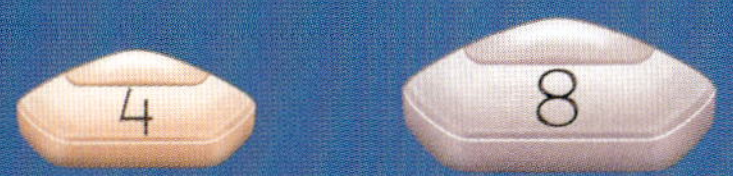

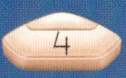
4 mg qd

8 mg qd

▶ **Important clinical considerations**

- **Liver monitoring:** Recommended at baseline, every 2 months for the first 12 months, and periodically thereafter. *Avandia* should not be initiated in patients with clinical evidence of active liver disease or ALT >2.5X the upper limit of normal

- **Fluid retention:** Since thiazolidinediones can cause fluid retention, which can exacerbate congestive heart failure, patients at risk (particularly those on insulin) should be watched for signs/symptoms of heart failure†

- **Hypoglycemia:** Patients receiving *Avandia* in combination with a sulfonylurea may be at risk, and a reduction in the sulfonylurea dose may be necessary

- **Anemia:** In clinical trials, the frequency was greater with the combination of *Avandia* plus metformin (7.1%) compared to metformin alone (2.2%). Lower pretreatment hemoglobin/hematocrit levels may have contributed to this higher reporting rate

† *Avandia* is not indicated for use in combination with insulin.

Please see Appendix A at the end of this book for complete prescribing information.

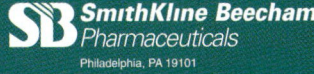
SmithKline Beecham Pharmaceuticals
Philadelphia, PA 19101

Bristol-Myers Squibb Company

Avandia is a registered trademark of SmithKline Beecham.
AV7636A   © SmithKline Beecham, 2000

Avandia®
rosiglitazone maleate
Redefining Type 2 Therapy

7.8	Bone and Mineral Metabolism 109		8.3	Bone and Mineral Metabolism 125	
	Biochemical Markers for Bone Turnover *109*			*Parathyroid Surgery* *125*	
	Calcium *110*		8.4	Diabetes Mellitus 125	
	Imaging: Bone Age *111*			*Exercise Regimens* *125*	
	Imaging: Bone Densitometry *111*			*Gene Therapy* *126*	
	Imaging: Bone Scan *112*			*Glucose Self-Monitoring* *127*	
	Imaging: Parathyroid Gland . . *112*			*Neuropathy* *128*	
	Parathyroid Screening *113*			*Nutritional Interventions* *128*	
7.9	Energy Metabolism 114			*Retinopathy* *129*	
	Diabetes: General Resources *114*			*Technological Developments in Insulin Delivery* *130*	
	Diabetes: Glucose *115*			*Transplantation: General Resources* *131*	
	Diabetes: Glucose, Fasting . . . *115*			*Transplantation: Biological Specimens* *132*	
	Diabetes: Glycated Hemoglobin *116*			*Transplantation: Pancreas and Islet Cell Transplantation* . . *132*	
	Diabetes: Insulin C-Peptide . . *116*		8.5	Metabolic Disease 133	
	Diabetes: Ketones *116*			*Gene Therapy* *133*	
	Diabetes: Oral Glucose Tolerance Test *117*			*Stem Cell Transplantation* . . . *134*	
	Diabetes: Stimulation Testing *117*		8.6	Neuroendocrine System 135	
	Diabetes: Urinalysis *118*			*Gene Therapy* *135*	
	Cholesterol and Lipoproteins *118*			*Pituitary Surgery* *135*	
	Metabolic Impairment Testing, General *119*			*Radiotherapy* *137*	
	Metabolic Testing: Amino Acid Analysis *121*		8.7	Pancreas 137	
	Metabolic Testing: Carnitine Analysis *121*		8.8	Thyroid Gland 138	
	Metabolic Testing: Magnetic Resonance Spectroscopy . . . *122*			*Antithyroid Agents* *138*	
	Metabolic Testing: Urine Organic Acid Analysis *122*			*Radioactive Iodine* *138*	
				Thyroid Surgery *139*	
8.	**THERAPEUTIC PROCEDURES AND SURGERY 123**		**9.**	**PHARMACOLOGY 141**	
			9.1	General Resources 141	
8.1	General Resources 123		9.2	Adrenal Glands 143	
8.2	Adrenal Glands 124			*Overview* *143*	
				Antiadrenal Agent: Aminoglutethimide *144*	
			9.3	Bone and Mineral Metabolism 144	
				Bisphosphonates *144*	
				Calcitonin *144*	

Over 5 Million Prescriptions Dispensed*

Impressive Glycemic Control That Lasts

▶ **Provides long-lasting control versus glyburide**

▶ **Enhances efficacy in combination with sulfonylureas or metformin**

▶ **Substantial reductions as monotherapy**

▶ **Important clinical considerations**

- **Liver monitoring:** Recommended at baseline, every 2 months for the first 12 months, and periodically thereafter. *Avandia* should not be initiated in patients with clinical evidence of active liver disease or ALT >2.5X the upper limit of normal

- **Fluid retention:** Since thiazolidinediones can cause fluid retention, which can exacerbate congestive heart failure, patients at risk (particularly those on insulin) should be watched for signs/symptoms of heart failure†

- **Hypoglycemia:** Patients receiving *Avandia* in combination with a sulfonylurea may be at risk, and a reduction in the sulfonylurea dose may be necessary

- **Anemia:** In clinical trials, the frequency was greater with the combination of *Avandia* plus metformin (7.1%) compared to metformin alone (2.2%). Lower pretreatment hemoglobin/hematocrit levels may have contributed to this higher reporting rate

* Scott-Levin SPA, August 2000.
† *Avandia* is not indicated for use in combination with insulin.

Please see Appendix A at the end of this book for complete prescribing information.

SB SmithKline Beecham Pharmaceuticals
Philadelphia, PA 19101

Bristol-Myers Squibb Company

Avandia is a registered trademark of SmithKline Beecham.

AV7636B   © SmithKline Beecham, 2000

Avandia®
rosiglitazone maleate
Redefining Type 2 Therapy

	Calcium *145*	
	Hormone	
	Replacement Therapy *145*	
	Parathyroid	
	Hormone Therapy *145*	
	Vitamin D *146*	
9.4	Cholesterol and	
	Lipoprotein Metabolism 147	
	Antilipemic Agents *147*	
9.5	Diabetes Mellitus 147	
	Overview *147*	
	Glucagon *148*	
	Insulin *149*	
	Oral Hypoglycemic Agents . . . *150*	
9.6	Metabolic Agents 151	
	Alkalinizing Agents *151*	
	Antigout Agents *152*	
	Enzyme Replacement	
	Therapy for	
	Metabolic Impairment *152*	
	Essential	
	Vitamins and Minerals *153*	
	Immunosuppressive Drugs . . . *154*	
	Minerals *154*	
9.7	Neuroendocrine System 155	
	Overview of Pituitary	
	Hormones and Analogs *155*	
	Bromocriptine *156*	
	Cosyntropin *156*	
	Gonadotropin-Releasing	
	Hormone and Analogs *156*	
	Growth Hormone *157*	
9.8	Obesity Medications 158	
9.9	Reproductive System 159	
	Androgen Therapy and	
	Complications of Therapy . . *159*	
	Gonadotropins *160*	
	Hormone Replacement	
	Therapy and	
	Complications of Therapy . . *160*	
	Oral Contraceptives *163*	

9.10	Thyroid Gland 163
	Overview *163*
	Antithyroid Agents *164*
	Thyroid Hormone *164*
9.11	Vascular System 164
	Antihypertensive Agents *164*

10. PATHOLOGY AND CASE STUDIES . . . 167

11. CLINICAL PRACTICE AND GUIDELINES 171

11.1	General Resources 171
11.2	Diabetes Mellitus 173

PART THREE TOPICAL RESOURCES AND ORGANIZATIONS

12. PUBLIC HEALTH AND POLICY TOPICS . . . 177

12.1	Advocacy 177
12.2	Diabetes Mellitus 178
	Economic Impact *178*
	Education and Support *178*
	Epidemiology *179*
	News *180*
	Organizations *181*
	Research *183*
	Statistics *184*
12.3	Estrogens, Environmental . . . 185
12.4	Hazards, Environmental 186
12.5	Legislation and Public Policy . 187
12.6	Screening/Prevention 188
	General Prevention Programs . *188*
	Cholesterol *188*
	Diabetes Mellitus *188*
	Hypertension *190*
	Obesity *191*
	Pediatric Screening *191*

	Thyroid Disease *192*
12.7	Patient Education and Support 193

13. SUBSPECIALTY TOPICS 199

13.1	Andropause 199
13.2	Drug Abuse, Endocrinologic and Metabolic Effects 199
13.3	Genetics. 200
13.4	Geriatric Endocrinology 202
13.5	Menopause 203
13.6	Osteoporosis in Men 204
13.7	Pediatric Endocrinology. 205
13.8	Reproductive Endocrinology 206

14. OTHER TOPICAL RESOURCES . . 209

14.1	Databases 209
14.2	Ethics 211
	Anabolic Steroid Abuse *211*
	Bioethics *212*
14.3	Informatics and Software 212

15. ORGANIZATIONS AND INSTITUTIONS . . . 215

15.1	Associations and Societies . . . 215
15.2	Foundations and Grant Support. 227
15.3	Selected Medical School Departments of Endocrinology and Metabolism. 229
15.4	Research Organizations 240
	Directories of Research Centers. *240*
	Individual Research Centers. . *241*
15.5	Selected Hospital Endocrinology and Metabolism Departments . . . 244

PART FOUR DISORDERS OF ENDOCRINOLOGY & METABOLISM

Alphabetical Listing. 257

16. GENERAL RESOURCES. . 261

17. NEUROENDOCRINE SYSTEM 263

17.1	Hypothalamic-Pituitary Axis Dysfunction. 263
	Diabetes Insipidus *263*
	Syndrome of Inappropriate ADH Secretion *264*
17.2	Pituitary Disorders: Conditions of Decreased Pituitary Functioning. 265
	Empty Sella Syndrome *265*
	Hypopituitarism *265*
	Growth Hormone Deficiency *266*
	Pituitary Apoplexy *267*
	Sheehan's Syndrome *268*
17.3	Pituitary Disorders: Conditions of Hormone-Secreting Pituitary Adenomas. 268
	Acromegaly *268*
	Cushing's Disease *269*
	Hyperprolactinemia and Galactorrhea *269*
17.4	Pituitary Disorders: Pituitary Tumors 270
	General Resources *270*
	Craniopharyngiomas *271*
17.5	Pineal Gland Disorders 271

18. THYROID GLAND 273

- 18.1 General Resources 273
- 18.2 Thyroid Hormone Deficiency 274
  - *Hypothyroidism, General*.... 274
  - *Congenital Hypothyroidism*.. 275
  - *Hashimoto's Thyroiditis* 277
  - *Myxedema Coma* 277
  - *Reidel's Thyroiditis* 278
  - *Subclinical Hypothyroidism*.. 278
- 18.3 Thyroid Hormone Excess ... 279
  - *Graves' Disease* 279
  - *Thyroid Storm* 280
  - *Subacute or deQuervain's Thyroiditis* ... 280
  - *Subclinical Thyroid Dysfunction* 281
  - *Thyrotoxicosis Factitia*...... 282
  - *Toxic Nodular Goiter (Plummer's Disease)* 282
- 18.4 Goiter 283
- 18.5 Thyroid Malignancy 284
- 18.6 Pregnancy and Thyroid Disorders...... 286
  - *General Resources* 286
  - *Hyperthyroidism* 287
  - *Hypothyroidism*........... 287
  - *Postpartum Thyroid Disease* . 288
- 18.7 Nonthyroidal Illness 288

19. ADRENAL GLANDS.... 291

- 19.1 General Resources 291
- 19.2 Adrenal Insufficiency....... 292
  - *General Resources* 292
  - *Addison's Disease* 293
  - *Adrenal Hemorrhage*....... 294
  - *Adrenoleukodystrophy (ALD)* 294
- 19.3 Adrenal Hormone Overproduction... 295
  - *General Resources* 295
  - *Congenital Adrenal Hyperplasia (CAH)* 295
  - *Hyperaldosteronism*........ 297
  - *Hypercortisolism: Cushing's Syndrome* 297
- 19.4 Adrenal Tumors........... 298
  - *General Resources* 298
  - *Aldosterone-Producing Adrenal Adenoma (Conn's Syndrome)* 299
  - *Non-Functioning Adrenal Incidentaloma* 299
  - *Pheochromocytoma*........ 300

20. GASTROINTESTINAL TRACT 301

- 20.1 General Resources 301
- 20.2 Neoplasms of the Pancreas .. 302
  - *General Resources* 302
  - *Gastrinoma (Zollinger-Ellison Syndrome)* 302
  - *Glucagonoma* 303
  - *Insulinoma* 303
  - *Vasoactive Intestinal Peptide Tumor (VIPoma)*... 304
- 20.3 Carcinoma of the Pancreas .. 304

21. FEMALE ENDOCRINOLOGY..... 307

- 21.1 General Resources 307
- 21.2 Amenorrhea 307
- 21.3 Hirsutism 308
- 21.4 Infertility 308
- 21.5 Menstrual Exacerbations of Medical Problems 309
- 21.6 Ovarian Cancer............ 309
- 21.7 Polycystic Ovary Syndrome .. 311
- 21.8 Premenstrual Syndrome..... 312
- 21.9 Uterine Bleeding Disorders .. 313

22. MALE ENDOCRINOLOGY 315

22.1 Androgen Abnormalities 315
22.2 Erectile Dysfunction 316
22.3 Gynecomastia 317
22.4 Infertility 318
22.5 Male Gonadal Disorders 319
   Cryptorchidism 319
   *Primary Hypogonadism:
      General Resources* 319
   *Primary Hypogonadism:
      Adult Leydig Cell Failure* ... 320
   *Secondary Hypogonadism:
      Kallman Syndrome* 320
22.6 Prostate Disorders 321
   General Resources 321
   *Benign Prostatic
      Hyperplasia (BPH)* 321
   Prostate Cancer 322
   Prostatitis 325
22.7 Testicular Cancer 326

23. DEVELOPMENT AND SEXUAL DIFFERENTIATION 327

23.1 Genetic Syndromes of
      Developmental Disorders ... 327
   Klinefelter's Syndrome 327
   Noonan's Syndrome 328
   Prader-Willi Syndrome 328
23.2 Precocious Puberty
      and Pubertal Delay 329
23.3 Sexual Differentiation 331
   General Resources 331
   *Androgen Insensitivity
      Syndrome (Male
      Pseudohermaphroditism)* ... 331
   *Congenital
      Adrenal Hyperplasia* 332
   *Female
      Pseudohermaphroditism* ... 332
   Hermaphroditism, General .. 332
   Klinefelter's Syndrome 333
   Turner's Syndrome 333

24. BONE AND MINERAL METABOLISM 335

24.1 Calcium,
      Phosphorus, and Vitamin D .. 335
   *Calcium Metabolism
      Disorders, General* 335
   Hypercalcemia 335
   Hypocalcemia 337
   Hyperphosphatemia 337
   Hypophosphatemia 337
   *Vitamin D
      Metabolism Disorders* 338
24.2 Bone
      Mineralization Disorders 338
   Osteomalacia 338
   Paget's Disease of the Bone .. 339
   Renal Osteodystrophy 339
   Rickets 340
24.3 Skeletal Dysplasias 340
24.4 Collagen Disorders 341
   Osteogenesis Imperfecta 341
24.5 Osteoporosis 342
24.6 Parathyroid Gland 343
   General Resources 343
   *Hyperparathyroidism:
      General* 344
   *Hyperparathyroidism:
      Adenoma* 345
   *Hyperparathyroidism:
      Carcinoma* 345
   Hypoparathyroidism 346
   Pseudohypoparathyroidism .. 346
24.7 Growth and Stature 346
   General Resources 346
   Short Stature: General 348

Short Stature:
Psychosocial Dwarfism 349
Short Stature:
Russell-Silver Syndrome . . . 350
Tall Stature 350

25. **VITAMIN AND TRACE MINERAL DEFICIENCIES 351**

26. **FLUID, ELECTROLYTE, AND ACID-BASE METABOLISM 353**

26.1 Magnesium
Metabolism Disorders 353

26.2 Potassium
Metabolism Disorders 354
Hyperkalemia 354
Hypokalemia. 354

26.3 Sodium and Water
Metabolism Disorders 355
General Resources 355
Hypernatremia 355
Hyponatremia 355

26.4 Disturbances of
Acid-Base Metabolism. 356
Metabolic Acidosis 356
Metabolic Alkalosis. 357

27. **DIABETES MELLITUS . . . 359**

27.1 General Resources 359

27.2 Type 1 Diabetes Mellitus 360

27.3 Type 2 Diabetes Mellitus 361
General Resources 361
Gestational Diabetes 362
Insulin Resistance 363

27.4 Complications 363
General Resources 363
Coronary Complications 364
Dermatologic Manifestations
of Diabetes 365

Diabetic
Foot Ulcers and Disease. . . . 365
Gastroparesis. 366
Ketoacidosis 366
Nephropathy 367
Neuropathy 368
Retinopathy. 369
Hyperglycemia, Hyperosmolar,
Nonketotic State 370
Hypoglycemia 370
Macrosomia 372
Organ Damage 372

28. **ENERGY METABOLISM . 373**

28.1 Obesity 373

28.2 Malnutrition 375

29. **LIPOPROTEIN AND CHOLESTEROL METABOLISM 377**

29.1 Hyperlipidemia 377
General Resources 377
Acquired Hyperlipidemia. . . . 379
Familial Lecithin Cholesterol
Acyltransferase Deficiency . . 379
Type I
Hyperlipoproteinemia 380
Type II
Hyperlipoproteinemia 380
Type III
Hyperlipoproteinemia 381
Type IV
Hyperlipoproteinemia 381
Type V
Hyperlipoproteinemia 382

29.2 Hypolipidemia. 382
General Resources 382
Abetalipoproteinemia 383
Hypobetalipoproteinemia . . . 383
Tangier Disease 384

30. METABOLISM, INBORN ERRORS 385

- 30.1 General Resources 385
- 30.2 Carbohydrate Metabolism ... 387
  - General Resources 387
  - Essential Fructosuria 387
  - Fructose-1,6-Bisphosphatase Deficiency 387
  - Galactokinase Deficiency 388
  - Galactosemia 388
  - Glycogen Storage Diseases: General .. 389
  - Glycogen Storage Diseases: Pompe Disease (Acid Maltase Deficiency) .. 389
  - Hereditary Fructose Intolerance 390
  - Mucopolysaccharidoses (MPS) and Related Diseases 391
  - UDPgalactose 4-Epimerase Deficiency 391
  - Pyruvate Carboxylase Deficiency 392
  - Pyruvate Dehydrogenase Complex Deficiency 392
- 30.3 Amino Acid Metabolism 393
  - General Resources 393
  - Alcaptonuria 393
  - Homocystinuria 394
  - Maple Syrup Urine Disease .. 394
  - Phenylketonuria (PKU) 395
  - Urea Cycle Disorders 395
  - Variant Forms of Hyperphenylalaninemia 396
- 30.4 Fatty Acid Oxidation and Carnitine 397
- 30.5 Purine and Pyrimidine Metabolic Disorders 398
- 30.6 Lysosomal Disorders 398
  - Lysosomal Storage Diseases, General 398
  - Cerebrotendinous Xanthomatosis 399
  - Fabry's Disease 399
  - Galactosylceramide Lipidosis (Krabbe's Disease) 400
  - Gaucher Disease 400
  - Generalized Gangliosidosis ... 402
  - Metachromatic Leukodystrophy 402
  - Niemann-Pick Disease 403
  - Refsum's Disease 403
  - Tay-Sachs Disease 404
  - Wolman's Disease 404
- 30.7 Peroxisomal Disorders 405
- 30.8 Carbohydrate-Deficient Glycoprotein Syndromes 405
- 30.9 Smith-Lemli-Opitz Syndrome 406
- 30.10 Porphyrias 406
  - General Resources 406
  - Acute Intermittent Porphyria .. 408
  - Congenital Erythropoietic Porphyria 408
  - Hereditary Coproporphyria ... 409
  - Porphyria Cutanea Tarda 409
  - Rarer Porphyrias 410
  - Variegate Porphyria 410

31. PARAENDOCRINE AND NEOPLASTIC SYNDROMES 411

- 31.1 Carcinoid Tumors and Carcinoid Syndrome 411
- 31.2 Medullary Thyroid Carcinoma 412
- 31.3 Multiple Endocrine Neoplasia . 412
- 31.4 Pheochromocytoma Syndromes 413
  - Neurofibromatosis (Recklinghausen's Disease) .. 413
  - Von Hippel Lindau Disease ... 414

32. POLYENDOCRINE DISORDERS.......... 415

32.1 Autoimmune Polyendocrinopathy......... 415

33. SYSTEMIC DISEASES: ENDOCRINE MANIFESTATIONS..... 417

33.1 Amyloidosis............... 417
33.2 HIV.................... 418
33.3 Malignancy............... 419

34. RARE DISORDERS..... 421

PART FIVE GENERAL MEDICAL WEB RESOURCES

35. REFERENCE INFORMATION AND NEWS SOURCES .. 425

35.1 Abbreviations and Acronyms............ 425
35.2 Abstract, Citation, and Full-text Search Tools... 425
35.3 General Medical Supersites.. 426
35.4 Government Information Databases..... 430
35.5 Government Organizations.. 431
Government Agencies and Offices....... 431
NIH Institutes and Centers .. 436
35.6 Guides to Medical Journals on the Internet..... 445
35.7 Health and Medical Hotlines.......... 451
35.8 Hospital Resources........ 451
35.9 Internet Newsgroups....... 451
35.10 Locating a Physician....... 452
35.11 Medical and Health Sciences Libraries.... 453
35.12 Medical Conferences and Meetings... 454
35.13 Medical Data and Statistics.. 456
35.14 Medical Dictionaries, Encyclopedias, and Glossaries............. 457
35.15 Medical Legislation........ 460
35.16 Medical News............ 461
35.17 Medical Search Engines and Directories..... 463
35.18 Pharmaceutical Information............... 471
35.19 Physician Directories....... 474

36. PROFESSIONAL TOPICS AND CLINICAL PRACTICE... 475

36.1 Anatomy and Surgery...... 475
36.2 Biomedical Ethics......... 477
36.3 Biotechnology............ 480
36.4 Chronic Pain Management .. 483
36.5 Clinical Practice Management...... 484
36.6 Genetics................. 487
36.7 Geriatrics................ 490
36.8 Grants and Award Guides... 491
36.9 Imaging and Pathology..... 492
36.10 Medical Informatics........ 496
36.11 Patent Searches........... 497

37. STUDENT RESOURCES.. 499

37.1 Fellowships and Residencies.. 499
37.2 Medical School Web Sites ... 500
37.3 Medical Student Resources .. 501

38. PATIENT EDUCATION AND PLANNING......505

- 38.1 Patient Resources..........505
- 38.2 Support Groups...........513
- 38.3 Medical Planning..........514
  - Blood Bank Information 514
  - Caregiver Resources........514
  - Chronic and Terminal Care Planning 515
  - Directing Healthcare Concerns and Complaints..516
  - Elder and Extended Care....518
  - End of Life Decisions 519
  - Hospice and Home Care 521
  - Medical Insurance and Managed Care 523
- 38.4 Nutrition and Physical Wellness 526
- 38.5 Online Drug Stores 528

39. WEB SITE AND TOPICAL INDEX ..531

Foreword

It is ironic that as physicians and their patients increasingly search for information and advice about healthcare on the World Wide Web, the guidance that they seek there often remains hard to find and, when located, may even prove to be unreliable. This new, rapidly expanding medium nonjudgmentally invites well-informed, creative sources of knowledge to compete with a haze of misinformation, personal and corporate self-interest, and just plain hocus-pocus—all of which can thwart the search for accurate, up-to-date answers. *Endocrinology & Metabolism: An Internet Resource Guide* is a first step to tame, or at least blaze a trail across, this Wild West.

The search for medical information has been one of the fastest growing sectors of the World Wide Web, on which it is now estimated that 25% of activity relates to medicine and health. A recent AMA study on physicians' use of the World Wide Web reported that 37% of physicians have used the Internet. Today's clinicians and clinical investigators have new search engines and databases that make their computers gateways to instantaneous fact-finding, journal searches, continuing medical education, clinical management, and referral. At the same time, their need for tools to organize this expanding world of information has also grown, particularly for knowledge in specific subspecialties. While general search and metasearch engines are useful, they often fail to provide the most efficient direction, unless one has already charted a course to the objective.

The areas of endocrinology and metabolism are well represented in all their dimensions on the Internet, where virtually every relevant journal, professional and lay association, medical school division, research program, and government agency has created its own Web site. This guide provides a detailed and fully indexed directory of these resources. Whether one is seeking specific articles through citation and full-text search tools or broader information about specific disorders and clinical issues, *Endocrinology & Metabolism: An Internet Resource Guide* enables medical professionals to locate the key facts and new developments.

Furthermore, this same body of information is available at a dedicated Web site (http://www.emedguides.com/endocrinology), so that every entry in this printed edition can also be consulted with the click of a mouse. The access code is 8029.

Time is one of a professional's most valuable commodities. Finding time to read and attend conferences while managing a clinical practice or pursuing research is more challenging than ever. This new book and its companion Web site offer timesaving guidance to identify needed information more efficiently from any office, clinic, laboratory, classroom, or home where a personal computer is at hand.

Readers, please help *Endocrinology & Metabolism: An Internet Resource Guide* remain the most comprehensive, authoritative, and up-to-date source directory of Web-based resources in endocrinology and metabolism. Send your suggested revisions so that this knowledge base can become even more useful to you and your colleagues.

Paul W. Ladenson, M.D.
E-mail: endocrinology@eMedguides.com

1. INTRODUCTION

1.1 Welcome to eMedguides

Welcome to eMedguides, the newest and largest online and in-print Internet directories for physicians, healthcare professionals, and advanced medical students, covering every major field in medicine!

As a user of this book, you now have a gateway to the extraordinary amount of information available on the Internet to help you find useful resources in your field, from electronic journals to selected Web sites on dozens of common and uncommon diseases and disorders.

We would like to thank our Consulting Medical Editor, Paul W. Ladenson, John Eager Howard Professor of Endocrinology and Metabolism and Director, Division of Endocrinology and Metabolism, Johns Hopkins University School of Medicine, for his valued assistance in this new project and for his many organizational and topical suggestions. In addition, we wish to thank Ruth Belin, M.D., in the same division at Johns Hopkins, for her hard work on this project. Our Consulting Medical Librarian, Karen Albert, Director of Library Services for the Fox Chase Cancer Center, also deserves thanks for her assistance in the development of the reference section of this volume.

We have approached the compilation of this directory from the point of view of both the professional practitioner and the researcher. Through the organization and indexing of topics, disorders, and associations and government agencies, we are able to lead you directly to the right destination on the Internet. Our medical compilers are trained professionals who have examined and evaluated Web sites in every category to provide you with a concise description and preview so that you will know ahead of time what you can expect to find.

This book has been divided into sections to help provide ease of access to material. The first part of this book is devoted solely to endocrinology and metabolism resources, including clinical information, disorder profiles, glossaries, current news sources, electronic journals, latest books, statistics, clinical studies, "supersites," therapies, and numerous topical resources.

The second part of the book is focused on the broad fields of medicine reference, clinical practice, and patient education. We have listed online databases and general medical resources, sources of current news and legislation, library access sites, government agencies in the health field, pharmaceutical data, student resources, and patient planning information.

Finally, a very extensive index is included, covering every topic, disorder, association, and Web site title, to make the fact-finding mission as efficient as possible.

How to Benefit Most from this Book

We realize that many physicians and other healthcare professionals may be overwhelmed by the extraordinary number of search engines to choose from, as well as the difficulty in finding very specific information that may appear only in a few locations on the Web. Our aim, therefore, has been to organize this book logically, topic by topic, giving descriptions of Web sites that we feel our readers will want to visit. To access a Web site, the user can type in the provided Web address (URL) or go straight to http://www.eMedguides.com where sites are listed just as they are in the book but with the added advantage of being in hyperlink form, which means that a simple mouse click will complete the connection to the desired site. *The access code included on the title page of this volume provides access to our Web site.*

Physicians and researchers may want to examine several of the unique resources in this volume. We have provided a list of the most recent books published in the past year in the specialty, which are all available at http://www.Amazon.com. Those readers who are interested in research can browse through our comprehensive journal section for access to thousands of articles and article abstracts every month. A further exploration can lead to medical libraries, university and nonprofit centers for research across the country, clinical studies currently underway in every phase, FDA trials of the latest drugs, and instant news sources for the latest breakthroughs.

Although much of the material in this book is intended for a professional, medical audience, key patient Web resources are also provided. Physicians may wish to refer patients to these sites. Many patient sites include up-to-date news and research and clear descriptions of diseases and their treatments.

Information on the Web is constantly changing, new sites and sources appear frequently while older sites get restructured, new books are published, new conferences scheduled, and major research progress is made every day. For this reason, *Endocrinology & Metabolism: An Internet Resource Guide* is always a work in progress. The print version will be published on an annual basis and the online version updated as new information appears.

The Benefits of Both Print and Online Editions

We feel that both the print and online editions of eMedguides can play an important role in the information gathering process, depending on the needs of the physician or health professional. The *print* edition is a "hands-on" tool, enabling the reader to thumb through a comprehensive directory, finding Web information and topical sources that are totally new and unexpected. Each page can provide discoveries of resources previously unknown to the reader that may never have been the subject of an online search. Without knowing what to expect, the reader can be introduced to useful Web site information just by glancing at the book at different times, looking through the detailed Table of Contents, or examining the extensive Index. This type of browsing is difficult to achieve online.

The *online* edition serves a different purpose. It provides "hot links" for each Web site, so the user can click on a topic and visit the destination instantaneously, without having to type the Web address into a browser. In addition, there are search features in this edition that can be used to find specific information quickly, and then the user can print out only what he or she wishes to use. The online edition will also have more frequent updates during the year.

Accessing the Online Edition

We encourage our readers to visit our Web site, through which readers can access any of the included sites with a simple click of the mouse. Our Web address is http://www.eMedguides.com. You will need a special access code that is included on the title page of this volume. By simply clicking on a specialty and typing in this code, the entire contents of the book can be browsed and then used as an online Internet guide. We will continually update the information in this volume on our Web site. Information will be posted on new books published in the field, newly announced conferences, and, of course, additional Web resources that become available and are of interest to physicians. You can also submit the names of other Web sites that you have discovered by e-mailing us at endocrinology@eMedguides.com.

We know that you will find the print and online versions of this volume to be useful Internet companions, always on hand to consult when you need to find timely medical information on the Internet.

1.2 Ratings and Site Selection

Site Selection Criteria

Our medical research staff has carefully chosen the sites for this guide. We perform extensive searches for all of the topics listed in our table of contents, and then select only the sites that meet established criteria. The pertinence and depth of content, presentation, and usefulness for physician and advisory purposes are taken into account.

The sites in this physician guide contain detailed reference material, news, clinical data, and current research articles. We also include and appropriately identify numerous sites that may be useful for patient reference. The large majority of our Web sites are provided by government, university, medical association, and research organizations. Sites operated by private individuals or corporations are only included if they are content-rich and useful to the physician. In these cases, we clearly identify the operator in the title and/or description of the site.

Ratings Guide

Those sites that are selected based on these criteria are subsequently rated on a scale of one star (✪) to three stars (✪✪✪). This rating only applies to the pool of sites that are in the guide; therefore, a one star site is considered worthy of inclusion but may not be outstanding.

A three-star site tends to have greater depth and more extensive information, or particularly hard-to-find resources.

In addition, if a site requires a fee, some fees, or a free registration/disclosure of personal information, we indicate this information next to the rating.

Abbreviations

See "Medical Abbreviations and Acronyms" under "Reference Information and News Sources" in Part 2 for Web sites that provide acronym translation. Below are a few acronyms you will find throughout this volume:

CDC	Centers for Disease Control and Prevention
CME	Continuing Medical Education
FAQ	Frequently Asked Questions
NIDDK	National Institute of Diabetes and Digestive and Kidney Diseases
NIH	National Institutes of Health
PDQ	Physician Data Query
URL	Uniform Resource Locator (the address of a Web site on the Internet)

1.3 Getting Online

The Internet is growing at a fantastic rate, but the vast majority of individuals are not yet online. What is preventing people from jumping on the "information highway"? There are many factors, but probably the most common factor is a general confusion about what the Internet is, how it works, and how to access it.

The following few pages are designed to clear up any confusion for readers who have not yet accessed the Internet. We will look at the process of getting onto and using the Internet, step by step. It is also helpful to consult other resources, such as the technical support department of the manufacturer or store where you bought your computer. Although assistance varies widely, most organizations provide startup assistance for new users and are experienced with guiding individuals onto the Internet. Books can also be of great assistance, as they provide a simple and clear view of how computers and the Internet work, and can be studied at your own pace.

What is the Internet?
The Internet is a large network of computers that are all connected to one another. A good analogy is to envision a neighborhood, with houses and storefronts, all connected to one another by streets and highways. Often the Internet is referred to as the "information superhighway" because of the vastness of this neighborhood.

The Internet was initially developed to allow people to share computers, that is, sublet part of their "house" to others. The ability to connect to so many other computers quickly and easily made this feasible. As computers proliferated, people used the Internet for sending information quickly from one computer to another.

For example, the most popular feature of the Internet is electronic mail (e-mail). Each computer has a mailbox, and an electronic letter can be sent instantly. People also use the Internet to post bulletins, or other information, for others to see. The process of sending e-mail or viewing this information is simple. A computer and a connection to the Internet are all you need to begin.

How is an Internet connection provided?
The Internet is accessed either through a "direct" connection, which is sometimes found in businesses and educational institutions, or through a phone line. Phone line connections are commonly used in small businesses and at home (although direct connections are becoming available for home use via cable and special phone lines). There are many complex options in this area; for the new user it is simplest to use an existing phone line to experience the Internet for the first time. After connecting a computer to a common phone jack, the computer can access the Internet. It will dial the number of an Internet provider, ask you for a user name and password, and give you access to the Internet. Keep in mind that while you are using the Internet, your phone line is tied up, and callers will hear a busy signal. Also, call waiting can sometimes interrupt an Internet connection and disconnect you from your provider.

Who provides an Internet connection?
There are many providers at both the local and national levels. One of the easiest ways to get online is with America Online (AOL). They provide software and a user-friendly environment through which to access the Internet. Because AOL manages both this environment and the actual connection, they can be of great assistance when you are starting out. America Online takes you to a menu of choices when you log in, and while

using their software you can read and send e-mail, view Web pages, and chat with others.

Many other similar services exist, and most of them also provide an environment using Microsoft or Netscape products. These companies, such as the Microsoft Network (MSN), Mindspring, and Earthlink, also provide simple, easy-to-use access to the Internet. Their environment is more standard and not limited to the choices America Online provides.

Internet connections generally run from $10-$20 per month (depending on the length of commitment) in addition to telephone costs. Most national providers have local phone numbers all over the country that should eliminate any telephone charges. The monthly provider fee is the only charge for accessing the Internet.

How do I get on the Internet?
Once you've signed up with an Internet provider and installed their software (often only a matter of answering basic questions), your computer will be set up to access the Internet. By simply double-clicking on an icon, your computer will dial the phone number, log you in, and present you with a Web page (a "home" page).

What are some of the Internet's features?
From the initial Web page there are almost limitless possibilities of where you can go. The address at the top of the screen (identified by an "http://" in front) tells you where you are. You can also type the address of where you would like to go next. When typing a new address, you do not need to add the "http://". The computer adds this prefix automatically after you type in an address and press return. Once you press return, the Web site will appear in the browser window.

You can also navigate the Web by "surfing" from one site to another using links on a page. A Web page might say "Click here for weather." If you click on this underlined phrase, you will be taken to a different address, where weather information is provided.

The Internet has several other useful features. e-mail is an extremely popular and important service. It is free and messages are delivered instantly. Although you can access e-mail through a Web browser (AOL has this feature), many Internet services provide a separate e-mail program for reading, writing, and organizing your correspondence. These programs send and retrieve messages from the Internet.

Another area of the Internet offers chat rooms where users can hold round table discussions. In a chat room you can type messages and see the replies of other users around the world. There are chat rooms on virtually every topic, although the dialog certainly varies in this free-for-all forum. There are also newsgroups on the Internet, some of which we list in this book. A newsgroup is similar to a chat room but each message is a separate item and can be viewed in sequence at any time. For example, a user might post a question about Lyme disease. In the newsgroup you can read the question, and then read the answers that others have provided. You can also post your own comments. This forum is usually not managed or edited, particularly in the medical field. Do not take the advice of a chat room or newsgroup source without first consulting your physician.

How can I find things on the Internet?
Surfing the Internet, from site to site, is a popular activity. But if you have a focused mission, you will want to use a search engine. A search engine can scan lists of Web sites to look for a particular site. We provide a long list of medical search engines in this book.

Because the Internet is so large and unregulated, sites are often hard to find. In the physical world it is difficult to find good services, but you can turn to the yellow pages or other resources to get a comprehensive list. Physical proximity is also a major factor. On the Internet, none of this applies. Finding a reliable site takes time and patience, and can require sifting through hundreds of similar, yet irrelevant sites.

The most common way to find information on the Internet is to use a search engine. When you go to the Web page of a search engine, you will be presented with two distinct methods of searching: using links to topics, or using a keyword search. The links often represent the Web site staff's best effort to find quality sites. This method of searching is the core of the Yahoo! search engine (http://www.yahoo.com). By clicking on Healthcare, then Disorders, then Lung Cancer, you are provided with a list of sites the staff has found on the topic.

The keyword approach is definitely more daring. By typing in search terms, the engine looks through its list of Web sites for a match and returns the results. These engines typically only cover 15% of the Internet, so it is not a comprehensive process. They also usually return far too many choices. Typing lung cancer into a search engine box will return thousands of sites, including one entry for every site where someone used the words lung cancer on a personal Web page.

Where do eMedguides come in?
eMedguides are organized sources of information in each major medical specialty. Our team of editors continually scour the Net, searching for quality Web sites that relate to specific specialties, disorders, and research topics. More importantly, of the sites we find, we only include those that provide professional and useful content. eMedguides fill a critical gap in the Internet research process. Each guide provides more than 500 Web sites that focus on every aspect of a single medical discipline.

Other Internet companies that lack our medical and physician focus have teams of "surfers" who can only cover a subject on its surface. Search engines, even medical search engines, return far too many choices, requiring hours of time and patience to sift through. With an eMedguide in hand, you can quickly identify the sites worth visiting on the Internet and jump right to them. At our site, http://www.eMedguides.com, you can access the same listings as in this book, and can simply click on a site to go straight to it. In addition, we provide continual updates to the book through the site and annually in print. Our editors do the surfing for you, and do it professionally, making your Internet experience efficient and fulfilling.

Taking medical action must involve a physician
As interesting as the Internet is, the information that you will find is both objective and subjective. Our goal is to expose our readers to Web sites on hundreds of topics-for informational purposes only. If you are not a physician and become interested in the ideas, guidelines, recommendations, or experiences discussed online, bring these findings to a physician for personal evaluation. Medical needs vary considerably, and a medical approach or therapy for one individual could be entirely misguided for another. Final medical advice and a plan of action must come only from a physician.

PART ONE

ENDOCRINOLOGY & METABOLISM WEB RESOURCES

2. QUICK REFERENCE

2.1 Endocrinology Disease Profiles

EndocrineWeb ◐ ◐
http://www.endocrineweb.com/index.html

Visitors to EndocrineWeb will find an introduction to endocrinology and endocrine surgery, as well as overviews of the thyroid, parathyroid, and adrenal glands. Sections devoted to diabetes, osteoporosis, and endocrine diseases of the pancreas are also available. The site also offers a search engine for finding useful resources throughout the EndocrineWeb domain, however, the physician search feature does not have objective criteria for inclusion.

Family Practice Notebook.com:
Hematologic, Electrolyte, and Metabolic Disorders ◐ ◐ ◐
http://www.vh.org/Providers/ClinRef/FPHandbook/05.html

Profiles of many endocrine and metabolic diseases are available from this source, including an overview of the disorder and discussions of etiology, evaluation, and treatment. Diseases listed include hyperthyroidism, thyroid storm, hypothyroidism, myxedema coma, thyroid enlargement, adrenal disease, and acid-base disorders. The site offers discussions of disorders in the metabolism of glucose, potassium, sodium, calcium, and magnesium. Electrolyte and metabolic formulas are also provided.

Healthtouch Online:
Endocrine, Hormonal, and Metabolic Disorders ◐ ◐
http://www.healthtouch.com

Endocrine disease profiles are provided by Healthtouch through the "Health Information" link at this home page. All health topics are listed alphabetically, including a section titled "Endocrine, Hormonal, and Metabolic Disorders." This section provides reprints of articles from several NIH institutes and other sources on acromegaly, Addison's disease, Cushing's syndrome, hyperparathyroidism, prolactinoma, Gaucher's disease, familial multiple endocrine neoplasia type 1, and Tay-Sachs disease.

NIDDK: Endocrine and Metabolic Diseases ◎ ◎ ◎
http://www.niddk.nih.gov/health/endo/endo.htm

This site provides links to NIDDK publications that describe a variety of endocrine disorders. Topics include acromegaly, Addison's disease, Cushing's syndrome, cystic fibrosis, familial multiple endocrine neoplasia, hyperparathyroidism, and prolactinoma. Other resources provided by this site include links to national endocrine organizations. Visitors can follow the "Health Information" link at this address to access a list of health topics by subject area, including diabetes, digestive diseases, kidney diseases, nutrition, urologic diseases, and weight loss and control.

2.2 Endocrinology Glossaries

Insulin-Free World Foundation: Glossary of Terms ◎ ◎
http://www.insulinfree.org/glossary.htm

Provided by the Insulin-Free World Foundation, this site contains a lengthy glossary primarily covering terms encountered in understanding diabetes.

National Institutes of Health (NIH): Diabetes Dictionary ◎ ◎
http://www.niddk.nih.gov/health/diabetes/pubs/dmdict/dmdict.htm

Prepared by the National Institutes of Health, this site contains a dictionary of diabetes-related terms designed for use by patients and the general public.

Reproductive Science Center Network: Glossary of Terms ◎ ◎
http://www.reproductivescience.com/glossary.htm

Maintained by the Reproductive Science Center Network, this site offers a concise glossary of infertility terms.

University of Maryland: Endocrinology Glossary ◎ ◎ ◎
http://www.umm.edu/endocrin/glossary.htm

An extensive glossary of terms related to all aspects of endocrinology has been made available by the University of Maryland School of Medicine at this Web site. Terms cover individual hormones, diseases, and anatomy and physiology.

2.3 Topical Search Tools

American Diabetes Association (ADA): Search Page ✪ ✪ ✪
http://www.diabetes.org/publications/adasearch/QUERY.ASP

The entire site of the American Diabetes Association may be searched from this page with either boolean or free-text entries. Information may also be obtained from professional publications, including *Clinical Diabetes* and *Diabetes Care*.

atEndocrine.com ✪ ✪
http://www.atendocrine.com/endocrine

Devoted entirely to the field of endocrinology, this search tool provides direct links to information on commonly searched terminology in the field, as well as the opportunity to perform an endocrinology-only Internet search. A direct connection to a Medline search designed for endocrinology is found, and the opportunities to create one's own custom Medline search engine or preferred journal list with search method are provided.

CliniWeb International: Search Tool ✪ ✪
http://www.ohsu.edu/cliniweb/search.html

A rich database of medical resources, including a strong representation of topics related to endocrinology and metabolism, may be searched through CliniWeb, a service of Oregon Health Science University. The initial search query asks for a topic, and the second display provides a listing of relevant resources in the database, each of which may then be accessed individually.

MEDLINEplus: Health Information Database ✪ ✪ ✪
http://www.nlm.nih.gov/medlineplus/medlineplus.html

A comprehensive database of health and medical information, MEDLINEplus serves a different purpose from its sister service, MEDLINE, which is a bibliographic search engine to locate citations and abstracts in medical journals and reports. MEDLINEplus offers the ability to search by topic and obtain full information rather than citations. One can search body systems, disorders and diseases, treatments and therapies, diagnostic procedures, side effects, and numerous other important topics related to personal health and medicine.

NIDDK Search Engine ✪ ✪ ✪
http://www.niddk.nih.gov

At the home page of the National Institute of Diabetes and Digestive and Kidney Disorders there is a very useful search engine that accesses information on numerous topics of interest to endocrinologists as well as patients and medical students. Articles and documents are presented and ranked by relevance, and document titles are accompanied by a content summary but can also be accessed in their entirety. Of additional value is an alphabetical index of health and medical topics related to endocrinology.

2.4 Endocrinology News

Diabetes Compilation Digest ◎ ◎
http://www.geocities.com/HotSprings/Resort/3146/digest/digest.htm
The Diabetes Compilation Digest provides a daily sampling of diabetes-related news and information on the Web. There are articles about prevention, trials, diet, alternative therapies, and new procedures.

Endocrine Disorders News at Doctor's Guide ◎ ◎
http://www.pslgroup.com/dg/endocrinenews.htm
Articles on hormone replacement therapy, new diabetes drugs, current surgical techniques, and FDA status information are provided at this Doctor's Guide listing. News from the American Diabetes Association, studies about osteoporosis care, and coverage of current discoveries in the field of endocrinology are included.

Endocrine Society: News ◎ ◎
http://www.endo-society.org/news_g/news.htm
Maintained by the Endocrine Society, this site offers news and facts related to the specialty. Current and recent headlines link to full-text versions of articles.

SciTalk.com: Diabetes News Center ◎ ◎
http://www.scitalk.com/diabetes/diabetes_news.cfm
Part of SciTalk.com, the Diabetes News Center offers links to diabetes news from Yahoo News, Excite News, and the Usenet Archive. There are also listings of Usenet groups where diabetes topics are discussed. Headlines from NewsWise.com are given with links to article summaries. Additionally, the site provides links to biopharmaceutical news items that relate to diabetes.

Yahoo! News Articles in Endocrinology ◎ ◎
http://search.news.yahoo.com/search/news?p=endocrine
Yahoo's search for articles related to endocrine research developments provides visitors with direct connections to PR Newswire information in endocrine-related drugs and research, as well as recent acquistions and up-to-date clinical trial details.

2.5 Conferences

Doctor's Guide: Medical Conferences and Meetings: Endocrine Disorders ○ ○ ○
http://www.pslgroup.com/dg/endocrine.htm

This easy-to-use site features a comprehensive listing of related conferences and meetings through the year 2003. The conference descriptions include subject reports, keywords, and valuable contact information.

MedicalConferences.com ○ ○ ○
http://www.medicalconferences.com

Visitors to this comprehensive source for medical conference listings can search for appropriate conferences by keyword, dates, and location. The site also provides a tool for registering for conferences, links to related sites with site profiles, answers to frequently asked questions, and contact details.

MediConf Online: Forthcoming Meetings ○ ○ (fee-based)
http://mediconf.de/scme/8007.HTM

MediConf Online provides an excellent directory of forthcoming meetings and conferences in every major medical specialty. The menu at this site enables the visitor to select the field of choice. For each meeting there is a listing including the dates, the contact telephone number, the contact e-mail address, and a link to the city where the visitor can learn about accommodations, weather, and other information.

Medmeetings ○ ○ ○
http://www.medmeetings.com

Requiring a free, one-time registration, Medmeetings.com allows visitors to search for meetings in their specialty, as well as specify meeting dates and locations desired. Lists returned to the user offer names of sponsoring organizations, conference names and dates, and links to registration and CME details. Instructions for adding a free basic meeting listing are offered.

2.6 Statistics

FedStats ○ ○ ○
http://www.fedstats.gov

Maintained by the Federal Interagency Council on Statistical Policy, this site provides fast facts and information from over 70 United States agencies, including the National Institute of Diabetes and Digestive and Kidney Diseases, the Agency for Healthcare Research and Quality, the Administration on Aging, the Health Care Financing

Administration, and the National Institutes of Health. In the "Briefing Room" visitors will find *Health, United States,* an online publication, presenting national trends in health statistic topics. Links to national programs responsible for the collection and dissemination of health-related statistics are available from the site, as well as a connection to CDC Wonder, which offers a single point of access to an assortment of guidelines and numeric health data of the Centers for Disease Control.

FedStats: One Stop Shopping for Federal Statistics ○ ○ ○
http://www.fedstats.gov

FedStats, maintained by the Federal Interagency Council on Statistical policy, serves as a comprehensive directory of statistical resources of interest to the public. The site offers an alphabetical index of topics, a site search engine, and a Fast Facts section for the latest economic and social indicators. Data access tools for locating specific statistics from federal agency databases, links to federal agencies supplying statistical resources, resources for kids, press releases, and links to sources of demographic statistics are also available.

National Center for Health Statistics (NCHS): Fast Stats A to Z ○ ○ ○
http://www.cdc.gov/nchs/fastats/Default.htm

The national government's vital and health statistics center offers statistical informaation regarding diabetes, ambulatory care, nutrition and nutrition monitoring, and other topics of interest. State-by-state numbers may be obtained from links at the site, with comprehensive data available for viewing or downloading in PDF format.

NIDDK: Diabetes Statistics ○ ○ ○
http://www.niddk.nih.gov/health/diabetes/pubs/dmstats/dmstats.htm

Provided by the National Institute of Diabetes and Digestive and Kidney Diseases, this site contains diabetes statistics, including prevalence of diabetes, incidence of diabetes, mortality rates, and prevalence of diabetes broken down by age, sex, and ethnicity. There are also discussions of types of diabetes, complications, cost, diagnostic criteria, and treatment. An appendix and references are found.

2.7 Clinical Studies and Trials

CenterWatch: Clinical Trials Listing Service ○ ○ ○
http://www.centerwatch.com/studies/listing.htm

Designed for both patients and healthcare professionals, this site provides an extensive listing of therapeutic clinical trials organized by disorder and is sponsored by both industry and government. Thirty-six endocrinology diseases are arranged alphabetically by type. The site is international in scope and provides data on more than 5,200 clinical trials that are actively recruiting patients. Keyword search–accessible, it also covers information on new FDA-approved drug therapies. Trials are listed by geographical region within each disorder.

CenterWatch: National Institutes of Health (NIH) Trials Listing ○ ○ ○
http://www.centerwatch.com/nih/index.htm

CenterWatch provides a convenient resource for accessing information on clinical trials at the NIH. These are clinical trials located at the Warren Grant Magnuson Clinical Center in Bethesda, Maryland. Trials are organized by disorder, with a short description provided for each entry. Under endocrinology, there are hundreds of government-sponsored studies, each with a full description.

ClinicalTrials.com ○ ○ ○ (free registration)
http://www.clinicaltrials.com

A compilation of patient information, community resources, and information for investigators is found at ClinicalTrials.com, a service of Pharmaceutical Research Plus, Inc. An investigator and trial registry, organized information on current clinical trials being conducted nationwide, and a specialized approach to connecting patients to relevant clinical trials being conducted are presented. Answers to Freqently Asked Questions, a clinical trials search engine, and details on FDA recently approved drugs are provided.

ClinicalTrials.gov ○ ○ ○
http://clinicaltrials.gov/ct/gui/c/r

The U.S. National Institutes of Health in conjunction with the National Library of Medicine present interested viewers with current information regarding clinical research studies. Visitors may search for individual studies by entering words or phrases or may find trials by searching for diseases, locations, treatments, or sponsor. Specific conditions may be browsed, and resource informaton on understanding clinical trials is presented.

2.8 Approved and Developmental Therapeutic Agents

CenterWatch: FDA Drug Approvals ○ ○ ○
http://www.centerwatch.com/drugs/druglist.htm

This clinical trials listing service provides a cataloging and descriptive profile of each new drug approved by the FDA in the last five years. Drugs are organized by year and by specialty. New endocrinology therapies for 2000 are described.

Pharmaceutical Research and Manufacturers of America (PhRMA): New Drugs under Development ○ ○ ○
http://www.phrma.org/webdb/phrmawdb.html

Hundreds of new drugs under development are listed at the PhRMA site. The publications in each area provide the product names, pharmaceutical company developers, indications, and status. A search feature allows the visitor to enter a disease name, indication, or drug name. There is a special section on diabetes and related disorders.

3. JOURNALS, ARTICLES, AND LATEST BOOKS

3.1 Abstract, Citation, and Full-text Search Tools

MEDLINE/PubMed at the National Library of Medicine (NLM) ◎ ◎ ◎
http://www.ncbi.nlm.nih.gov/PubMed

PubMed is a free MEDLINE search service providing access to 11 million citations with links to the full text of articles of participating journals. Probably the most heavily used and reputable free MEDLINE site, PubMed permits advanced searching by subject, author, journal title, and many other fields. It includes an easy-to-use "citation matcher" for completing and identifying references, and its PreMEDLINE database provides journal citations before they are indexed, making this version of MEDLINE more up-to-date than most.

Search the Endocrine Society Journals Online ◎ ◎ ◎
http://endo.endojournals.org

All journals or specific journal selection searches may be conducted at this page, which returns visitors articles from 1996 through the most current issues. Users may specify sort results and may specify simple or qualified search options for a return of articles from *Endocrinology, Endocrine Reviews, Molecular Endocrinology*, and *The Journal of Clinical Endocrinology and Metabolism*.

Society for Endocrinology Search Page ◎ ◎ ◎
http://journals.endocrinology.org/search/search.asp

Abstracts of *Endocrine Related Cancers,* the *Journal of Endocrinology,* and the *Journal of Molecular Endocrinology,* may be searched from this site. Visitors may search by author name, title or abstract contents, and publication date. The full text articles of *Endocrine Related Cancers* may be freely downloaded in PDF format.

WebMedLit: Endocrinology ○ ○ ○
http://webmedlit.silverplatter.com/topics/endocrin.html

Extremely efficient access to professional publications is provided at this WebMedLit address. By typing in keywords, visitors are returned an extensive listing of article abstracts from professional journals in the specialty, with best matches displayed first. The full text of each article may be accessed directly from the site, and a special feature of the page allows visitors to subscribe to e-mail updates of current articles in the field. As with PubMed searches, the WebMedLit search results provide visitors with a connection to similar article listings for each citation shown.

3.2 Journals on the Internet

Selected Articles and Commentaries

Endocrinology Review Articles and Commentaries ○ ○
http://journals.endocrinology.org/RevArtCom.htm

From the Society for Endocrinology, this site offers a selection of free, full-text reviews and commentaries from the Society's major endocrinology journals. Bibliographic details are available as a PDF file, and links to a collection of chosen archived articles may, additionally, be accessed.

Individual Journal Web Sites

The following journals may be accessed on the Internet. Our table of information for each journal identifies content that is accessible free-of-charge or with a free registration, and also identifies content that requires a password and fee for access. We have indicated if back issues are accessible. Journals are listed in alphabetical order by title.

Acta Diabetologica
http://link.springer.de/link/service/journals/00592/index.htm

Publisher	Springer–Verlag, back issues available
Free resources	Table of Contents, Abstracts
Pay resources	Articles

Advances in Contraception
http://kapis.www.wkap.nl/kapis/CGI-BIN/WORLD/journalhome.htm?0267-4874

Publisher	Kluwer, back issues available
Free resources	Table of Contents
Pay resources	Abstracts, Articles

American Journal of Clinical Nutrition
http://www.ajcn.org
- Publisher: American Society for Clinical Nutrition, HighWire Press, back issues available
- Free resources: Table of Contents, Abstracts
- Pay resources: Articles

American Journal of Obstetrics and Gynecology
http://www1.mosby.com/scripts/om.dll/serve?action=searchDB&searchDBfor=home&id=ob
- Publisher: Mosby, back issues available
- Free resources: Table of Contents, Abstracts
- Pay resources: Articles

Amino Acids
http://link.springer.de/link/service/journals/00726/index.htm
- Publisher: Springer–Verlag, back issues available
- Free resources: Table of Contents, Abstracts
- Pay resources: Articles

Andrologia
http://www.blackwell-synergy.com/issuelist.asp?journal=and
- Publisher: Blackwell Science, back issues available
- Free resources: Table of Contents, Abstracts
- Pay resources: Articles

Annals of Nutrition and Metabolism
http://www.karger.ch/journals/anm/anm_jh.htm
- Publisher: Karger, back issues available
- Free resources: Table of Contents, Abstracts
- Pay resources: Articles

Annual Reviews of Nutrition
http://biomedical.AnnualReviews.org/current/11.shtml
- Publisher: Annual Reviews, back issues available
- Free resources: Table of Contents, Abstracts
- Pay resources: Articles

Archives of Andrology
http://www.tandf.co.uk/journals/tf/01485016.html
    Publisher   Taylor and Francis, back issues available
    Free resources   Table of Contents
    Pay resources   Abstracts, Articles

Best Practice and Research
Clinical Endocrinology and Metabolism
http://www.harcourt-international.com/journals/beem
    Publisher   Harcourt International, back issues available
    Free resources   Table of Contents, Abstracts
    Pay resources   Articles

Biological Signals and Receptors
http://www.karger.ch/journals/bsi/bsi_jh.htm
    Publisher   Karger
    Free resources   Table of Contents, Abstracts
    Pay resources   Articles

Biology of Reproduction
http://www.biolreprod.org
    Publisher   Society for the Study of Reproduction, back issues available
    Free resources   Table of Contents, Abstracts
    Pay resources   Articles

Bone
http://www.elsevier.com/inca/publications/store/5/2/5/2/3/3
    Publisher   Elsevier Science, back issues available
    Free resources   Table of Contents
    Pay resources   Abstracts, Articles

Canadian Journal of Diabetes Care
http://endocrine.medscape.com/CDA/CJDC/public/journal-CJDC.html
    Publisher   Medscape, back issues available
    Free resources   Table of Contents, Abstracts
    Pay resources   Articles

Clinical Chemistry
http://www.clinchem.org
- Publisher — HighWire Press, back issues available
- Free resources — Table of Contents, Abstracts
- Pay resources — Articles

Clinical Diabetes
http://www.diabetes.org/ClinicalDiabetes
- Publisher — American Diabetes Society, back issues available
- Free resources — Table of Contents, Abstracts
- Pay resources — Articles

Clinical Drug Investigations
http://endocrine.medscape.com/adis/CDI/public/journal.CDI.html
- Publisher — Medscape, back issues available
- Free resources — Table of Contents, Abstracts
- Pay resources — Articles

Clinical Endocrinology
http://www.blacksci.co.uk/~cgilib/jnlpage.bin?Journal=CEND&File=CEND&Page=aims
- Publisher — Blackwell Science, back issues available
- Free resources — Table of Contents
- Pay resources — Abstracts, Articles

Clinical Nutrition
http://www.harcourt-international.com/journals/clnu
- Publisher — Harcourt International, back issues available
- Free resources — Table of Contents, Abstracts
- Pay resources — Articles

Clinical Transplantation
http://www.munksgaarddirect.dk/usr/munksgaard/mdenglish.nsf?OpenDatabase
- Publisher — Munksgaard, back issues available
- Free resources — Table of Contents
- Pay resources — Abstracts, Articles

Current Opinion in Endocrinology and Diabetes
http://www.biomednet.com/cgi-bin/members1/shwtoc.pl?J:end

    Publisher   Lippincott, Williams and Wilkins, back issues available

    Free resources   Table of Contents, Abstracts

    Pay resources   Articles

Current Problems in Obstetrics, Gynecology, and Fertility
http://www1.mosby.com/scripts/om.dll/serve?action=searchDB&searchDBfor=home&id=og

    Publisher   Mosby, back issues available

    Free resources   Table of Contents, Abstracts

    Pay resources   Articles

Cytokine and Growth Factor Reviews
http://www.elsevier.com/inca/publications/store/8/6/8

    Publisher   Elsevier Science, back issues available

    Free resources   Table of Contents, Abstracts

    Pay resources   Articles

Diabetes
http://www.diabetes.org/Diabetes

    Publisher   American Diabetes Society, back issues available

    Free resources   Table of Contents, Abstracts

    Pay resources   Articles

Diabetes Care
http://www.diabetes.org/DiabetesCare/default.asp

    Publisher   American Diabetes Society, back issues available

    Free resources   Table of Contents, Abstracts

    Pay resources   Articles

Diabetes Forecast
http://www.diabetes.org/diabetesforecast

    Publisher   American Diabetes Society, back issues available

    Free resources   Table of Contents, Abstracts

    Pay resources   Articles

Diabetes, Obesity and Metabolism
http://www.blackwell-science.com/~cgilib/
jnlpage.bin?Journal=DOM&File=DOM&Page=aims

Publisher	Blackwell Science, back issues available
Free resources	Table of Contents
Pay resources	Abstracts, Articles

Diabetes Research and Clinical Practice
http://www.sciencedirect.com/science?_ob=JournalURL&_cdi=5015&_version=1&_urlVersion=0&_userid=0&md5=e96a270c9be230de923825ddc3b3f5c4

Publisher	Elsevier, back issues available
Free resources	Table of Contents
Pay resources	Abstracts, Articles

Diabetes Reviews
http://www.diabetes.org/DiabetesReviews

Publisher	American Diabetes Society, back issues available
Free resources	Table of Contents, Abstracts
Pay resources	Articles

Diabetes Spectrum
http://www.diabetes.org/DiabetesSpectrum

Publisher	American Diabetes Society, back issues available
Free resources	Table of Contents, Abstracts
Pay resources	Articles

Diabetes/Metabolism Reviews
http://www.interscience.wiley.com/jpages/0742-4221

Publisher	Wiley, back issues available
Free resources	Registration Required to access Table of Contents and Abstracts
Pay resources	Articles

Diabetic Medicine
http://www.blackwell-synergy.com/issuelist.asp?journal=dme

Publisher	Blackwell Science, back issues available
Free resources	Table of Contents, Abstracts
Pay resources	Articles

Diabetologia
http://link.springer.de/link/service/journals/00125/index.htm

    Publisher   Springer–Verlag, back issues available

    Free resources   Table of Contents, Abstracts

    Pay resources   Articles

Digestive Diseases and Sciences
http://www.wkap.nl/journalhome.htm/0163-2116

    Publisher   Kluwer, back issues available

    Free resources   Table of Contents

    Pay resources   Abstracts, Articles

Endocrine and Metabolic Drug Reviews
http://pharminfo.com/pubs/msb/msbendo.html

    Publisher   Pharmaceutical Information Associates, Ltd., back issues available

    Free resources   Table of Contents, Abstracts, Articles

    Pay resources   None

Endocrine Research
http://www.dekker.com/e/p.pl/0743-5800

    Publisher   Marcel Dekker, back issues available

    Free resources   Table of Contents, Abstracts

    Pay resources   Articles

Endocrine Reviews
http://edrv.endojournals.org

    Publisher   Endocrine Society, back issues available

    Free resources   Table of Contents, Abstracts

    Pay resources   Articles

Endocrine-Related Cancer
http://journals.endocrinology.org/erc/erc.htm

    Publisher   Society for Endocrinology, back issues available

    Free resources   Table of Contents, Abstracts

    Pay resources   Articles

Endocrinology
http://www.endojournals.org
- Publisher: Endocrine Society, back issues available
- Free resources: Table of Contents, Abstracts
- Pay resources: Articles

Endocrinology and Metabolism
http://ajpendo.physiology.org
- Publisher: American Physiological Society, back issues available
- Free resources: Table of Contents, Abstracts
- Pay resources: Articles

European Journal of Contraception and Reproductive Care
http://www.parthpub.com/contra/home.html
- Publisher: Parthenon Publishing Group, back issues available
- Free resources: Table of Contents
- Pay resources: Abstracts, Articles

European Journal of Endocrinology
http://www.eje.org
- Publisher: European Federation of Endocrine Societies, back issues available
- Free resources: Table of Contents, Abstracts
- Pay resources: Articles

European Journal of Obstetrics and Gynecology and Reproductive Biology
http://www.elsevier.nl:80/inca/publications/store/5/0/5/9/6/1
- Publisher: Elsevier Science, back issues available
- Free resources: Table of Contents
- Pay resources: Abstracts, Articles

European Menopause Journal
http://endocrine.medscape.com/PMSI/EMJ/public/journal.EMJ.html
- Publisher: Medscape, back issues available
- Free resources: Table of Contents, Abstracts
- Pay resources: Articles

Fertility and Sterility
http://www.elsevier.com/locate/fertilsteril
- Publisher: Elsevier Science, back issues available
- Free resources: Table of Contents, Abstracts, Articles
- Pay resources: None

Frontiers in Endocrinology
http://www.apnet.com/www/journal/fn.htm
- Publisher: Academic Press, back issues available
- Free resources: Table of Contents, Abstracts
- Pay resources: Articles

Frontiers in Neuroendocrinology
http://www.apnet.com/www/journal/fn.htm
- Publisher: Academic Press, back issues available
- Free resources: Table of Contents, Abstracts
- Pay resources: Articles

General and Comparative Endocrinology
http://www.apnet.com/www/journal/gc.htm
- Publisher: Academic Press, back issues available
- Free resources: Table of Contents, Abstracts
- Pay resources: Articles

Growth Hormone and IGF Research
http://www.churchillmed.com/online/GrowthHormone/JHome.html
- Publisher: Churchill Livingstone, back issues available
- Free resources: Table of Contents, Abstracts
- Pay resources: Articles

Gynecological Endocrinology
http://www.parthpub.com/gynend/home.html
- Publisher: Parthenon Publishing Group, back issues available
- Free resources: Table of Contents
- Pay resources: Abstracts, Articles

Hormone and Metabolic Research
http://www.thieme.com/onGILJMAEEEGDH/display/761
- Publisher   Thieme Journals
- Free resources   Table of Contents
- Pay resources   Abstracts, Articles

Hormone Research
http://www.karger.ch/journals/hre/hre_jh.htm
- Publisher   Karger, back issues available
- Free resources   Table of Contents, Abstracts
- Pay resources   Articles

Hormones and Behavior
http://www.apnet.com/www/journal/hb.htm
- Publisher   Academic Press, back issues available
- Free resources   Table of Contents, Abstracts
- Pay resources   Articles

Human Reproduction
http://humrep.oupjournals.org
- Publisher   Oxford University Press, back issues available
- Free resources   Table of Contents, Abstracts
- Pay resources   Articles

Journal of Assisted Reproduction and Genetics
http://www.wkap.nl/journalhome.htm/1058-0468
- Publisher   Kluwer, back issues available
- Free resources   Table of Contents
- Pay resources   Abstracts, Articles

Journal of Bone and Mineral Metabolism
http://link.springer.de/link/service/journals/00774/index.htm
- Publisher   Springer–Verlag, back issues available
- Free resources   Table of Contents, Abstracts
- Pay resources   Articles

Journal of Bone and Mineral Research
http://www.blacksci.co.uk/~cgilib/jnlpage.bin?Journal=XJBMR&File=XJBMR&Page=aims
- Publisher: Blackwell Science, back issues available
- Free resources: Table of Contents
- Pay resources: Abstracts, Articles

Journal of Cerebral Blood Flow and Metabolism
http://www.jcbfm.com
- Publisher: Lippincott, Williams, and Wilkins, back issues available
- Free resources: Table of Contents
- Pay resources: Abstracts, Articles

Journal of Clinical Endocrinology and Metabolism
http://jcem.endojournals.org
- Publisher: Endocrine Society, back issues available
- Free resources: Table of Contents, Abstracts
- Pay resources: Articles

Journal of Diabetes and its Complications
http://www.elsevier.com/inca/publications/store/5/0/5/7/7/0
- Publisher: Elsevier Science, back issues available
- Free resources: Table of Contents
- Pay resources: Abstracts, Articles

Journal of Endocrinological Investigation
http://www.kurtis.it/endoinv.htm
- Publisher: Italian Society of Endocrinology, back issues available
- Free resources: Table of Contents, Abstracts
- Pay resources: Articles

Journal of Endocrinology
http://journals.endocrinology.org/JOE/joe.htm
- Publisher: Society for Endocrinology, back issues available
- Free resources: Table of Contents, Abstracts
- Pay resources: Articles

Journal of Genetic Counseling
http://www.wkap.nl/journalhome.htm/1059-7700
- Publisher: Kluwer, back issues available
- Free resources: Table of Contents
- Pay resources: Abstracts, Articles

Journal of Human Nutrition and Dietetics
http://www.blackwell-science.com/PRODUCTS/JOURNALS/JNLTITLE.HTM
- Publisher: Blackwell Science, back issues available
- Free resources: Table of Contents
- Pay resources: Abstracts, Articles

Journal of Inherited Metabolic Disease
http://www.wkap.nl/journalhome.htm/0141-8955
- Publisher: Kluwer, back issues available
- Free resources: Table of Contents
- Pay resources: Abstracts, Articles

Journal of Molecular Endocrinology
http://journals.endocrinology.org/JME/jme.htm
- Publisher: Society for Endocrinology, back issues available
- Free resources: Table of Contents, Abstracts
- Pay resources: Articles

Journal of Neuroendocrinology
http://www.blackwell-science.com/~cgilib/jnlpage.bin?Journal=JNEUR&File=JNEUR&Page=aims
- Publisher: Blackwell Science, back issues available
- Free resources: Table of Contents
- Pay resources: Abstracts, Articles

Journal of Nutritional Biochemistry
http://www.elsevier.com/inca/publications/store/5/2/5/0/1/3
- Publisher: Elsevier Science, back issues available
- Free resources: Table of Contents
- Pay resources: Abstracts, Articles

Journal of Peptide Research
http://www.munksgaarddirect.dk/usr/munksgaard/mdenglish.nsf?OpenDatabase
- Publisher   Munksgaard, back issues available
- Free resources   Table of Contents
- Pay resources   Abstracts, Articles

Journal of Pineal Research
http://www.munksgaarddirect.dk/usr/munksgaard/mdenglish.nsf?OpenDatabase
- Publisher   Munksgaard, back issues available
- Free resources   Table of Contents
- Pay resources   Abstracts, Articles

Journal of Reproductive Medicine
http://www.jreprodmed.com
- Publisher   Science Printers and Publishers, Inc., back issues available
- Free resources   Table of Contents
- Pay resources   Abstracts, Articles

Mineral and Electrolyte Metabolism
http://www.karger.ch/journals/mem/mem_jh.htm
- Publisher   Karger, back issues available
- Free resources   Table of Contents, Abstracts
- Pay resources   Articles

Molecular and Cellular Endocrinology
http://www.sciencedirect.com/science?_ob=JournalURL&_cdi=4946&_version=1&_urlVersion=0&_userid=0&md5=8222aaa7f64b75595dc3836c900678e8
- Publisher   Elsevier, back issues available
- Free resources   Table of Contents
- Pay resources   Abstracts, Articles

Molecular Endocrinology
http://mend.endojournals.org
- Publisher   Endocrine Society, back issues available
- Free resources   Table of Contents, Abstracts
- Pay resources   Articles

Molecular Genetics and Metabolism
http://www.academicpress.com/mgm
- Publisher: Academic Press, back issues available
- Free resources: Table of Contents, Abstracts
- Pay resources: Articles

Molecular Human Reproduction
http://molehr.oupjournals.org
- Publisher: Oxford University Press, back issues available
- Free resources: Table of Contents, Abstracts
- Pay resources: Articles

Molecular Reproduction and Development
http://www3.interscience.wiley.com/cgi-bin/jtoc?ID=37692
- Publisher: Wiley, back issues available
- Free resources: Table of Contents, Abstracts
- Pay resources: Articles

Neuroendocrinology
http://www.karger.ch/journals/nen/nen_jh.htm
- Publisher: Karger, back issues available
- Free resources: Table of Contents, Abstracts
- Pay resources: Articles

Nutrition
http://www.elsevier.com/inca/publications/store/5/2/5/6/1/4
- Publisher: Elsevier Science, back issues available
- Free resources: Table of Contents
- Pay resources: Abstracts, Articles

Nutrition, Metabolism, and Cardiovascular Diseases
http://www.medikal.it
- Publisher: Medikal Press, back issues available
- Free resources: Table of Contents
- Pay resources: Abstracts, Articles

Nutrition Research
http://www.elsevier.com/inca/publications/store/5/2/5/4/8/3
- Publisher   Elsevier Science, back issues available
- Free resources   Table of Contents
- Pay resources   Abstracts, Articles

Osteoporosis International
http://link.springer.de/link/service/journals/00198/index.htm
- Publisher   Springer–Verlag, back issues available
- Free resources   Table of Contents, Abstracts
- Pay resources   Articles

Pituitary
http://www.wkap.nl/journalhome.htm/1386-341X
- Publisher   Kluwer, back issues available
- Free resources   Table of Contents
- Pay resources   Abstracts, Articles

Practical Diabetes International
http://www3.interscience.wiley.com/cgi-bin/jtoc?ID=70003726
- Publisher   Wiley, back issues available
- Free resources   Table of Contents, Abstracts
- Pay resources   Articles

Prostaglandins and Other Lipid Mediators
http://www.elsevier.nl/inca/publications/store/5/2/5/0/1/9
- Publisher   Elsevier Science, back issues available
- Free resources   Table of Contents, Abstracts
- Pay resources   Articles

Prostaglandins, Leukotrines, and Essential Fatty Acids
http://www.harcourt-international.com/journals/plef
- Publisher   Harcourt Publishers Ltd., back issues available
- Free resources   Table of Contents, Abstracts, Articles
- Pay resources   None

Prostate
http://www3.interscience.wiley.com/cgi-bin/jtoc?ID=34304
- Publisher: Wiley, back issues available
- Free resources: Table of Contents, Abstracts
- Pay resources: Articles

Psychoneuroendocrinology
http://www.sciencedirect.com/science?_ob=JournalURL&_cdi=5154&_version=1&_urlVersion=0&_userid=0&md5=c83bcf859eac48b3dfb9b9f342747e7c
- Publisher: Elsevier, back issues available
- Free resources: Table of Contents
- Pay resources: Abstracts, Articles

Reproduction, Fertility and Development
http://www.publish.csiro.au/journals/rfd
- Publisher: CSIRO Publishing, back issues available
- Free resources: Table of Contents, Abstracts
- Pay resources: Articles

Reproductive Health Matters
http://www.blackwell-science.com/PRODUCTS/JOURNALS/JNLTITLE.HTM
- Publisher: Blackwell Science, back issues available
- Free resources: Table of Contents
- Pay resources: Abstracts, Articles

Reproductive Medicine Review
http://www.journals.cup.org/owa_dba/owa/ISSUES_IN_JOURNAL?JID=RMR
- Publisher: Cambridge University Press, back issues available
- Free resources: Table of Contents, Abstracts
- Pay resources: Articles

Reviews in Endocrine and Metabolic Disorders
http://www.wkap.nl/journalhome.htm/1389-9155
- Publisher: Kluwer, back issues available
- Free resources: Table of Contents
- Pay resources: Abstracts, Articles

Sexual Dysfunction
http://www.blackwell-synergy.com/issuelist.asp?journal=sdy

Publisher	Blackwell Science, back issues available
Free resources	Table of Contents, Abstracts
Pay resources	Articles

Steroids
http://www.sciencedirect.com/science?_ob=JournalURL&_cdi=5165&_version=1&_urlVersion=0&_userid=0&md5=ad99a6b44fb2ed9097e6eb4037775b3c

Publisher	Elsevier, back issues available
Free resources	Table of Contents
Pay resources	Abstracts, Articles

The Endocrinologist
http://www.theendocrinologist.org

Publisher	Lippincott Wiliams and Wilkins, back issues available
Free resources	Table of Contents
Pay resources	Abstracts, Articles

Thyroid
http://www.thyroid.org/journal/journal.htm

Publisher	Mary Ann Liebert, Inc., back issues available
Free resources	Table of Contents
Pay resources	Abstracts, Articles

Transplant International
http://link.springer.de/link/service/journals/00147/index.htm

Publisher	Springer–Verlag, back issues available
Free resources	Table of Contents, Abstracts
Pay resources	Articles

Transplantation
http://www.wwilkins.com/TP

Publisher	Lippincott, Williams and Wilkins, back issues available
Free resources	Table of Contents, Abstracts
Pay resources	Articles

Trends in Endocrinology and Metabolism
http://www.sciencedirect.com/science?_ob=JournalURL&_cdi=4949&_version=1&_url
Version=0&_userid=0&md5=4fe2bf13b9dcc19b9297e950c23b53ac

Publisher	Elsevier, back issues available
Free resources	Table of Contents
Pay resources	Abstracts, Articles

World Diabetes
http://www.who.int/ncd/dia

Publisher	World Health Organization, back issues available
Free resources	Table of Contents, Articles
Pay resources	None

3.3 Books on Endocrinology Published in 1999/2000

The following listing contains books published during the past 12 months in the fields of endocrinology and metabolism. The books are categorized under major topics, although many books contain material that extends beyond the highlighted subject. All of these books may be purchased through Amazon at http://www.amazon.com.

The following topics appear below, in order:

General Resources
Clinical Endocrinology
Diabetes, General
Diabetes, Nutrition
Diabetic Complications
Diagnostics
Disorders
Endocrine Oncology
Environmental Endocrinology
Epidemiology and Prevention
Genetics
Growth Hormone Therapy
Hormone Replacement Therapy
Menopause
Neuroendocrinology
Pediatric Endocrinology
Physiology
Reproductive Endocrinology
Therapeutics

General Resources

The Year Book of Endocrinology 2000 (Year Book of Endocrinology, 2000), John D. Bagdade. Mosby-Year Book, 2000, ISBN: 0323015026.

Clinical Endocrinology

1999 Year Book of Endocrinology, John D. Bagdade. Mosby-Year Book, 1999, ISBN: 081519627X.

Atlas of Clinical Endocrinology, Stanley G. Korenman (Editor). Blackwell Science Inc.. 1999, ISBN: 0632043970.

Atlas of Clinical Endocrinology, Volume IV: Neuroendocrinology and Pituitary Disease, David Heber (Editor). Blackwell Science Inc., 2000, ISBN: 0632044055.

Basic & Clinical Endocrinology, Francis S. Greenspan. Appleton & Lange, 2000, ISBN: 083850597X.

Basic Endocrinology: An Interactive Approach, J. Matthew Neal. Blackwell Pub., 1999, ISBN: 0632044292.

Diabetes (Atlas of Clinical Endocrinology, Vol. 2), C. Ronald Kahn (Editor). Blackwell Science Inc., 1999, ISBN: 0632043997.

Diabetes: Emergency and Hospital Management, Simon R. Page, George M. Hall. B M J Books, 1999, ISBN: 0727912291.

Endocrinology and Metabolism (Clinical Medicine Series), Aldo Pinchera(Editor), Lewis Braverman (Editor). McGraw Hill Text, 2000, ISBN: 0077095200.

Endocrinology of the Heart (Contemporary Endocrinology Vol. 21), Leonard Share (Editor). Humana Press, 1999, ISBN: 0896037266.

Endocrinology of the Lung: Development and Surfactant Synthesis (Contemporary Endocrinology), Carole R. Mendelson (Editor). Humana Press, 2000, ISBN: 0896036766.

Management of Ed: Focus on Sildenafil: A Diabetologist's/Endocrinologist's Approach (Pharmanual), C. E. Morgensen (Editor). Pharma Libri Pub., 1999, ISBN: 0919839541.

Medical and Surgical Management of Adrenal Diseases, Joseph C. Cerny. Lippincott, Williams & Wilkins, 1999, ISBN: 0683303449.

Molecular and Cellular Endocrine Pathology (Principles of Medical Biology, Vol. 10A, 10B), Lucia Stefaneanu (Editor), Hironobu Sasano (Editor), Kalman Kovacs (Editor). Lippincott-Raven Publishers, 1999, ISBN: 041211271X.

Mosby's Color Atlas and Text of Diabetes and Endocrinology, Peter E. Belchetz, Peter Hammond. Mosby-Year Book, 2000, ISBN: 0723431043.

Post-Transcriptional Processing and the Endocrine System (Frontiers of Hormone Research, Vol. 25), Shern L. Chew (Editor). 1999, ISBN: 3805568495.

Research Methodologies in Human Diabetes, Carl Erik Mogensen, E. Standl, Walter DeGruyter. 2000, ISBN: 3110145553.

The Endocrine Response to Acute Illness (Frontiers of Hormone Research, Vol. 24), R. C. Jenkins (Editor), Richard J. M. Ross (Editor). S. Karger Publishing, 1999, ISBN: 3805568223.

Transgenics in Endocrinology (Contemporary Endocrinology), Martin Matzuk(Editor), et al. Humana Press, 2000, ISBN: 0896037649.

Diabetes, General

101 Nutrition Tips for People with Diabetes, Patti B. Geil, M.S., R.D., Lea Ann Holzmeister, R.D. American Diabetes Assn., 1999, ISBN: 1580400280.

American Diabetes Association Complete Guide to Diabetes: The Ultimate Home Diabetes Reference, Elizabeth A. Walker, et al. American Diabetes Assn., 2000, ISBN: 1580400388.

Coping with Diabetes: A Guide to Living with Diabetes for You and Your Family, Robert H. Phillips. Avery Pub. Group, 1999, ISBN: 0895299232.

Current Review of Diabetes, Simeon I. Taylor (Editor). Current Medicine, 1999, ISBN: 1573401323.

Diabetes, Lynne Jerreat. Whurr Publishers, 1999, ISBN: 1861560990.

Diabetes (Lucent Overview Series), Gail Stewart. Lucent Books, 1999, ISBN: 1560065273.

Diabetes Mellitus, Campbell, Lebovitz. Health Press, 2000, ISBN: 1899541888.

Diabetes Mellitus: A Practical Handbook, Sue K. Milchovich, Barbara Dunn-Long. Bull Pub. Co., 1999, ISBN: 092352147X.

Diabetes Patient Education Manual, Simon B. Weavers (Editor), Judy Marcus (Editor). Aspen Publishers, Inc., 1999, ISBN: 0834212757.

Diabetes (Perspectives on Disease and Illness), Judith Peacock. Lifematters, 2000, ISBN: 0736802770.

Diabetes (Understanding Illness), Sue Vander Hook. Smart Apple Media, 2000, ISBN: 1583400230.

Evidence-Based Diabetes Management, Hertzel C. Gerstein, R. Brian Haynes. BC Decker Inc., 2000, ISBN: 1550091247.

Experimental Models of Diabetes, John H. McNeil (Editor). CRC Press, 1999, ISBN: 0849316677.

Living with Diabetes, Jenny Bryan. Raintree/Steck Vaughn, 1999, ISBN: 0817255753.

Living with Diabetes: What You Really Need to Know, Rob Buckman, et al. Lebhar-Friedman Books, 2000, ISBN: 086730796X.

Staged Diabetes Management: A Systematic Approach to the Prevention, Detection, and Treatment of Diabetes and Its Complications, R. S. Mazze (Editor). International Diabetes Center. 1999, ISBN: 1885115555.

The Diabetes Annual 12, S. M. Marshall (Editor), P. D. Home (Editor), R. A. Rizza (Editor). Elsevier Science Ltd., 1999, ISBN: 0444828966.

The Diabetes Cure: A Medical Approach That Can Slow, Stop, Even Cure Type 2 Diabetes, Vern S. Cherewatenko, Paul Perry (Introduction). Cliff Street Books, 1999, ISBN: 0060192100.

The Diabetes Problem Solver: Quick Answers to Your Questions about Treatment and Self-Care, Nancy Touchette, Ph.D. American Diabetes Assn., 1999, ISBN: 1580400094.

The Diabetes Sourcebook: Today's Methods and Ways to Give Yourself the Best Care, Diana W. Guthrie, Richard A. Guthrie. Lowell House, 1999, ISBN: 0737300841.

The Diabetic Male's Essential Guide to Living Well, Hank Belopavlovich, Joseph Juliano. Henry Holt & Company, Inc., 1999, ISBN: 0805038841.

Type 2 Diabetes, Gerald M. Reaven, Terry Kristen Strom. Merit Publishing International, 2000, ISBN: 1873413173.

Type 2 Diabetes: Prediction and Prevention (Wiley Practical Diabetes Series), Graham Hitman (Editor). John Wiley & Sons, 1999, ISBN: 0471985953.

Diabetes, Nutrition

101 Nutrition Tips for People with Diabetes, Patti B. Geil, M.S., R.D. Lea Ann Holzmeister R.D. CDE, Patti B. Geil. American Diabetes Assn., 1999, ISBN: 1580400280.

101 Tips for Improving Your Blood Sugar,, Sherrye Landrum (Editor). American Diabetes Assn., 1999, ISBN: 1580400264.

American Diabetes Association's Guide to Medical Nutrition Therapy for Diabetes (Clinical Education Series), Marion J. Franz (Editor), John P. Bantle (Editor) American Diabetes Assn.. 1999, ISBN: 158040006X.

Complete Diabetic Cookbook, Mary Jane Finsand, Edith White. Black Dog & Leventhal Pub., 1999, ISBN: 1579120644.

New Diabetic Cookbook, Kristi Fuller (Editor). Better Homes and Gardens Books, 1999, ISBN: 0696207923.

The Other Diabetes: Living and Eating Well with Type 2 Diabetes, Elizabeth Hiser. William Morrow & Company, 1999, ISBN: 0688153291.

What to Eat when Your Doctor Says It's Diabetes, Carolyn Leontos. American Diabetes Assn, 1999, ISBN: 0945448988.

Diabetic Complications

Diabetes and the Eye, Hamish Towler, Julian Patterson, Susan Lightman. B. M. J. Books, 1999, ISBN: 0727913816.

Hypoglycaemia in Clinical Diabetes (Diabetes in Practice), Brian M. Frier (Editor), B. Miles Fisher (Editor). John Wiley & Sons, 1999, ISBN: 0471982644.

Levin and O'Neal's the Diabetic Foot, John H. Bowker, Michael A. Pfeifer. Mosby-Year Book, 2000, ISBN: 155664471X.

Mechanisms in Progression of Renal Disease: Kidney & Blood Pressure Research, J. Floege (Editor). S. Karger Publishing, 1999, ISBN: 3805568762.

Nephropathy in Type 2 Diabetes (Oxford Clinical Nephrology Series), Ivan Rychlik (Editor), Eberhard Ritz (Editor). Oxford Univ. Press, 1999, ISBN: 019262945X.

The Diabetes Eye Care Sourcebook, Donald S. Fong, M.D., Robin Demi Ross, M.D. Lowell House, 1999, ISBN: 0737301333.

Diagnostics

Atlas of Planar and Spect Bone Scans, Lawrence G. Holder, M.D., et al. Dunitz Martin Ltd., 2000, ISBN: 1853174696.

Biophosphates in Bone Disease: From the Laboratory to the Patient, Herbert Fleisch. Academic Press, 2000, ISBN: 0122603702.

Diagnosis and Management of Pituitary Tumors, Kamal Thapar (Editor), Kalman Kovacs (Editor), Bernd Scheithauer (Editor). Humana Press, 1999, ISBN: 0896034038.

Handbook of Diagnostic Endocrinology (Contemporary Endocrinology), Janet E. Hall(Editor), Lynette Nieman (Editor). Humana Press, 2000, ISBN: 0896037576.

Standardization of Growth Hormone Measurement Evidence-Based Medicine (Hormone Research, 51/1), M. B. Ranke (Editor), J. Dowie (Editor). S. Karger Publishing, 1999, ISBN: 3805568983.

Disorders

Adrenal Disorders (Contemporary Endocrinology), George P. Chrousos (Editor), A. N. Margioris (Editor). Humana Press, 2000, ISBN: 0896034119.

Androgen Disorders in Women: The Most Neglected Hormone Problem, Theresa Cheung, Theresa C. Leung. Hunter House, 1999, ISBN: 0897932609.

Atlas of Diseases of the Kidney, Tomas Berl (Editor), Joseph V. Bonventre (Editor), Robert W. Schrier. Blackwell Science Inc., 1999, ISBN: 0632043857.

Autoimmune Endocrinopathies (Contemporary Endocrinology, Vol. 15), Robert Volpe (Editor). Humana Press, 1999, ISBN: 0896036804.

Dynamics of Bone and Cartilage Metabolism,, Markus J. Seibel (Editor), Simon P. Robins (Editor), John P. Bilezikian (Editor). Academic Press Inc., 1999, ISBN: 0126348405.

Endocrine Tumors, Orio H. Clark, et al. B. C. Decker Inc., 2000, ISBN: 1550091344.

Graves' Disease: Pathogenesis and Treatment, Basil Rapoport, Sandra M. McLachlan. Kluwer Academic Publishers, 2000, ISBN: 0792377907.

Handbook of Fluid, Electrolyte and Acid-Base Disorders, Leonard G. Feld. Butterworth-Heinemann, 2000, ISBN: 0750699574.

Heart, Kidney and Renal Failure (Mineral and Electrolyte Metabolism, 25/2), Natale Gaspare De Santo (Editor), Luigi Iorio (Editor). S. Karger Publishing, 1999, ISBN: 3805568592.

Hemochromatosis: Genetics, Pathophysiology, Diagnosis, and Treatment, Corwin Q. Edwards(Editor), James C. Barton. Cambridge Univ. Press, 2000, ISBN: 0521593808.

Hormone Resistance Syndromes (Contemporary Endocrinology, Vol. 14), J. Larry Jameson (Editor). Humana Press, 1999, ISBN: 0896036529.

Hypertension: A Companion to Brenner & Rector's the Kidney, Suzanne Oparil (Editor), Michael A. Weber (Editor). W. B. Saunders Co., 1999, ISBN: 0721677649.

Inborn Metabolic Diseases: Diagnosis and Treatment, J. Fernandes (Editor), et al. Springer–Verlag, 2000, ISBN: 354065626X.

Insulin Resistance: The Metabolic Syndrome X (Contemporary Endocrinology Vol. 12), Gerald M. Reaven (Editor), Ami Laws (Editor). Humana Press, 1999, ISBN: 0896035883.

Physical Activity and Obesity, Claude Bouchard (Editor). Human Kinetics Pub., 2000, ISBN: 0880119098.

Renal Pathophysiology (Pathophysiology Series), Louis J. Riley. Fence Creek Pub., 1999, ISBN: 1889325031.

The Osteoporotic Syndrome: Detection, Prevention, and Treatment, Louis V. Avioli (Editor). Academic Press, 2000, ISBN: 0120687054.

The Thyroid Sourcebook for Women, M. Sara Rosenthal. Lowell House, 1999, ISBN: 073730264X.

Thyroid Cancer: Clinical Management, L. Wartofsky (Editor). Humana Press, 1999, ISBN: 0896034291.

Thyroid Disease: The Facts (Oxford Medical Publications), R. I. S. Bayliss, W. M. G. Tunbridge. Oxford Univ. Press, 1999, ISBN: 0192629468.

Thyroid Disorders, Tony Smith. Dorling Kindersley Publishers, 1999, ISBN: 078944173X.

Endocrine Oncology

Endocrine Oncology (Contemporary Endocrinology), Stephen P. Ethier (Editor). Humana Press, 2000, ISBN: 0896036219.

Endocrinology of Breast Cancer (Contemporary Endocrinology, Vol. 11), Andrea Manni (Editor). Humana Press, 1999, ISBN: 0896035913.

Environmental Endocrinology

Advances in the Analysis of Environmental Endocrine Disruptors (American Chemical Society Symposium Series), Larry Keith, Tammy Jones, Larry Needham. American Chemical Society, 1999, ISBN: 084123650X.

Endocrine Disruptors: Effects on Male and Female Reproductive Systems, Rajesh K. Naz (Editor). CRC Press, 1999, ISBN: 0849331641.

Environmental Endocrine Disrupters: An Evolutionary Perspective, Louis J. Guillette, Jr. (Editor), D. Andrew Crain (Editor). Hemisphere Pub., 2000, ISBN: 1560325712.

Hormonal Chaos: The Scientific and Social Origins of the Environmental Endocrine Hypothesis, Sheldon Krimsky, Lynn Goldman. Johns Hopkins Univ. Press, 1999, ISBN: 0801862795.

Hormonally Active Agents in the Environment, National Research Council, Committee on Hormonally Active Agents in The Environment. National Academy Press, 1999, ISBN: 0309064198.

Epidemiology and Prevention

Preventing Diabetes: Theory, Practice, and New Approaches, Dan Cheta. John Wiley & Sons, 1999, ISBN: 0471999148.

The Epidemiology of Diabetes Mellitus, Jean M. Ekoe (Editor), et al. John Wiley & Sons, 2000, ISBN: 047197448X.

Genetics

Gene Engineering in Endocrinology (Contemporary Endocrinology (Vol. 22), Margaret A. Shupnik (Editor). Humana Press, 2000, ISBN: 0896037185.

The Genetics of Endocrine Disorders (Contemporary Endocrinology), Maria I. New (Editor). Humana Press, 2000, ISBN: 089603786X.

Geriatrics

Diabetes Mellitus in the Elderly, James W. Cooper (Editor). Haworth Press, 1999, ISBN: 0789006820.

Growth Hormone Therapy

Challenges in Growth Hormone Therapy, John P. Monson (Editor). Blackwell Science Inc., 1999, ISBN: 0632051647.

Human Growth Hormone: Research and Clinical Practice (Contemporary Endocrinology), Roy G. Smith, Michael O. Thorner. Humana Press, 1999, ISBN: 0896035050.

Hormone Replacement Therapy

DK Healthcare: Hormone Replacement Therapy, Miriam Stoppard. DK Pub. Merchandise, 1999, ISBN: 0789437562.

Estrogen: How and Why It Can Save Your Life, Adam Romoff, Ina L. Yalof. Golden Books Pub. Co., 1999, ISBN: 1582380120.

Hormone Replacement Therapy: A Guide for Primary Care (Oxford Medical Publications), Sally Hope (Editor), Janet Brockie, Margaret Rees. Oxford Univ. Press, 1999, ISBN: 0192629565.

Hormone Replacement Therapy and the Brain: A Clinical Perspective on the Role of Estrogen, Victor Henderson. Parthenon Pub. Group, 1999, ISBN: 1850700788.

Hormone Replacement Therapy (Contemporary Endocrinology, Vol. 13), A. Wayne Meikle (Editor), Wayne A. Meikle (Editor). Humana Press, 1999, ISBN: 0896036014.

Mechanisms and Biological Significance of Pulsatile Hormone Secretion: No. 227: Novartis Foundation Symposium (Ciba Foundation Symposia Series, 227), Johannes D. Veldhuis, et al. John Wiley & Sons, 2000, ISBN: 0471999180.

Menopause and Hormone Replacement Therapy: A Simple but Complete Guide for Today's Busy Woman, Dr. Sharon Lunz. S. L. Publishers/Sharon Lunz, 1999, ISBN: 0966998502.

The Estrogen Alternative: What Every Woman Needs to Know about Hormone Replacement Therapy and Serms, the New Estrogen Substitutes, Steven R. Goldstein, Laurie Ashner. Putnam Pub. Group, 1999, ISBN: 0399144536.

The Estrogen Answer Book: 150 Most-Asked Questions about Hormone Replacement Therapy, Ruth S. Jacobowitz. Little Brown & Co., 1999, ISBN: 0316458082.

Menopause

Menopause: Endocrinology and Management (Contemporary Endocrinology, Vol. 18), David B. Seifer (Editor), Robert Wood Johnson (Editor). Humana Press, 1999, ISBN: 0896036774.

Smart Medicine for Menopause: Hormone Replacement Therapy and Its Natural Alternatives, Sandra Cabot. Avery Pub. Group, 1999, ISBN: 089529897X.

Neuroendocrinology

An Introduction to Behavioral Endocrinology, Randy J. Nelson. Sinauer Assoc., 1999, ISBN: 0878936165.

Neurosteroids: A New Regulatory Function in the Nervous System (Contemporary Endocrinology, Vol. 21), Etienne-Emile Baulieu (Editor), Michael Schumacher (Editor), Paul Robel. Humana Press, 1999, ISBN: 089603545X.

Steroid-Hormone-Dependent Organization of Neuroendocrine Functions (Neuroscience Intelligence Unit), Vladimir Patchev, O. F. X. Almeida. R. G. Landes Co., 1999, ISBN: 1570595550.

Pediatric Endocrinology

Living with Juvenile Diabetes: A Family Guide, Victoria Peurrung. Hatherleigh Press, 2000, ISBN: 1578260574.

Molecular and Cellular Pediatric Endocrinology (Contemporary Endocrinology, Vol. 10), Stuart Handwerger (Editor). Humana Press, 1999, ISBN: 0896034062.

Pediatric Nephrology, T. Martin Barratt (Editor), Ellis D. Avner (Editor), William Harmon (Editor). Lippincott, Williams & Wilkins, 1999, ISBN: 0683300555.

Physiology

Endocrine Physiology, Balint Kacsoh, M.D. McGraw-Hill, 2000, ISBN: 0070344329.

Handbook of Physiology: A Critical, Comprehensive Presentation of Physiological Knowledge and Concepts: Section 7: The Endocrine System: Hormonal, Jack Kostyo (Editor), H. Maurice Goodman (Editor). Oxford Univ. Press, 1999, ISBN: 0195113055.

Handbook of Physiology: The Endocrine Pancreas and Regulation of Metabolism (No. 7, Vol. 2), Leonard S. Jefferson(Editor), Alan D. Cherrington (Editor). Amer. Physiological Society, 2000, ISBN: 0195113268.

Human Brain Stem Vessels: Including the Pineal Gland and Information on Brain Stem Infarction, Henri M. Duvernoy. Springer–Verlag, 1999, ISBN: 3540643494.

Ims: Endocrine System, Goodman. Fence Creek Pub., 2000, ISBN: 1889325325.

Principles of Molecular Regulation, P. Michael Conn (Editor), et al. Humana Press, 2000, ISBN: 0896036308.

Recent Progress in Hormone Research: Proceedings of the 1998 Conference (Vol. 54), P. Michael Conn (Editor). Endocrine Society, 1999, ISBN: 1879225336.

Textbook of Endocrine Physiology, James E. Griffin (Editor), Sergio R. Ojeda (Editor). Oxford Univ. Press, 2000, ISBN: 0195135415.

The Bone and Mineral Manual: A Practical Guide, Michael Kleerekoper (Editor), Michael McClung (Editor), Ethel Siris (Editor). Academic Press, 1999, ISBN: 0124126502.

Reproductive Endocrinology

Adolescent Gynecology and Endocrinology: Basic and Clinical Aspects (Annals of the New York Academy of Sciences, Vol. 816), George Creatsas (Editor), George Mastorakos (Editor), George P. Chrousos. New York Academy of Sciences, 1999, ISBN: 0801862159.

Clinical Gynecologic Endocrinology and Infertility: Self Assessment and Study Guide, David B. Seifer, Leon Speroff. Lippincott, Williams & Wilkins, 1999, ISBN: 0683303813.

Endocrinology and Management of Reproduction and Fertility: Practical Diagnosis and Treatment (Contemporary Endocrinology), Daniel Spratt (Editor), Nanette Santoro (Editor). Humana Press, 2000, ISBN: 0896035549.

Reproductive Endocrinology (Atlas of Clinical Gynecology, Vol. 3), Daniel R. Mishell (Editor). Appleton & Lange, 1999, ISBN: 0838503195.

Reproductive Endocrinology: Physiology, Pathophysiology, and Clinical Management, Samuel S. C. Yen (Editor), Robert B. Jaffe (Editor), Robert L. Barbieri. W. B. Saunders Co., 1999, ISBN: 0721668976.

Sex-Steroid Interactions with Growth Hormone (Serono Symposia USA), Johannes D. Veldhuis (Editor), Andrea Giustina (Editor). Springer–Verlag, 1999, ISBN: 0387988106.

The Young Woman at the Rise of the 21st Century: Gynecological and Reproductive Issues in Health and Disease (Annals of the New York Academy of Sciences), G. Creatsas (Editor), et al. New York Academy of Sciences, 2000, ISBN: 1573312274.

What Your Doctor May Not Tell You about Premenopause: Balance Your Hormones and Your Life from Thirty to Fifty, John R. Lee, Virginia Hopkins, Jesse Hanley. Warner Books, 1999, ISBN: 0446673803.

Therapeutics

Advances in Metabolism (Vol. 12), Viktor Mutt (Editor). Academic Press, 2000, ISBN: 0120273128.

Advances in Metabolism (Vol. 13/000), Levine (Editor). Academic Press, 2000, ISBN: 0120273136.

Advances in Research and Applications (Vitamins and Hormones, Vol. 58), Gerald Litwack (Editor). Academic Press, 2000, ISBN: 0127098585.

Growth Hormone (Endocrine Updates, 4), Bengt-Ake Bengtsson (Editor). Kluwer Academic Pub., 1999, ISBN: 0792384784.

Radiation and Thyroid Cancer, G. Thomas (Editor), A. Karaoglou (Editor), E. D. Williams (Editor). World Scientific Publishing Company, 1999, ISBN: 9810238142.

Therapeutic Outcome of Endocrine Disorders: Efficacy, Innovation and Quality of Life (Serono Symposia USA), Brian Stabler(Editor), Barry B. Bercu (Editor). Springer–Verlag, 2000, ISBN: 0387989625.

Vitamins and Hormones, Vol. 59, Gerald Litwack. Academic Press, 2000, ISBN: 0127098593.

4. CONTINUING MEDICAL EDUCATION (CME)

4.1 CME Resources

Accreditation Council for Continuing Medical Education (ACCME) ◐ ◐

http://www.accme.org

The ACCME offers voluntary accreditation to providers of continuing medical education who are interested in being recognized further for their high standards and quality. At the ACCME Web site, visitors will discover necessary information regarding all aspects of the accreditation process, as well as the current activities of the organization regarding communications and quality control protocols.

American Medical Association (AMA): CME Locator ◐ ◐ ◐

http://www.ama-assn.org/iwcf/iwcfmgr206/cme

The American Medical Association CME locator provides convenient access to over 2,000 activities sponsored by CME providers that are either accredited by the Accreditation Council for Continuing Medical Education (ACCME) or approved by the American Medical Association. CME selections of United States, Canadian, and international conferences, seminars, workshops, and home study courses are contained in the database. By customizing a search through the selection of a specialty, location, and date, visitors are returned a locator result set, which provides access to course objectives, registration information, and related Web address, where applicable.

CME Unlimited ◐ ◐ ◐

http://www.landesslezak.com/cgi-bin/start.cgi/cmeu/index.htm

This nonprofit division of the Audio-Digest Foundation specializes in producing audio CME programs for delivery to physicians and allied healthcare professionals on a subscription basis. It provides a high-quality selection of over 6,000 continuing medical education products from medical associations, institutions, and societies via audio, video, and CD-ROM. The offerings at this Web site include 13 specialty series and two jointly sponsored activities, with audio materials of medical symposia, review courses, and specialty meetings readily available. Each course listing includes its description, sponsor, target audience, accreditation, objectives, and faculty in addition to a list of currently available formats.

CMEWeb ○ ○ (fee-based)
http://www.cmeweb.com/#pdr

CMEWeb is an online resource for participation in electronic CME courses. It is provided by American Health Consultants, a commercial group accredited by the Accreditation Council for Continuing Medical Education (ACCME). CME resources are only available to registered members of the site, and registration requires a fee.

Cyberounds ○ ○
http://www.cyberounds.com/links/home.html

Cyberounds is an online, interactive forum moderated by distinguished professionals. It is available for use by physicians, medical students, and other selected healthcare professionals. All users must register to access resources at the site. Registration is free of charge but restricted to healthcare professionals. Continuing medical education opportunities, an online bookstore, links to quality sites relevant to a variety of specialties, and additional educational resources are available.

Ed Credits ○ ○ (some features fee-based)
http://www.edcredits.com

Ed Credits offers opportunities for CME credits for medical and other professionals. Registration is available for an annual fee, and any number of courses can be taken within this time. Material for the courses is available for free on the Web site, but registration is necessary to take the tests and to receive certificates.

Medical Computing Today: CME Sites ○ ○ ○ (some features fee-based)
http://www.medicalcomputingtoday.com/0listcme.html

Medical Computing Today provides a site that presents an alphabetical listing of currently available category I CME credit offerings listed by the Accreditation Council for Continuing Medical Education (ACCME). Principal areas of specialty covered at each of 85 sites are listed and directions for searching the text via Netscape Navigator are viewable. Alphabetical navigation bars throughout the text also provide visitors the opportunity to successfully locate educational materials of their choosing. CME descriptions, credits, and associated costs are included in CME entries. Registration for CME credit may be completed online.

Medical Matrix: CME Courses Online ○ ○ ○ (some features fee-based)
http://www.medmatrix.org

Medical Matrix's CME Courses Online is a resource for continuing medical education on the World Wide Web, with 39 accessible CME credit listing sites. General learning modules are available via the Virtual Lecture Hall Health Professionals CME, Health-

Gate CME Courses, and Medscape's Online Articles for CME Reviews. The Cleveland Clinic Foundation, the National Institutes of Health, and Virtual Hospital Online all provide opportunities to access Internet-based CME courses, often with immediate feedback on performance. A multitude of top-rated CME modules and interesting feature sites include the Interactive Patient, which provides users with the opportunity to view a simulated online patient, request history, perform exams, and review diagnostic data. Credit fees vary by organization site.

National Institutes of Health (NIH): Continuing Education
http://text.nlm.nih.gov/nih/upload-v3/Continuing_Education/cme.html

This continuing medical education site, sponsored by NIH and the Foundation for Advanced Education in the Sciences, invites users to participate in an online experiment in distance learning. Visitors can access consensus statements, details of the CME course, and a CME exam on a variety of health topics.

4.2 Selected Medical School CME Programs

Baylor College of Medicine: Online Continuing Medical Education
(free registration)
http://www.baylorcme.org

Registered visitors to this site can access online CME lectures. Features available in the presentation modules include audio accompaniments to each slide; an index of slide topics; a search tool; access to PubMed for literature searches; a discussion forum organized by topic; and a concluding continuing medical education test. Answers to common technical questions about the online lectures are also available.

Columbia University: Center for Continuing Education in the Health Sciences
http://cpmcnet.columbia.edu/dept/cme

This home page offers resources for professionals interested in CME programs through Columbia Presbyterian Medical Center. Visitors will find a calendar of events, a brochure request form, a description of CME activities, and a mission statement.

Cornell University Joan and Sanford I. Weill Medical College Office of Continuing Medical Education
http://www.med.cornell.edu/cme/index.html

The Office of Continuing Medical Education at Cornell University offers listings of weekly departmental Grand Rounds at both New York Presbyterian Hospital and the Hospital for Special Surgery. Contact details, weekly dates, and weekly times are posted for each department offering rounds. This site also lists contact details.

Harvard Medical School Department of Continuing Education ○ ○ ○
http://www.med.harvard.edu/conted

Resources provided by the home page of the Harvard Medical School Department of Continuing Education include a list of hospitals, medical groups, and health centers offering CME programs; contact details; travel and housing details; and directories of specific CME programs. Visitors can search the directory of courses by topic, specialty, or date. Online registration forms are available. Information and online registration forms for home study programs are also found at the site.

Johns Hopkins Office of Continuing Medical Education ○ ○ ○
http://www.med.jhu.edu/cme

Visitors to this address will find comprehensive resources related to CME programs at Johns Hopkins University. The site offers a calendar of events, a site search engine for locating relevant CME programs, a listing of special programs available by appointment only, and information on graduate certificate programs. Information on distance education, video programs on CD-ROM, and Webcast courses is also available. Readers of these newsletters can receive CME credit through completion of a test at the conclusion of the newsletter.

University of Chicago: Center for Continuing Medical Education ○ ○
http://www.uchicago.edu/bsd/cme

The Center for Continuing Medical Education offers this calendar of conferences, seminars, and other opportunities for CME credit through the University of Chicago. Titles, dates, and location details are provided. Street address and contact details for the center are also available.

University of Pennsylvania Health System: Continuing Medical Education ○ ○
http://www.med.upenn.edu/cme

CME resources offered through the University of Pennsylvania Health System are listed through this home page. A calendar of events lists 1999 conferences, seminars, grand rounds, mini-fellowships, and ongoing lecture series. Online CME programs are also available from the site. Additional information about the CME program includes a mission statement, a summary of goals, and accreditation details.

Washington University Continuing Medical Education ○ ○
http://cme.wustl.edu

Information on CME programs at Washington University is available from this site. Visitors can search a directory of seminars by specialty and date. Information on program logistics and travel arrangements is also available. The site also offers links to related programs throughout the university, as well as contact details.

Yale University School of Medicine
Office of Postgraduate and Continuing Medical Education ◎ ◎ ◎
http://info.med.yale.edu/CME

Professionals interested in CME at Yale University School of Medicine will find a mission statement; a current schedule of CME courses; a Yale-New Haven Medical Center weekly schedule of events; and subscription details for *The Medical Letter/Yale School of Medicine CME Program,* a publication providing two annual exams for CME credit based on the previous six months' issues of *The Medical Letter on Drugs and Therapeutics.*

5. OVERVIEW SITES

5.1 Supersites

About.com: Thyroid Disease and Endocrinology ○ ○ ○
http://thyroid.about.com/health/thyroid/msub27.htm

About.com is an extensive source of information on medical topics. The section addressing thyroid disease and other endocrinology issues provides articles and information summaries on numerous topics, such as menopause, hormone rhythms, and individual disorders. The sidebar has a listing of more than 25 topics, including diseases, drugs, support groups, issues, and diagnostic tests. By utilizing the strong search engine, under the general topic of endocrinology, or on any specific subtopic, an additional set of resources, articles, and links can be found.

EndocrineWeb ○ ○
http://www.endocrineweb.com

EndocrineWeb provides a searchable patient education site about endocrine disorders and endocrine surgery. Articles on the specialty areas of endocrinology, endocrine surgery, thyroid and parathyroid glands, adrenal glands, diabetes, and osteoporosis are provided, with colorful illustrations at each site, and links to diagnosis and treatment details for both consumer and professional reference.

Hardin Meta Directory of
Internet Health Services: Endocrinology and Diabetes ○ ○ ○
http://www.lib.uiowa.edu/hardin/md/endocrin.html

The Hardin Meta Directory offers professionals and other interested visitors access to some of the largest link listings in endocrinology on the Internet. New York's Online Access to Health, diabetic-only link listings, MEDLINEPlus Health Information from the National Library of Medicine, and Emory University's MedWeb links in endocrinology are just a handful of the large number of listings provided. SciCentral's endocrinology and diabetes connection and Martindale's Health Science Guide offer visitors excellent starting points for research in the medical specialty.

Karolinska Institutet: Endocrine Diseases ○ ○ ○
http://www.mic.ki.se/Diseases/c19.html

A wide range of general resources, such as case studies and tutorials in endocrinology and site listings devoted to specific endocrine disorders, can be found through this comprehensive Internet directory. Diseases listed include diabetes mellitus, diabetic ketoacidosis and other complications, Wolfram syndrome, endocrine gland neoplasms, adrenal gland diseases, autoimmune polyendocrinopathies, breast diseases, pituitary diseases, parathyroid diseases, thyroid diseases, and gonadal disorders. Each group of disorder connections includes an assortment of general disease information, fact sheets from disorder-specific organizations, clinical guidelines for practitioners, and pathology and case studies.

Medical Matrix ○ ○ (free registration)
http://www.medmatrix.org

Medical Matrix is a directory of professionally reviewed medical sites on the Internet. Visitors will find Internet sources for news, full-text articles, abstracts, online textbooks, practice guidelines, case studies, pathology and clinical images, continuing medical education resources, patient education materials, directories, classified advertisements, and discussion forums. Free registration is required for access to the site.

MedMark: Endocrinology ○ ○ ○
http://www.medmark.org/endo/endo2.html

This tremendous one-stop site contains an exceptional number of links to sites related to endocrinology. Connection categories include major endocrinology associations and societies, research centers and laboratories, academic divisions, sites related to education and training in the specialty, consumer information, practice guidelines, professional journals, and current news and topics in the field.

Medscape: Diabetes and Endocrinology ○ ○ ○
http://endocrine.medscape.com/Home/Topics/endocrinology/endocrinology.html

This site provides an array of information for healthcare professionals. Interesting connections include a Web-enabled documentation tool for clinicians, a CME center, a journal room, treatment updates, and a listing of expert-authored reports from key meetings in endocrinology. Today's diabetes and endocrinology news, case studies, and a general information library are all found, providing diagnostic, nutritional, exercise, statistical, and other disease management information. An upcoming conference listing and state-of-the-art treatment strategies in endocrinology are provided.

Medscout:
Endocrine, Nutritional, Metabolic, and Immunity Disorders ○ ○ ○
http://medscout.com/diseases/endocrine/index.htm

This site provides resources within a number of endocrinology categories, including professional associations and disorder organizations, as well as major endocrinology Internet sites. Clinical guidelines, fact sheets, and articles on disorders of the thyroid, the adrenal glands, and diabetes may be accessed from the site, with an even distribution between professionally oriented and consumer-oriented material.

5.2 General Resources

CliniWeb International: Endocrine Diseases ○ ○ ○
http://www.ohsu.edu/cliniweb/C19/C19.html

CliniWeb provides a wide range of research resources on various endocrine topics via preformatted PubMed query links. Article abstracts can be obtained in a number of ways, including reviews, therapeutics, and diagnosis on adrenal gland diseases, diabetes, endocrine gland neoplasms, gonadal disorders, parathyroid diseases, and pituitary diseases. Other resources, such as clinical guidelines, information from the Centers for Disease Control and Prevention, and professional journal articles, are found.

Endocrine Cafe ○ ○ ○
http://www.endocrinecafe.com

This Web site provides an excellent resource for endocrinologists, clinicians, patients, and consumers seeking information on endocrinology and related topics. Academic resources and laboratories, endocrinology societies, prominent journals, and educational guidelines are all accessible from the main page. For the patient seeking to locate a practicing endocrinologist, a list is provided.

Endocrinology.com ○
http://www.endocrinology.com

Endocrinology.com is an extensive Web site devoted to all aspects of this medical specialty. The public resource section offers a set of links to several endocrinology organizations which are intermixed with private site listings. Other sections offer information on thyroid, parathyroid, adrenal, and pituitary disorders, as well as information on sexual dysfunction and weight management. Patient case studies can be examined, and a professional directory can be consulted. The site offers forums on major disorders for message postings. The site focus is on patient education and public awareness.

HealthWeb: Endocrinology ◉ ◉ ◉
http://www.galter.nwu.edu/hw/endo

A collaborative effort of the health sciences libraries of the Committee on Institutional Cooperation (CIC) and the National Network of Libraries of Medicine of the Greater Midwest Region, HealthWeb maintains a collection of endocrinology-related resources. A General Resources section contains links to valuable databases and general sites. The publications connection offers links to guidelines and fact sheets, electronic textbooks and journals, and newsletters and upcoming events in the specialty. Additionally, an educational resources section lists links to atlases and images, case studies, textbooks, and lectures. Visitors can also browse links to organizations, patient information sheets, and resources specific to diabetes.

PharmInfoNet: Endocrine Disease and Diabetes Center ◉ ◉
http://www.pharminfo.com/disease/endocrine.html

Visitors to this site will find an interesting assortment of professional and consumer-oriented information related to diabetes, as well as additional endocrinology disorders. The *Medical Sciences Bulletin* link reviews new drugs for the treatment of endocrine disease and diabetes, and a medical meetings section offers electronic highlights from major scientific meetings in the field. Professional and patient discussion groups, patient resource sites and FAQs, and links to specific disease resources are offered. A special section on endocrine disease and diabetes products and services is found.

5.3 National Institute of Diabetes and Digestive and Kidney Diseases (NIDDK)

NIDDK Web Site Features

National Institute of Diabetes and Digestive and Kidney Diseases (NIDDK) ◉ ◉ ◉
http://www.niddk.nih.gov

The National Institute of Diabetes and Digestive and Kidney Diseases (NIDDK) supports a wide range of clinical and basic science investigations in metabolic diseases and diabetes, inborn errors of metabolism, endocrine disorders, mineral metabolism, digestive diseases, nutrition, urology and renal diseases, and hematology. The NIDDK home page offers a mission and history of the institute, staff directories, event calendars, employment notices, and news briefs. Visitors will also find details of NIDDK extramural funding programs, intramural laboratories, clinical trials funded by NIDDK, and health education programs. The site also offers links to databases of health information relevant to the institute's specialties, as well as reports to Congress, Coordinating Committee descriptions, and strategic plans.

NIDDK: Clinical Trials

http://www.niddk.nih.gov/patient/patient.htm

Clinical trials resources found at this site include descriptions of selected clinical trials funded by NIDDK and links to additional details. The site also provides links to the NIH clinical trials database (ClinicalTrials.gov), a database of clinical trials from the NIH Warren Grant Magnuson Clinical Center, and a NIH Rare Diseases Clinical Research Database.

NIDDK: Health Education Programs

http://www.niddk.nih.gov/health/edu.htm

Details of NIDDK Health Education Programs are available from this address, including the National Diabetes Education Program (NDEP), the Weight Control Information Network (WIN), the National Diabetes Information Clearinghouse (NDDIC), and the National Kidney and Urologic Diseases Information Clearinghouse (NKUDIC). Links to program home pages are available, as well as brief descriptions of each project.

NIDDK: Health Information

http://www.niddk.nih.gov/health/health.htm

NIDDK offers a variety of consumer health publications, including Spanish-language publications, easy-to-read publications, statistics, and directories of professional and voluntary organizations. Health publications describing specific diseases are also available, listed both alphabetically and by subject area. Visitors will also find publications lists and order forms and a link to the Combined Health Information Database (CHID).

NIDDK: Research Funding Opportunities

http://www.niddk.nih.gov/fund/fund.htm

Encompassing both intramural and extramural research activities and funding, this site provides one-stop access to all of the division's coordinated research endeavors and funding details. Career development and a tutorial on grant and contract applications are available, as well as grant review information and NIDDK-sponsored educational event connections. Of special interest are connections to seven Diabetes and Endocrinology Research Centers funded by the NIH that focus on biomedical research, as well as links to four research and training-oriented locations.

NIDDK: Special Reports, Planning, Coordination, and Testimony

http://www.niddk.nih.gov/federal/planning.htm

Visitors to this section of the site will find NIDDK Coordinating Committee overviews, reports to Congress, testimony from the NIDDK director concerning the Fiscal Year 2001 budget, and strategic plans.

NIDDK: Welcome
http://www.niddk.nih.gov/welcome/welcome.htm

This welcome section offers a description of the institute, an overview of organizational structure, NIH maps, a searchable staff directory, NIDDK scientist biographies, calendars of extramural program conferences and other events, employment listings, and both current and archived news briefs.

Intramural Research

NIDDK: Laboratories
http://www.niddk.nih.gov/intram/intram.htm

Information available through the NIDDK intramural research home page includes an overview of research and training within NIDDK, profiles of senior scientists' research projects, descriptions of research interests of individual NIDDK laboratories and branch descriptions , training opportunities, and scientific databases and resources.

Extramural Research

NIDDK: Division of Diabetes, Endocrinology, and Metabolic Diseases (DEM)
http://www.niddk.nih.gov/fund/divisions/DEM/DEMintro.htm

This extramural NIDDK division offers funding and support for basic and clinical research in diabetes, endocrinology, metabolic diseases, and cystic fibrosis. Training and career development funding is also available. This site provides information on research opportunities and programs, a list of request for applications RFAs and Program Announcements, profiles of upcoming DEM initiatives, conference notices and conference reports, additional special reports, NIH announcements and information on extramural grant funding, descriptions of ongoing clinical trials, details of informational research resources for investigators, and links to related organizations.

NIDDK: Division of Digestive Diseases and Nutrition (DDN)
http://www.niddk.nih.gov/fund/divisions/DDN/DDNintro.htm

Resources provided by the DDN site include RFAs and Program Announcements, a directory of core research centers, a profile of the Training and Career Development Program, information on clinical trials, details of Small Business Innovation Research and Small Business Technology Transfer programs, meeting notices, special reports, links to special committees, and links to related sites. A DDN program booklet available at the site offers details of program areas, contacts, and application procedures for research grants.

NIDDK: Division of Nutrition Research Coordination (DNRC)
http://www.niddk.nih.gov/federal/dnrc.htm

The DNRC home page offers a calendar of nutrition meetings and conferences, nutrition education materials, a list of activities planned for National Nutrition Month, and NIH Nutrition Coordinating Committee (NCC) meeting minutes.

Health Education Programs

National Diabetes Information Clearinghouse ○ ○ ○
http://www.niddk.nih.gov/health/diabetes/ndic.htm

The National Diabetes Information Clearinghouse is a service of the National Institute of Diabetes and Digestive and Kidney Diseases. They offer responses to inquiries about diabetes by fax, mail, and e-mail. They also provide online fact sheets and publications on a variety of topics related to the disorder. There are links to other resources, including a newsletter, a directory of diabetes organizations, and a federally sponsored diabetes education program.

National Kidney and Urologic Diseases Information Clearinghouse ○ ○ ○
http://www.niddk.nih.gov/health/kidney/nkudic.htm

The National Kidney and Urologic Diseases Information Clearinghouse is part of the National Institute of Diabetes and Digestive and Kidney Diseases. They offer responses to inquiries about kidney and urologic diseases by fax, mail, and e-mail. They also offer online publications on a variety of related topics including glomerual diseases, good pasture syndrome, hematuria, hemodialysis, high blood pressure, nephrotic syndrome in adults, and many other topics. There are also links to Spanish publications and statistics.

NIDDK: Diabetes Research and Training Center's Demonstration and Education Divisions ○ ○
http://www.niddk.nih.gov/health/diabetes/pubs/drtc/index.htm

From the National Institute of Diabetes and Digestive and Kidney Diseases, this site contains an article on Diabetes Research and Training Centers Demonstration and Education Divisions. The site gives a general overview of the Centers' objectives and includes information about current research and development projects and health professional education programs. There is a list of specific programs available for download, as well as information about staff members and other programs.

Weight-control Information Network (WIN) ○ ○ ○
http://www.niddk.nih.gov/health/nutrit/win.htm

An information service of the National Institute of Diabetes and Digestive and Kidney Diseases, the Weight-control Information Network (WIN) offers science-based information about obesity. Their site offers links to online publications, including brochures, conference proceedings, and fact sheets. There is also information about clinical nutrition research centers and clinical nutrition research units. There is a newsletter and links to related sites.

5.4 Other Government Agencies and Programs

Centers for Disease Control and Prevention (CDC): Division of Diabetes Translation ○ ○ ○
http://www.cdc.gov/diabetes

Conferences, diabetes FAQs, details regarding the National Diabetes Education Program, and state-based control programs are provided at this page of the National Center for Chronic Disease Prevention and Health Promotion of the Centers for Disease Control (CDC). Diabetes research articles, statistics, links, press releases, and the CDC's position paper on the diagnosis and classification of diabetes are easily accessible. Publications may be ordered from the site's product listing.

Diabetes Caucus ○ ○
http://www.house.gov/nethercutt/diabetes.htm

The Congressional Diabetes Caucus, one of the most influential congressional health-related organizations, offers details on its goals and achievements for promotion of research into diabetes and complications of the disease. Links to information on the Insulin Dependant Diabetes Trust, information about beef insulin and import and the Center for Drug Evaluation and Research, and summaries of facts and long-term disease consequences are provided.

Health Resources and Services Administration (HRSA): Division of Transplantation ○ ○
http://www.hrsa.gov/osp/dot

The Health Resources and Services Administration's Division of Transplantation gives federal oversight and financial support to organ procurement, allocation, and transplantation. Their site includes information about the division and its legislative and regulatory activities. There is information on the following branches of the division: bone marrow transplantation branch; public and professional education branch; and the operations and analysis branch.

National Glycohemoglobin Standardization Program ◎ ◎
http://web.missouri.edu/~diabetes/ngsp.html

This site offers information about the National Glycohemoglobin Standardization Program. There is data bout the relationship between glycohemoblobin (GHB) and blood glucose, as well as information about programs and federal studies.

Veterans Health Administration Diabetes Program ◎ ◎
http://www.va.gov/health/diabetes/default.htm

The Veteran's Health Administration's clinical guidelines for diabetes management, diabetes mellitus information for veterans, related links, and connections to information on benefits, facilities, and special programs are provided.

PART TWO

BIOLOGICAL, DIAGNOSTIC, AND THERAPEUTIC RESOURCES

6. ANATOMY AND PHYSIOLOGY

6.1 General Principles

American Medical Association (AMA): The Endocrine System ◎ ◎
http://www.ama-assn.org/insight/gen_hlth/atlas/newatlas/endo.htm
From the American Medical Association, this site provides a diagram of the endocrine system, with definitions and brief information on the adrenal glands, hypothalamus, ovaries and testicles, pancreas, parathyroid glands, pineal body, pituitary gland, thymus gland, and thyroid gland.

Endocrine System Anatomy ◎ ◎
http://calloso.med.mun.ca/~tscott/endo/endotut.htm
This site offers a tutorial on the endocrine glands, with a section on principles of organization that includes an image of the thyroid gland. Sections on the pancreas and adrenal gland include information on the development, gross anatomy, histology, and clinical anatomy of each. Images are provided.

Furman University: The Endocrine System ◎ ◎
http://www.furman.edu/~dhaney/es.htm
This site offers a tutorial on the endocrine system. The introduction includes a comparison to the nervous system and an overview of hormone classifications. Sections on amine hormones and steroid hormones, the central endocrine systems, peripheral endocrine systems, the thyroid gland, and the adrenal gland are offered.

Indiana State University Terre Haute Center for Medical Education: Medical Biochemistry Tutorial ◎ ◎ ◎
http://web.indstate.edu/thcme/mwking/home.html
This site for medical biochemistry offers links to a wide variety of topics on the biochemistry of metabolic processes. Glycogen metabolism, metabolism of lipids, and other fuel metabolic process tutorials are accessible. Hormones and their receptors,

signal transduction, and the biochemistry of diabetes mellitus are included. Additional links lead to online lecture notes covering muscular biochemistry, the processes of inborn errors of metabolism, vitamins and coenzymes, and other medical biochemistry topics including chemistry review material and the basics of biomolecules.

Indiana University: School of Medicine: The Endocrine System ✪ ✪ ✪
http://histo.ipfw.indiana.edu/histo-embryo/endocrine.html

Written by a professor of the Indiana University School of Medicine, this site provides an outline of the histology and embryology of the 'traditional' endocrine glands. There is a listing of general characteristics, as well as sections on the pituitary gland, thyroid gland, pharyngeal hypophysis, parathyroid glands, adrenal gland, pineal body, islets of Langerhans, testes, and ovaries.

Memorial University of Newfoundland: The Endocrine Glands ✪ ✪
http://calloso.med.mun.ca/~tscott/endo/endotut.htm

Images and text provide a detailed overview of the fetal development, gross anatomy, histology, and clinical anatomy of the endocrine glands at this address. Visitors can read descriptions of the pituitary, thyroid, parathyroid, pancreas, and adrenal glands, as well as other endocrine tissue. Corresponding images are available for highlighted terms.

On-Line Biology Book: The Endocrine System ✪ ✪ ✪
http://gened.emc.maricopa.edu/bio/bio181/BIOBK/BioBookENDOCR.html

This endocrine system overview begins with an introduction to endocrine evolution and presents review of hormone classes, endocrine system negative feedback cycles, and mechanisms of hormone action. Following the hormone review, there is a lesson on the basics of endocrine system problems related to hormone overproduction, underproduction, and nonfunctional receptors. The interrelationship between the nervous system and the endocrine system, as well as hormone production and release by the various endocrine organs, are presented. Other chemical messengers, such as prostaglandins, circadian rhythms, and other biological cycles, conclude the review.

University of California Davis: Endocrine System Tutorial ✪ ✪ ✪
http://bio2000.ucdavis.edu/bis10/endocrine/endocrine.htm

Written by a professor at the University of California, this site offers information on the endocrine system, with a comprehensive table listing human hormones. Details on source and mechanism of action are provided, as well as a link to a diagram indicating how water soluble and non-water soluble hormones act on target cells. Endocrine gland function is reviewed.

6.2 Hormones

Biochemical Categories

Illinois State Academy of Science: Endocrinology Databases ◎ ◎
http://www.il-st-acad-sci.org/data2.html

Databases available at this site offer normal ranges of pituitary hormones, steroid hormones, thyroid hormones, insulin-like growth factors, and other hormones present in both humans and animals. Conversion tables for hormones and concentration units, a table outlining steroid nomenclature, and links to other databases are also available.

Indiana State University Terre Haute Center for Medical Education: Peptide Hormones ◎ ◎
http://web.indstate.edu/thcme/mwking/peptide-hormones.html

Maintained by the Terre Haute Center for Medical Education, this site contains a tutorial on peptide hormones. There is a descriptive table of peptide hormones as well as discussions of the structure and function of hormones, receptors for peptide hormones, and the basics of peptide hormones. Discussions of the growth hormone family, the glycoprotein hormone family, and the pro-opiomelanocortin family are found, as well as information about vasopressin, oxytocin, parathyroid hormone, calcitonin, and gastrointestinal peptide hormones.

Indiana State University Terre Haute Center for Medical Education: Steroid Hormones ◎ ◎
http://web.indstate.edu/thcme/mwking/sterhorm.html

This site, maintained by the Terre Haute Center for Medical Education, provides an introduction to the steroid hormone class and discussions on several topics, including reactions of steroid hormone synthesis, steroid hormones of the adrenal cortex, regulation of adrenal steroid synthesis, and gonadal steroid hormones.

Pharmacology Central: Peptide Hormones ◎
http://www.pharmcentral.com/peptides.htm

From Pharmacology Central, this site offers diagrams and discussions of peptide hormones, endorphins and substance P, vasopressin and giractide, the angiotensin system, insulin, growth hormones, gonadal peptides, and other peptides.

**University Institute of Psychiatry Division of Clinical
Psychopharmacology: Steroid Hormone Metabolism**
http://matweb.hcuge.ch/matweb/endo/
Reproductive_health/Steroid_hormone_metabolism.html

A tutorial on steroid hormone metabolism is found at this site, with an introduction and sections on structure, nomenclature, and classification of steroid hormones. Steroid hormone biosynthesis, steroid hormones in the blood, steroid interaction with target tissues, and steroid inactivation and catabolism are reviewed.

**University of North Carolina, Chapel Hill School of
Public Health: Peptide/Protein Hormones and Their Receptors**
http://www.sph.unc.edu/courses/nutr110-001/ha092998.html

This site offers a tutorial on peptide and protein hormones and their receptors. Definitions and a table listing the characteristics of hormones are provided, along with sections describing synthesis and secretion, growth hormone, prolactin, pancreatic hormones, and G-protein-linked receptors.

Endocrine Rhythms

Endocrine Society: Endocrinology and Hormone Rhythms
http://www.endo-society.org/pubaffai/factshee/hormnrhy.htm

Produced by the Endocrine Society, this site offers consumer information about endocrinology and hormone rhythms. There are short sections on the importance of hormone rhythms, disorders of hormone rhythms, and the role of endocrinology.

Feedback Control in Endocrine Systems

Colorado State University: Endocrine Activity
http://arbl.cvmbs.colostate.edu/hbooks/pathphys/endocrine/basics/control.html

Maintained by Colorado State University, this site offers information about the control of endocrine activity. There is an introduction and a section on feedback control of hormone production. Hormone profiles and a graph showing concentrations over time are presented.

Mechanisms of Action

Colorado State University: Hormone Action
http://arbl.cvmbs.colostate.edu/hbooks/pathphys/endocrine/moaction/index.html

As a service of Colorado State University, this site provides information about the mechanisms of hormone action, with a general overview and index to related information at the site. Topics discussed include hormonal influences on target cells, changes in target cells, hormones with cell surface receptors, and hormones with intracellular receptors.

Colorado State University: Hormones, Receptors, and Target Cells
http://arbl.cvmbs.colostate.edu/hbooks/pathphys/endocrine/basics/hormones.html

This university Web link offers specific details on hormone receptors and target cells, accompanied by explanatory diagrams. Definitions and information on endocrine action, paracrine action, autocrine action, agonists, and antagonists are offered.

University of Miami Department of Biology: Hormones and Chemical Messages
http://fig.cox.miami.edu/~lfarmer/BIL265/endocrine.HTM

This site offers detailed text and images describing hormones and chemical messages created by the endocrine system. The article discusses cell signaling, types of chemical messages, hormone receptors, antagonistic effects of hormones, and neuroendocrine secretion.

Synthesis, Storage, and Release

Colorado State University: Hormone Chemistry, Synthesis, and Elimination
http://arbl.cvmbs.colostate.edu/hbooks/pathphys/endocrine/basics/chem.html

A review of structural groupings, illustrations of chemical compounds, and other information on hormone molecules are provided at the introductory page, with links to the principle hormone groupings found.

University of South Dakota: Mechanisms of Action: Hormone Synthesis
http://courses.usd.edu/biol427001/syn.html

An outline of hormone synthesis, receptor regulation, and hypothalamus-hypophysial communication is presented as part of this online course material.

6.3 Neuroendocrine System

General Resources

Brain Tumor Foundation of Canada: Neuroendocrine Function
http://www.btfc.org/english/handbooks/pediatric/pchp13.html
Maintained by the Brain Tumor Foundation of Canada, this site contains a chapter on neuroendocrine function. There is a table that lists individual hormones and their functions, in addition to sections on disorders of growth, disorders of sexual development, and weight loss and obesity.

British Neuroendocrine Group
http://www.neuroendo.org.uk
Current and archived organization newsletters provide details on research into neuroendocrine function and disease, research opportunity information, and contacts and details for meetings and symposiums in growth hormone research, steroid receptors, and other neuroendocrine topics. The *Journal of Neuroendocrinology* may be accessed from the site, and visitors will find abstracts, full-text articles, and reprints in PDF format. The "Neuroendocrinology Briefings" page offers online articles, courtesy of the British Neuroendocrine Group, that promote awareness to both specialists and nonspecialists with regard to current, diverse topics in the field. Some of the presentations available include environmental estrogens, leptin and obesity, stress and hormones, sex hormones and mood, sex differences in the brain, and biological timekeeping.

International Neuroendocrine Federation
http://www.isneuro.org
The International Neuroendocrine Foundation, formerly the International Society of Endocrinology, provides information on the upcoming International Congress of Neuroendocrinology as well as membership details at this organization Web page. A listing of additional upcoming events is provided and includes a pituitary disease workshop and an international meeting on steroids and the nervous system. The objectives of the International Neuroendocrine Federation, which include promoting research and education in neuroendocrinology throughout the world, are outlined.

Neurotransmitters and Hormones
http://www.lurking.demon.co.uk/mind/chemical.htm
An introduction to neurotransmitters and hormones is available from this site. There are profiles of epinephrine, insulin, melatonin, norepinephrine, serotonin, and testosterone.

Northeastern University Pharmacology: Catecholamines ◎ ◎
http://155.33.221.112/neuroanatomy/cyberclass/pharmacology/Catecholamine.htm

Information about the catecholamines is provided at this site. There is an overview and sections on a family of neurotransmitters, catecholamine receptor agonists and antagonists, and the degradation of catecholamines.

Society for Behavioral Neuroendocrinology ◎ ◎
http://www.sbne.org

Connections to society meetings and membership information and a link to the organization's official professional journal are found at this site of the Society for Behavioral Neuroendocrinology. The organization's mission of providing an investigative forum for the advancement of the understanding between behavior and neuroendocrine function is presented. Visitors are encouraged to visit related neuroendocrine Web sites or access related journals at this NeuroRing Web site.

Society for Neuroscience (SFN) ◎ ◎ ◎
http://www.sfn.org

The site index at this home page of the Society for Neuroscience offers details on registration for the organization's annual meeting and allows viewers to scroll through public information on conditions, clinicians, and related links. Three society publication links are accessible from the site, in addition to legislative news and a connection to the Website of Recent Neuroscience. At this innovative connection, visitors will find specifics on recent advancements in neuroscience technology and details about an effort to archive neuroscientific research history. One of the SFN publications, *Brain Briefings,* offers short articles on neuroscience topics explaining how recent discoveries have paved the way for clinical applications across a variety of medical specialties.

Hypothalamic-Pituitary Hormones and Function

Colorado State University: Hypothalamus and Pituitary Gland ◎ ◎
http://arbl.cvmbs.colostate.edu/hbooks/pathphys/endocrine/hypopit/index.html

Maintained by Colorado State University, this site provides an introduction to the hypothalamus and pituitary axis. An index of related information available at the site includes functional anatomy of the hypothalamus and pituitary gland, an overview of hypothalamic and pituitary hormones, anterior pituitary hormones, and posterior pituitary hormones.

Finch University of Health Sciences/Chicago Medical School: Anterior Pituitary Hormones ◉ ◉

http://www.finchcms.edu/Pharmacology/snyderslides/antpit/index.htm

This site contains a slide presentation on anterior pituitary hormones and includes discussion of growth hormone secretion, somatostatin, prolactin, adrenocorticotrophic hormone, thyrotropin, gonadotropins, clomiphene, and other hormones.

Finch University of Health Sciences/Chicago Medical School: Posterior Pituitary Hormones ◉ ◉

http://www.finchcms.edu/Pharmacology/snyderslides/postpit/index.htm

This site contains a slide presentation on posterior pituitary hormones. There are 25 slides on various topics, including oxytocin, vasopressin, and posterior pituitary hormones.

Hebrew University School of Medicine Department of Endocrinology: Pituitary Gland ◉ ◉ ◉

http://info.md.huji.ac.il/pituitary

Written by Dr. Benjamin Glaser of the Department of Endocrinology at Hebrew University School of Medicine, this site offers lecture notes on the pituitary gland. Topics discussed include anatomy of the pituitary and anterior pituitary gland. Information on growth hormone, prolactin, and hormone-secreting anterior pituitary tumors is found, and tables and figures are included.

Illinois State Academy of Science: Pituitary Hormone Levels in Humans ◉ ◉

http://www.il-st-acad-sci.org/hormone1.html

Normal ranges for pituitary hormone levels in humans are listed in table form at this address, including plasma adrenocorticotropin, circulating lutropin, follicular fluid prolactin, serum prolactin, urinary prolactin, fasting serum somatotropin, serum thyrotropin, and plasma vasopressin. Reference ranges for pituitary hormones in neonates, infants, children, and adolescents are also listed. A list of reference citations is also provided.

Integrated Medical Curriculum: Anterior Pituitary ◉ ◉ ◉

http://www.imc.gsm.com/integrated/hponline/HumnPhys/program/section5/5ch2/5ch2line.htm

This site offers an outline of a chapter on the anterior pituitary. Topics discussed in the chapter include the anatomy of the pituitary gland, anterior pituitary hormones, control of synthesis and secretion of pituitary hormones, mechanism of action of anterior pituitary hormones, and actions of anterior pituitary hormones. Items in the outline hyperlink to related text, tables, and diagrams.

King's College Division of Physiology: Pituitary and Hypothalamus ◎ ◎ ◎

http://www.umds.ac.uk/physiology/banks/pithorm.html

Maintained by King's College Division of Physiology, this site offers a tutorial on the pituitary and hypothalamus. Sections on the anterior pituitary, growth hormone and its actions, abnormalities in growth hormone release, prolactin, adrenocorticotrophic hormone, alpha melanocyte-stimulating hormone, the posterior pituitary, arginine vasopressin, and oxytocin are offered.

Tulane University: Posterior Pituitary ◎

http://www.mcl.tulane.edu/classware/pathology/Medical_pathology/pituitary/12posterior_pit.html

An outline of posterior pituitary disorders is found at this site. There is information on antidiuretic hormone (ADH) deficiency, including causes, and information on diabetes insipidus. Information on the syndrome of inappropriate ADH secretion (SIADH) is, additionally, included.

University of Colorado Department of Psychology: Hypothalamus and Its Hormonal Role ◎ ◎

http://psych.colorado.edu/~biopsych/heather/hypo2.html

This site describes the hypothalamus and its hormonal role. There is a table listing neurohypophyseal hormones and their function, as well as information on hypothalamic substances that stimulate or inhibit the release of anterior pituitary hormones.

University of Kansas School of Medicine Medical Pharmacology Learning Modules: Hypothalamic and Pituitary Hormones ◎ ◎

http://www.kumc.edu/research/medicine/pharmacology/mgordon/Endocrine/Hypothalamic/framehypo.htm

A thorough technical overview of hypothalamic and pituitary hormones is available from this online tutorial, including a list of learning objectives for the medical student. Information is presented in outline form and includes an overview of the endocrine function and production of hypothalamic and pituitary hormones. Hormones of the anterior pituitary gland and related hormones are discussed, including corticotrophin-releasing hormone, thyroid-releasing hormone, thyroid-stimulating hormone, gonadotropin-releasing hormone, luteinizing hormone-releasing hormone, follicle stimulating hormone, and dopamine. Hormones of the posterior pituitary gland are also presented, including vasopressin and synthetic desmopressin. Practice questions and case studies are also available.

University of Kansas School of Medicine
Medical Pharmacology Learning Modules: Gonadal Hormones

http://www.kumc.edu/research/medicine/pharmacology/
mgordon/Endocrine/Gonadal/framegonadal.htm

Information related to gonadal hormones is provided in this extensive teaching tutorial, including estrogens, progestins, hormonal contraception, selective estrogen receptor modulators (SERM), progesterone antagonists, ovulation-inducing agents, androgens and anabolic steroids, and antiandrogens. Pharmacologic effects, clinical uses, and adverse effects are presented in outline form. Practice questions and case studies are also available.

University of Michigan: Anterior Pituitary Physiology

http://141.214.232.16/osteo/pitphysout/index.htm

This site offers a tutorial on anterior pituitary physiology. There are diagrams and discussions of the hypothalamic-pituitary-thyroid axis, hypothalamic-pituitary-adrenal axis, hypothalamic-pituitary-growth hormone axes, hypothalamic-pituitary-gonadal axes, and rhythms in endocrinology.

University of Texas Southwestern Medical Center
Department of Pathology: Pituitary Gland

http://pathcuric1.swmed.edu/ScribeService/Resources/
path/objectives/Endocrine/endocrine-Pituitar.html

This site offers a tutorial on the pituitary, with a section on gross anatomy and discussion of the portal blood system and its role in disease. Diagrams and images are included.

University of Virginia
Health System: Posterior Pituitary Hormones

http://avery.med.virginia.edu/medicine/basic-sci/
pharm/dab_lab/docs/course/adh_oxy/index.htm

This site contains a slide presentation on posterior pituitary hormones. The table of contents includes 16 slides on vasopressin, diabetes insipidus, oxytocin, uterine motility agents, and recapitulation.

Washington University School of Medicine:
Hypothalamus and Autonomic Nervous System

http://thalamus.wustl.edu/course/hypoANS.html

Maintained by the Washington University School of Medicine, this site contains a tutorial on the hypothalamus and autonomic nervous system. There are definitions of terms, diagrams, images, and tables of information.

Pineal Gland and Melatonin Physiology

Harvey Mudd College: Pineal Gland
http://www.cs.hmc.edu/~steve/psych53/bio.html
Biology of the pineal gland, melatonin, and phase therapy for the sleep-wake cycle are included at this site. There are hyperlinks to definitions of terms used in the text, as well as a glossary and reference listing.

Kimball's Biology Pages: Melatonin and the Pineal Gland
http://www.ultranet.com/~jkimball/BiologyPages/P/Pineal.html
Discussion of the function of the pineal gland and its principle hormone is found at this site of Kimball's Biology Pages. Information on synthesis and release of melatonin and links to a graphic and further details on the circadian cycle are provided.

6.4 Thyroid Gland

Colorado State University: Thyroid and Parathyroid Glands
http://arbl.cvmbs.colostate.edu/hbooks/pathphys/endocrine/thyroid/index.html
Provided by Colorado State University, this site contains an introduction to the thyroid and parathyroid glands and an index to related information at the site. Information includes articles on the functional anatomy of the thyroid and parathyroid glands, chemistry of thyroid hormones, synthesis and secretion of thyroid hormones, mechanism of action, control of thyroid hormone synthesis and secretion, calcitonin, and parathyroid hormone. There are also supplemental articles on thyroid hormone receptors and related topics.

Illinois State Academy of Science: Thyroid Hormone Levels in Humans
http://www.il-st-acad-sci.org/hormone2.html
Maintained by the Illinois State Academy of Science, this site provides links to information on thyroid hormone levels in humans. Details are provided on serum calcitonin, total serum thyroxine, free serum thyroxine, total serum triiodothyronine, free serum triiodothyronine, serum reverse triiodothyronine, serum thyroxine uptake, ovarian follicular fluid, serum free thyroid hormone indices, serum thyroglobulin, and serum thyroxine. References are included.

6.5 Adrenal Glands

Colorado State University: Adrenal Gland
http://arbl.cvmbs.colostate.edu/hbooks/pathphys/endocrine/adrenal/index.html

Maintained by Colorado State University, this site offers an introduction to the adrenal gland and an index of related information. Information on adrenal physiology is offered on the functional anatomy of the adrenal gland, the adrenal medullary hormones, and adrenal steroids. Advanced histological presentations are provided.

Colorado State University: Glucocorticoids
http://arbl.cvmbs.colostate.edu/hbooks/pathphys/endocrine/adrenal/gluco.html

From Colorado State University, this site offers information on glucocorticoids. Topics include cortisol and glucocorticoid receptors, the physiologic effects of glucocorticoids, control of cortisol secretion, and disease states.

Colorado State University: Mineralocorticoids
http://arbl.cvmbs.colostate.edu/hbooks/pathphys/endocrine/adrenal/mineralo.html

From Colorado State University, this site offers information on mineralocorticoids. Included are an overview and discussions of aldosterone and mineralocorticoid receptors, physiologic effects of mineralocorticoids, control of aldosterone secretion, and disease states. There are hyperlinks to other topics mentioned in the text.

EndocrineWeb: Adrenal Disorders and Treatments
http://www.endocrineweb.com/adrenal.html

From EndocrineWeb, this site offers illustrated information about adrenal glands. A general overview of basic function and a list of indications for surgical removal of adrenal glands are provided. There are also links to specific disorders and treatments related to the adrenal gland.

Kimball's Biology Pages: Adrenal Glands
http://www.ultranet.com/~jkimball/BiologyPages/A/Adrenals.html

Part of Kimball's Biology Pages, this site contains a tutorial on the adrenal cortex. An organ overview and sections on glucocorticoids, mineralocorticoids, androgens, Addison's disease and Cushing's syndrome, and the adrenal medulla are provided. Chemical illustrations and hyperlinks to definitions of terms used in the text are found.

Rensselaer Polytechnic Institute: Adrenal Cortex
http://www.rpi.edu/dept/naturalsci/parsons/LECT31/31Lect.html

This site offers a tutorial on the adrenal cortex, with review of basic adrenal gland anatomy, major steps in synthesis, sources of cholesterol, and the action of adrenocorticotrophic hormone (ACTH) on adrenal cells. Mineralocorticoid and glucocorticoid effects and actions are reviewed.

6.6 Kidney

Parts and Workings of the Human Kidney ◎ ◎ ◎
http://www.clark.net/pub/nhp/med/kidney/basics.html#Bowman's

Information for this page, taken from the computer program *Body Works 3.0*, offers visitors complete information on the anatomy and physiology of the human kidneys, with text and images provided in an easily navigable format.

The Kidney: Structure and Function ◎ ◎
http://www.bhs.berkeley.k12.ca.us/departments/
Science/anatomy/anatomy97/urinary/html/kidney.html

This portion of a urinary system tutorial offers visitors online views of the kidney, excerpted from *The Human Body in Health and Disease,* as well as a detailed analysis of kidney structure and function.

6.7 Gastrointestinal Tract

Colorado State University: Gastrointestinal Hormones ◎ ◎ ◎
http://arbl.cvmbs.colostate.edu/hbooks/pathphys/endocrine/gi/index.html

Maintained by Colorado State University, this site provides an introduction to gastrointestinal hormones and an index to information located at the site. There are links to information about gastrin, secretin, and motilin. Articles are found on enteroglucagon and glucagon-like peptides, gastric inhibitory peptide, and vasoactive intestinal peptide.

Kimball's Biology Pages: Gastrointestinal Hormones ◎ ◎
http://www.ultranet.com/~jkimball/BiologyPages/G/GutHormones.html

From Kimball's Biology Pages, this site offers information about hormones of the gut. Five hormones, including gastrin, secretin, cholecystokinin, somatostatin, and neuropeptide Y, are discussed, with hyperlinks to term definitions found.

6.8 Reproductive Organs

Ovaries and Female Reproductive Tract

AMA Health Insight:
Atlas of the Body: Female Reproductive System
http://www.ama-assn.org/insight/gen_hlth/atlas/newatlas/femrep.htm

Everyday health information is offered at this page of the American Medical Association, which focuses on the process of fertilization. A labeled figure of the female reproductive system and basic terminology are presented for consumer reference.

University of Kansas
Medical Center: Female Reproductive System
http://www.kumc.edu/instruction/medicine/anatomy/histoweb/female/female.htm

In-depth review of anatomy, physiology, and cell biology is presented at this Kansas University Medical Center site. Descriptions, tables, and micrographic images of the ovary, corpus luteum, and uterus are available, with an expanded view feature provided.

Testes

AMA Health Insight:
Atlas of the Body: Male Reproductive System
http://www.ama-assn.org/insight/gen_hlth/atlas/newatlas/male.htm

Male reproductive anatomy is presented as a service of Emory University and the American Medical Association at this AMA Health Insight Web address. A labeled illustration of the male reproductive tract and basic terminology are reviewed, with a link to the Atlas of the Human Body home page offered.

Texas Tech University Health Sciences Center Department of
Cell Biology and Biochemistry: Male Reproductive System
http://www.grad.ttuhsc.edu/courses/histo/notes/malerep.html

This site offers a general discussion of the male reproductive system, presented in language suitable for patients, consumers, and students. Discussions and illustrations describe testes compartmentalization, the seminiferous tubules, the interstitial area, the overall hormonal regulatory scheme, the duct system, and accessory glands, with educational objectives listed.

6.9 Bone and Mineral Metabolism

Bone Physiology

Cancer Institute of Long Island: Mineral and Bone Metabolism
http://www.cancerinst.sunysb.edu/shtm/lectures/HAD411/MINBONSLD/index.htm
This site contains a slide presentation on mineral and bone metabolism. The table of contents lists more than 45 slides on various topics including Paget's disease, bone resorption markers, bone structure, osteoporosis, hypocalcaemia, and hypercalcemia.

Merck: Bone Physiology/Metabolism
http://www.merck.com/pro/osteoporosis/inde28.htm
This portion of the *Merck* Osteoporosis Education System presents three modules on bone physiology and metabolism, including calcium homeostasis, other systemic and local factors involved in bone, and a bone remodeling discussion. Calcium balance, parathyroid hormone, vitamin D metabolic effects, and the role of calcitonin are detailed, with links provided to illustrative figures. Osteoblastic and osteoclastic functions and their regulation are reviewed, and the continuous bone destruction and renewal process is described, emphasizing its major events.

Calcium, Vitamin D, and Parathyroid Hormone

Colorado State University: Calcitonin
http://arbl.cvmbs.colostate.edu/hbooks/pathphys/endocrine/thyroid/calcitonin.html
Created by Colorado State University, this site offers information about the hormone calcitonin. A general definition and discussions of the physiologic effects of calcitonin on the bone and kidney are provided. There are also discussions of the control of calcitonin secretion and disease states.

University of Iowa Department of Physiology and Biophysics: Mineral Metabolism
http://galileo.physiology.uiowa.edu/lectures/fellows/lecture6/lecture6.htm
This site offers lecture notes on mineral metabolism. Major topics include the anatomy of parathyroid glands, physiological effects of PTH, calcitonin, and vitamin D. Diagrams are included.

Parathyroid Gland Anatomy and Physiology

Crump Institute for Biological Imaging: Parathyroid Embryology, Anatomy, Histology, and Function ◐ ◐

http://www.crump.ucla.edu/NM-Mediabook/
TCL_files/topic.asp?topic_id=1033&system_id=402

Parathyroid embryology, anatomy, histology, and function are described in this brief article. The description includes a detailed overview of cellular structures and normal body locations.

EndocrineWeb: Your Parathyroid ◐ ◐ ◐

http://www.endocrineweb.com/parathyroid.html

From EndocrineWeb, a portion of this site is devoted to the normal and abnormal function of the parathyroid glands. Hyperparathyroidism, symptoms of disease processes, diagnosis, and treatment of disease are also found at this complete parathyroid tutorial.

Jefferson Health System: The Parathyroid Glands ◐

http://www.jeffersonhealth.org/diseases/endo/paragla.htm

A discussion of parathyroid anatomy and function is available from this address. Links are available to related endocrinology resources, as well as similar resources on related topics.

University of Texas Southwestern Medical Center Department of Pathology: Parathyroid ◐ ◐

http://pathcuric1.swmed.edu/ScribeService/Resources/
path/objectives/Endocrine/endocrine-Parathyr.html

This site offers a tutorial on the parathyroid, with sections on embryology and anatomy, histology, parathyroid hormone, and physiology. Images are included.

6.10 Energy Metabolism

Cellular Metabolism: General

University of South Australia: Introductory Metabolism Module ◐ ◐ ◐

http://www.roma.unisa.edu.au/08366/h&p2carb.htm

A complete introduction to carbohydrate metabolism is outlined at this site, including glucose catabolism, glycogen and glucose interconversion, and utilization of glucose in the fed and fasting states. Diagrams throughout the text illustrate the Cori cyc

Cellular Metabolism: Carbohydrate

Indiana State University Terre Haute Center for Medical Education: Glycogen
http://web.indstate.edu/thcme/mwking/glycogen.html

An introduction to glucose and discussions of glycogen breakdown, regulation of glycogen catabolism, glycogen synthesis and its regulation, and the clinical significance of glycogen metabolism are reviewed at this educational site.

Indiana State University Terre Haute Center for Medical Education: Non-Glucose Carbons in Glycolysis
http://web.indstate.edu/thcme/mwking/fruc_gal.html

Maintained by the Terre Haute Center for Medical Education, this site offers information about the metabolism of major non-glucose sugars. There are discussions of fructose, galactose, mannose, and glycerol metabolisms.

Cellular Metabolism: Lipid

Indiana State University Terre Haute Center for Medical Education: Fatty Acids
http://web.indstate.edu/thcme/mwking/lipid-synthesis.html

Information about fatty acids is reviewed at this site, including discussions of fatty acid synthesis, origin of acetyl-CoA for fat synthesis, regulation of fatty acid synthesis, elongation and desaturation of fatty acids, triacylglyceride synthesis, phospholipid structures, phospholipid metabolism, plasmalogen synthesis, sphingolipid metabolism, clinical significance of sphingolipids, eicosanoid metabolism, cholesterol and bile acid synthesis, and fatty acid oxidation.

Kansas University Medical Center: Lipid Metabolism
http://www.kumc.edu/AMA-MSS/study/lipids.htm

This study of lipid metabolism may be downloaded in its entirety from the Web site. Fatty acid oxidation and synthesis, lipid metabolism, and absorption and lipid transport are reviewed. Lipids as metabolic fuels are summarized, including fuel reserves; synthesis of triacylglycerol, its regulation and insulin; and lipolysis. Additional details on ketone bodies and their utilization are provided.

Cellular Metabolism: Protein

Amino Acid Metabolism
http://www.bmb.leeds.ac.uk/illingworth/metabol/amino.htm

Amino acids essential in human nutrition, amino acid degradation pathways, and the urea cycle are reviewed at this site of the University of Leeds. Separate sections cover porphyrin metabolism and amino acid biochemistry. Diagrams at this page demonstrate the central role of glutamate and the transaminase mechanism, and a table at the site outlines amino acid degradation.

Cholesterol and Lipoprotein Metabolism

Indiana State University
Terre Haute Center for Medical Education: Cholesterol
http://web.indstate.edu/thcme/mwking/cholest.html

This site provides an introduction to cholesterol and discussions of metabolism, biosynthesis, regulation, and utilization of cholesterol. Bile acid synthesis and the clinical significance of bile acids are reviewed.

Indiana State University
Terre Haute Center for Medical Education: Lipoproteins
http://web.indstate.edu/thcme/mwking/lipoprot.html

From the Terre Haute Center for Medical Education, this site provides information on lipoproteins, including discussions of intestinal uptake of lipids, composition of lipoprotein complexes, the clinical significance of lipoprotein metabolism, hyperlipidemias, hypolipidemias, and pharmacologic interventions.

Metabolic Regulation

Cell Biology Tutorials: Cell Metabolism
http://mindquest.net/biology/cell-biology/outlines/ec8guide.html

A discussion of ATP and its conversion to energy, elementary metabolism terminology, and basic information on metabolic pathways are found, including glycolysis, gluconeogenesis, and glycogenolysis. Cellular respiration, the Krebs cycle, ketogenesis, and several other processes in cellular metabolism are detailed.

Indiana State University
Terre Haute Center for Medical Education: Glycolysis ◎ ◎ ◎
http://web.indstate.edu/thcme/mwking/glycolys.html

Maintained by the Terre Haute Center for Medical Education, this site offers links to information on energy derived from glycolysis, images of the pathway of glycolysis, anaerobic glycolysis, regulation of glycolysis, metabolic fates of pyruvate, lactate metabolism, ethanol metabolism, the entry of non-glucose carbons into glycolysis, glycogen metabolism, and regulation of blood glucose levels.

Integration and Regulation of Fuel Metabolism ◎ ◎ ◎
http://med.inje.ac.kr/lrc/Simpo/Nutrition/Nutrition_2.htm

The interrelationship of carbohydrate, lipid, and protein metabolism; the central role of the liver in metabolism; and tissue-specific metabolism during the feed-fast cycle are explained and illustrated in detail at this site. Figures depict overviews of lipid metabolism, pathways of amino acid and fatty acid metabolism in the liver, and the flow of substrates among tissues and organs during fasting and starvation states. System integration and homeostasis are discussed, as well as interchanges of amino acids and their metabolites among body organs and tissues.

New York University: Insulin Receptor Signaling ◎ ◎
http://www.med.nyu.edu/Research/E.Skolnik-res.html

Authored by a professor from the New York University School of Medicine, this site contains an article on insulin receptor signaling. A diagram and list of related publications are included.

Pancreatic Anatomy and Physiology

Colorado State University: Endocrine Pancreas ◎ ◎ ◎
http://arbl.cvmbs.colostate.edu/hbooks/pathphys/endocrine/pancreas/index.html

Maintained by Colorado State University, this site provides an introduction to the endocrine pancreas and an index of related information at their site. Core information at the site includes functional anatomy of the endocrine pancreas, insulin synthesis and secretion, physiologic effects of insulin, and glucagon. An article discussing the structure of insulin is accessible.

Glucagon.com ◎ ◎
http://www.glucagon.com

Authored by a physician of Toronto General Hospital, this site provides information about glucagon and the glucagon-like peptides, with articles provided on glucagon, glucagon gene, and gut endocrine cells. Highlights of recent publications and information on meetings and research reagents are provided. There are links to related sites of interest.

Seoul National University
College of Medicine: Endocrine Pancreas ○ ○ ○

http://osk.snu.ac.kr/Lecture/Pancreas/Pancreas.html

This site offers information on the pancreas, with one section providing a comprehensive overview of the endocrine pancreas and associated diseases. Review topics include embryology, anatomy, physiology, tumors, insulinoma, glucagonoma, gastrinoma, and VIPoma. Publication abstracts and a case study are included.

University of California Berkeley:
Molecular and Cell Biology: Endocrine Pancreas ○ ○

http://mcb.berkeley.edu/courses/mcb135e/pancreas.html

This site provides information on the endocrine pancreas. There are sections on the structure and function of the pancreas and the secretion and actions of insulin.

University of Manchester: Insulin and Glucagon ○ ○ ○

http://www.teaching-biomed.man.ac.uk/student_projects/2000/mnby7lc2/default.htm

Presented as a service of the University of Manchester, this collection of pages offers an animated presentation of insulin and glucagon production, with the purpose of the islets of Langherhans of the exocrine pancreas reviewed. Schematic illustrations, pages describing alpha and beta cell functions, and factors affecting the secretion of insulin and glucagon are provided, with the delicate balance of the process discussed. A diagram accessible at the site summarizes the process, and the metabolic effects of insulin and glucagon are addressed.

7. DIAGNOSTICS AND MONITORING

7.1 General Endocrinology Tests

General Resources

Adam.com: Hormones ○ ○ ○
http://www.adam.com/dir/Tests/Lab/Blood/Hormones/Hormones.htm
Each hormone link listed offers connections to alternative names, how testing for the hormone is performed, and specific endocrine disorders that can be determined through the hormone tests. Information is offered on over 30 hormone result interpretations, and pertinent drug leaflets accompany many of the connections.

Central Laboratory Services: Endocrinology ○ ○
http://128.147.36.130/Procedures/Endocrinology/Procedures/default.asp
Central Laboratory Services provides access to information on 25 endocrinology urine and serum laboratory procedures and screens at this site. Test details may be viewed by either selecting from the pull down menu or clicking on a chosen endocrinology procedure. Although the information contained at the site is geared toward laboratory professionals, the procedure principles, limitations of procedure, and clinical significance portions of the text may be useful for physicians and other healthcare practitioners.

Great Smokies Diagnostic Laboratory: Laboratory Assessments ○ ○ ○
http://www.gsdl.com/assessments
Nutritional, endocrinology, and metabolic assessments are included in this laboratory's testing protocols, and connections to each specialty Web section offer visitors the opportunity to peruse a variety of revolutionary and less well known profiles and analyses in disorders of endocrinology and metabolism. Links to specific tests offer in-

depth reviews of the tests' applications, answers to frequently asked questions, and sample reports.

Interpretation of Laboratory Test Profiles ○ ○ ○
http://www.neosoft.com/~uthman/lab_test.html

Brief analysis of a wide range of laboratory tests is found at this site, authored by a diplomate of the American Board of Pathology. Interpretations of increases and decreases in sodium, potassium, chloride, CO2 content, anion gap, glucose, blood urea nitrogen, creatinine, uric acid, inorganic phosphorus, calcium, iron, alkaline phosphatase, and a host of hormone and other levels are reviewed. Blood cell counts, lipid assessment, and detailed information on diabetes mellitus diagnostic criteria are found, for a comprehensive overview of basic laboratory pathology.

University of Pittsburgh Department of Medicine: Screening Tests for Common Medical Management ○ ○
http://www.upmc.edu/endodocs/NScreeni.htm

A listing of diagnostic/screening tools for a variety of diseases of the thyroid, endocrine pancreas, adrenal gland, anterior and posterior pituitary, and gonads are listed at this site, according to suspected disorder. A page listing of normal values for common endocrine tests is accessible.

Genetic Tests

Cancer and Genetics: Multiple Endocrine Neoplasia ○ ○ ○
http://www.cancergenetics.org/men.htm

A case study from the Cancer and Genetics Web site offers details about a case of familial medullary thyroid carcinoma and multiple endocrine neoplasia (MEN) II. Glands affected in the various MEN syndromes, historical family information, discussion of inheritance patterns, other features in MEN II mutations, and additional genetic considerations are first introduced. An optimal assessment of risk according to the Bayesian analysis is reviewed, and two examples illustrate the essence of Bayesian calculations. Outlines of indirect testing with tumor markers, direct DNA mutation testing, and an individual DNA testing link are found at this interesting and thorough presentation, which is accompanied by colorful, animated illustrations. DNA analysis topics include molecular tools, amplifying gene sequence, and analyzing gene sequences with southern blotting and DNA sequencing.

GeneTests ○ ○ (free registration)
http://www.genetests.org

Funded in part by the National Library of Medicine, GeneTests is a genetic testing resource that includes a directory of genetics laboratories, a directory of genetics clinics, and information about genetic counseling and testing. Information about genetic testing includes an overview and discussions of uses of genetic testing, ancillary services, genetics consultations, and ordering genetic testing. Free registration is required for access to the site.

HealthGate: Lipoprotein Phenotyping ⊙
http://www.healthgate.com/tests/test214.shtml

From HealthGate, this site contains a profile of lipoprotein phenotyping, a blood test that determines the classification of hyperlipoproteinemia or hypolipoproteinemia. The profile offers information about patient preparation, the test itself, post-test care, and reading the results.

HealthGate: Sex Chromatin ⊙
http://www.healthgate.com/tests/test310.shtml

Offered by HealthGate, this site contains a profile of sex chromatin, a tissue analysis that screens for abnormal sexual development. The test aids in the assessment of an infant with ambiguous genitalia and determines how many Y chromosomes are present. The profile provides information about patient preparation, the test itself, post-test care, and interpreting the results.

MEDLINEplus Health Information: Genetic Testing/Counseling ⊙ ⊙ ⊙
http://www.nlm.nih.gov/medlineplus/genetictestingcounseling.html

Governmental and additional resources on genetic and prenatal testing are provided at this MEDLINEplus site, with site selections provided by the National Library of Medicine. A link to the National Institutes of Health's primary research organization in genetic testing is found at the site, and a variety of connections to basic information sheets, glossaries, directories, print publications, research endeavors, and disease screening details are provided. Specific discussions on osteogenesis imperfecta and Prader-Willi syndrome may be accessed, as well as an assortment of genetic testing discussions from reputable disorder-specific and research organizations.

National Institutes of Health (NIH):
Task Force on Genetic Testing ⊙ ⊙ ⊙
http://www.med.jhu.edu/tfgtelsi

The Final Report of the Task Force on Genetic Testing of the National Human Genome Research Institute includes principles of prenatal and carrier testing, safety compliance and effectiveness of genetic testing in clinical practice, and laboratory quality principles. A chapter on genetic testing for rare, inherited disorders is found, with details on the Metabolic Information Network research registry. The task force's goals of expanding providers' knowledge of genetic testing and removing of obstacles to educational improvements are emphasized.

National Tay-Sachs and Allied
Health Diseases Association, Inc.: Genetic Testing ◎ ◎
http://www.ntsad.org/ntsad/intromap.htm#Testing

Contact information and test types for laboratories providing genetic testing worldwide are provided at this organization subsite. A discussion of carrier detection, genetic sampling techniques, and information on intensive educational campaigns to provide mass screening to at-risk communities are provided.

University of Texas M.D. Anderson
Cancer Center: Genetic Testing for Endocrine Tumors ◎ ◎
http://endocrine.mdacc.tmc.edu/genetic.html

Details on the availability of genetic testing of endocrine tumors, including multiple endocrine neoplasias, Von Hippel Lindau disease, and neurofibromatosis, are found at this university subsite. A connection to the Von Hippel Lindau Family Alliance Page highlights DNA testing for the disease, as well as sources of DNA testing worldwide. The national neurofibromatosis link offers a search engine that returns news, articles, and research on DNA testing with appropriate search terms. Contact information for other genetic testing laboratories is also available.

Overview of Dynamic Tests in Endocrinology

Inter Science Institute:
Hypothalamic-Pituitary Axis and Releasing Factor Tests ◎ ◎ ◎
http://www.interscilsa.com/hparf.html

This site contains information related to the hypothalamic-pituitary axis and releasing factor tests, with dynamic challenge protocols for antidiuretic hormone, growth hormone, beta-luteinizing hormone, and prolactin found. There are profiles of several tests, including the hypothalamic hormone screen, growth hormone axis, gonadotropin axis, comprehensive hypothalamic-pituitary axis, and comprehensive hypothalamic-pituitary-thyroid-steroid axis. Individual profiles include information about specific tests, patient preparation, and specimen requirements.

Poole Hospital: Endocrine Dynamic Function Tests ◎ ◎ ◎
http://www.poolehos.org/pathgp/edft/edfts.htm

Information on dynamic function tests of the anterior pituitary, posterior pituitary, and adrenal glands are available at this address, as well as glucose tolerance tests and miscellaneous procedures, such as the pentagastrin stimulation test for medullary thyroid carcinoma screening. Aims, indications, contraindications, procedural outlines, sampling, and guidelines to interpretation are outlined for each diagnostic procedure.

7.2 Hypothalamic-Pituitary Testing

General Resources

Manual of Use and Interpretation of Pathology Tests: Hypopituitarism ◎ ◎
http://www.rcpa.edu.au/pathman/hypopitu.htm

This page of the electronic version of the pathology manual explains diagnosis and evaluation of hypopituitarism by assessment of target gland or pituitary hormones. Tests of value, initial presentation of singular hormone deficiency in panhypopituitarism, alpha subunit, a listing of functioning and nonfunctioning tumors, and several other causes of abnormalities are listed, as a service of the Royal College of Pathologists of Australia.

Massachusetts General Hospital and Harvard Medical School: Clinically Non-functioning Pituitary Adenomas: Characterization and Diagnosis ◎ ◎ ◎
http://neurosurgery.mgh.harvard.edu/e-f-933.htm

A case presentation with laboratory features and other recent advances in the ability to diagnose pituitary adenomas are found at this address. Advances in radioimmunoassay, immunocytochemical, and molecular biology techniques, allowing for detailed characterization of tumor type, are discussed. Explanations of commonly detected serum hormone levels and the general availability of more sensitive and specific glycoprotein hormone free subunit assays are provided.

Oncology: Pituitary Adenomas: Current Methods of Diagnosis and Treatment ◎ ◎ ◎
http://intouch.cancernetwork.com/journals/oncology/o9706b.htm#Diagnosis

After a background presentation on the signs and symptoms of benign pituitary adenomas, visitors are able to view a listing of the hormonal syndromes associated with these tumors and are presented with an overview of the endocrinologic work-up. Adrenocorticotrophic hormone screenings, growth hormone hypersecretion, prolactin levels, TSH, and gonadotropin elevations should be assessed for diagnostic and baseline purposes. Neurological evaluation, surgical diagnosis, and additional sections on management are provided.

Antidiuretic Hormone Testing

Manual of Use and Interpretation of Pathology Tests: Antidiuretic Hormone (ADH) Plasma
http://www.rcpa.edu.au/pathman/antidiur.htm

Specimen details and interpretation of results in conjunction with plasma osmlality are briefly outlined at the site.

Pathophysiology of the Endocrine System: Antidiuretic Hormone (Vasopressin)
http://arbl.cvmbs.colostate.edu/hbooks/pathphys/endocrine/hypopit/adh.html

The physiologic effect of antidiuretic hormone and variables in its control are reviewed, with discussion of plasma osmolarity in connection with plasma concentration of antidiuretic hormone. Discussion of disease states related to antidiuretic hormone level or inability to respond to the hormone are discussed.

Follicle-Stimulating Hormone

HealthGate: Follicle-Stimulating Hormone (FSH)
http://www.healthgate.com/tests/test59.shtml

Part of HealthGate, this site contains a profile of blood follicle-stimulating hormone, a blood test used to diagnose the cause of early puberty in boys and girls. It also helps confirm diagnosis of infertility and menstruation disorders and may determine the cause of underdeveloped sexual organs. The profile includes estimated cost of the test, patient time, and reliability of results. There is information about patient preparation, risks and precautions, and the sensory factors of the test itself. Also found are details regarding post-test care and test results.

Growth Hormone

HealthGate: Growth Hormone
http://www.healthgate.com/tests/test65.shtml

From HealthGate, this site contains a profile of blood growth hormone, a blood test that helps diagnose dwarfism, chronic acromegaly and gigantism, and pituitary tumors. The test also helps evaluate human growth hormone therapy. The profile offers information about the cost of the test, patient time, and reliability of results. It also discusses pre-testing procedures, the test itself, follow-up care, and reading the test results.

Somatomedin C (IGF-1): Adult Growth Hormone Deficiency ◐ ◐
http://www.aalrl.com/IGF-1.htm

The decline in human growth hormone secretion as one ages and testing principles for somatomedin C reduction are outlined at this Web address. Laboratory changes seen in this syndrome and somatomedin C (IGF-1) as the best indicator of adult growth hormone deficiency in an outpatient setting are discussed.

Prolactin

Central Laboratory Services: Prolactin Procedure ◐ ◐
http://128.147.36.130/Procedures/Endocrinology/Procedures/ProlactinAxSYMdata.htm

A test for the quantitative determination of prolactin in human serum or plasma is found at this laboratory Web site. Although geared toward laboratory professionals, the site includes valuable review of procedure principles and clinical significance of hyperprolactinemia and decreased prolactin levels.

Imaging

Kyoto University Hospital:
The Pituitary: Magnetic Resonance Imaging Protocols ◐ ◐
http://www.mipg.upenn.edu/~miki/PAPER/pitsyllabus.html

Magnetic resonance imaging protocols of the pituitary gland are discussed at this online article, which was presented at an annual meeting of the International Society for Magnetic Resonance in Medicine (ISMRM). The importance of obtaining high-resolution images, as well as an emphasis on countermeasures for phase-shift, magnetic susceptibility, and chemical shift artifacts, are discussed. Imaging findings for pituitary adenomas and magnetic resonance imaging of other pituitary lesions are reviewed.

Inferior Petrosal Sinus Sampling

Massachusetts General Hospital:
Bilateral Inferior Petrosal Sinus Sampling in Cushing's Syndrome ◐ ◐ ◐
http://neurosurgery.mgh.harvard.edu/e-f-932.htm

The diagnostic problems in Cushing's syndrome are introduced at this site of Massachusetts General Hospital and Harvard University, where recent advances in the diagnostic workup of Cushing's syndrome patients are discussed. The use of bilateral petrosal sinus sampling (BIPSS) and its ability to determine with certainty the correct location of hormone excess are reviewed. Rare difficulties in the ability to localize and lateralize are outlined and include incorrect catheter placement and anomalous venous drainage. Complications of the procedure, although infrequent, are summarized.

Vanderbilt University Medical Center: Inferior Petrosal Sinus Sampling ◎ ◎
http://www.pituitarycenter.com/html/article1.html

Patients suspected of having a pituitary tumor and Cushing's syndrome may be candidates for inferior petrosal sinus sampling. The procedure is detailed at the site, with information on catheter insertion, blood sample collection, and corticotrophin-releasing hormone administration. Ratios obtained and use of results are explained. Other resources at the site include details on additional tests of pituitary function, answers to FAQs, and a specialized case of the month. Additional, archived cases and laboratory results are included.

Stimulation Testing

Adam.com: Growth Hormone Stimulation Test ◎ ◎
http://www2.adam.com/ency/article/003377.htm

Information on the growth hormone stimulation test, otherwise known as the arginine test, is presented at this site of the adam.com encyclopedic database. Test preparation, associated risks, and value interpretation are presented.

Clinical Uses of Corticotropin-Releasing Hormone in the Evaluation of Patients with Cushing's Syndrome ◎ ◎ ◎
http://neurosurgery.mgh.harvard.edu/e-f-942.htm

Harvard University and Massachusetts General Hospital collaborate to bring Web visitors this testing guideline on the investigational use of corticotropin-releasing hormone (CRH). The hormone currently under evaluation for clinical use, clinical indications for the peptide, and its key uses in Cushing's syndrome evaluation are reviewed.

Endocrine Society: Comparison Between Insulin-Induced Hypoglycemia and Growth Hormone Secretion Tests for the Diagnosis of GH Deficiency in Adults ◎ ◎ ◎
http://jcem.endojournals.org/cgi/content/full/83/5/1615?searchid=976311599891_3765

An online article from the *Journal of Clinical Endocrinology and Metabolism* discusses the reliability of the insulin tolerance test for the diagnosis of adult growth hormone deficiency, as well as a more potent stimulus of growth hormone (GH) secretion in diagnosis. Review of alternative provocative tests of GH secretion with an emphasis on appropriate cut-off limits, and the comparative reliability of the tests, is presented.

Inter Science Institute: Growth Hormone Challenge ◎ ◎
http://www.interscilsa.com/book/indi05.html#48

This site offers a growth hormone challenge protocol for arginine stimulation. The protocol includes specimen requirements, stimulus, expected response, interpretation, and contraindications.

Vanderbilt University Medical Center: Arginine Infusion Test ◎ ◎
http://www.pituitarycenter.com/html/test.html

A procedural outline is presented at the site, as well as concise information on interpretation. Additional tests of pituitary function are accessible at the same page.

Vanderbilt University Medical Center: Low Dose ACTH Stimulation Test ◎ ◎
http://www.pituitarycenter.com/html/test2.html#2

The low dose adrenal insufficiency test for diagnosis of central adrenal insufficiency is found at this subsite of Vanderbilt Medical Center's testing pages. An explanation of serum cortisol levels and their meaning is found. Connections to information on additional pituitary function tests, FAQs, and an online case of the month are included.

Vanderbilt University Medical Center: TRH Stimulation of TSH Test ◎ ◎
http://www.pituitarycenter.com/html/test4.html#1

This infrequently used test is explained in terms of procedure and interpretation at the site. Its importance in differentiating between thyroid disease type and assessing the efficacy of thyroxine therapy is reviewed. Visitors may access a case of the month at the site, archives of related cases, and additional tests of pituitary function.

Suppression Testing

Adam.com: Dexamethasone Suppression Test ◎ ◎
http://www.adam.com/ency/article/003694.htm

Adam.com's encyclopedic articles include this review of the dexamethasone suppression test, which includes discussion of two ways to administer the test, test preparation for patients, and test purpose. Drugs that may affect results are listed, and a link to normal values and abnormal result meanings is found.

HealthGate: Growth Hormone Suppression Test ◎
http://www.healthgate.com/tests/test183.shtml

From HealthGate, this site provides a profile of growth-hormone suppression, a blood test that assesses elevated levels of growth hormone, confirms diagnosis of gigantism in children, and suggests diagnosis of acromegaly in adults. The profile includes information about cost of the test, patient time, and reliability of results. There are also discussions of pre-testing preparation, the test itself, post-test care, and results.

Manual of Use and Interpretation of Pathology Tests: Dexamethasone Suppression Test (Overnight) ○

http://www.rcpa.edu.au/pathman/dexamet2.htm

Information on this initial investigation of Cushing's syndrome includes specimen requirements and other diagnoses to rule out when failure to suppress occurs.

Vanderbilt University Medical Center: Oral Glucose Suppression Test for Growth Hormone Secretory Dynamics ○ ○

http://www.pituitarycenter.com/html/test3.html

Indications for the oral glucose tolerance test, procedural details, and value result interpretation are reviewed at this site of the Vanderbilt Medical Center. The possibility and meaning of false positive results are mentioned.

7.3 Thyroid Gland

General Resources

Thyroid Disease Manager: Evaluating Thyroid Function and Anatomy ○ ○ ○

http://thyroidmanager.bsd.uchicago.edu/FunctionTests/thyfunc.htm

The online Thyroid Disease Manager, provided as a service of the University of Chicago, offers access to four lectures at this site regarding thyroid disease diagnosis. Complete tutorials on evaluation of thyroid hormones and related substances, ultrasonography of the thyroid, fine needle aspiration biopsy, and isotope scanning are offered. Each article discusses technical aspects, normal thyroid imaging, and results; and several case examples of diseased thyroid tissue, as evidenced by the respective imaging or other diagnostic modality, are accessible. Sonography in the patient with thyroid cancer, sonography in conjunction with fine needle aspiration biopsy, and complete review of total hormone measurements, free thyroid hormone tests, and thyroid-specific autoantibodies are found.

Thyroid Disease Manager: Evaluation of Thyroid Function in Health and Disease ○ ○

http://www.thyroidmanager.org/Chapter6/6-text.htm

From the Thyroid Disease Manager, this site contains a chapter on the evaluation of thyroid function in health and disease. The chapter provides a table listing all tests of thyroid function. Clinical descriptions are given for the tests and result interpretation tables are found.

Thyroid Disease Manager: Tests Assessing the Effects of Thyroid Hormones on Body Tissues ◎ ◎ ◎
http://www.thyroidmanager.org/Chapter6/Ch-6-5.htm

Measurement of hormonal supply via parameters other than thyroid gland activity is reviewed at this online tutorial, providing insight into a more complete picture of thyroid disease effects. Basal metabolic rate result interpretation, photomotogram and its diagnostic value, tests related to cardiovascular function, and details on miscellaneous biochemical and physiological changes related to thyroid function on other body systems are provided.

Imaging

HealthGate: Thyroid Ultrasonography ◎
http://www.healthgate.com/tests/test334.shtml

Maintained by HealthGate, this site offers information about thyroid ultrasonography, an examination used to study the structure of the thyroid, differentiate between cystic tumors and solid tumors, and monitor the size of the thyroid gland. The profile includes information about patient preparation, the test itself, post-test care, and reading the results.

Nuclear Imaging Tests of the Thyroid ◎ ◎ ◎
http://www.wramc.amedd.army.mil/departments/nuclear/williams/nucmed/Endocrine/Thyroid/Imaging%20Tests/Nuclear%20Imaging%20Tests.html

The techniques of radioactive iodine uptake for thyroid gland assessment, its indications, and factors affecting thyroid iodine uptake are reviewed at this educational page. Etiologies resulting in increased and decreased radioactive iodine uptake value are listed, and additional procedures are explained, including the thyroid suppression test, the TSH stimulation test, and the Percholate washout test. Contraindications to thyroid scanning and pregnancy are reviewed.

Santa Monica Thyroid Diagnostic Center ◎ ◎
http://www.thyroid.com

Patient information, physician pages, nuclear medicine diagnosis, and thyroid ultrasound reviews are included at this comprehensive page dedicated solely to thyroid disease diagnosis. The ultrasound Web page describes four reasons why ultrasound is preferred, and the nuclear medicine page briefly discusses PET, CT, and MRI thyroid scans. A bookstore at the site allows for online ordering of patient and medical textbooks on thyroid pathophysiology. Internet article links are accessible, including practice guidelines in diagnosis.

University of California Los Angeles:
Nuclear Medicine Protocols: Thyroid Uptake and Scan ◐ ◐

http://laxmi.nuc.ucla.edu:8000/NM-Mediabook/protocols/thyscan.html

This measure of thyroid function is outlined at the site, with sections presented on patient preparation, radiopharmaceutical dose factors, positioning for imaging, and additional preparatory protocols.

University of California Los Angeles:
Nuclear Medicine Protocols: Total Body Scan ◐ ◐

http://laxmi.nuc.ucla.edu:8000/NM-Mediabook/protocols/totbody.html

This useful procedure, for determination of the completeness of thyroidectomy and for identification of any metastases, is reviewed in terms of clinical indications, patient procedure, radiopharmaceutical and dose factors, acquisition parameters, and positioning and imaging details.

University of Texas Health Science Center:
Thyroid and Parathyroid Nuclear Medicine ◐ ◐ ◐

http://radiology.uthscsa.edu/rad/williams/thyroid.htm

Thyroid function, fetal and neonatal thyroid function, and additional physiology discussions introduce this tutorial on thyroid and parathyroid nuclear imaging. Radionuclides and their dose and indications are reviewed, in addition to four nuclear imaging tests of the thyroid and scintigraphic and non-scintigraphic parathyroid imaging. The pathophysiology, clinical findings, specific imaging, and treatment for most thyroid disorders and parathyroid diseases are included.

University of Texas Health Science Center:
Thyroid Nuclear Medicine ◐ ◐ ◐

http://wwwmed.medic.ukm.my/nucmed/NucMed/thy02.htm

The characteristics of several radionuclides in the diagnosis of thyroid disease are reviewed at this site, with dosage, indications, and diagnostic technique reviewed. The radioactive iodine uptake test, factors affecting uptake, indications, and etiologies resulting in abnormal results are enumerated. The thyroid suppression test, TSH stimulation test, and the Perchlorate washout test are described.

Immunoassays

Immunoassays: Thyroid Autoimmunity ◐ ◐

http://www.biocode.be/pages/products/immunoas/autoimmu/immuauto.htm

Immunoassays for diagnosing thyroid autoimmune disease are listed at this site, with links offered to information on eight individual tests. Sample information and normal test values are provided. A link is provided to a general discussion on endocrine autoimmunity and thyroid disease.

Thyroid Disease Manager: Thyroid Autoantibodies ◉ ◉ ◉
http://www.thyroidmanager.org/Chapter6/Ch-6-6.htm

Techniques developed for the measurement of thyroid autoantibodies, thyroid-stimulating immunoglobulins, thyroid stimulation assays, thyroid growth-promoting assays, and other useful tests in the diagnosis of thyroid dysfunction are discussed at this site. A discussion of cell-mediated immunity in autoimmune thyroid disease and methods of its measurement are included.

Thyroid Biopsy

American Foundation of Thyroid Patients: Fine Needle Aspiration Biopsy of the Thyroid ◉ ◉
http://www.thyroidfoundation.org/aspiration.htm

An excerpt from the newsletter Thyroid USA offers visitors a discussion of fine needle aspiration biopsy of the thyroid. Information on accuracy of the test and classification of results is provided.

EndocrineWeb: Thyroid Nodule Biopsy ◉ ◉ ◉
http://www.endocrineweb.com/fna.html

At the EndocrineWeb reference visitors will find this page dedicated to providing accurate, easy-to-understand information on the safety and efficacy of the thyroid biopsy procedure for definitive diagnosis of thyroid nodules. Features that favor a benign thyroid nodule, features that increase the suspicion of malignancy, and links to pages on the thyroid scan and thyroid ultrasound are offered. This colorful site contains additional coverage of relevant terminology and access to the basics of thyroid nodules.

HealthGate: Thyroid Biopsy ◉
http://www.healthgate.com/tests/test333.shtml

Information about the thyroid biopsy is offered at the site, with information about cost, time, and reliability of the test. There is also information about patient preparation, the test itself, post-test care, and reading the results.

Thyroid Foundation of Canada: Fine Needle Aspiration Biopsy of Thyroid Nodules ◉ ◉
http://home.ican.net/~thyroid/Articles/EngE12B.html

The Thyroid Foundation of Canada's assortment of educational articles includes this online paper on fine needle aspiration biopsy of thyroid nodules. The similarities between the procedure and core needle biopsy are explained, and patient tolerability and other advantages are discussed. Instructions for patients undergoing core needle biopsy are found.

Thyroid Function Tests

Inter Science Institute: Thyroid Tests ◎ ◎
http://www.interscilsa.com/tts.html

This site offers dynamic challenge protocols for thyroid stimulating hormone, with profiles of eight diagnostic tests related to the thyroid also provided. These include the hypothyroid profile, hyperthyroid profile, medullary carcinoma of the thyroid, and hypothalamic-pituitary-thyroid axis evaluations.

University of Missouri Health Sciences Center: Thyroid Function Tests ◎ ◎
http://www.muhealth.org/~daveg/thyroid/thy_test.html

This site offers profiles of thyroid function tests. Details for interpretation of the antithyroid antibodies, TSH, free T4, total T4, and resin T3 uptake are found, in addition to other thyroid function tests. Diseases and conditions that will produce abnormal levels are discussed.

7.4 Adrenal Glands

ACTH Stimulation Test

Adam.com: ACTH (Cortrosyn) Stimulation Test ◎ ◎
http://thirdage.adam.com/ency/article/003696.htm

Adam.com's encyclopedic Web reference provides an overview of the adrenocorticotrophic (ACTH) stimulation test at this site, which includes details on test preparation, special considerations regarding cortisol levels at different periods of the day, normal values after ACTH stimulation, and possible diagnoses with abnormal results. Links to specific diseases diagnosed by this test are found.

Prolonged ACTH Stimulation Test ◎
http://members.aol.com/Richstott/Lonsyn.htm

Patient preparations and cautionary measures with regard to performing this test on Cushing's disease patients are outlined at the site. Blood sample procedures and result interpretation are found, for a simple introduction to the prolonged ACTH test and its principles.

Vanderbilt University
Medical Center: Traditional ACTH Stimulation Test ◉ ◉
http://www.pituitarycenter.com/html/test3.html#2

An explanation of the traditional ACTH stimulation test with Cortrosyn is outlined at the site, with procedural steps and interpretation details provided. Links to additional pituitary diagnostics, a case of the month, and archived cases with laboratory values are included.

Dexamethasone Suppression Testing

Vanderbilt University Medical Center:
Dexamethasone Suppression Tests ◉ ◉
http://www.pituitarycenter.com/html/article4.html

Several variations of the dexamethasone suppression tests, the basis for their use, and procedures for the overnight, low-dose; the formal, 2-day high-dose; and other tests are discussed. A case of the month may be accessed, as well as case archives.

Hormones

Manual of Use and Interpretation of
Pathology Tests: Adrenocorticotrophic Hormone (ACTH) Plasma ◉
http://www.rcpa.edu.au/pathman/adrenoc3.htm

A description of plasma level testing of adrenocorticotrophic (ACTH) hormone is found in this online manual. Reference interval, purpose of investigation, and corticosteroid excess interpretation are summarized.

Manual of Use and Interpretation of
Pathology Tests: Cortisol (Plasma or Serum) ◉
http://www.rcpa.edu.au/pathman/cortisol.htm

The reference interval, testing purpose, and specimen collection information are briefly reviewed at this online pathology manual page.

Postgraduate Medicine:
Assessment of Adrenal Glucocorticoid Function ◉ ◉ ◉
http://www.postgradmed.com/issues/1998/07_98/hasinski.htm

Issues in the assessment of hypoadrenalism and hyperadrenalism are reviewed by a professor of endocrinology and metabolism at the Allegheny University of the Health Sciences. Options for testing critical adrenal functions and current information on interpreting test outcomes and accurate diagnosis are provided. The main difficulties in recognizing adrenal insufficiency and its assortment of symptoms, base screening tests, corticotropin-dependent and corticotropin-independent causes of Cushing's syndrome, and determination of hypercortisolism are reviewed. The dexamethasone suppression test and scanning techniques are discussed.

Hypertension Evaluation, Adrenal

Central Laboratory Services: Urine Catecholamines Procedure ◎ ◎
http://128.147.36.130/Procedures/Endocrinology/Procedures/UrineCatecholaminesData.htm

Principles of the procedure and clinical significance of the test are reviewed at this laboratory Web site. Although geared toward laboratory personnel, the site offers valuable review of catecholamine-secreting neurochromaffin tumor, pheochromocytoma, paraganglioma, and neuroblastoma diagnosis.

HealthGate: Catecholamines ◎
http://www.healthgate.com/tests/test48.shtml

Provided by HealthGate, this site contains a profile of blood catecholamines, a test used to rule out pheochromocytoma in people with hypertension, as well as distinguish between adrenal-medulla and other catecholamine-producing tumors. The synopsis includes cost, patient time, and reliability of results. There is information about preparation, the test itself, follow-up, and results.

Inter Science Institute:
Hypertension, Corticosteroid, and Mineralocorticoid Tests ◎ ◎
http://www.interscilsa.com/hcm.html

Offered by the Inter Science Institute, this site provides information about hypertension, corticosteroid, and mineralocorticoid tests, with dynamic challenge protocols for aldosterone-renin, aldosterone-cortisol, catecholamines, cortisol, ACTH-cortisol, and 11-deoxycortisol-cortisol. Profiles of screens for hypertension, adrenal-renal function, mineralocorticoid screen, pituitary-adrenal screen, corticosteroid screen, tetrahydrocorticosteroids, and tetrahydromineralocorticoids are outlined.

University of Michigan
Department of Internal Medicine:
Testing for Pheochromocytoma ◎
http://www.vhl.org/profinfo/96aspheo.htm

Diet prior to testing and proper preservation of samples are stressed at this site, which discusses diagnosis of pheochromocytoma by 24-hour urine testing and plasma testing. Specific information for patients on vanillyl mandelic acid testing and catecholamines, metanephrines, epinephrine, and norepinephrine dietary considerations are reviewed, as well as additional collection considerations.

Imaging

Adrenal Imaging ◉ ◉ ◉
http://www.mamc.amedd.army.mil/williams/NucMed/
Genitourinary/Adrenal%20imaging/Contents.htm

Disease processes and neoplasms imaged by meta-iodobenzylguanidine (MIBG) are reviewed at this site's links, and access to details on the pharmacology, indications, and technique associated with MIBG is found. The clinical presentation, radiographic findings, and scintigraphic findings of pheochromocytoma and neuroblastoma are discussed. Disorders imaged with the cholesterol analog, NP-59, are also reviewed, and the pharmacology, non-suppressed exam, and dexamethasone suppression exam are explained. Radiographic and scintigraphic findings in Conn's syndrome and other evaluation details are introduced.

Armed Forces Institute of Pathology Lecture Series: Adrenal Imaging in Adults ◉ ◉
http://www.radpath.org/syllabus/GU/Wagner/ADRENAL1.html

This course syllabus provides an outline of the pathophysiology of adrenal disease, with microscopic and macroscopic pathology and CT and MRI findings. Non-contrast CT, contrast-enhanced CT, and opposed phase MRI notes are included.

Boston University Medical Center: An On-Line Adrenal Imaging Teaching Program ◉ ◉ ◉
http://www.mcqs.com/adrenal.htm

A downloadable file found at this site offers visitors case histories, exam details, and questions regarding appropriate diagnostic procedures and decisions. Immediately after answering the clinical management questions, visitors are presented with correct answers and rationale, accompanied by imaging examples. Users may adjust the level of difficulty of the tutorial by sliding the appropriate marker at the top of the screen.

EndocrineWeb: X-Ray Tests for Adrenal Gland Tumors ◉ ◉
http://www.endocrineweb.com/adrtest.html

Four primary imaging modalities for tumor imaging of the adrenal glands are presented at the site, accompanied by CT, MRI, and MIBG scan images and explanations.

Urine Free Cortisol

Central Laboratory Services: Urinary Free Cortisol Procedure
http://128.147.36.130/Procedures/Endocrinology/Procedures/ACS180UrineFreeCortisol.htm

Provided as a service of Central Laboratory Services, this site explains the principle of the procedure, its clinical significance, specimen information, reagent materials, and other laboratory details and procedures. Information on accuracy, limitations of the procedure, and textbook references are provided.

HealthGate: Urine Free Cortisol
http://www.healthgate.com/tests/test364.shtml

General information on urine free cortisol testing, test purpose, patient preparation, and a test description are found at this online brochure, courtesy of HealthGate.com's guide to medical testing.

7.5 Kidney

Blood Urea Nitrogen

Blood Urea Nitrogen (BUN)
http://www.rnceus.com/renal/renalbun.html

Blood urea nitrogen alterations are discussed at this fact sheet, which includes reference values for BUN and causes of elevated and decreased BUN. The use of the test as a general index of glomerular function is mentioned.

Lexi-Comp Clinical Reference Library: Urea Nitrogen, Blood
http://informatics.drake.edu/lth/html/chapter/mono/ch020700.htm

The meaning of the blood urea nitrogen (BUN) measurement, as well as the interpretation of increased and decreased values, is outlined at this site. Reference ranges, clinical uses, and limitations with regard to sensitivity are discussed. Related links and similar discussions on the BUN/creatinine ratio, creatinine clearance, serum creatinine, and additional tests are accessible, with each providing a detailed clinical profile.

Creatinine

HealthGate: Creatinine
http://www.healthgate.com/tests/test53.shtml

From HealthGate, this site offers a profile of blood creatinine, a blood test that determines the presence and severity of suspected kidney disease and screens for kidney damage. The profile includes estimated cost, patient time, and reliability of results. There is information about risks and precautions, patient preparation, and sensory factors involved in the procedure. There is also information about equipment used, post-test care, and results.

Imaging

HealthGate: Renal Angiography
http://www.healthgate.com/tests/test296.shtml

A profile of renal angiography, an X-ray examination used to evaluate kidney structures and blood vessels, to determine the cause of hypertension, and to evaluate chronic kidney disease, is found at this HealthGate Web site, which also provides information about cost, time, and test reliability. Visitors will, additionally, find information about preparation, the test itself, follow-up care, and reading the results.

HealthGate: Renal Computed Tomography
http://www.healthgate.com/tests/test297.shtml

From HealthGate, this site contains a profile of renal computed tomography, a structural test used to detect kidney disease, including kidney stones, tumors, obstructions, abnormalities, infections, and fluid accumulation around the kidney. The profile includes information about patient preparation, the test itself, post-test care and activity, and test results.

HealthGate: Renal Ultrasonography
http://www.healthgate.com/tests/test298.shtml

Provided by HealthGate, this site offers a profile of renal ultrasonography, a test that determines the size, shape, and position of the kidneys. The test also evaluates and determines the location of urinary obstructions and abnormal accumulations of fluid and assesses complications following a kidney transplant. The profile provides information about pre-testing procedures, the test itself, follow-up care, and reading test results.

HealthGate: Renal Venography ⊙
http://www.healthgate.com/tests/test299.shtml

From HealthGate, this site offers a profile of renal venography, an X-ray examination used to detect blood clots in kidney veins, kidney-vein compression, vein abnormalities and defects, and imperfect kidney development. The test assesses kidney tumors, and the profile includes information about patient preparation, the test itself, and reading the results.

HealthGate: Retrograde Ureteropyelography ⊙
http://www.healthgate.com/tests/test302.shtml

Provided by HealthGate, this site offers a profile of retrograde ureteropyelography, an X-ray examination that outlines the kidney and ureters and detects the presence of kidney stones, tumors, abscesses, blood clots, and strictures. The profile includes information about test preparation, the test itself, follow-up care, and reading the results.

7.6 Gastrointestinal Tract

Imaging

McMahon Archives: Endoscopic Ultrasound Imaging Modality for a Variety of Pancreatic Diseases ⊙ ⊙
http://www.mcmahonmed.com/wworks/MAGAZINES/gastro/archived/gen0699-11a.htm

The use of endoscopic ultrasound in pancreatic disease and its superiority to conventional imaging modalities are discussed at this news article, which also discusses current studies in endoscopic ultrasound, its potential for significant impact in diagnosis of pancreatic masses, and additional diagnostic reviews.

Philipps University Marburg: Modern Imaging Procedures in the Diagnostics of Pancreatic Disease ⊙ ⊙
http://www.chirurgie.cz/sborniky/kv/kv_42.htm

Imaging modalities to answer questions regarding disease staging, differential diagnosis, complications, therapeutic plan, and functional status are listed at this electronic table. Specific disease entities and pathways to follow in diagnosis are reviewed for pancreatitis, carcinoma, and other pancreatic tumors.

Tests

HealthGate: Amylase ○
http://www.healthgate.com/tests/test38.shtml
Provided by HealthGate, this site provides a profile of blood amylase, a blood test used to diagnose acute pancreatitis. The profile includes cost of the test, patient time, and reliability. There is information given about the purpose of the test, patient preparation, sensory factors, post-testing procedures, test results, and drug interactions.

HealthGate: Lipase ○
http://www.healthgate.com/tests/test213.shtml
This site contains a profile of lipase, a blood test used to diagnose pancreatic diseases and acute pancreatitis. The profile offers information about the cost of the test, the time it takes, and the reliability of the results. Preparation instructions, a description of the test, post-test care information, and information on reading the results are found.

HealthGate: Urine Amylase ○
http://www.healthgate.com/tests/test353.shtml
As a service of the HealthGate database, this site provides information on urine amylase, a urine test that evaluates function of the pancreas and salivary glands. The test helps diagnose acute pancreatitis and confirms the diagnosis of chronic pancreatitis and salivary-gland disorders. The profile includes information about patient preparation, the test itself, post-test care and activity, and result interpretation.

Inter Science Institute: Pancreatic Tests ○ ○ ○
http://www.interscilsa.com/gi.html
Maintained by the Inter Science Institute's Gastrointestinal (G.I.) Hormones Laboratory, this site offers protocols and information about numerous pancreatic function tests. Test protocols are included for calcitonin, cholecystokinin, gastric inhibitory polypeptide, gastrin, glucagon, insulin, motilin, and pancreatic polypeptide screening. There are also profiles of the watery diarrhea screen, the G.I. neuroendocrine screen, the diabetes screen, the insulin insensitivity screen, the Ulcer/Zollinger-Ellison screen, the comprehensive G.I. work-up, and the pancreatic function screen.

Laboratory Corporation of America: C-Peptide, Serum ○
http://www.labcorp.com/datasets/labcorp/html/chapter/mono/sr001400.htm
In addition to reviewing collection and storage information for obtaining proper samples, this site discusses the uses of C-peptide testing in the evaluation of hypoglycemia and for the diagnosis of insulin-secreting neoplasms. Causes of false negative or false positive results are considered.

Lexi-Comp Clinical Reference Library: Gastrin, Serum

http://informatics.drake.edu/lth/html/chapter/mono/ch011000.htm

Diagnosis of Zollinger-Ellison syndrome based on basal gastrin levels, reference range and critical values, and testing limitations are outlined at this site. Additional causes of elevated gastrin levels, preference of a fasting specimen, and details on the secretin test, calcium infusion, and differential diagnosis are discussed. Notes on related endocrine tumors in multiple endocrine neoplasia are included.

Manual of Use and Interpretation of Pathology Tests: Gastrin, Serum

http://www.rcpa.edu.au/pathman/gastrin_.htm

Specimen information, testing application, and result interpretation are concisely reviewed at the site, with details on the possible need for additional diagnostic tests.

7.7 Reproductive Glands

Gonadal Hormone Tests

HealthGate: Estrogens

http://www.healthgate.com/tests/test55.shtml

As a service of the HealthGate database, this site offers a profile of blood estrogens, a test used to determine if female hormone secretion is normal. The profile includes an estimated cost of the test, patient time, and reliability of results. There is information about preparation, the test itself, post-test care, and reading the results.

HealthGate: Testosterone Testing

http://www.healthgate.com/tests/test329.shtml

Provided by HealthGate, this site contains a profile of testosterone, a blood test used to diagnose early sexual development in boys. It is also used to confirm the diagnosis of deficient activity of the testes or ovaries and evaluate male infertility. The profile includes information about cost, time, and reliability of the test, as well as patient preparation details, facts about the test itself, follow-up care, and test results.

HealthGate: Total Urine Estrogens

http://www.healthgate.com/tests/test339.shtml

At this address, visitors will find a profile of total urine estrogens, a urine test used to evaluate ovarian function. The test helps determine the cause of amenorrhea, confirms the diagnosis of testicular tumors, and assesses fetal development and placental function. The profile includes information about patient preparation, the test itself, post-test care, and interpreting the results.

Inter Science Institute:
Reproductive Endocrinology and Gonadal Steroid Tests ○ ○ ○

http://www.interscilsa.com/regs.html

Dynamic challenge protocols and 18 gonadal steroid profile tests may be accessed from this site of the Inter Science Institute. The dynamic challenge protocols detail the tests measured and time of collection, as well as interpretive information and contraindications. Each gonadal steroid profile lists its included tests and provides several individual links to test details. The clinical significance of each hormonal measurement is discussed.

Imaging

Healthcare Solutions Group
On-Line CME Credits: Ultrasound of the Testis and Scrotum ○ ○

http://www.healthcare.agilent.com/mpgcme/article7.html

Written by a consultant radiologist at the Freeman Hospital, this site provides information about ultrasound of the testis and scrotum. There is information about instrumentation, the use of the doppler in the scrotum, indications, exam tips and techniques, and the normal scrotum and flow. Ultrasound images are provided.

Virtual Hospital: Pelvic Imaging ○ ○

http://www.vh.org/Providers/TeachingFiles/
NormalRadAnatomy/Text/PelvImagtitle.html

Radiographic images of the pelvis, computed tomography images, and magnetic resonance examples are presented at this Virtual Hospital module. Visitors may also link to a transvaginal ultrasound of the ovaries image. Normal radiologic anatomy is presented, with enlargeable, labeled graphics.

7.8 Bone and Mineral Metabolism

Biochemical Markers for Bone Turnover

European Calcified Tissue Society: Biochemical Markers of
Bone Metabolism: Clinical Uses in Osteoporosis ○ ○ ○

http://www.ectsoc.org/reviews/004_garn.htm

The recent improvements in specificity of biochemical markers of bone metabolism are discussed at this article, which examines the major consequences of osteoporosis, outlines biochemical markers of bone turnover, and reviews the assessment of bone resorption. The future of disease-specific markers with an increasing knowledge base, clinical uses of bone markers in osteoporosis, and review of longitudinal and cross-sectional studies of bone markers and bone loss are presented. Bone markers and osteoporotic fractures are an additional topic of discussion. Visitors will also discover a useful table of diagnostic tests for predicting hip fracture, as well as a discussion of the importance of bone markers in ongoing monitoring. References are accompanied by PubMed abstract links.

Osteovision: Major Biochemical Markers of Bone Turnover

http://www.osteovision.ch/slides/33.html

Adapted from a clinical endocrinology journal, this site lists formation and resorption bone markers and discusses their use in the assessment of osteoporosis. By advancing to the next slide in the series, visitors will find further details in assessment applications of the rate of bone turnover.

Postgraduate Medicine: Biochemical Markers of Bone Turnover

http://www.postgradmed.com/issues/1998/10_98/rosen.htm

This article from *Postgraduate Medicine* describes the physiology of bone turnover and presents a table outlining the biochemical markers of bone turnover. Serum and urine markers of bone formation and their clinical value are thoroughly reviewed. The monitoring of bone loss and the effects of therapy with biochemical markers is examined. Potential limitations of biochemical markers, including variations in marker measurements, are reviewed.

Calcium

Adam.com: Serum Calcium

http://www.adam.com/ency/article/003477.htm

An overview of serum calcium testing is prepared for consumers at this address, with an additional link to normal values and what abnormal results may indicate. By clicking on any one of the listed conditions, visitors will learn more about lower-than-normal levels and above-normal indications. A listing of additional diseases that may require serum calcium testing is presented.

Manual of Use and Interpretation of Pathology Tests: Calcium: Plasma or Serum

http://www.rcpa.edu.au/pathman/calcium_.htm

Specimen information and the applications of serum calcium measurement are presented at this one-page review of the test. Differentiation between total, corrected, and ionized calcium is mentioned in the interpretation details.

Imaging: Bone Age

HealthGate: Bone Age ○
http://www.healthgate.com/dph/html/chapter/mono/xr124100.shtml

This professional research tool offers clinicians a basic review of the indications and standard radiographs associated with bone age testing. References are provided for this pediatric endocrinology test.

Parents' Common Sense Encyclopedia: Bone Age ○
http://sleeptight.com/EncyMaster/B/bone_age.html

A simple introduction to the bone age assessment test to determine relative maturity of a child's skeletal system is described at this online information sheet. Determination of glandular abnormalities and other purposes of the test, such as growth potential determination, are reviewed.

Imaging: Bone Densitometry

Bone Mineral Density Testing: Incorporating BMD into Your Practice ○ ○ ○
http://www.bonemeasurement.com//hcp/bmd_testing/incorporate_practice.html

Details on consideration of a baseline BMD measurement, the importance of early diagnosis, bone mass measurements and technologies, and answers to frequently asked questions by healthcare professionals are examined at the site. Details on interpreting reports from various BMD technologies and manufacturers are provided and accompanied by tables on T-score interpretations. Other information on device selection and incorporating BMD into a professional practice is found.

Imaginis: Diagnosis of Osteoporosis with Bone Mineral Density Measurement ○ ○
http://www.imaginis.net/osteoporosis/osteo_diagnose.asp

Overviews of dual energy X-ray absorptiometry, ultrasound methods, and other bone mineral density test types are presented at the site. Accuracy of the tests, patients recommended for bone mineral density measurements, Medicare guidelines for bone densitometry, and concise information on T-score and Z-score results, established by the World Health Organization, are presented.

Major Bone Mass Measurement Techniques ○ ○
http://www.osteovision.ch/slides/28.html

A listing and discussion of several techniques for the measurement of bone mass are found at this site, with a brief overview of differences in applications and precision. By advancing to further slides, visitors will find in-depth information on dual energy X-ray absorptiometry, important indications for bone mass measurements, and expression of bone mineral density.

Stanford University: Bone Mineral Density Applet ○ ○ ○
http://www-stat-class.stanford.edu/pediatric-bones

Gender- and ethnic-specific curves for bone mineral density, obtained from normative data, may be displayed at the site, with methods of calculation explained and a description of the included sample provided. Directions for deriving standard deviation scores for areal and volumetric bone mineral density with use of the applet are found.

Imaging: Bone Scan

Brooke Army Medical Center:
Bone Imaging: Metabolic Bone Disease ○ ○
http://www.nmc.dote.hu/williams/NucMed/BONE09.HTM

A bone scan for the purpose of detecting advanced disease in hyperparathyroidism is reviewed at this site of the Brooke Army Medical Center. Diffusely increased skeletal activity in secondary hyperparathyroidism and osteomalacia is briefly discussed, and diffusely increased osseous activity in hyperthyroidism and various observations in different stages of Paget's disease are reviewed. Illustrated case reports of Paget's disease and osseous sarcoidosis are available from the site.

Imaging: Parathyroid Gland

EndocrineWeb: Preoperative Localization of Parathyroid Tumors ○ ○
http://www.endocrineweb.com/localization.html

The preferred method for identifying diseased parathyroid tissue when necessary and information on additional imaging modalities are presented at this site of the EndocrineWeb database. Links to detailed technical information on sestamibi scanning, a 3-D reconstructed SPECT scan video, and pages on CT scans and ultrasound for parathyroid imaging are available.

EndocrineWeb: Sestamibi Scanning Technical Details ○ ○ ○
http://www.endocrineweb.com/howsesta.html

The procedural aims of sestamibi scanning for parathyroid disease are summarized at this page of EndocrineWeb's disorders and surgery Web site. Details on this localizing and functional study, examination time, patient preparation, and radiopharmaceutical dose and technique of administration are outlined. Critical information on patient position, image field, and views is offered. Acquisition protocol and delayed images and performance of SPECT imaging are presented. Additional pages and images of

SPECT scans are accessible, as is information on other imaging modalities for detection of hyperactive parathyroids.

EndocrineWeb: Tests for Parathyroid Localization ○

http://www.endocrineweb.com/MRICAT.html

Tests for localization of parathyroid tumors are briefly discussed at the page and include use of the CT scan, MRI, and ultrasound under occasional circumstances. In-depth review of the preferred, preoperative sestamibi scan is available from a direct connection at this site.

Parathyroid Scan ○

http://www.derriford.co.uk/nucmed/leaflets/Specific/Parathyroid.htm

Information on a nuclear medicine parathyroid scan is found at this outpatient leaflet, especially useful for consumer reference. Questions and answers are provided regarding the test's purpose, its safety, preparation requirements, side effects, and procedures used. General information on nuclear medicine scans in children and adults is accessible at the appropriate link.

University of California Los Angeles:
Nuclear Medicine Protocols: Parathyroid Imaging ○ ○

http://laxmi.nuc.ucla.edu:8000/NM-Mediabook/protocols/parathy2.html

The sestamibi protocol for parathyroid scanning is outlined in detail at the page, with sections included on patient preparation, radiopharmaceutical and dose factors, acquisition parameters, and appropriate technique.

Parathyroid Screening

HealthGate: Parathyroid Hormone (Parathormone; PTH) ○

http://www.healthgate.com/tests/test77.shtml

From HealthGate, this site gives a profile of blood parathyroid hormone, a blood test used in the evaluation of suspected parathyroid disease. The profile gives an estimated cost of the test, patient time for the test, and result reliability. Information about the test includes a discussion of sensory factors, equipment used, and testing procedures. Additional details about preparation, post-test care, and result interpretation are found.

National Institutes of Health (NIH): Consensus Development
Conference Statement: Hyperparathyroidism ○ ○

http://isis.nlm.nih.gov/nih/cdc/www/82txt.html

The manuscript at this page addresses panel findings for hyperparathyroidism diagnosis, as well as the relationship between diagnosis in an asymptomatic patient and further management. The full text of the consensus panel includes discussion of the most accurate and cost-effective method of diagnosing hyperparathyroidism, with total serum calcium and other pertinent data derived from multiphasic screening results.

7.9 Energy Metabolism

Diabetes: General Resources

American Diabetes Association (ADA): Clinical Practice Recommendations 2000: Tests of Glycemia in Diabetes ○ ○ ○

http://journal.diabetes.org/FullText/Supplements/DiabetesCare/Supplement100/s80.htm

This position statement from the American Diabetes Association offers a professional overview of proper monitoring of glycemic status in patients with diabetes. Recommendations are provided for blood glucose testing by patients, blood glucose testing by healthcare providers for routine outpatient management of diabetes, urine testing, and glycated protein testing. Reference citations are provided.

Diabetes Mellitus: Understanding Laboratory Tests ○ ○

http://www.well-net.com/diabetes/dmunderstandinglabtests-1.html

Laboratory tests determining high blood glucose levels are reviewed at the site, including serum glucose monitoring and urine glucose monitoring. A brief discussion of those at risk for diabetes and outlines of the diagnoses based on the oral glucose tolerance test, random plasma glucose test, and fasting plasma glucose test are found.

HeliosHealth.com: Diabetes Type 2, Diagnosis ○ ○

http://www.helioshealth.com/diabetes/diagnosis.html

Simple explanations of blood tests used to diagnose diabetes are outlined at the site, for convenient consumer reference.

NIDDK: National Diabetes Clearinghouse: Diabetes Diagnosis ○ ○

http://www.niddk.nih.gov/health/diabetes/pubs/diagnosis/diagnosis.htm

An overview of diagnostic criteria for type 1 and type 2 diabetes is provided mainly for consumers and patients at this address, including information on new glucose levels criteria and risk factors for diabetes. The site also provides a link to the Combined Health Information Database (CHID) for additional resources.

Ray Williams Institute of Paediatric Endocrinology: Diagnostic Criteria for Diabetes in Childhood and Adolescence ◎ ◎
http://www.rwi.nch.edu.au/apegbook/diabnew2.htm#E9E2

The basis for diagnostic criteria of the World Health Organization study group on diabetes mellitus is outlined at this Web page, with indications for the oral glucose tolerance test and interpretation criteria. By accessing the table of contents, visitors may view an assortment of topic chapters on diagnosis and management.

Diabetes: Glucose

Lexi-Comp Clinical Reference Library: Glucose, Random ◎ ◎
http://informatics.drake.edu/pth/html/chapter/mono/ch011400.htm

Specimen details, reference ranges, possible abnormal results, and use of the random glucose test are referenced at this page. Establishment of uniform quality control procedures, evaluation of glycated hemoglobin and self-monitoring, and other related topics are briefly discussed.

Mediconsult.com: Random Plasma Glucose ◎
http://216.94.120.154/mc/mcsite.nsf/conditionnav/
diabetes~treatment~basics~diagnostic~randomplasma

A concise description of the test and purpose of random plasma glucose screening is found at this site of Mediconsult.com. The diagnostic testing link leads visitors to additional physician-ordered diagnostic tests.

Diabetes: Glucose, Fasting

HealthGate: Fasting Plasma Glucose ◎ ◎
http://www.healthgate.com/tests/test159.shtml

HealthGate's testing profiles include this page on fasting plasma glucose purposes, risks and precautions, and other test details. Post-test care, normal value range, and indications of high and low blood sugar levels are reviewed.

Lexi-Comp Clinical Reference Library: Glucose, Fasting ◎ ◎ ◎
http://informatics.drake.edu/lth/html/chapter/mono/ch011300.htm

This test book chapter contains details on the use of the fasting glucose test, including its purpose, patient preparation details, and standard reference ranges. A discussion of test limitations cautions readers that certain diagnoses may be missed and presents other details on misleading test results. Testing methodology, causes of high glucose, dangers of hypoglycemia, and three major hypoglycemic categories are reviewed.

Additional clinical details on the use of the test in infants and children are presented. Links at the top of the document lead visitors to related testing information.

Diabetes: Glycated Hemoglobin

Diabetes Care: Biological Variation of Glycated Hemoglobin ◎ ◎ ◎
http://www.diabetes.org/diabetescare/1998-02/PG261.htm

The implications of biological variation of glycated hemoglobin for diabetes screening is reviewed at this page of the online *Diabetes Care* publication. The evaluation discusses the potential use of glycated hemoglobin as a screening tool for type 2 diabetes. The importance of the tool in the assessment of glycemic control is reviewed.

Interpreting Glycated Hemoglobin Levels ◎
http://hiru.mcmaster.ca/dem/docs/patient/9000007.htm

This journal adaptation provides clinicians with information on the clinical application of glycated hemoglobin levels, including diabetes mellitus diagnosis and self-monitoring. A table at the site designates high levels and target range.

Lexi-Comp Clinical Reference Library: Glycated Hemoglobin ◎ ◎
http://informatics.drake.edu/lth/html/chapter/mono/ch011700.htm

Overall, consistent glycemic control can be measured with glycated hemoglobin testing, which is fully reviewed at this test book chapter. Reference range, critical values, limitations of glycated hemoglobin levels, and methodology are reviewed. Possible causes of misleading low and high levels are mentioned.

Diabetes: Insulin C-Peptide

HealthCentral: Insulin C-Peptide ◎
http://www.healthcentral.com/peds/top/003701.cfm

Details on performing C-peptide testing in adults and children are provided at this site of the HealthCentral database. Test preparation, normal values, and purpose and abnormal result meanings are displayed.

Diabetes: Ketones

Ketone Site: What Every Healthcare Professional Should Know ◎ ◎
http://www.statsite.com/ketofaq.htm

A discussion on ketone testing and its importance as a measure of metabolic control is found at this Web page, with a distinction made between urinary and blood ketone testing. Specific information on beta-hydroxybutyrate to accurately monitor ketosis and developing ketoacidosis is provided. Beta-hydroxybutyrate versus traditional dipstick acetoacetate testing is compared.

Lexi-Comp Clinical Reference Library: Ketone Bodies, Blood ◐ ◐
http://informatics.drake.edu/pth/html/chapter/mono/ch013300.htm
Collection methods, a range indicating severe ketosis, and test uses are listed, including ketoacidosis resulting from diabetes mellitus, starvation, glycogen storage diseases, infantile organic acidemias, and additional metabolic disorders. Testing limitations, such as false negatives and false positives, are discussed, and additional information about specific indications of test results is provided.

Diabetes: Oral Glucose Tolerance Test

Broomfield Hospital:
Glucose Tolerance Testing Diagnostic Criteria ◐
http://www.broombio.demon.co.uk/guidelines/glucosetolerance.html
Diagnostic criteria for diabetes mellitus with glucose tolerance testing is found at the site, with indications for the procedure outlined. Uses for modified glucose tolerance testing are listed.

HealthGate: Oral Glucose Tolerance Test (OGTT) ◐ ◐
http://www.healthgate.com/tests/test240.shtml
General information on the oral glucose tolerance test is provided at the site, with preprocedural recommendations, details about what to expect, and immediate post-test care. Test result interpretation facts, drugs that may affect results, and other factors to consider before performing the test are listed.

Diabetes: Stimulation Testing

Canterbury Health: Insulin Tolerance Test (ITT) ◐ ◐
http://www.chl.govt.nz/chlabs/endo/insutole.htm
A consumer information brochure at the site describes the aims of the test and the normal hormonal response to the test. Procedure for insulin administration, test safety and risks, and a summary of what to expect are included.

HealthGate: Insulin Tolerance Test ◐
http://www.healthgate.com/tests/test202.shtml
From HealthGate, this site offers a profile of insulin tolerance, a blood test that confirms diagnosis of several disorders, including growth-hormone deficiency, an-

drenocorticotropic-hormone deficiency, primary and secondary adrenal insufficiency, and pituitary impairments. The profile offers information about pre-testing procedures, the test itself, follow-up care, and reading the results.

Diabetes: Urinalysis

Complete Guide to Medical Tests: Abnormal Findings of Routine Urinalysis ◎ ◎

http://life-and-love.icq.thriveonline.oxygen.com/medical/library/article/003579res.html

Thriveonline presents an appendix of the *Complete Guide to Medical Tests,* which depicts several commonly observed and microscopic findings of the urinalysis and what each particular finding may indicate. Specific gravity, appearance and odor, pH, proteins and sugars, ketones, and blood cells in the urine suggest a variety of disease states, including inborn metabolism errors, kidney disease, and diabetes.

Internet Pathology Laboratory: Urinalysis ◎ ◎ ◎

http://www-medlib.med.utah.edu/WebPath/TUTORIAL/URINE/URINE.html

Macroscopic and microscopic urinalysis are reviewed at this site of the University of Utah. Information is provided on direct measures of observation, urine dipstick chemical analysis, and the methodology and examination of a microscopic sample. Links to images of the presence of red blood cells in the urine, pyuria, and oval fat bodies are found, as well as microscopic viewing of a variety of cast types and urine crystal formation. Methods of urine collection are presented.

Cholesterol and Lipoproteins

American Diabetes Association (ADA): Detection and Management of Lipid Disorders in Diabetes ◎ ◎ ◎

http://www.diabetes.org/diabetescare/Supplement/s96.htm

A consensus statement for the testing and management of lipoprotein risk factors associated with diabetes mellitus is found at this publication, courtesy of the American Diabetes Association. The report answers questions regarding the relationship between lipid levels and cardiovascular disease in diabetes mellitus, the goals of antilipemic and other therapies for lipid disorders in diabetes, and future research directions.

Baylor College of Medicine Lipid Laboratory: Test Profiles ◎ ◎

http://www.bcm.tmc.edu/medicine/athero/LipidLab/profiles.html

Among the leaders in preventive, predictive, and diagnostic testing, this clinical laboratory provides a listing of its 20 lipoprotein test profiles, with each synopsis offering alternative test names, specimen collection, methodology, and expected values.

HealthGate: Phospholipids Test ○
http://www.healthgate.com/tests/test256.shtml

Part of HealthGate, this site contains a profile of phospholipids, a blood test that helps evaluate fat metabolism and confirm the diagnosis of hypothyroidism, diabetes mellitus, nephrotic syndrome, pancreatitis, jaundice, and hypolipoproteinemia. The profile provides information about patient preparation, the test itself, post-test care, and results.

HealthGate: Total Cholesterol Test ○
http://www.healthgate.com/tests/test338.shtml

Maintained by HealthGate, this site offers information about total cholesterol, a blood test that helps determine the risk of heart disease, evaluates fat metabolism, and confirms the diagnosis of nephrotic syndrome, pancreatitis, liver disease, hyperthyroidism, and hypothyroidism. The profile includes information about patient preparation, the test itself, post-test care, and interpreting the results.

Metabolic Impairment Testing, General

British Inherited Metabolic Diseases Group Homepage and U.K. Directory ○ ○ ○
http://www.ssiem.org.uk/bimdg.html

A comprehensive index of diseases, metabolites, and enzymes is presented at this directory to laboratories, offering a reference for listings of specific metabolic assays; assays for carbohydrate, amino acid, and organic acid disorders; enzyme assays for lysosomal storage disorders; tests for mitochondrial disorders; porphyrins and haem; and a host of additional metabolic disease tests. By clicking on the link to tests required, visitors are given alphabetical assay listings and an Online Mendelian Inheritance in Man (OMIM) link, which provides literature on the particular deficiency.

Case Western Reserve University Center for Inherited Disorders of Energy Metabolism (CIDEM): General Test Information ○ ○ ○
http://www.cwru.edu/med/CIDEM/assaygen.htm

From Case Western Reserve University, this site offers information about tests of various categories and their clinical applications in diagnosing mitochondrial metabolism disorders. The CIDEM testing laboratories offer information on metabolites in body fluids, enzyme assays, mitochondrial oxidative phosphorylation, and mitochondrial DNA and other mutational analyses. Specific tests are listed and described under each category.

Inter Science Institute: Pediatric and Enzyme Deficiency Tests ◎ ◎
http://www.interscilsa.com/ped.html

This site offers profiles of pediatric and enzyme deficiency tests. Profiles are included for the following: 21a-hydroxylase deficiency, 11b-hydroxylase deficiency; 3b-hydroxysteroid dehydrogenase deficiency; 17a-hydroxylase deficiency; 17, 20 desmolase deficiency; 5a-reductase deficiency; aromatase deficiency; 18-hydroxylase deficiency; and 20, 22 desmolase deficiency.

Lexi-Comp Clinical Reference Library: Phenylalanine, Blood ◎ ◎
http://informatics.drake.edu/lth/html/chapter/mono/ch016900.htm#ch016900

A description of the phenylalanine blood test, its purpose, and patient preparation are described at this online fact sheet. Reference range, possible panic range, and the possibility of false negative results are reviewed. An in-depth discussion of the importance of successful detection of phenylketonuria (PKU) is found, with a review of classical PKU and its variants.

Metabolic Screening and Biochemical Genetics ◎ ◎ ◎
http://www.rch.unimelb.edu.au/biochem/metsamps.htm#umet

This index of metabolic disorder tests allows individuals to go directly to any of nearly 40 blood and urine screens. Amino acid analysis, carnitine screening, lysosomal enzyme testing, mucopolysaccharide screen, and fatty acid analyses are but a handful of the tests accessible. Included are descriptions of their purposes, special considerations with regard to results, and specimen collection information.

Royal Children's Hospital Division of Laboratory Services: Metabolic Disorders and Tests for Their Investigation ◎ ◎
http://www.rch.unimelb.edu.au/biochem/metcond.htm

A listing of metabolic disorders and tests for their investigation is found at this site, with links to the appropriate tests found within each disorder paragraph. Purposes of specific metabolic tests accessed and sample collection information are provided.

Royal Children's Hospital: Introduction to Metabolic Testing ◎ ◎ ◎
http://www.rch.unimelb.edu.au/biochem/metinfo2.htm

Visitors to this Web address will find an in-depth article that provides a review of the vast array of inborn errors of metabolism. Information on enzymes and biochemical pathways, metabolic testing procedures, the urine metabolic screen, and amino acid and organic acid measurement is provided. Discussion of specialized methods of accurately determining concentrations and implications in treatment are found.

Metabolic Testing: Amino Acid Analysis

Great Smokies Diagnostic Laboratory: Amino Acid Analysis
http://www.gsdl.com/assessments/aminoacids/index.html

A description of amino acid analysis at this laboratory is provided, with explanation of its use in diagnosis of nutritional deficits, metabolic impairments, and amino acid transport disorders. The application guide offers a four-page article on dietary protein metabolism. Frequently asked questions on solving diagnostic mysteries in amino acid analysis and healthy body chemistry are answered, and an amino acid analysis sample report is accessible.

Lexi-Comp Clinical Reference Library: Amino Acid Screen, Plasma
http://informatics.drake.edu/lth/html/chapter/mono/ch001600.htm#ch001600

The plasma screen for amino acids is described at this fact sheet, which provides a synopsis of the test's purpose, patient preparation, limitations, and methodology. Special considerations with regard to testing time, specific details on cystinuria and other diseases, and a table outlining the relevant enzymes, clinical findings, and laboratory findings of several congenital disorders of amino acid metabolism are found.

Lexi-Comp Clinical Reference Library: Amino Acid Screen, Qualitative, Urine
http://informatics.drake.edu/lth/html/chapter/mono/ch001650.htm

Commonly included amino acids, a brief discussion of urinary amino acid excretion in metabolic diseases, and patient preparation details are reviewed.

Metabolic Testing: Carnitine Analysis

Case Western Reserve University Center for Inherited Disorders of Energy Metabolism (CIDEM): Carnitine Analysis
http://www.cwru.edu/med/CIDEM/carninfo.htm

From Case Western Reserve University, this site offers information about carnitine screening and analysis. There is also information about the quantitative acylcarnitine urine profile and the quantitative acylcarnitine plasma or tissue profile. Diagrams are provided.

Metabolic Testing: Magnetic Resonance Spectroscopy

University of California San Francisco: The Future of Magnetic Resonance Spectroscopy and Spectroscopic Imaging ○ ○ ○
http://www.sf.med.va.gov/mrs/PAPERS/Futrmrs.htm

From the magnetic resonance unit of the Department of Veterans Affairs Medical Center in San Francisco comes this article regarding the future of magnetic resonance spectroscopy (MRS), which allows for metabolic imaging. Problems still to overcome in its development and a discussion of the possible applications for these techniques in clinical research and diagnosis are reviewed, including tumor diagnosis, muscle metabolism, and tumor response therapy.

Metabolic Testing: Urine Organic Acid Analysis

Marquette General Health System: Organic Acids Screen, Urine ○
http://www.mgh.org/lab/CATALOG/TESTS/5065.HTM

Specimen information, testing method, and reference ranges for organic acids are concisely presented at this hospital laboratory Web site.

MetaMetrix: Organic Compounds in Urine Metabolic Profiling to Assess Functional Nutrient Deficiencies, Gut Dysbiosis, and Toxicity ○ ○ ○
http://metametrix.com/articles/artcl_uoa.htm

This article, excerpted from *Natural Medicine,* offers a thorough discussion of urinary organic acid analysis for metabolic profiling, as well as a quick reference guide to abnormal findings in urine organic acid tests. In-depth review of compounds contained in this profile is provided. Specific vitamin deficiency indicators and testing for compounds derived from dietary protein, fat, and carbohydrates are reviewed.

8. THERAPEUTIC PROCEDURES AND SURGERY

8.1 General Resources

About.com: Endocrine Surgery ◎ ◎ ◎
http://surgery.about.com/health/surgery/msubendocrine.htm

Various articles at this About.com subsite provide details regarding endocrine surgery generally, operations of the thyroid, postoperative treatment, and parathyroid protocols. Tumor localization techniques, minimally invasive procedures, surgical approaches to the adrenal gland, and details about pheochromocytoma are included article topics. Other articles include review of a technique for endoscopic pituitary tumor removal and the treatment of adrenal cancer by surgery.

Johns Hopkins Medical Institutions: Endocrine Surgery Web ◎ ◎
http://www.path.jhu.edu/endocrine

An overview of endocrine surgery, clinical and basic research currently being conducted, and an online chat for exchange of information are provided at this Johns Hopkins subsite.

Temple University School of Medicine: Principles of Endocrine Surgery ◎ ◎
http://blue.vm.temple.edu/~pathphys/surgery/endocrine_surgery.html

Types of endocrine surgery, an outline of hypersecretory endocrinopathies, and a disease example are summarized. Diagnosis, pathology, and surgical strategy for primary hyperparathyroidism are presented.

University of Michigan: Review of Endocrine Surgery ◎ ◎
http://www.med.umich.edu/lrc/coursepages/M3/surgery/EndocrineReview.html

Indications for surgery, diagnosis, and operation type are reviewed at the online table, which outlines benign and malignant thyroid disease, primary hyperparathyroidism, pituitary tumors, and tumors of the endocrine pancreas. The workup for diseases of the adrenal gland that require surgical intervention is reviewed.

8.2 Adrenal Glands

Adrenal Surgery: A Clinical Study on Incidentalomas, Aldosteronomas, and Laparoscopic Adrenalectomy ◎ ◎
http://ethesis.helsinki.fi/julkaisut/laa/kliin/vk/siren/sisallys.html

This academic dissertation from Helsinki University Central Hospital offers a review of the current literature describing adrenal surgery, followed by a thorough discussion of the investigation on which this dissertation was based. The paper describes patient demographics; retrospective, prospective, and follow-up studies; techniques and protocols; and results of the investigation. A discussion, conclusion, summary, and reference citations are also provided.

EndocrineWeb: Laparoscopic Adrenalectomy ◎ ◎
http://www.endocrineweb.com/laparo.html

EndocrineWeb's educational pages provide visitors with an in-depth look at this laparascopic approach to adrenal surgery. Details on this preferred operation are reviewed, providing a case example that is well-suited to a minimally invasive technique. Illustrations at the site provide close-up depictions of steps of the technique. Candidates for the laparoscopic method are defined.

EndocrineWeb: Surgical Approaches to the Adrenal Gland ◎ ◎
http://www.endocrineweb.com/adrsurg.html

Well-recognized surgical approaches to adrenal surgery are reviewed at this address, including standard trans-abdominal, thoraco-abdominal, and laparoscopic adrenalectomy methods. A discussion of the decision involved in choosing appropriate techniques and a link to a fully illustrated page on the laparoscopic method are found. Factors that determine which adrenal procedure will be performed are outlined.

8.3 Bone and Mineral Metabolism

Parathyroid Surgery

EndocrineWeb: Minimally Invasive Parathyroid Surgery ◎ ◎ ◎
http://www.endocrineweb.com/minimalpara.html

The technique known as minimally invasive radioguided parathyroidectomy (MIRP), which utilizes intraoperative nuclear mapping, is discussed at EndocrineWeb's endocrinology and surgery pages. Details on its introduction in 1996 are found, and more information from the surgeon who pioneered the operation may be accessed. EndocrineWeb provides a link directly from this site to a complete compilation of photos, which illustrate the MIRP procedure step-by-step. Numerous potential advantages to this alternative surgery and its potential candidates are discussed. Another useful link connects visitors to a flowchart outlining a popular approach to the preoperative workup for primary hyperparathyroidism. A separate page regarding scientific publications on radioguided minimally invasive parathyroidectomy is provided.

EndocrineWeb: Parathyroid Surgery: The Standard Technique ◎ ◎
http://www.endocrineweb.com/standardpara.html

The standard technique for parathyroid gland removal is reviewed at this address, and information on the standard bilateral neck exploration is summarized. An overview of the standard surgery concludes the article.

8.4 Diabetes Mellitus

Exercise Regimens

American Diabetes Association (ADA): Diabetes and Exercise ◎ ◎ ◎
http://www.diabetes.org/DiabetesCare/Supplement/s30.htm

The importance of physical activity as a key ingredient in diabetes management is stressed at this position statement of the American Diabetes Association. Separate discussions of exercise programs in type 1 and type 2 diabetes are found, emphasizing special precautions in type 1 and exercise as adjunct therapy for glycemic control improvement in type 2.

American Diabetes Association (ADA): Exercise: Just the FAQs ⊙ ⊙ ⊙

http://www.diabetes.org/exercise

An exercise profile of the month offers stories on personally tailored exercise routines for diabetics, and FAQs about exercise also provide general information regarding the importance of exercise for people with diabetes. A diabetes exercise quiz and the opportunity to order the American Diabetes Association publication, *The Fitness Book,* are found. Additional exercise information is offered in the form of fact sheets, related *Diabetes Forecast* articles, and details on the Tour de Cure and America's Walk for Diabetes.

Barbara Davis Center for Childhood Diabetes: Exercise and Diabetes ⊙ ⊙

http://www.uchsc.edu/misc/diabetes/chap12.html

Maintained by the Barbara Davis Center for Childhood Diabetes, this site contains a chapter on exercise and diabetes. Discussions are included on the importance of exercise in diabetics, managing exercise in people with diabetes, choosing an exercise program, and nutrition with exercise.

Diabetic Gourmet: Gestational Diabetes and Exercise ⊙

http://diabeticgourmet.com/articles/00articles/17.shtml

An article from an online diabetes magazine offers consumers information on daily exercise programs in pregnancy. Information on warm-ups and target heart rates is found, as well as precautions for patients taking insulin during pregnancy. Special information on insulin administration where diet and exercise fail to control blood sugar levels is offered.

Physician and Sportsmedicine: Exercise for Osteoporosis ⊙ ⊙

http://www.physsportsmed.com/issues/1998/02feb/katzpa.htm

The article, authored by a professor at the University of Pennsylvania, functions as a recommendation guide for exercise therapy, with information on weight-bearing exercise, resistance training, and other essentials of exercise therapy for patients with osteoporosis.

Gene Therapy

Gene Therapy Approaches for Diabetes and its Complications ⊙ ⊙

http://www.niddk.nih.gov/fund/reports/gene_therapy_summ.htm

This report of the NIDDK summarizes preliminary results of new technology surrounding gene therapy approaches, as recently researched by investigators. Topics for a previously held scientific session are reviewed and include progress in the areas of gene therapy approaches for expressing Insulin, for immunomodulation, for cell-based therapies, and for complications. A summary of recommendations for developing new therapeutic strategies is provided.

McGill University: Gene Could Lead to New Therapy for Diabetes ◐ ◐
http://www.mcgill.ca/media/releases/1999/march/diabetes

Identification of a gene that could lead to new therapies for type 2 diabetes and obesity is the focus of this McGill University media release. Review of a recently published article on cell sensitivity to insulin from the *American Journal of Science* and information on a gene that may lead to a decline in insulin's ability to regulate glucose levels are examined.

Glucose Self-Monitoring

American Diabetes Association (ADA): Self-Monitoring of Blood Glucose ◐ ◐ ◐
http://www.diabetes.org/diabetescare/Supplement/s62.htm

A *Diabetes Care* supplement found at this page contains a review of the American Diabetes Association Consensus Conference on dealing with issues surrounding self-monitoring. A discussion of the epidemiology of self-monitoring, future research goals, potential indications for self-monitoring, and review of the current technology and system limitations are provided.

International Diabetes Federation: Guidelines to Type 1 Diabetes: Self-Monitoring of Blood Glucose ◐ ◐
http://www.diabetesguidelines.com/health/dwk/pro/guidelines/type1/3_3.htm

Use and assessment of self-monitoring and achieving effective self-monitoring are outlined at this page of the European Diabetes Policy Group. The guidelines emphasize evaluation of self-test results, regular assessment of skills, appropriate training and technique review, and regular result recording. Patterns of testing, according to need, are listed.

Words in a Row: Diabetes Control and Complications Trial (DCCT) ◐ ◐
http://www.wordsinarow.com/chapter1.html

An overview of the importance of aggressive, long-term blood glucose management, as concluded from the results of the Diabetes Control and Complications Trial (DCCT), is presented at this page. Those patients that received intensive diabetes education and checked their blood glucose levels four or more times per day, adjusting insulin dosages accordingly, avoided diabetic complications far more often than those not in the intensely managed group. Additional details of the study and further details on the benefits of self-monitoring are summarized.

Neuropathy

Current and Future Therapies of Diabetic Neuropathy
http://www.uspharmacist.com/NewLook/DisplayArticle.cfm?item_num=145

From U. S. Pharmacist, this site contains an article on current and future therapies in neuropathy. Included are a general overview and sections on pathophysiology, strict glycemic control, autonomic neuropathy, sensory motor neuropathy, and diabetic neuropathic foot ulceration. References are provided.

Nutritional Interventions

American Diabetes Association (ADA): Dietary Recommendations for Persons with Diabetes
http://www.hry.info.gifu-u.ac.jp/~diabetes/dietary/mtable2.html

Dietary recommendations from the American Diabetes Association are reviewed in table format at this site, including information on specific nutrients, sugar substitutes, sodium, and alcohol.

American Diabetes Association (ADA): Nutrition Recommendations and Principles for Diabetes Mellitus
http://www.diabetes.org/DiabetesCare/Supplement197/s14.htm

These clinical practice recommendations of the American Diabetes Association review medical nutritional therapy as an integral part of total diabetes management. Goals of medical nutrition therapy, nutrition therapy in both type 1 and type 2 diabetes, protein and other nutrient requirements, and special considerations with regard to micronutrients, alcohol, sodium, fiber, and nonnutritive sweeteners are discussed. Also included are historical perspectives of nutrition recommendations and nutrition recommendations specific to pregnant diabetics.

Dietary Management of Diabetes Working Group
http://www.clininfo.health.nsw.gov.au/NSWhealth/NSWHEALTH1/nwgroup.htm

Medical professionals from prominent endocrinology divisions have collaborated to present this *Principles of Lifestyle and Nutritional Management of Diabetes* document. By clicking on the contents links, visitors are taken to a listing of six principles of dietary and other lifestyle management techniques and a link to additional useful resources for diabetic patients. Small, regular meals; consistent physical activity; fat intake reduction; smoking control; and other recommendations of the group may be viewed. Each discussion includes the physiological benefits of applying the principle and adds practical advice for instituting each suggestion.

Dietary Management of Individuals with Metabolic Disorders: Mead Johnson Special Metabolic Diets ◎ ◎ ◎
http://www.meadjohnson.com/metabolics/metabolichandbook.html

As a service of Mead Johnson products, this Web site contains information on diets specifically limited in various offending nutrients for those with metabolic disease. Access to information on these supplements provides useful details on the patient's requirements for growth and development. Descriptions of special metabolic diets and nutritional/metabolic modules, a metabolic centers directory, and clinical articles on the special dietary requirements of patients with urea cycle disorders, galactosemia, maple syrup urine disease, hereditary tyrosinemia, and other metabolic disorders are accessible. Dietary management tips are offered at a special page, as a service of New York University Metabolic Disease Center.

NIDDK: I Have Diabetes: What Should I Eat? ◎ ◎ ◎
http://www.niddk.nih.gov/health/diabetes/pubs/nutritn/what/index.htm

This site contains a patient education pamphlet for newly diagnosed patients, offering nutritional guidelines and details on maintaining good eating habits. An overview of diabetic control through healthy eating and sections on food groups and the food pyramid are found.

Treating Diabetes with Good Nutrition: Dietary Guidelines ◎ ◎
http://www.cyberdiet.com/modules/diabetes/outline.html

Dietary guidelines to include in an overall treatment regimen for diabetes are reviewed at this Mediconsult article, which speaks specifically about lowering the glycemic effect of all foods. Attention to consumption of carbohydrates, insulin activity and blood sugar control, suggestions for keeping carbohydrate absorption gradual, and consumption of legumes in conjunction with carbohydrate-rich foods are discussed.

Retinopathy

Diabetic Retinopathy Foundation: Treatment of Retinopathy ◎ ◎
http://www.retinopathy.org/info04.htm

This site offers consumer-oriented discussions of treatments for early and advanced stages of retinopathy. Prevention of retinopathy through glucose control is also discussed, and links are available to explanations of several terms. Illustrations depicting focal and pan-retinal laser photocoagulation are also provided.

Technological Developments in Insulin Delivery

Diabetes Monitor: Devices for Glucose Monitoring
http://www.diabetesmonitor.com/other-3a.htm

Links to information on blood glucose meters are found at this site and include a wide variety of monitoring system and product Web sites. Connections are available to sites offering new noninvasive and minimally invasive monitoring instruments that may eliminate lancets. Other sites and software to enable diabetics to monitor blood sugar readings and maintain overall control are provided.

Insulin Pumpers
http://www.insulin-pumpers.org

This organization Web site provides support and educational materials to diabetics of all ages interested in insulin pump therapy. This site provides answers to frequently asked questions about insulin pumps, instructional information on how to use insulin pumps, a printable diabetes log book, a directory of physicians who prescribe insulin pumps, and chat forums. Links are provided to the home pages of several insulin pump manufacturers, information on carbohydrate content of various foods, and additional information on diabetes and insulin pumps.

NIDDK: Devices for Taking Insulin
http://www.niddk.nih.gov/health/diabetes/summary/altins/altins.htm

Courtesy of the NIDDK, this article offers information on devices for taking insulin, including insulin pens, insulin jet injectors, external insulin pumps, implantable insulin pumps, insulin patches, and the inhaled insulin delivery system. Contact information for additional resources is found.

NIDDK: Noninvasive Blood Glucose Monitors
http://www.niddk.nih.gov/health/diabetes/summary/noninmet/noninmet.htm

From the National Institute of Diabetes and Digestive and Kidney Diseases, this site contains an article on noninvasive blood glucose monitors. The article discusses FDA inspection and lists some noninvasive techniques being studied.

On-line Diabetes Resources: Meters
http://www.cruzio.com/~mendosa/meters.htm

This site contains a list of more than 20 providers of glucose monitoring systems. For each manufacturer, a concise description is presented of the system offered, including explanations of calibration and the technology utilized. A Web link is provided for each manufacturer, and links to informative articles and other related resources are also available.

Ray Williams Institute of Paediatric Endocrinology: Devices for Insulin Delivery ○ ○
http://www.rwi.nch.edu.au/apegbook/diabne33.htm#E9E33

Descriptions of insulin syringe types, insulin pen information, automatic injection devices, and jet injectors and pumps are concisely reviewed at the site. Illustrations of each are shown, including an automatic injector that is especially useful for pediatric patients.

UTHealth.com: Devices to Take Insulin ○ ○ ○
http://www.citihealth.com/layout.cfm?hc=0&Body=Articles/00003754

Currently available insulin administration devices are discussed at this site, including insulin pens, insulin jet injectors, and external insulin pumps. Insulin methods of delivery currently under development are mentioned, such as implantable insulin pumps and the continuous administration of the insulin patch. Visitors may view the results of updated information of the Combined Health Information Database to discover the latest information on alternative methods of insulin delivery.

Transplantation: General Resources

American Society of Transplant Physicians (ASTP) ○
http://www.a-s-t.org/index.htm

This professional society serves physicians and scientists and promotes research, patient care, advocacy, and education. Information concerning bylaws, CME, meetings, ethics, officers, membership, job postings, publications, and certification is provided. A restricted section for members provides committee reports, slide lectures, a newsletter, CME transcripts, and a member directory. Preregistration for meetings is also possible via the site.

American Society of Transplant Surgeons (ASTS) ○ ○
http://www.asts.org

The American Society of Transplant Surgeons exists to promote education and research related to organ and tissue transplantation. This site contains the bylaws of the organization and information on membership, training programs, annual meetings, awards, and fellowships. Sections describing public policy activities and ethics are also available.

Insulin-Free World Foundation: Articles About Immunology ○ ○ ○
http://www.insulinfree.org/articimm.htm

From the Insulin-Free World Foundation, this site lists articles related to immunology. There are more than 40 articles related to immune regulation, endothelium, transcription, immune responses, receptor families, graft rejection, gene therapy, and other topics.

TransWeb ◎ ◎ ◎
http://www.transweb.org

TransWeb offers information about transplantation and donation. The site offers profiles of recipients and candidates. There are answers to questions about transplantation and donation, as well as a quiz revealing myths and a multimedia guide to the transplant process. A reference desk offers links to transplant centers around the world as well as connections to articles, books, journals, magazines, publications, educational sites, organizations, government agencies, and registries.

Transplantation: Biological Specimens

American Association of Tissue Banks ◎ ◎
http://www.aatb.org

The American Association of Tissue Banks was founded to aid the availability of transplantable human tissues. Its site offers information about the organization, a fact page on organ and tissue donations, and answers to frequently asked questions. Information is provided about accreditation, personnel certification, training courses, and annual meetings. A list of accredited tissue banks is also available.

Transplantation: Pancreas and Islet Cell Transplantation

Insulin-Free World Foundation ◎ ◎ ◎
http://www.insulinfree.org

Information about the current state of pancreas and islet cell transplantation is the focus of the Insulin-Free World Foundation. Visitors will find islet trial details, articles about pancreas transplantation, and a directory of pancreas transplant centers. Helpful contact information for transplant candidates, scientific abstracts, and facts and statistics about islet transplants are all provided. Sections dedicated to engineered cells and xenotransplantation, related immunology information, and an islet trials registration and update service are additionally accessible at this site dedicated to providing up-to-date research and details on curing diabetes.

International Islet Transplant Registry ◎ ◎
http://www.med.uni-giessen.de/itr

The International Islet Transplant Registry is based at the Faculty of Medicine of the University of Giessen, Germany, and functions as a repository for data collection and computer entry on islet auto-, allo-, and xenotransplants performed worldwide. Their site offers scientific data analysis results in the form of archived newsletters. Links to news and additional publications, organ transplantation details, diabetes research, and other selected sources are provided.

International Pancreas and Islet Transplant Association (IPITA) ◎ ◎
http://www.jr2.ox.ac.uk/ipita

IPITA is dedicated to encouraging research, providing a forum for the exchange of relevant information, and promoting contacts between researchers. The site provides information about the association, including upcoming meetings, officers, constitution, and bylaws. Other resources include a discussion board, an e-mail list, and links to related sites.

Islet Foundation ◎ ◎ ◎
http://www.islet.org

The Islet Foundation is dedicated to finding a cure for diabetes. This home page offers a table of contents with articles on many aspects of diabetes and islet cell research, as well as information about upcoming and recent conferences, research news, clinical trials, and working groups. There are links to scientific articles and conference reports. There are also links to related sites, a message forum, and advocacy information.

NIDDK: Pancreatic Islet Transplantation ◎ ◎
http://www.niddk.nih.gov/health/diabetes/summary/pancisl/pancisl.htm

Maintained by the NIDDK, this site offers an article on pancreatic islet transplantation. There is information on obtaining enough viable islets and preventing rejection, as well as contact details for obtaining additional information.

8.5 Metabolic Disease

Gene Therapy

Journal of Gene Medicine Website ◎ ◎ ◎
http://www.wiley.co.uk/genetherapy

The *Journal of Gene Medicine* Web site provides access to the Wiley genetics information Web site, the new genomics community Web site, and up-to-date listings and information on clinical trials in gene therapy. Colorful pie charts illustrate protocols and patients by continent, and details on specific diseases addressed are found. Protocols on familial hypercholesterolemia, Gaucher's disease, mucopolysaccharidoses, purine metabolic disorders, and cancers are included. Some clinical result citations and abstracts may be accessed, in addition to current and archived journal abstracts.

National Institutes of Health (NIH): Pilot Studies on Gene Therapy Vectors for Metabolic Diseases ○ ○
http://research.uth.tmc.edu/PATEXT/par97002.htm

The National Institute of Diabetes and Digestive and Kidney Diseases presents the full description of a program to provide awards for research into the basic mechanisms and cellular activity involved in metabolic diseases. Eligibility requirements and a comprehensive discussion of the objectives of the program are provided.

University of Minnesota Gene Therapy Program ○ ○
http://www.peds.umn.edu/Centers/gene

The University of Minnesota Institute of Human Genetics offers details of its research and a link to news on a clinical trial of gene therapy for Hunter syndrome. Information on the Gene Therapy for Metabolic Disorders Program, access to the mucopolysaccharidosis (MPS) databases, details on gene therapy research staff, and related links on gene therapy are all accessible from this site.

University of Pennsylvania Health System: Institute for Human Gene Therapy ○ ○ ○
http://www.med.upenn.edu/ihgt/info/links1.html

The University of Pennsylvania Health System provides this excellent starting point for gene therapy research, including introductory information on advances in gene therapy and a guide to genomics in disease and therapy. Recent articles from *Scientific American*, an additional series of articles from the *Philadelphia Inquirer*, and surveys of progress and technique advancements in the field are available at this interesting assortment of connections. An additional section offers links to the related field of bioethics. Attention to specific diseases is found, as well as prominent publications that focus on genetic therapy innovations.

Stem Cell Transplantation

International Society for Mannosidosis and Related Diseases, Inc.: Bone Marrow Transplants ○ ○ ○
http://www.mannosidosis.org/bmtinfo.htm

This therapy for the alpha mannosidosis and the ogligosaccharide family of diseases is discussed, with links to transplant centers that have performed the procedure and connections to several transplantation resources and links. Connections include the Fairview Medical Center, which presents an interesting article on hematopoietic stem cell transplantation for storage diseases and offers a PDF version of the center's latest newsletter. Other research, clinical trials, and bone marrow transplant program information from Duke University Medical Center and the University of Connecticut is accessible from the site.

Stem Cell Transplantation Moves Front and Center ◎ ◎
http://www.bhpharmacy.com/Merchant/journal/journalarticles.html

Promising stem cell transplant therapy is the focus of this article, which reviews some high hopes that researchers have for this treatment. Attention to a study on recent stem cell transplantation in patients with osteogenesis imperfecta is found, and the ideas behind stem cell transplantation in this disease are summarized. Problems with autologous transplantation and hopes for homologous transplantation are presented.

8.6 Neuroendocrine System

Gene Therapy

Journal of Molecular Endocrinology: Gene Therapy Strategies for the Treatment of Pituitary Tumors ◎ ◎
http://journals.endocrinology.org/jme/022/jme0220009.htm

An article abstract discussing potential therapeutic nucleic acids and recent advances in the field is provided. The full text of this article, authored by clinicians at the University of Manchester, may be downloaded in PDF format for a comprehensive review of the evidence recently gained from clinical trials.

Pituitary Surgery

FAQs in Endocrinology: Surgery for Pituitary Adenomas ◎ ◎
http://members.xoom.com/_XMCM/endocrine/pitsurgery.htm

The diagnosis and management of pituitary adenomas are discussed at this site, including a detailed discussion of transphenoidal craniotomy.

Johns Hopkins Brain Tumor Radiosurgery: Pituitary Tumor ◎ ◎
http://www.med.jhu.edu/radiosurgery/trial/pit/nf_pit.html

Important options for pituitary surgery are briefly discussed at this Johns Hopkins Web site, and a connection to a pituitary adenoma online consultation is found. Discussions on microsurgical resection of pituitary adenomas, stereotactic radiosurgical technique, and a consultation data questionnaire to submit online are provided. A subscription to the *Johns Hopkins Brain Tumor Newsletter*, which provides coverage of new developments in pituitary adenomas, is available free of charge at the site.

London Radiosurgical Centre: Practice Guidelines: Pituitary Adenomas ◎ ◎

http://www.radiosurgery.co.uk/doc_pitu.htm

A discussion of current practice for pituitary adenoma surgery and radiotherapy is presented at the site, with practice guidelines accessible for PETscanning and radiosurgery, craniopharyngioma, and metastases. Data that demonstrate the efficacy of radiosurgery for pituitary adenomas, and studies that report the results of current radiosurgical techniques in Cushing's syndrome and acromegaly are presented. Results are reviewed, with evidence of a faster decline in secretory hormone with radiosurgery than with radiotherapy discussed, as well as the implications of this evidence.

Massachusetts General Hospital: History of Stereotactic Radiosurgery ◎ ◎

http://neurosurgery.mgh.harvard.edu/hist-pb.htm

Early experiences with pituitary radiosurgery and the evolution of treatment and imaging in proton radiosurgery are outlined at this site of Massachusetts General Hospital and Harvard University. The department provides further details on the principles and development of beam delivery and patient positioning.

Massachusetts General Hospital: Long-term Mortality and Morbidity after Transsphenoidal Surgery for Pituitary Adenomas ◎ ◎

http://neurosurgery.mgh.harvard.edu/e-s-961.htm

A review of the long-term morbidity and mortality of patients following transsphenoidal surgery is provided at this site of Massachusetts General Hospital and Harvard Medical School. Pathology and mortality by tumor type, major surgical complications, causes of death, and disability details are discussed and displayed via charts and figures. A link to the Pituitary Tumor Center homepage provides access to information on stereotactic proton radiosurgery and the center's research study details.

University of Pittsburgh: Endoscopic Transsphenoidal Pituitary Surgery ◎ ◎

http://www.neuronet.pitt.edu/groups/ctr-innov/endopit.htm

Facts about minimally invasive transsphenoidal pituitary surgery through a nostril for pituitary adenomas, prolactinomas, acromegaly, and Cushing's disease are presented at this site. The conventional versus the minimally invasive methods are discussed, favoring an endoscopic approach. Schematic drawings at the site demonstrate techniques of endoscopic pituitary therapy. Intraoperative endoscopic images are displayed in full color, in addition to preoperative and corresponding postoperative axial, coronal, and sagittal MRI images.

Radiotherapy

Radiotherapy.com ○ ○ ○
http://www.radiotherapy.com

More than 25 radiotherapy-related organization links may be accessed from this site, including the American College of Radiology and the American Society of Therapeutic Radiology and Oncology. The news page index at the site offers information on radiotherapy in cancer trials, as a service of the National Cancer Institute, and current review of androgen suppression methods in the treatment of advanced prostatic cancer. Several online journals related to radiotherapy are accessible from the site, in addition to an assortment of radiotherapy practice guidelines. Thyroid, head and neck, testis, and gynecological cancer clinical practice guidelines lists are available. A large listing of radiotherapy departmental links are provided, as well as a listing of related educational Internet sites.

8.7 Pancreas

CancerBACUP: Understanding Cancer of the Pancreas: Surgery ○ ○
http://www.bacup.org/info/pancreas.htm

A patient information brochure on surgical interventions in pancreatic cancer is found at the site. Sections of the document briefly review procedural and postprocedural considerations. Connections to further details on types of treatments used, radiotherapy, and chemotherapy are included.

OncoLink: Metastatic Insulin-secreting Carcinoma of the Pancreas: Clinical Course and the Role of Surgery ○ ○
http://www.oncolink.net/pdq_html/cites/00/00742.html

The role of surgical intervention in pancreatic, insulin-secreting carcinoma is reviewed at this abstract, courtesy of the University of Pennsylvania Cancer Center. Recurrence rate, median survival, and other details on this treatment of choice are summarized.

Surgical Experience with Pancreatic and Peripancreatic Neuroendocrine Tumors ○ ○
http://www.ssat.com/97ddw/ddw9.htm

A retrospective review of patient files with functioning and nonfunctioning tumors is presented in summary format at this site, with preoperative localization details, common operative procedures performed, and postoperative complications. Mortality rate and predictors of negative outcome for patients with malignancies, as well as overall morbidity and mortality of surgically treated patients are discussed.

8.8 Thyroid Gland

Antithyroid Agents

Family Practice Notebook.com: Antithyroid Drugs
http://www.fpnotebook.com/END94.htm

Indications and dosages of antithyroid drugs in Graves' disease and thyroid storm are outlined at the site. A listing of adverse events is included, and links to further information on aplastic anemia, thyrotoxicosis, and thyroid storm are found.

Radioactive Iodine

Family Practice Notebook.com: Thyroid Radioiodine
http://www.fpnotebook.com/END95.htm

Indications for radioactive iodine administration and additional details on efficacy and follow-up treatment are found at this site.

New York Thyroid Center:
Radioactive Iodine for Testing and Treatment
http://cpmcnet.columbia.edu/dept/thyroid/RAI.html

FAQs regarding radioactive iodine (RAI) administration for the treatment of various thyroid conditions are found at this electronic fact sheet. General instructions and information on what to expect for RAI scanning and additional radioactive iodine administration are presented. Outpatient RAI treatment, inpatient treatment, and details on a low iodine diet are presented. Measures to take to reduce unnecessary radiation exposure to other persons are listed.

Nucmednet Featured Procedure:
Treating Thyroid Disease with Radioactive Iodine
http://www.nucmednet.com/thyroid_therapy.htm

Treatment of diseased thyroid tissue with radioactive iodine is the focus of this Nucmednet article, which emphasizes precautions of the therapy and different dosages in the treatment of Graves' disease and toxic nodular goiter. The use of radioactive iodine in a total body scan following surgery in order to identify low levels of iodine concentrated by thyroid cancers is discussed. Treating remaining cancer with ablation, additional whole-body studies, and expected outcomes are reviewed.

University of California
Los Angeles: Radioiodine Ablative Therapy ◎ ◎
http://laxmi.nuc.ucla.edu:8000/NM-Mediabook/protocols/ablative.html

An outline of postoperative radioiodine ablative therapy protocols is presented at this site of the University of California Los Angeles, with sections included on indications, radiopharmaceutical and dosage factors, and dosage administration notes. A prior thyroid uptake scan, withholding of thyroid replacement medication, and other considerations in patient preparation of therapeutic sodium iodide administration are listed.

Thyroid Surgery

AACE Clinical Practice Guidelines
for the Management of Thyroid Carcinoma ◎ ◎ ◎
http://www.tsh.org/ptinfo/guidecan.html

Clinical guidelines for thyroid cancer management are provided as a service of the American Association of Clinical Endocrinologists and the American College of Endocrinology at this page. Evolved treatment strategies and management modalities used by the majority of the thyroid practice community are presented. A contemporary consensus and dissenting opinion are expressed in the document.

About.com: Types of Thyroidectomy ◎ ◎
http://surgery.about.com/health/surgery/library/weekly/aa020699.htm

About.com provides this article, which offers a brief account of the different types of thyroid procedures. General descriptions of total thyroidectomy, hemi-thyroidectomy, lobectomy, nodulectomy, and additional operations are found. Recommended Web site links are included.

Endocrine Search: Endoscopic Thyroidectomy ◎ ◎
http://www.endocrinesearch.com/images/endoscop1.htm

General information on this laparoscopic procedure is provided at the site, with an outline of proper patient selection and contraindications. Included links allow visitors to read details regarding technique and to view a list of references.

EndocrineWeb: Thyroid Operations ◎ ◎
http://www.endocrineweb.com/surthyroid.html

Surgical options for thyroid disease, depending on specific clinical problem, are reviewed at this EndocrineWeb site, which specializes in providing general, comprehensive information on endocrine disease and surgery. Reasons for choosing lobectomies, sub-total thyroidectomies, and total thyroidectomies are reviewed. Surgical technique, the relationship of the thyroid to the voice box and caution to be exercised, and the use of fine needle aspiration biopsy are presented. Potential complications, although rare, are reviewed.

ScienceDaily Magazine:
Surgical Experience Improves Thyroidectomy Outcome ◎ ◎
http://www.sciencedaily.com/releases/1998/10/981007154239.htm

Research updates from *ScienceDaily Magazine* include this release from Johns Hopkins Medical Institutions, which discusses the relationship of surgical experience to thyroidectomy outcomes. Objective, useful evidence for the advancement of clinical care is presented.

Thyroid Disease Manager: Surgery of the Thyroid Gland ◎ ◎ ◎
http://www.thyroidmanager.org/Chapter21/21-frame.htm

An up-to-date resource for thyroid disease management, this portion of the site offers surgical anatomy, indications for thyroidectomy, preoperative preparatory techniques, and surgical approaches to thyroidectomy. Complications of thyroidectomy, such as thyroid storm and wound hemorrhage, are addressed at this work, sponsored in part by a grant from the Nathan and Frances Goldblatt Society for Cancer Research.

Thyroid-Cancer.net ◎ ◎ ◎
http://www.thyroid-cancer.net

Provided as a service of the Johns Hopkins Thyroid Tumor Center, this page contains access to surgical treatment information for thyroid nodules and cancer. Specific clinical situations are addressed in terms of surgical outcome, other potential treatments, innovative techniques, and plenty of answers to Frequently Asked Questions.

University of Texas
M.D. Anderson Cancer Center: Your Care Path ◎ ◎
http://endocrine.mdacc.tmc.edu/educational/thyroidectomy.htm

An educational guide to thyroid cancer surgery is provided at this site and includes a procedural description, patient preparation, recovery, and home care. Risk factors and diagnostic tests prior to surgery to check for cancer spreading are reviewed.

Vesalius Clinical Folios: Thyroidectomy ◎ ◎ ◎
http://vesalius.com/graphics/cf_procedures/thy_ect/cfpr_thy_ect1.asp

The pages at Vesalius Clinical Folios use graphics accompanied by text to explain thyroidectomy procedures. Thumbnails provide listings of related images in the image archive and can be used as an index to the related narrative. An interactive presentation of anatomic layers using ShockWave or QuickTime technology is incorporated into the site, as well as a quiz that allows visitors to identify labeled structures using drag and drop icons.

9. PHARMACOLOGY

9.1 General Resources

About.com:
Hormones and Drugs Affecting the Endocrine System ◎ ◎ ◎
http://pharmacology.miningco.com/health/pharmacology/msubend.htm
A pharmacology guide from About.com provides consumer and professional reference to specific drug information, articles and links on oral contraceptives, antidiabetic therapy, hormone replacement, thyroid disease treatments, and several connections to information on growth hormone, hypogonadism, and infertility treatments. Links to online pharmacies, drug companies, and new drug approval databases are accessible at the left sidebar menu. The subject library provides additional pages on contraceptive information specifically geared toward professionals.

Kansas University Medical Center: Pharmacology:
Basic Pharmacology, Autonomic Nervous System, Endocrine ◎ ◎ ◎
http://www.kumc.edu/AMA-MSS/study/pharm1.htm
This downloadable study guide provides a review of basic pharmacologic principles, with equations, routes of administration, drug permeation, biotransformation, and pharmacokinetic topics. Information on catecholamine synthesis and autonomic receptors and a primer on therapeutic hormones and other medication administration are provided.

Oregon Health Sciences University: Hormone Antagonists ◎ ◎
http://medir.ohsu.edu/cliniweb/D27/D27.505.440.450.html
From CliniWeb International, this site offers links to PibMed documents related to hormone antagonists. Specific antagonists indexed include aldosterone antagonists, androgen antagonists, antithyroid agents, estrogen antagonists, insulin antagonists, leukotriene antagonists, and prostaglandin antagonists.

PCS Health Systems: Hormones ○ ○
http://www.druglist.com/xiii.htm#XIII. HORMONES

This summary of hormonal drugs offers general prescribing guidelines and drug descriptions for health professionals. Specific drug recommendations are available, as well as clinical details, precautions, and possible side effects. Drug topics include adrenal corticosteroids, thyroid replacement and antithyroid agents, androgens, growth hormones, gonadotropin releasing agonists, gonadotropin inhibitors, and ovulation inducing agents.

PharmInfoNet: Endocrine Disease and Diabetes Center ○ ○ ○
http://pharminfo.com/disease/endocrine.html

PharmInfoNet's Endocrine Disease and Diabetes Center offers patient information, expert advice, and links to related sites. Resources include endocrine disease and diabetes review articles, news from medical meetings, professional and patient discussion groups, and lists of products and services. Extensive patient information includes diabetes statistics, answers to frequently asked questions, and a glossary of terms. Links are available to resources on benign prostatic hyperplasia, diabetes, fertility disorders, Gaucher's disease, hormone deficiencies, hyperparathyroidism, hypogonadism, menopause, nutritional disorders, obesity, osteoporosis, and premenstrual syndrome. Links to information on 17 related drugs, news groups, mailing lists, and other Internet resources are also provided.

University of California Los Angeles: Introduction to Endocrine Pharmacology, Hypothalamic and Pituitary Hormones ○ ○ ○
http://www.medsch.ucla.edu/https/pharm/99lectures/chaudhuri/phintro.htm

An outline of introductory pharmacology of the endocrine system is presented at this site of the University of California Los Angeles. Information on hormone use, drugs that affect the endocrine glands, and drugs that affect target tissue receptors for hormones is found. The physiology and use of gonadotropin-releasing hormone (GnRH), gonadatropin-releasing hormone analogues, follicle-stimulating hormone (FSH), leutinizing hormone (LH), human menopausal gonadotropin (HMG), human chorionic gonadotropin (HCG), somatotropin, prolactin, adrenocorticotropic hormone, and hormones of the posterior pituitary are reviewed, and a list of particularly important drugs is provided.

University of Oklahoma College of Pharmacy: A First Course in Pharmacokinetics and Biopharmaceutics ○ ○ ○
http://157.142.72.143/gaps/pkbio/pkbioF.html

A review of basic pharmacokinetics and biopharmaceutics is presented at this electronic tutorial, which allows for keyword searches of material. Funded in part by the American Association of Colleges of Pharmacy, the lesson provides analysis of urine data, routes of drug administration, pharmacokinetics with oral dosing, and calculation of bioavailability parameters. Physiological factors that may affect oral absorption, formulation solutions, and routes of excretion are outlined. Other topics discussed include metabolic reactions, drug distribution patterns, and clinical applications in drug monitoring, pediatrics, and geriatrics. JavaScript online calculators are accessible.

9.2 Adrenal Glands

Overview

Cancer Medicine: Corticosteroids ○ ○ ○
http://intouch.cancernetwork.com/canmed/Ch072/072-0.htm

The online *Cancer Medicine* publication offers review of hormones of the adrenal cortex, with chapters on pharmacokinetics, steroid synthesis, pharmaceutical derivatives, and the physiologic and pharmacologic effect of these substances. Corticosteroids in the treatment of neoplasms, mechanisms of glucocorticoid action, and a complete reference listing are provided.

Family Practice Notebook.com: Systemic Corticosteroid ○ ○
http://www.fpnotebook.com/END72.htm

Dosing details for systemic corticosteroids are found at this page, with specific information for a pediatric population and high, low, and medium potency equivalent dosages. The relative anti-inflammatory potency for the various agents, relative mineralocorticoid potency, half-life, and a guideline for osteoporosis prevention with long-term steroids are detailed.

University of Kansas School of Medicine Medical Pharmacology Learning Modules: Adrenocorticosteroids ○ ○ ○
http://www.kumc.edu/research/medicine/pharmacology/
mgordon/Endocrine/Adrenocort/frameadreno.htm

This learning module offers a valuable pharmacologic overview of adrenocorticosteroids. Topics include the physiology of adrenocorticosteroids, primary adrenocorticosteroid functions, pharmacodynamics of natural and synthetic glucocorticoids, glucocorticoids and adrenal disorders, glucocorticoids for nonadrenal disorders, adverse effects of glucocorticoids, commonly used glucocorticoids, mineralocorticoids, adrenal androgens, adrenocortical drug antagonists, and mineralocorticoid antagonists. Practice questions and case studies are also available.

Antiadrenal Agent: Aminoglutethimide

Mayo Clinic: Aminoglutethimide ◐ ◐
http://mayohealth.org/usp/html/202026.htm

Aminoglutethimide, an antiadrenal and antineoplastic drug, is summarized in this fact sheet. A description of the drug is followed by prescribing precautions, proper dosage and use, precautions during use, side effects, and additional important details.

9.3 Bone and Mineral Metabolism

Bisphosphonates

Doctor's Guide: Bisphosphonates May Reduce Metastases ◐
http://www.pslgroup.com/dg/15007A.htm

An article related to metastases that originate in the breast and settle in bones offers an update on this relatively new drug class. The potential of bisphosphonates for stopping bone metastases from developing and discussion of recent evidence in favor of administration of the drug are reviewed.

University of Washington: Bisphosphonates ◐ ◐
http://courses.washington.edu/bonephys/opbis.html

Indications, contraindications, and the use of alendronate in osteoporosis are addressed at this tutorial on the bisphosphonate drug class. Its potentials in blocking resorption and a summary of results of the Fracture Intervention Trial are provided. The text provides answers to alendronate dosing, safety, and fracture incidence. The drug's use in the elderly is reviewed, and further connections to the mechanisms of action of bisphosphonates and to additional references are provided. Illustrations at the site depict the anti-resorptive potency of various bisphosphonates.

Calcitonin

MEDLINEplus Health Information: Calcitonin ◐ ◐ ◐
http://www.nlm.nih.gov/medlineplus/druginfo/calcitoninsystemic202106.html

The National Library of Medicine offers this presentation of systemic calcitonin usage, which details the drug category; its proper use as an antihypercalcemic, bone resorption inhibitor, and its use in osteoporosis therapy; precautions to exercise while using; and rare and more common side effects.

Calcium

Canadian Medical Association Journal:
Prevention and Management of Osteoporosis: Calcium Nutrition ○ ○ ○
http://www.cma.ca/disease/osteo_p1/no4.htm

This special supplement, authored by a professor at the University of Toronto Metabolic Bone Clinic, offers recommendations on appropriate calcium level intake in light of recent studies. Options for obtaining correct amounts of calcium, based on review of controlled, randomized, and prospective studies, and pharmaceutical calcium supplementation recommendations are provided. Further information on adequate vitamin D dosing and obtaining requirements through food sources is provided, and the need for further research on calcium supplementation in adolescents is considered.

Johns Hopkins Bayview Medical Center: Clinical Nutrition: Calcium ○
http://www.jhbmc.jhu.edu/NUTRI/calcihealth.html

This consumer information sheet on calcium supplementation provides review of the function of calcium, recommended daily allowances, and dietary sources, as a service of the hospital's Clinical Nutrition Department.

Hormone Replacement Therapy

EndocrineWeb: Estrogen Replacement After Menopause ○
http://www.endocrineweb.com/osteoporosis/estrogen.html

Hormone replacement therapy after menopause for the prevention of osteoporosis is discussed at this page of the EndocrineWeb site. Information is provided on designer estrogens and when to begin therapy.

Parathyroid Hormone Therapy

Calcitonin in the Prevention and Treatment of Osteoporosis ○ ○ ○
http://www.ectsoc.org/reviews/008_genn.htm

Calcitonin's efficacy in its ability to inhibit osteoclastic activity in bone calcitonin, calcitonins available for clinical use, routes of administration, and recent results of a study that established significant reduction in vertebral fracture incidence are reviewed. Other clinical studies, a somewhat heterogeneous response profile, hormone resistance in some patients, and other discussion on calcitonin's indications are provided. Most reference citations are accompanied by links to their related PubMed entries.

Project AWARE: Parathyroid Hormone Restores Almost Full Bone Mass to Women with Osteoporosis ◎ ◎
http://www.project-aware.org/resource/Inthenews/parathyroid_osteoporosis.html

A recently updated news article discusses the discovery of the effective use of parathyroid hormone as a treatment for osteoporosis. Bone mineral density and biochemical markers for bone loss are reviewed, and comparisons are made between the prospects of parathyroid hormone and hormone replacement therapy. Promising results with PTH, which stimulates the formation of osteoblasts, are revealed.

Vitamin D

Canadian Medical Association: Vitamin D Metabolites and Analogs in the Treatment of Osteoporosis ◎ ◎ ◎
http://www.cma.ca/disease/osteo_p1/no8.htm

A special supplement of the *Canadian Medical Association Journal* provides readers with in-depth information on vitamin D metabolism and function, studies on the current state of knowledge on its effects on the skeletal system, and review of the latest clinical trials of vitamin D in the treatment of osteoporosis. Summary of the benefits, harm, and costs of therapy, along with recommendations with regard to further research and future study are presented.

Oregon Health Sciences University: Studying Vitamin D as Treatment for Prostate Cancer ◎
http://www.eurekalert.org/releases/ohsu-svd111199.html

Review of recent research at Oregon Health Sciences University is presented at this news release, which outlines a study funded by the National Institutes of Health to discover the possible role of vitamin D in the treatment of prostate cancer.

Osteovision: Vitamin D and Analogues in the Treatment of Osteoporosis ◎
http://www.osteovision.ch/slides/66.html

This concise lesson considers the importance of vitamin D, its toxic effects, and a brief discussion on its deficiency, supplementation in the elderly, and potent vitamin D analogues. An additional slide in the series offers review of the cumulative probability of fracture in the elderly, according to calcium and vitamin D intake.

9.4 Cholesterol and Lipoprotein Metabolism

Antilipemic Agents

American Heart Association (AHA): Cholesterol-Lowering Drugs
http://www.americanheart.org/Heart_and_Stroke_A_Z_Guide/choldr.html

Cholesterol target goals of therapy, risk factors in addition to out-of-range levels, and a discussion of drugs commonly used to treat blood lipid disorders, where exercise, diet, and other lifestyle measures are inadequate, are presented at this AHA information sheet. Common side effects, less commonly prescribed medications, and links to other pages of this online guide are presented. Visitors may access related information on drug approvals, generic substitutions, cholesterol screening, and statistics, and several position statements of the AHA are provided.

Temple University
School of Medicine: Antihyperlipidemic Agents
http://blue.temple.edu/~tupharm/medcourse/Hyperlipid/index.htm

A slide presentation at this site, authored by James L. Daniel, offers visitors information on antilipemic agents, with information presented on lipoprotein metabolism, types of hyperlipidemias, and therapeutic uses and benefits of drugs used in their treatment.

9.5 Diabetes Mellitus

Overview

Diabetes Specialist: Treatment of Diabetes Mellitus
http://www.aboutdiabetes-endocrinology.com/1_dia/dm04_treatment.htm

An overview of the pharmacology of diabetes mellitus treatment is presented at the site, with summaries of oral medications and a separate connection to a page dedicated solely to insulin therapy. Goals of therapy, specific preparations and insulins, and insulin administration tools are reviewed. Practical issues surrounding intensive insulin therapy are addressed.

Michigan Diabetes Outreach Network: Pharmacologic Treatment of Diabetes ◐ ◐
http://www.diabetes-midon.org/Chapters/QuickCh5.htm

An online project of the Michigan Diabetes Outreach Network offers professionals quick reference information on the pharmacologic management of diabetes mellitus. A link to insulin and type 2 diabetes management, and details regarding sulfonylureas, metformin, alpha glucosidase inhibitors, thiazolidinediones, and repaglinide are found at this address. Dosing, precautions, and other administration details are available for browsing in both text and table format.

University of Kansas School of Medicine Medical Pharmacology Learning Modules: Diabetes ◐ ◐ ◐
http://www.kumc.edu/research/medicine/pharmacology/mgordon/Endocrine/Diabetes/framediabetes.htm

This valuable learning module offers an extensive discussion of diabetes and related pharmacologic therapies. An overview of diabetes includes a description of the islets of Langerhans, properties of type 1 diabetes and clinical presentation, and properties of type 2 diabetes. A description of insulin includes details of physiologic secretion and degradation, as well as a summary of endocrine effects of insulin on the liver, muscle, and adipose tissue. The tutorial also offers pharmacologic details of different types of insulin preparations, oral hypoglycemics, and glucagon. Information is presented in a concise, outline format. Practice questions and case studies are, additionally, presented.

Glucagon

Glucagon: Insulin "Antidote" ◐
http://www.minimed.com/files/glucagon_antidote.htm

A professor of medicine at the University of Southern California Los Angeles reviews the findings of a British study, which found that a very low percentage of insulin-dependent diabetics keep glucagon at home. The importance of an emergency glucagon kit and family education are stressed.

Regional Emergency Medical Services Council: Glucagon ◐
http://www.nycremsco.org/protocols/drugs/Glucagon.htm

A description of glucagon and its use, indications, adverse reactions, and dosage and administration are concisely reviewed at this protocol of the Regional Emergency Medical Services Council of New York City.

Insulin

American Diabetes Association (ADA): Position Statement: Insulin Administration ○ ○ ○
http://www.diabetes.org/diabetescare/Supplement/s31.htm

This position statement of the American Diabetes Association discusses the various types and species of insulin and their different pharmacologic properties. Storage of vials, proper inspection prior to administration, insulin mixing, and additional topics related to insulin usage are introduced. Subcutaneous insulin administration, injection technique and procedures, and injection site selection are reviewed. Dosing, self-monitoring, and other details regarding insulin and effective metabolic control are summarized.

Clinica Diabetologica: Insulin Types ○ ○
http://www.clinidiabet.com/educ_en/1d05_en.htm

The duration and action of the various insulin types and the most commonly used commercial mixtures are listed at this site in a colorful, easy-to-read format. By accessing the site index, visitors can also gain entry to pages on injection site selection, factors influencing insulin's effect, factors that may increase insulin resistance, and specific information on the new ultrafast insulin. Drugs that may affect blood glucose levels are listed at a pharmacy link found at the site index, in addition to a review of glycosylated hemoglobin, information on the insulin pump, and other educational material.

Diabetes Care: Insulin Administration ○ ○ ○
http://journal.diabetes.org/FullText/Supplements/DiabetesCare/Supplement100/s86.htm

From the Clinical Practice Recommendations 2000 of the American Diabetes Association comes this article describing insulin types, storage, mixing, and syringes. Syringe alternatives, such as jet injectors, and injection techniques with respect to dose preparation, injection procedures, and injection site selection are reviewed. Additional discussion on appropriate dosages, self-monitoring tips, and hypoglycemia reactions are found.

Postgraduate Medicine: Insulin Therapy ○ ○ ○
http://www.postgradmed.com/issues/1997/02_97/sym_intr.htm

The three in-depth articles accessible from this site of *Postgraduate Medicine* focus on insulin analogues and the clinical use of insulin. A cursory review of pharmacology, with discussion of short-acting, long-acting, and hepatospecific analogues, is provided in the first article. The second article offers information on lispro and postprandial glucose level control, with practical prescribing advice and the rationale behind its introduction. Lastly, an all-inclusive review of the insulin use in type 2 diabetics is found, including insulin monotherapy, combination therapy, and lispro use.

Ray Williams Institute of Paediatric Endocrinology: Types of Insulin Preparations ◐ ◐

http://www.rwi.nch.edu.au/apegbook/diabne23.htm#E9E23

Ultra-short-acting, short-acting, intermediate-acting, long-acting, and mixed insulin preparations are reviewed at this electronic document, with onset of action, peak of action, duration of action, and available preparations listed. Schematic profiles of duration of action are viewable at the site.

Oral Hypoglycemic Agents

Diabetes Spectrum: Pharmacological Properties and Clinical Use of Currently Available Agents ◐ ◐ ◐

http://www.diabetes.org/DiabetesSpectrum/98v11n4/pg211.htm

Diabetes Spectrum offers review of management objectives in type 2 diabetes mellitus, with discussion of sulfonylurea agents, metformin, and additional diabetic agents. Pharmacologic differences among the agents are presented, and a table outlines targets for metabolic control and body mass index in type 2 diabetes patients. Pancreatic and extrapancreatic effects of sulfonylureas; pharmacologic effect on insulin levels, lipids, and body weight; and glycemic control with monotherapy and combination therapy are presented. Comprehensive profiles of side effects are included for each drug.

Lexi-Comp Informatics Library: Hypoglycemic Agents Comparison, Oral ◐ ◐

http://informatics.drake.edu/pth/html/appendix/section/hf602100.htm

A comparison of oral hypoglycemic agents is made at an online chart at this page, which lists equivalent dosages, daily dosages, usual regimen, duration of action, onset, half-life, and additional pharmacologic parameters.

Polycystic Ovary Syndrome: Metabolic Challenges and New Treatment Options ◐ ◐ ◐

http://macmcm.com/asrm/asrm98-pos.htm

Present treatment strategies of polycystic ovary syndrome (PCOS) and the option of prescribing an insulin-sensitizing agent are discussed at this electronic article. The relationship between insulin resistance and PCOS is explored, although not fully understood. Attempts at answers to questions regarding empirical use of insulin-sensitizing agents, time for institution of therapy, and their routine use for ovulation induction are made, with recent studies supporting their use in PCOS management.

University of California
Los Angeles: School of Medicine: Hypoglycemic Agents
http://www.medsch.ucla.edu/https/pharm/99lectures/chaudhuri/phhypogl.htm

From the University of California, Los Angeles School of Medicine, this site offers information about hypoglycemic agents. Topics include glucose homeostasis and the diabetic state, hormones responsible for blood glucose homeostasis, chemistry of insulin, mechanism of action of insulin, diabetes mellitus, pharmacological actions of insulin, side effects, preparation and dosage, oral hypoglycemic agents, and drug interactions.

University of Chicago:
Evaluation of New Oral Hypoglycemic Agents
http://dacc.bsd.uchicago.edu/drug/Bulletins/n0896.html

An evaluation of acarbose, glimepiride, and metformin is provided at this site of the University of Chicago Medical Center. Included are the mechanisms of action and pharmacology of these three newer antidiabetic agents. Combination therapy in non-insulin dependent diabetes mellitus (NIDDM), such as acarbose with insulin therapy and long-term patient follow-up, are reviewed. Contraindications in therapy and potential adverse effects of oral antidiabetics are summarized at an online table, and warnings and precautions with respect to lactic acidosis, renal function, and drug interactions are presented. Comparative pharmacokinetic parameters are shown, as well as comparative costs of agents.

9.6 Metabolic Agents

Alkalinizing Agents

RxMed: Sodium Bicarbonate
http://www.rxmed.com/monographs/sodiumb.html

Details of sodium bicarbonate pharmacology are available from this fact sheet, including mechanisms of action, indications, parenteral administration, contraindications, precautions, drug interactions, adverse effects, overdose symptoms and treatment, and proper dosage. Details of use as a urinary alkalinizer and for treatment of acidosis associated with chronic renal failure and general acidosis are also available.

Antigout Agents

E-Doc: Colchicine
http://www.edoc.co.za/medilink/actives/264.html

Prescribing information for colchicine, a common antigout drug, is available from this resource. Mechanism of action, indications, contraindications, dosage, side effects, and precautions are listed.

Family Practice Notebook.com: Allopurinol
http://www.fpnotebook.com/RHE54.htm

The antigout medication allopurinol is described at this address, including indications, precautions, mechanism of action, dosage, and adverse effects. Links are available to summaries of highlighted terms.

Infomed Drug Guide: Allopurinol
http://www.infomed.org/100drugs/allotoc.html

The pharmacology, indications, adverse reactions and interactions, contraindications and precautions, and risk groups for adverse effects due to allopurinol are listed at this address. Reference citations are also provided.

Enzyme Replacement Therapy for Metabolic Impairment

Canadian Medical Association Journal: Enzyme Replacement Therapy for Gaucher's Disease
http://www.cma.ca/cmaj/vol-159/issue-10/1273.htm

This article of the *Canadian Medical Association Journal* focuses on the recent development of enzyme replacement therapy in the treatment of Gaucher's disease. The study analyzes indications for treatment and selection of patients, demographic details, study with regard to the financial impact of the treatment, and future challenges in enzyme replacement therapy.

Enzyme Replacement Therapy
http://www-biol.paisley.ac.uk/Courses/Enzymes/glossary/Replace.htm

Aside from the treatment of enzyme deficient states, the use of enzyme replacement therapy in the treatment of inborn errors of metabolism is examined at this site. The reasoning that administration of enzymes might be beneficial in decreasing abnormal amounts of substrate due to inadequacies of lysosmal enzymatic catabolism is introduced. A connection to a discussion on therapeutic enzymes reviews a broad variety of specific uses, including replacement for metabolic deficiencies.

Gauchers Association:
Effect of Low-dose Enzyme Replacement Therapy on Bones ○ ○
http://www.gaucher.org.uk/bones_zi.htm

Discussion of recent research that demonstrates the efficacy of low-dose enzyme replacement therapy in Gaucher disease with severe bone involvement is found at the site. Confirmation of bone improvement with the therapy and credence to the theory that low-dose regimens may be as effective as high doses are topics of discussion. An abstract of the original article may be accessed from a connection at the site, as well as the entire article in PDF format and related commentary.

Essential Vitamins and Minerals

American Dietetic Association (ADA):
Vitamin and Mineral Supplementation ○ ○ ○
http://www.eatright.org/asupple.html

This position statement details the research on the relationship between diet and disease and the current state of knowledge with regard to epidemiological studies and scientific hypotheses about particular nutrients for optimal health. Public interest in dietary supplementation, recent research on identified nutrients and antioxidant components, recommended nutrient intake and nutrient supplementation in the United States, and the need for strong scientific evidence based on controlled clinical trials are reviewed. Circumstances for which supplementation is indicated, food fortification, and discussion of toxicities and adverse interactions are included.

Environmed Research, Inc.:
Minerals: Essential Knowledge in Nutrition ○ ○
http://www.nutramed.com/nutrition/calcium_magnesium.htm

The role of calcium concentration in osteomalacia and osteoporosis, measuring bone mineral density, the use of biophosphanates and other minerals in treatment, and specific details on calcium treatment and absorption are presented. Ratio ranges of mineral combinations, magnesium deficiency and supplementation, and additional nutritional considerations in mineral deficient states and supplementation are provided.

Washington University: Nutrients and Solubility ○ ○ ○
http://wunmr.wustl.edu/EduDev/LabTutorials/Vitamins/vitamins.html

This tutorial offers a thorough overview of nutrients and the physiologic mechanisms of nutrient solubility. Topics include vitamins and minerals as essential dietary components, the molecular basis for water solubility and fat solubility of vitamins, structures and functions of key vitamins, effects of artificial fats on vitamin solubility, and quantitative measures of mineral solubility. Calcium in the body is also discussed, including the solubility and absorption of calcium and the control of calcium levels.

Immunosuppressive Drugs

Baylor College of Medicine
Transplantation Primer: Immunosuppression Medicine ⊙ ⊙ ⊙
http://www.bcm.tmc.edu/transplant/drugs/text.html

From the *Transplantation Primer*, this site offers information about immunosuppressant medicine. The table of contents includes a historical background and discussion of approaches to immunosuppression. Sections on purine analogs, pyrimidine analogs, folic acid antagonists, alkylating agents, antibiotics, and cyclosporin are found, as well as discussion of several lymphocyte depleting agents. Blood transfusions and complications of immunosuppressive therapy are reviewed. Comments regarding future progress in immunosuppression are found, involving full preservation of immunocompetence.

Insulin-Free World Foundation: Pharmaceutical Information ⊙ ⊙ ⊙
http://www.insulinfree.org/idrugs.htm

From the Insulin-Free World Foundation, this site contains links to articles about immunosuppressive medications. Articles are listed by drug, with generic names and manufacturers provided. Manuscripts regarding strategies to block organ rejection, press releases, scientific pharmacologic details, and additional information on organ transplantation and advances in immunosuppressive therapies are provided. Details pertaining to therapies specifically geared toward successful implantation of islet cells are found.

New Developments in Transplantation Medicine ⊙ ⊙
http://206.1.96.39/pubs/news/0597a.htm

Immunosuppressant agents in clinical transplantation are discussed at this site of *New Developments in Transplantation Medicine*. A summary of new immunosuppressive agents is presented in table format, and significant benefits and side effects are reviewed. Several questions that remain to be answered regarding available options for post-transplant recipients are introduced at this CME journal site.

Minerals

RxMed: Sodium Chloride ⊙ ⊙
http://www.rxmed.com/monographs/sod-chlo.html

Prescribing details for sodium chloride are presented in this general monograph. Topics include pharmacology, indications, topical use, contraindications, warnings, use in children, drug interactions, adverse effects, overdose symptoms, overdose treatment, and dosage.

9.7 Neuroendocrine System

Overview of Pituitary Hormones and Analogs

Diabetes Web: Vasopressin ⊙
http://www.cs.odu.edu/~wild/DiabetesWeb/education/posterior.html
Replacement vasopressin for treatment of a common cause of diabetes insipidus is reviewed at this encyclopedic entry, provided as a service of *Encyclopedia Britannica*.

Finch University of Health Sciences/Chicago Medical School: Posterior Pituitary Hormones ⊙ ⊙
http://www.finchcms.edu/Pharmacology/snyderslides/postpit/index.htm
Vasopressin secretion and action, an outline of clinical uses, other agents used in the treatment of diabetes insipidus, and the clinical uses of oxytocin are presented in a concise format at this sequence of slides.

Hypothalamic and Other Peptide Hormones ⊙ ⊙ ⊙
http://intouch.cancernetwork.com/canmed/Ch071/071-0.htm
Cancer Medicine offers visitors online access to all 17 chapters of this publication, which reviews the analogs of peptide hormones, current uses of hormone antagonists, and details on the treatment of tumors with various peptide analogs. Specific uses in cases of exocrine pancreatic cancer, breast cancer, epithelial ovarian cancer, and gastric tumors are reviewed, with inhibitory effects of certain agents and review of experimental observation and administration.

Overview of Hypothalamic and Pituitary Hormones ⊙ ⊙ ⊙
http://arbl.cvmbs.colostate.edu/hbooks/pathphys/endocrine/hypopit/overview.html
Overview information on anterior and posterior pituitary hormones is presented at this page provided by Colorado State University. Illustrative figures and tables provide details on individual hormones, major target organs, and major physiologic effects. Linking to any one of the eight pituitary hormone pages allows access to in-depth information on individual hormone secretion, receptors, and related figures. Classical negative feedback loop in the secretion of hormones, in-depth review of physiologic effects, control of hormone secretion, and pharmaceutical uses are discussed.

Virtual Drugstore: Desmopressin ⊙
http://www.virtualdrugstore.com/insipidus/desmopressin.html
The mechanism of action and use of desmopressin are reviewed at the site. Further details on side effects, special precautions, and drug interactions are found. A short list of references is provided.

Bromocriptine

MEDLINEplus Health Information: Bromocriptine ○ ○ ○
http://www.nlm.nih.gov/medlineplus/druginfo/bromocriptinesystemic202094.html

Brand names, drug categories, and additional general information on bromocriptine therapy are provided at this reference of the National Library of Medicine. Visitors to the site will find review of the drug, including its use as a growth hormone suppressant and infertility therapy adjunct. Proper use and dosing, precautions while taking the medication, and more common and less common side effects are introduced.

Neurosurgical Focus: Bromocriptine Therapy for Prolactin: Secreting Pituitary Adenomas ○ ○
http://www.neurosurgery.org/journals/online_j/july96/4.html

Authored by professors of the University of Virginia Health Sciences Center, this site contains a review of the management of prolactin-secreting pituitary adenomas. The ways in which bromocriptine therapy can control prolactinomas, discussion of efficacy, and accompanying guidelines for initiating and maintaining bromocriptine treatment are presented. Alternatives where drug intolerance is found and other adjustments in the medical management schedule are presented.

Cosyntropin

Lexi-Comp Clinical Reference Library: Cosyntropin ○ ○
http://informatics.drake.edu/patch_f/html/chapter/mono/hf033200.htm

Diagnosis with cosyntropin is reviewed at this fact sheet, provided as a service of an online medical reference database. Its use, precautions, adverse reactions, mechanism of action, and usual dosage are described. Reference range, test indications, and patient information are concisely reviewed, and a pronunciation link is found.

Gonadotropin-Releasing Hormone and Analogs

Family Practice Notebook.com: Gonadotropin-Releasing Hormone Agonist ○
http://fpnotebook.com/GYN78.htm

This family medicine resource offers concise information on GnRH agonists, including indications, mechanisms of action, efficacy, and adverse events.

Fertilitext: Gonadatropin-releasing Hormone: GnRH ◎
http://fertilitext.org/gonadotr.html

The use of gonadotropin-releasing hormone (GnRH) for women who fail to ovulate for any number of clinical reasons is discussed at this online text. Hormone benefits, routes of administration, and differences between GnRH and human menopausal gonadotropins are mentioned.

Nafarelin Acetate ◎
http://www.drugref.com/members/database/ndrhtml/nafarelinacetate.html

The mechanism of action and uses of this GnRH are outlined at the site, with information on contraindications, special concerns, adverse events, and dosages for both endometriosis and central precocious puberty stated.

Growth Hormone

Adult Hormone Growth Deficiency Therapy ◎ ◎
http://www.hgfound.org/adulthormonetherapy.htm

The diagnostic criteria for adult growth hormone deficiency and hormone replacement therapy are discussed. The goals of somatotropin replacement therapy are reviewed.

Evolution of Growth Hormone Therapy ◎ ◎
http://www.optioncare.com/growthhormone/background.htm

The introduction of synthetically produced growth hormone, natural sequence products, and other developments in growth hormone therapy are discussed. Manufacturer links and the recent approval of an adult indication for growth hormone therapy are introduced.

Human Growth Foundation: Growth Hormone Treatment ◎ ◎
http://www.hgfound.org/growthhormone.html

Discussions of physical and psychological effects of growth hormone therapy, pros and cons of treatment, expense of the hormones, and other considerations and recommendations regarding the decision to institute such therapy are offered.

Massachusetts General Hospital: Growth Hormone Replacement in Adults ◎ ◎ ◎
http://neurosurgery.mgh.harvard.edu/e-f-944.htm

This site offers an article on recent advances in recombinant human growth hormone replacement therapy in adults. There is an overview of growth hormone deficiency syndrome, as well as a summary of recombinant human growth hormone therapy. Sections on body composition, lipid metabolism, bone density, and cardiovascular function are included, as is a section on side effects and future directions. References are provided.

Massachusetts General Hospital Neuroendocrine Center: Advances in Recombinant Human Growth Hormone Therapy ○ ○ ○
http://neurosurgery.mgh.harvard.edu/e-f-944.htm

The etiology of acquired growth hormone deficiency and the novel therapeutic approach of recombinant human growth hormone therapy in adults is discussed, with regard to its effects on lipid metabolism, exercise capacity, and recent investigation into its relation to bone density. Future directions in growth hormone replacement therapy research, such as determination of long-term effects, are considered.

Society for Endocrinology: Adult Growth Hormone Replacement ○ ○ ○
http://www.endocrinology.org/SFE/gh.htm

Growth hormone deficiency, more appropriately named somatotrophin deficiency, and the consequences of its declined secretion in adulthood are discussed at this in-depth article. Information on clinical and metabolic features of adult somatotrophin deficiency, psychological symptoms, diagnosis, and the clinical efficacy of supplementation with growth hormone are discussed. Several conclusions, drawing upon a review of the published literature, are outlined, including significant improvements in body composition parameters, well-being, and quality of life. Dosing, side effects, and cost considerations are presented, as well as details on patient selection criteria.

9.8 Obesity Medications

About.com: Prescription Drugs for the Treatment of Obesity ○ ○
http://pharmacology.tqn.com/health/pharmacology/library/weekly/bl980401.htm

The table of contents at this site includes articles on medications that promote weight loss, single drug and combination drug treatments, and potential risks and benefits about pharmacotherapeutic treatments. The entire About.com site may be searched, or visitors may, alternatively, check the "New Drug Approvals" database or "Drugs in the News" for further information.

Obesity Meds and Research News ○ ○ (some features fee-based)
http://www.obesity-news.com/newdrugs.htm

Non-subscriber access is available at this site to articles on clinical trials, pipeline drugs, and recently rejected drugs for the treatment of obesity. Gene discoveries, other journal articles, and the opportunity to subscribe online to the full text of *Obesity Meds and Research News* are provided at the site. Articles and monographs of drugs currently in use and OTC preparation information may be accessed, although much material requires a user subscription.

PharmInfoNet: Obesity Information ○ ○ ○
http://pharminfo.com/disease/obesity/obesity_info.html

Drugs used in the treatment of obesity, research news from current medical meetings, and an online archive of articles from the *Medical Sciences Bulletin, MedWatch News,* and other reputable publications are found. Background information on drug therapy of obesity may be displayed and contains access to press releases on new drugs, statistics related to obesity, and an e-mail LISTSERV for discussion of the latest research. A review of pharmacotherapy in obesity weighs the risks and benefits of drugs used in obesity treatment.

9.9 Reproductive System

Androgen Therapy and Complications of Therapy

Cancer Medicine:
Hormones and Etiology of Cancer: Prostate Cancer ○ ○ ○
http://intouch.cancernetwork.com/CanMed/Ch014/014-5.htm

Studies of prostate cancer and circulating levels of testosterone and hormonal risk determinants are reviewed at this site, with hormonal pathways in prostate cancer causation illustrated and discussed. The androgen receptor gene and its possible role in prostate carcinogenesis, endocrine manipulation with administration of estrogens and leutinizing hormone-releasing hormone agonists, and well-established disease risk factors for prostatic cancer are presented.

MEDLINEplus Health Information: Androgens (Systemic) ○ ○ ○
http://www.nlm.nih.gov/medlineplus/druginfo/androgenssystemic202036.html

Brand names, drug categories, and medication description and dosage forms are all introduced at this site of the National Institutes of Health. Proper use of various forms of the medication, precautions, dosing, side effects, and the importance of acknowledging the presence of other medical problems before using the medication are discussed.

PersonalMD.com: Male Hormones Linked to Prostate Cancer ○ ○
http://www.personalmd.com/news/a1996123107.shtml

A report from researchers at the University of Wisconsin Comprehensive Cancer Center explores the role of male sex hormones in regulating cell activity. The ability of androgens to activate antioxidants and the understanding of how reduced levels of male hormones in older men may influence prostate cancer risk are examined. Review of a commentary on the study, published in the *Journal of the National Cancer Institute,* is found.

PowerPak Pharmacy Online Continuing Education: Androgen Replacement Therapy for Male Hypogonadism ◐ ◐ ◐

http://www.powerpak.com/CE/Androgen

The learning objectives of this module include being able to compare and contrast the clinical features of prepubertal and adult onset hypogonadism, contrasting the differing pathophysiologies, knowing the disorders associated with hypogonadism, and stating the potential benefits and risks of androgen therapy. Disease manifestations, goals of androgen therapy, and overviews of currently available pharmacology options are discussed. New and upcoming therapies, pharmacokinetics, clinical study reviews, and discussions of several important considerations in androgen therapy are found. Also presented are case studies, including a Klinefelter's patient and a patient with diabetes, as well as a 20 question review.

Gonadotropins

Institute for Reproductive Medicine and Science of Saint Barnabas: Common Questions about Human Menopausal Gonadotropins ◐ ◐

http://www.sbivf.com/menogona.htm

Answers to commonly asked questions regarding human menopausal gonadotropins (HMG) are answered at this Web site fact sheet, which explains the hormones' purposes in ovulation induction. Differences in preparations, routes of administration, and relevant terminology are defined. Risks of HMG therapy, information on risk minimization, and answers to other FAQs are provided.

Mayo Clinic Scottsdale Center for Reproductive Medicine: Side Effects of Gonadotropins ◐ ◐

http://www.mayo.edu/mcs/Medical_Specialties/Reproductive_Medicine/Gonadotropins.html

Side effects associated with gonadotropins are discussed in this clinical fact sheet, including ovarian hyperstimulation (OHSS), multiple gestation, ectopic pregnancies, birth defects, adnexal torsion, and ovarian cancer.

Hormone Replacement Therapy and Complications of Therapy

BioCognizance.com: Elevated Sex Hormones are Breast Cancer Risk ◐ ◐

http://www.biocognizance.com/_bcforum/00000284.htm

A discussion of the association between serum hormone levels and breast cancer is found at this study review, sponsored in part by the National Institutes of Health.

Levels of bioavailable estradiol and unbound testosterone, with a gradient of risk observed across increasing concentrations, are observed. The results of the study presented indicate that these hormones may be used successfully as a clinical measure of risk identification. Intervention to reduce risk for breast cancer is reviewed, with goals of the Women's Health Initiative presented and additional risk factors for breast cancer discussed.

Cancer Medicine: Hormones and Etiology of Cancer ○ ○ ○
http://intouch.cancernetwork.com/CanMed/Ch014/014-0.htm

Chapter 14 of this *Cancer Medicine* edition provides review of the convincing clinical and epidemiological evidence of the relationship between hormones and the etiology of breast, endometrial, ovarian, prostate, and several additional metastatic diseases. Hypothesized relationships between hormones and cancer are illustrated and discussed, with comprehensive summaries of consistently documented existing data and established risks reviewed.

Froedtert Hospital and Medical College: Hormones and Breast Cancer ○ ○
http://www.froedtert.com/grandrounds/marapr97/page2.html

This volume of Froedtert's Grand Rounds presentation includes discussion of the relationship between pregnancy and breast cancer, the effect of pregnancy termination on breast cancer risk, and the influence of physiologic estrogen and progestin levels in the risk of relapse. The issue of subsequent pregnancy in women with a breast cancer history and the use of hormone replacement therapy in this group are topics reviewed.

Louisiana State University Medical Center: The Menopausal Patient and Hormone Replacement Therapy ○ ○
http://lib-sh.lsumc.edu/fammed/grounds/menopaus.html

A clinical overview of menopause and the use of hormone replacement therapy is available in this article. A definition of menopause and premature menopause is followed by details of physiology, an estrogen deficiency state caused by menopause, hot flashes, osteoporosis, psychological symptoms, and genital and breast atrophy. Estrogen and hormone replacement therapies are described, including associated benefits and risks. Possible increased risks of breast cancer and endometrial cancer are described, and proper patient selection for hormone replacement therapy is also discussed. Dosage and administration of estrogen and progesterone are discussed, and alternative therapies are also summarized for a comprehensive overview of the pros and cons of this treatment.

National Cancer Institute MedNews:
Menopausal Hormone Replacement Therapy ◐ ◐
http://www.meb.uni-bonn.de/cancernet/600310.html

Provided by the National Cancer Institute and redistributed at this address by the University of Bonn Medical Center, this article offers a professional discussion of menopause, including symptoms and health effects. The health benefits and concerns associated with hormone replacement therapy are also discussed, including mention of a National Cancer Institute clinical trial determining if hormone replacement therapy increases a woman's risk of endometrial cancer. The future of hormone replacement therapy is also discussed, including details of other National Institutes of Health studies and important health considerations when choosing to begin hormone replacement therapy.

OncoLink: Hormones and Cancer ◐ ◐ ◐
http://www.oncolink.upenn.edu/causeprevent/hormones

The University of Pennsylvania Cancer Center provides access to articles containing information about the impact of hormones on cancers of the breast, ovary, cervix, endometrium, and prostate. Several OncoLink articles detail effective and ineffective treatment, the risk of oral contraceptives, and news and FAQs relating to ovarian cancer and ovulatory stimulation, progestin in oral contraceptives, and postmenopausal hormone replacement therapy. Resources from the National Cancer Institute, the North American Menopause Society, and MedScape are also available.

Progesterone Advocates Network:
Ovarian, Uterine, Cervical Cancer, and Hormones ◐
http://www.progestnet.com/documents/ovarian_cancers.html

The hormonal imbalances that may result in ovarian, uterine, and cervical cancers are discussed at this site of the Progesterone Advocates Network. The relative risk of ovarian cancer fatality and its relation to estrogen replacement therapy, the unopposed estrogen present in premenopausal women, and the link between oral contraceptives and endometrial/cervical cancers are reviewed. The role of progesterone in counteracting estrogen's growth stimulation is introduced.

Reuters Health Information:
High Level of Estrogen Increases Breast Cancer Risk ◐ ◐
http://www.wcn.org/news/98/Sep/ep09098a.asp

A case control study at Harvard Medical School reveals that estrogen levels may be tied to an increased risk of breast cancer among postmenopausal women. This Reuters Health Information headline presents research findings, as published in the *Journal of the National Cancer Institute*, that provide strong evidence for reducing the levels of endogenous estrogens as a means of breast cancer prevention.

Oral Contraceptives

McKinley Health Center: Pill Interactions with Other Drugs ◐ ◐
http://www.uiuc.edu/departments/mckinley/health-info/sexual/birthcon/oral-dru.html

This fact sheet offers an overview of oral contraceptive interactions with seizure medications, antifungal medications, antibiotics, and other common medications. The relative significance of interactions, adverse effects, and clinical recommendations are listed in table form.

9.10 Thyroid Gland

Overview

About.com: Thyroid Drugs ◐ ◐ ◐
http://thyroid.about.com/health/thyroid/msub9.htm

Articles, information, and Web sites on Synthroid, Armour, Thyrolar, and antithyroid medications are provided at this About.com compilation. A review of thyroid hormone replacement, recent research published in the *New England Journal of Medicine* regarding supplementation and cognitive functioning, Synthroid lawsuit details, and an article on the stability and potency problems in certain preparations are found. Guidelines for patients taking thyroid medications are presented, as are detailed product literature and related psychopharmacology.

University of Kansas School of Medicine: Medical Pharmacology Learning Modules: Thyroid and Antithyroid Drugs ◐ ◐
http://www.kumc.edu/research/medicine/pharmacology/mgordon/Endocrine/Thyroid/framethyroid.htm

Topics presented in this comprehensive teaching module include thyroid physiology and pharmacology, thyroid histology, physiological effects of triiodothyronine and thyroxine, symptoms associated with hyperthyroidism and hypothyroidism, thyroid hormone synthesis and release, regulation of thyroid function, and specific thyroid diseases. Practice questions and case studies are also available.

Antithyroid Agents

Thyroid Disease Manager: Hyperthyroidism Management with Antithyroid Drugs ◐ ◑
http://thyroidmanager.bsd.uchicago.edu/algorithms/algorithm15.htm

Algorithms provided by the University of Chicago Thyroid Disease Manager include this chart of antithyroid management protocol for hyperthyroidism. Treatment timetables and recommendations on continuation, increasing, and decreasing of dosages are illustrated.

Thyroid Hormone

American Thyroid Association: Thyroid Hormone Treatment ◐ ◑
http://www.thyroid.org/patient/brochur8.htm

An online brochure explains how the proper dosage of thyroid hormone is chosen by physicians and offers facts concerning the differences between synthetic and desiccated preparations. Symptoms of too little or too much thyroid hormone and other consumer-oriented information are presented.

Washington State Department of Health: Brief Review of Thyroid Hormone Regulation and Biological Effects of Thyroid Hormone ◐ ◑
http://www.doh.wa.gov/phl/newborn/review97.htm

Identification of over- or undertreatment of congenital hypothyroidism is the focus of this article, which discusses the basics of thyroid hormone regulation for consumer education or professional review. Basic treatment goals, including maintenance of T4 levels in the high normal range during the first three years of life, are presented.

9.11 Vascular System

Antihypertensive Agents

Alpha and Beta Blockers ◐ ◑
http://www.hypertensionmeds.com/abb.html

Alpha-and beta-blocking antihypertensives are reviewed at this pharmacology site, with select package insert access and generic, brand, and classification listings provided. Chapters on pharmacology, adverse reactions, precautions, and dosage and administration are included.

Infomed Drug Guide: Spironolactone
http://www.infomed.org/100drugs/spitoc.html

The pharmacology, indications, adverse reactions, contraindications, and risk groups associated with this aldosterone antagonist are presented as a service of the Infomed drug index. Sections provide concise review of the drug's effects, uses for primary hyperaldosteronism, and indications for other manifestations of secondary hyperaldosteronism. Additional recognized indications and a reference listing are offered.

10. PATHOLOGY AND CASE STUDIES

DigiDoc Medical Software Endocrinology Cases ○ ○
http://icarus.med.utoronto.ca/digidoc/digiendo.html
A computed tomography image in Graves' ophthalmology, radiography of acromegaly, diabetic retinopathy, and other interesting images are found at this DigiDoc Web site. Case questions and answers accompany some images.

Frontiers in Bioscience: A Tumor Atlas and Knowledge Base ○ ○ ○
http://www.bioscience.org/atlases/tumpath/tumpath.htm
This online knowledge base includes several tumors of the adrenal, thyroid, and parathyroid gland. By accessing the instructions link, visitors are explained the options for using the tumor atlas with or without a split screen. Use of the tumor tutorial without a split screen allows visitors to find information at various sites using the online resource or visualizing the appearance of tumors. Images and information may be seen by clicking the appropriate text or body organ location. A split screen atlas allows browsing with an index on the left and information and images on the right. Classifications of disease, risk factors, laboratory tests, diagnosis, clinical features, and TNM staging information are found in the endocrine system section. Separate access to text and images of the female and male reproductive system is also provided.

GeoCities: Med Files Case Studies in Endocrinology ○ ○ ○
http://www.geocities.com/HotSprings/2255/endocrine.html
The case studies and teaching files found at this Med Files site include medical management overviews of diabetes, non-insulin dependent diabetes, diabetic ketoacidosis, and teaching modules on specific thyroid diseases. Several case presentations, courtesy of Tulane University, are found, including files on precocious puberty, hirsutism, and hypertension. Miscellaneous cases include acromegaly, hyperparathyroidism, and Cushing's syndrome.

Internet Pathology Library: Diabetes Mellitus ○ ○ ○
http://www-medlib.med.utah.edu/WebPath/TUTORIAL/DIABETES/DIABETES.html

From the Internet Pathology Library of the University of Utah, this site contains a tutorial on diabetes mellitus. Images and descriptions of normal islets of Langerhans, microscopic insulitis, and microscopic deposition of amyloid may be viewed. Several other educational slides are available relating to renal, ocular, and atherosclerotic complications of diabetes mellitus. Diabetic ketoacidosis and its relation to mucormycosis is demonstrated at an online microscopic stained image.

Internet Pathology Library: Endocrine Pathology Index ○ ○ ○
http://www-medlib.med.utah.edu/WebPath/ENDOHTML/ENDOIDX.html

Provided by the University of Utah, the main tutorial menu offers an index of images related to all aspects of endocrine pathology. Included are 23 images of normal and diseased thyroid tissue, eight images of the pituitary, seven images of the parathyroid and its diseases, 25 images of the adrenal gland, and seven images of islets of Langerhans. Each link connects users to close-up gross and histologic depictions, accompanied by detailed image explanations.

Loyola University Medical Education Network: A Clinical Evaluation of the Thyroid in Health and Disease ○ ○
http://www.meddean.luc.edu/lumen/MedEd/medicine/endo/thyroid.htm

Prepared by a clinician of Loyola University Medical Center, this site provides useful clinical evaluation of the thyroid in health and disease. Individual slide presentations are available on the thyroid gland, hypothyroidism, hyperthyroidism, thyroid nodule, and thyroid malignancy.

Mallinckrodt Institute of Radiology (MIR) and Washington University Medical Center: MIR Nuclear Medicine Teaching File ○ ○ ○
http://gamma.wustl.edu/home.html

Cases without diagnoses, cases with diagnoses, and a search engine for teaching file cases are found at this site of Washington University Medical Center's nuclear medicine teaching files. Thyroid, parathyroid, testicular, renal, bone, and octreotide scintigraphy cases and evaluations for metastatic disease are accessible. Visitors will find main images, second images, a similar case search, and full history and diagnostic information included in each teaching file.

MatWeb: Pituitary Imaging Abnormalities ○ ○ ○
http://matweb.hcuge.ch/matweb/
Selected_images/pituitary__abnormalities_imaging.htm

Abnormalities viewable from this Web site include empty sella syndrome, multiple endocrine neoplasia type 1, pituitary adenoma, pituitary hypoplasia, prolactinoma, and other pathology images of the pituitary gland. Eleven reputable sources are listed, including the *New England Journal of Medicine,* the University of Kansas Medical Center, and Michigan State University. This collection contains one or more diagnostic images for each entry, clinical details of the cases, findings, discussions, and links to related information.

MatWeb: Selected Medical Images: Adrenal Abnormalities ✪ ✪ ✪
http://matweb.hcuge.ch/matweb/
Selected_images/adrenal__abnormalities_imaging.htm

Adrenal abnormalities in this image compilation include adrenal cortical adenomas, adrenal hemorrhage, congenital adrenal hyperplasia, and pheochromocytoma. A brief history, one or more images for each diagnosis, findings, and follow-up details are provided in these cases. Related links, contributing cases, references, general discussions, teaching file links, a similar case search connection, and the opportunity to view previously made comments about each case are just some of the features offered.

MatWeb: Selected Medical Images: Thyroid Abnormalities ✪ ✪ ✪
http://matweb.hcuge.ch/matweb/
Selected_images/thyroid__abnormalities_imaging.htm

Cold nodule of the thyroid, follicular adenoma, goiter, Graves' disease, hypothyroidism, subacute thyroiditis, and seven additional diagnoses are available for viewing at this site of the MATWEB database. One or several images are available for each diagnosis, with each view accompanied by a pull-down legend.

Penn State: Case Studies in Endocrinology ✪ ✪
http://www.collmed.psu.edu/endo/clincorr/clinmain.htm

The Milton S. Hershey Medical Center College of Medicine presents two case studies in endocrinology at this site, including virilizing tumors of the adrenal gland and postpartum autoimmune thyroid syndrome. Each clinical case study offers a thorough history and examination discussion, as well as the laboratory presentation, pathophysiology review, treatment, and differential diagnosis.

Tulane University Medical Center Department of Pathology and Laboratory Medicine: Case Studies in Endocrine Disorders ✪ ✪
http://www.mcl.tulane.edu/classware/pathology/
medical_pathology/endocrine_cases/casesTop.html

Cases found at this site cover evaluation of the pituitary, thyroid, parathyroid, adrenal, and reproductive endocrinology topics. Each of seven cases contains brief information on patient history and results of the physical exam, and correct answers regarding patient diagnosis and laboratory evaluations are accessible.

University of Texas Southwestern Medical Center Department of Pathology: Endocrine Masses

http://pathcuric1.swmed.edu/ScribeService/Resources/path/objectives/Endocrine/endocrine-Masses.html

This site contains a tutorial on endocrine masses, with medullary carcinoma, follicular carcinoma, papillary carcinoma, and multinodular goiter discussed in terms of their clinical and pathological findings. Images accompany each descriptive outline.

Urbana Atlas of Pathology: Endocrinology Section

http://www.med.uiuc.edu/PathAtlasf/framer/path2.html

Supported by the University of Illinois College of Medicine at Urbana-Champaign, the site offers numerous pathology images. The site includes descriptions and images of colloid goiter, thyroiditis, thymoma, and pheochromocytoma. Normal and abnormal pituitary images and an adenoma of the thyroid may be viewed.

Walter Reed Army Medical Center: Endocrine Nuclear Imaging

http://160.151.63.50/cgi-win/nuclear.exe?oEnd

Six clinical scenarios of the thyroid gland include details regarding the physical exam and several enlargeable images. The "Answer Page" offers a diagnostic conclusion, findings, a discussion with differential diagnosis, and links and references to further reading.

11. CLINICAL PRACTICE AND GUIDELINES

11.1 General Resources

American Association of Clinical Endocrinologists (AACE): Clinical Practice Guidelines ◎ ◎ ◎

http://www.aace.com/clinguideindex.htm

This site provides an index of clinical guidelines and position statements from the American Association of Clinical Endocrinologists. Guidelines for treatment of lipid disorders, diabetes mellitus, obesity, hypogonadism, thyroid carcinoma, hyperthyroidism and hypothyroidism, postmenopausal osteoporosis, thyroid nodule, and male sexual dysfunction are found. Additional practice information on the use of growth hormone in adults and the management of menopause are provided. Most information is available in either HTML or PDF format.

American Thyroid Association: Thyroid Disease Guidelines for Physicians ◎ ◎ ◎

http://www.thyroid.org/members/guidline.htm

Three guidelines for the diagnosis and management of thyroid disease are available from the American Thyroid Association at this address. Guidelines describe the use of laboratory tests in thyroid disorders, the treatment of patients with hyperthyroidism and hypothyroidism, and the treatment of patients with thyroid nodules and well-differentiated thyroid cancer. Full-text versions of the guidelines are accessible at the site.

MedPharm: Learning Modules for Endocrinology
http://www.medfarm.unito.it/education/endo.html

MedPharm provides links to 16 sources of learning modules related to endocrinology at this address. Modules include case studies in endocrine disorders, AACE thyroid treatment guidelines, thyroid testing guidelines, guidelines on complications of diabetes mellitus, diabetic neuropathy diagnosis guidelines, and osteoporosis clinical practice guidelines. Additional documents describe hyperthyroidism, hypothyroidism, familial multiple endocrine neoplasia, papillary microcarcinoma, the pathology of diabetes mellitus, and male factor infertility.

Medstudents: Endocrinology
http://www.medstudents.com.br/endoc/endoc.htm

Visitors to this address will find teaching articles written by senior medical students in the field of endocrinology. Article topics include Cushing's syndrome, osteoporosis, Grave's disease, hypothyroidism, anorexia nervosa, and Kallmann syndrome.

National Guideline Clearinghouse (NGC): Endocrine Disease Guidelines
http://www.guideline.gov/BROWSE/mesh_tree.asp?Leftkey=39109&Rightkey=39420&LevelNum=3

From the National Guideline Clearinghouse, this site offers links to guidelines on endocrine diseases. Eighty guidelines are available, and subtopics include diabetes mellitus, adrenal gland diseases, parathyroid diseases, endocrine gland neoplasms, gonadal disorders, thyroid diseases, and breast diseases. The site is fully searchable and may be browsed by disease type, treatment, or organization. The site may be customized by visitors who wish to compile their own online guideline collections.

University of Alabama School of Library and Information Studies: Endocrinology Clinical Resources (some features fee-based)
http://www.slis.ua.edu/cdlp/unthsc/clinical/endocrinology/index.htm

Endocrinology Internet resources are available through this directory, which contains a collection of clinical material by disease subtopic, as well as general endocrinology clinical resources. Professional material on adrenal diseases, breast disorders, diabetes, calcium disturbances, obesity, ovarian disorders, parathyroid diseases, pituitary diseases, and thyroid diseases is provided in the form of online textbook chapters, a variety of clinical practice guidelines, pathology indices, clinical trials details, and governmental documents. Some online texts may require a user subscription, although a wide variety of free clinical material is available.

11.2 Diabetes Mellitus

American Association of Clinical Endocrinologists (AACE): Clinical Practice Guidelines for Management of Diabetes Mellitus ○ ○ ○

http://www.aace.com/clinindex.htm

Developed by the AACE and the American College of Endocrinology, a guide to diabetes management is available from the site's Clinical Practice Guidelines link in PDF format. A year 2000 update to the original guideline adds new evidence for management and treatment of diabetes mellitus types I and II, with an emphasis on type II self-management. A systematic multidisciplinary approach is employed to achieve normal serum glucose levels, and basic requirements for implementation of the program, such as active patient participation, are stressed. Initial assessment guidelines and laboratory evaluations are reviewed, and an assessment of the patient knowledge base and motivation is presented. Patient-physician communication, as well as additional steps in assessment and follow-up are discussed in this online management model. Visitors may also access additional clinical guidelines, a clinical research database, and the Fellow Clinical Corner.

American Diabetes Association (ADA): Clinical Practice Recommendations 2000 ○ ○ ○

http://journal.diabetes.org/CareSup1Jan00.htm

The entire text of the Clinical Practice Recommendations 2000 of the American Diabetes Association may be accessed from the site on a chapter-by-chapter basis. An online search utility may be utilized or visitors may opt to directly access specific text chapters. Screening recommendations, the implications of the Diabetes Control and Complications Trial, nutrition recommendations, diabetes mellitus and exercise, management of dyslipidemia, preconception care, testing, hospital admission, and insulin administration are only a handful of the sections available. A summary of revisions, a position statement, and the Report of the Expert Committee on the Diagnosis and Classification of Diabetes Mellitus are provided.

Clinical Practice Guidelines: Diabetes ○ ○ ○

http://medicine.ucsf.edu/resources/guidelines/guidedm.html

Clinical guidelines valuable to physician practice, major diabetes studies, journal articles, textbooks, and access to patient education handouts are all provided at this comprehensive medical resource for family physicians and endocrinologists, compiled by the University of California, San Francisco. Guidelines include those of the National Guidelines Clearinghouse, the American Diabetes Association, and the 2000 Clinical Practice Recommendations of the *Diabetes Care* publication. Other major endocrine practice association guidelines are accessible, as well as discussions of the University Group Diabetes Program, the Diabetes Control and Complications Trial, and additional study articles, editorials, and PubMed abstracts. A multitude of online algorithms and textbook chapters focusing on diagnosis, therapy, and major challenges in current diabetes care are accessible.

Diabetes Care: Hospital Admission Guidelines for Diabetes Mellitus ○ ○ ○

http://www.diabetes.org/DiabetesCare/supplement/s37.htm

Guidelines for determining when a patient requires hospitalization are presented at this site and include a listing of situations appropriate for inpatient treatment and an analysis of the acute metabolic complications of diabetes. Guidelines in cases of uncontrolled diabetes and requirements for admission based on common complications and other acute medical conditions are reviewed, as a service of the American Diabetes Association.

Diagnosing Diabetes ○ ○

http://www.jr2.ox.ac.uk/Bandolier/band39/b39-4.html

A diagnostic review provides visitors with background information on the significance of glycosylated hemoglobin values, the World Health Organization data for interpretation of glucose tolerance tests, and the use of other variables in the diagnosis of diabetes.

# PART THREE

TOPICAL RESOURCES AND ORGANIZATIONS

12. PUBLIC HEALTH AND POLICY TOPICS

12.1 Advocacy

Center for Reproductive Law and Policy (CRLP)
http://www.crlp.org

The Center for Reproductive Law and Policy is a public policy organization that promotes women's reproductive rights. This home page offers information about activities in the United States and the status of reproductive rights around the world. Links to publications, press releases, and a newsletter are also available.

Insulin Dependent Diabetes Trust U.S. (IDDT U.S.)
http://www.diabetes.pair.com

The IDDT U.S. advocates for the informed choice of treatments for diabetic patients, including the continued production of natural animal insulin. This site offers updates on the latest diabetes news, suggestions on finding pork or beef insulin, notices of new glucose monitoring systems, contact details, and links to related sites.

Insulin-Free World Foundation: Government Relations
http://www.insulinfree.org/govrelations.htm

From the Insulin-Free World Foundation, this site provides links to information about diabetes advocacy and government relations. Links are included to legislative documents, the Department of Health and Human Services, the National Institutes of Health, the National Institute of Diabetes and Digestive Kidney Disease, Medicare, and state health insurance departments. Visitors will also find information on contacting senators and congressmen, details of advocacy campaigns, summaries of government funding, and overviews of current health policy.

12.2 Diabetes Mellitus

Economic Impact

University of Pittsburgh: Diabetes Health Economics Study Group ○ ○ ○
http://www.pitt.edu/~tjs/diabecon.html

The Diabetes Health Economics Study Group was created to promote discussion and raise awareness of the rising costs of diabetes treatment. Resources at the site include a directory of persons working in the area, a bibliography of papers on the topic, estimates of the cost of diabetes, economic evaluation studies in literature, online publications, and presentations and slides. Links to general diabetes resources, journals, international agencies, non-governmental organizations, and conference listings are provided.

Education and Support

Children with Diabetes ○ ○
http://www.childrenwithdiabetes.com

Children with Diabetes is a support and information network for children and families affected by diabetes. The site features up-to-date headlines related to the disorder, as well as clinical, nutritional, and research review. News and advocacy links may be accessed at this searchable site.

Diabetes Digest ○ ○
http://www.diabetesdigest.com

This online version of *Diabetes Digest* provides information for diabetics. General information includes an overview of the condition, a discussion of different types of diabetes, and a description of symptoms, treatment, care, and prevalence. Information on oral medications, insulin, glucose meters and testing, and nutrition is found, as well as an online newsletter and links to popular articles from the newsstand edition of the magazine.

Diabetes Knowledge ○ ○
http://people.ne.mediaone.net/dclc/home.html

Intended for parents of children with diabetes, this site offers advocacy information, access to recent news articles and information, and tips on applying the Individuals with Disability Education Act on behalf of their children. Product information, links to related sites, and personal page links are found.

Eli Lilly: Managing Your Diabetes: Patient Education Program ◎ ◎
http://diabetes.lilly.com/index.html

Provided by Eli Lilly, this site offers patient information on managing diabetes. Information about the disorder includes a general overview and discussions of diabetes types, blood sugar control, complications, and related problems. A section on diabetes management includes information on treatment plans, stages of care, traveling, and foot care. Meal planning and links to other diabetes sites are offered.

Epidemiology

American Diabetes Association (ADA): Council on Epidemiology and Statistics ◎ ◎
http://www.diabetes.org/councils/epidemiology/epi.html

The ADA Council on Epidemiology and Statistics offers clinical news, professional education, and research news regarding the epidemiology of diabetes and the application of epidemiological methods to the etiology and pathogenesis of diabetes and its complications. The *Professional Section Quarterly* editions are available online. Information on both postgraduate courses and research symposiums on epidemiological topics is provided.

Centers for Disease Control and Prevention (CDC): Division of Diabetes Translation ◎ ◎ ◎
http://www.cdc.gov/diabetes/index.htm

This site of the Centers for Disease Control and Prevention (CDC) provides information on the preventive aims of the division and offers access to *Diabetes at a Glance 2000,* a publication discussing CDC programs and opportunities for diabetes prevention. The National Hispanic/Latino Diabetes Initiative for Action, the National Diabetes Laboratory, and other endeavors of the CDC in preventing diabetic illness are presented at this public health resource. Connections to state-based programs, the Diabetes Today public health training program, and the Diabetes Surveillance Report of 1999 are accessible from the site. Also provided is a listing of this CDC division's initiatives and their respective Web sites, which aim to strengthen public health surveillance, conduct applied translational research, and develop state-based diabetes control programs.

NIDDK: Diabetes in African American Populations ◎ ◎
http://www.niddk.nih.gov/health/diabetes/pubs/afam/afam.htm

From the NIDDK, this site provides information on diabetes in African Americans, with sections on incidence, risk factors, effects on young people, effects on pregnant women, and complications. An explanation of how the NIDDK is specifically addressing the problem of diabetes in the African American population is provided.

NIDDK: Diabetes in American Indians and Alaska Natives ◐ ◐
http://www.niddk.nih.gov/health/diabetes/pubs/amindian/amindian.htm

From the National Institute of Diabetes and Digestive and Kidney Diseases, this site contains an index of information about diabetes in American Indians and Alaska natives, including specific demographic information and details regarding the division's related research.

NIDDK: Diabetes in Asian and Pacific Islander Americans ◐ ◐
http://www.niddk.nih.gov/health/diabetes/pubs/asianam/asianam.htm

This NIDDK Web address offers an informational brochure on diabetes in Asian and Pacific Islander Americans. There are details surrounding incidence, risk factors, pregnancy, cardiovascular health, complications, and current research. References are included.

NIDDK: Diabetes in Hispanic Americans ◐ ◐
http://www.niddk.nih.gov/health/diabetes/pubs/hispan/hispan.htm

Hispanic Americans are the focus of this fact sheet, which answers commonly asked questions relating to diabetes in this population. Major studies of diabetes in Hispanic Americans and information about incidence, risk factors, Hispanic youth, pregnant women, complications, and current research are provided. References and resources from the National Diabetes Information Clearinghouse are found.

World Health Organization (WHO): Diabetes ◐ ◐
http://www.who.int/ncd/dia

The Diabetes Programme of the World Health Organization (WHO) is responsible for providing member states with recommendations regarding strategic monitoring and prevention of diabetes. Landmarks in the development of the WHO Diabetes Programme, links to collaborating centers, global partners, internal and related external publications, and news are offered.

News

American Diabetes Association (ADA): In the News ◐ ◐ ◐
http://www.diabetes.org/ada/new.asp

Recent and continuously updated news items are accessible at this link of the American Diabetes Association. The current Scientific Session Online, articles from the press, legal and legislative updates, and access to Yahoo!'s diabetes headlines are provided. New medications, statements of the American Diabetes Association, and *In the News* archives are all available at this timely diabetes headline resource.

Diabetes News ○ ○
http://www.diabetesnews.com

The Diabetes News home page offers information on new diabetes products and islet cell transplantation as well as reports on current research in other related areas. Access to current and back issues of *Diabetes Forecast,* a health and wellness magazine of the American Diabetes Association, is provided.

Diabetes News Home ○ ○
http://www.diabetesnews.com

Diabetes News Home offers updated news articles related to diabetes. The full text of each article is provided. There is a link to archived articles, each of which is presented chronologically.

Diabetes News Library ○
http://personal.inet.fi/koti/peter.granholm/DIABET.HTM

The Diabetes News Library offers links to diabetes news sites, search engines, libraries, advice sites, dictionaries, and related articles and information.

Joslin Diabetes Center: Diabetes News ○ ○ ○
http://www.joslin.org/news/inthenews.html

The latest news in diabetes prevention, diagnosis, treatment, and cure is provided at this subsite of the Joslin Diabetes Center. Current and recently archived articles pertaining to glucose monitoring systems, research published in major medical journals, and other authoritative sources of discovery are provided. News releases on the FDA-approved laser device for obtaining blood samples, early results of clinical trials, Medicare updates, and practice guideline revisions are all included. Breaking news on investigational drugs, genetic links, and the latest on worldwide research of islet transplants are found.

Organizations

American Association of Diabetes Educators ○ ○
http://www.aadenet.org

The American Association of Diabetes Educators is a multidisciplinary organization composed of healthcare professionals who care for and educate diabetes patients. Their site provides information about diabetes legislation and advocacy issues, with details regarding CME meetings and conferences provided. Products available for purchase at the site include professional education resources, patient education materials, and patient products. A list of participating educators and contact information is found.

American Diabetes Association (ADA) ○ ○ ○
http://www.diabetes.org

The American Diabetes Association provides research, information, and advocacy in an effort to improve the lives of diabetic patients. The site features diabetes in the news and current association headlines, in addition to advocacy and detailed disorders reviews. Facts and figures, special information for the newly diagnosed patient, and educational material for teachers and healthcare providers are accessible. Links to MEDLINE searches, as well as the association's professional journal, are found.

Canadian Diabetes Association ○ ○
http://www.diabetes.ca

Promoting health through diabetes research, education, and advocacy, the Canadian Diabetes Association offers information for consumers and professionals alike, with general information about diabetes, prevalence statistics, and current research initiatives. A clinical and scientific section of the site offers information for clinicians, and a diabetes educator section is found. Links to publications, information about conferences and events, awards, and the clinical practice guidelines of the association are found.

Diabetes UK ○ ○
http://www.diabetes.org.uk

Diabetes UK, formerly the British Diabetic Association provides education, support, and news on the latest in diabetes research and advocacy. Professional conference and course information, publications, and association reports are found at the site, in addition to sections on healthy eating and living for diabetic patients.

International Diabetes Federation ○ ○
http://www.idf.org

The International Diabetes Federation works to improve the lives of people with diabetes, providing information about the disorder, its management and treatment, and the organization's activities, events, and publications.

International Society for Pediatric and Adolescent Diabetes ○ ○ ○
http://www.ispad.org

The International Society for Pediatric and Adolescent Diabetes is a professional organization of doctors and scientists in the field providing information about scientific meetings, membership, and educational activities of the society. Consensus guidelines for managing insulin-dependent patients, abstracts from annual meetings, and links to articles authored by society members may be viewed. Topical coverage of ketoacidosis and the significance of glycosylated hemoglobin values is found at this searchable site.

Juvenile Diabetes Foundation (JDF) International ○ ○
http://www.jdf.org

Providing diabetes research support, patient education, and advocacy, the JDF maintains a Web site with extensive resources for the diabetes community. There is a news section with article summaries as well as the full-text articles, a section providing clinical trial information, and additional features devoted to daily care and living with diabetes, questions and answers on important topics, and new book summaries. A broad range of additional information is available through the Links Section, leading the visitor to other resources within the JDF and from government agencies as well as research and treatment centers. Useful reports on abstracts on research topics are accessed through the Research Section.

National Diabetes Education Initiative ○ ○ ○
http://www.ndei.org

The National Diabetes Education Initiative is an educational program designed for endocrinologists, diabetologists, primary care physicians, and other healthcare professionals. Its searchable site offers a news section with late-breaking developments in the field, a literature section with abstracts from recent journal articles, and clinical guidelines for diabetes care. Noteworthy events, clinical data on diabetes, and highlights from annual conferences are accessible, in addition to details on related continuing medical education.

Research

Diabetes Center of the Albert Einstein College of Medicine ○ ○
http://medicine.aecom.yu.edu/diabetes/DC.htm

The Diabetes Center is committed to research into the causes and treatment of diabetes, development and evaluation of new techniques in education and healthcare delivery, and rendering of patient care and education. There is information about the Diabetes Research and Training Center, the Diabetes Clinical Research Unit, and the Montefiore-Einstein Clinical Diabetes Center.

Diabetes Education and Research Center ○ ○
http://www.libertynet.org/diabetes

A nonprofit organization, the Diabetes Education and Research Center provides worldwide service to diabetes patients. Their site provides information about the center, answers to frequently asked questions, and information about classes and events. Links to archived news articles and related sites are found.

Diabetes Institutes Foundation ◎ ◎
http://www.dif.org

The Diabetes Institutes Foundation supports research at the Leonard R. Strelitz Diabetes Institutes of Eastern Virginia Medical School. The site provides information about the foundation, their supporters, and the patients they have treated. Links to diabetes and nutrition topics, special event details, and related sites are offered.

Insulin-Free World Foundation ◎ ◎ ◎
http://www.insulin-free.org

The Insulin-Free World Foundation provides comprehensive information on the current state of diabetes research. Articles specific to type 1 and type 2 diabetes, diabetes facts and statistics, and details regarding a current diabetes prevention trial are found. Interesting coverage of pancreas transplantation, islet cell replacement, immunology, and mechanical solutions is offered, as is a discussion regarding the political and economical aspects of discovering a cure.

Statistics

Insulin-Free World Foundation: Diabetes Facts and Statistics ◎ ◎ ◎
http://www.insulinfree.org/factsgen.htm

From the Insulin-Free World Foundation, this site offers facts and statistics about diabetes. Statistics include diabetes death rates, statistics from the National Institute of Diabetes and Kidney Diseases, and statistics from the Department of Health and Human Services. Also provided are a list of urgent reasons to cure diabetes, a national diabetes fact sheet, and an overview of diabetes and its impact.

Insulin-Free World Foundation: Facts and Statistics about Islets ◎ ◎
http://www.insulinfree.org/factsisl.htm

Provided by the Insulin-Free World Foundation, this site offers facts and statistics about islets. The site contains 1999 Islet Transplant Registry statistics, islet transplant records from 1996, and the International Islet Transplant Registry from 1996. There are also statistics related to glucose control with functioning islets.

Insulin-Free World Foundation: Pancreas Facts and Statistics ◎ ◎
http://www.insulinfree.org/factspan.htm

The Insulin-Free World Foundation provides facts and statistics about pancreas transplantation at this subsite. Transplant statistics from the International Pancreas Transplant Registry, information about the average cost of a transplant, the total number of transplants in 1998, and the number of worldwide pancreas transplants from the beginning of the procedure's implementation through 1996 are offered. From the United Network for Organ Sharing, the site provides facts and statistics about transplantation and transplant reports and studies.

NIDDK: Diabetes Statistics ◎ ◎ ◎
http://www.niddk.nih.gov/health/diabetes/pubs/dmstats/dmstats.htm

Provided by the National Institute of Diabetes and Digestive and Kidney Diseases, this site contains diabetes statistics, including prevalence of diabetes, incidence of diabetes, mortality rates, and prevalence of diabetes broken down by age, sex, and ethnicity. There are also discussions of types of diabetes, complications, cost, diagnostic criteria, and treatment. An appendix and references are found.

12.3 Estrogens, Environmental

Center for Bioenvironmental Research of Tulane and Xavier Universities: Environmental Estrogens and Other Hormones ◎ ◎ ◎
http://www.tmc.tulane.edu/ecme/eehome

From the Center for Bioenvironmental Research of Tulane and Xavier universities, this site offers a comprehensive resource for information on environmental estrogens and other hormones. The site offers links to news articles and announcements related to environmental hormones, educational fact sheets on environmental estrogens and other chemicals, research briefs, answers to frequently asked questions, links to related sites, notices of upcoming conferences, conference summaries, and a searchable bibliography of citations and abstracts from scientific articles describing environmental hormone research. Visitors can also access a timeline of important milestones in environmental hormone research and media articles discussing environmental hormones and related topics.

Tulane University: Environmental Estrogens and Other Hormones ◎ ◎ ◎
http://www.som.tulane.edu/ecme/eehome

Maintained by the Center for Bioenvironmental Research of Tulane and Xavier Universities, this site provides information about natural compounds and synthetic chemicals that mimic natural estrogens. The table of contents includes an overview of estrogen and a definition of environmental estrogen. There are discussions of modes of action, sources of environmental estrogen, their effects, environmental estrogens versus hormones, and phytoestrogens. There is also information about the hormone system, evidence of danger, and interpreting the findings. There are news articles and links to related sites.

12.4 Hazards, Environmental

Endocrine Disruptors Research Initiative ◉ ◉ ◉
http://www.epa.gov/endocrine

This site introduces the hypothesis that environmental chemicals interact with the human endocrine system to create a variety of health hazards. This site chronicles the efforts of the Endocrine Disruptor Working Group of the National Science and Technology Council's Committee on the Environment and Natural Resources in investigating this hypothesis. Fact sheets, research publications, and listings of upcoming meetings are detailed, and visitors can search the Federal Research Project Inventory for 1996 and the Global Research Project Inventory for 1998. Additionally, the site provides listings of participating agencies and links to related sites.

Endocrine/Estrogen Letter ◉ ◉
http://www.eeletter.com

A global press newsletter, the *Endocrine/Estrogen Letter* seeks to provide accurate, unbiased information about issues related to endocrine disrupters. Subscription to the newsletter, published every two weeks, is available for a fee. Visitors may view recent articles and sample issues at the site, as well as access related academic and scientific pages on endocrine disrupters, environmental activist groups, government sites, journals, phytoestrogen sites, and information on brominated flame retardant material.

Environmental Protection Agency: Endocrine Disruptor Screening Program ◉ ◉
http://www.epa.gov/scipoly/oscpendo

Maintained by the Environmental Protection Agency Office of Science Coordination and Policy, this site provides information about the endocrine glands and hormones and how certain chemicals may affect the endocrine system. Information about the Endocrine Disruptor Screening Program and the current status of implementation is reviewed. Controversy surrounding endocrine disruptors and an overview of plans for appropriate regulatory action are summarized.

Physicians for Social Responsibility: Endocrine Disruptors ◉ ◉
http://www.psr.org/edpage.htm

Articles on endocrine disrupters and the current state of this scientific debate offer information on environmental effects on reproductive function, regulatory actions intended to protect public health, and access to a current publication that explores the effects of synthetic chemicals on the endocrine system. A connection to the Environmental Protection Agency's related advisory committee is found, and research updates provide news on the International Programme on Chemical Safety (IPCS).

World Wildlife Fund (WWF) Canada: Endocrine Disrupting Chemicals ⊙ ⊙ ⊙

http://www.wwfcanada.org/hormone-disruptors

The WWF Canada Web Guide to Endocrine Disrupting Chemicals offers information about the functions of the endocrine system and potential endocrine disrupters. The site features a listing of these chemicals, including various herbicides, fungicides, insecticides, and industrial chemicals and contaminants. The site also describes the effects of disrupters on reproduction, in addition to their hazardous effects on immune function, cancer, brain development, and behavior. Information is provided about efforts to overcome this problem, and links to related publications are accessible.

12.5 Legislation and Public Policy

Endocrine Society: Public Affairs ⊙ ⊙ ⊙

http://www.endo-society.org/pubaffai/pubaffai.htm

Maintained by the Endocrine Society, this site offers links to public affairs news related to the discipline. Current and recent headlines link to full-text versions of articles, and society press releases are accessible, including commentary from the society addressed to the FDA, the House Appropriations Subcommittee, and the National Institutes of Health. Media advisories, national statements and recommendations, and additional testimony of the organization are found.

Health Resources and Services Administration (HRSA): Legislative and Regulatory Activities ⊙ ⊙

http://www.hrsa.gov/osp/dot/legislative.htm

Maintained by the Health Resources and Services Administration, this site offers information about legislative and regulatory activities surrounding organ tissue procurement and transplantation. A fact sheet on improving the nation's organ transplantation system, a news brief, and a chronology of recent events related to the subject matter are found.

12.6 Screening/Prevention

General Prevention Programs

**Centers for Disease Control
and Prevention (CDC): Division of Diabetes Translation** ○ ○ ○
http://www.cdc.gov/diabetes/index.htm
This site of the CDC provides information on the preventive aims of the division and offers access to *Diabetes at a Glance 2000,* a publication discussing CDC programs and opportunities for diabetes prevention. The National Hispanic/Latino Diabetes Initiative for Action, the National Diabetes Laboratory, and other endeavors of the CDC in preventing diabetic illness are presented at this public health resource. Connections to state-based programs, the Diabetes Today public health training program, and the Diabetes Surveillance Report of 1999 are accessible from the site. Connecting to the projects link takes visitors to a complete listing of this CDC division's initiatives and their respective Web sites that aim to strengthen public health surveillance, conduct applied translational research, and develop state-based diabetes control programs.

Cholesterol

Cholesterol Screening in Asymptomatic Adults, Revisited ○ ○ ○
http://www.acponline.org/journals/annals/01mar96/garber.htm
The American College of Physicians-American Society of Internal Medicine assesses the role of serum lipid level screening in adults with this analysis of clinical trials, supplemented by data from the Framingham Heart Study. Populations most likely to benefit from cholesterol screening, treatment effectiveness, and the association of cholesterol and all-cause mortality are discussed. Other aspects of screening reviewed include persons with familial hypercholesterolemia, the potential role of other tests in discovering high-risk lipid profiles, cost-effectiveness of screening, and the frequency with which screening should be administered. References and a connection to a cross-referenced clinical guideline for lipid profile screening are found.

Diabetes Mellitus

allHealth.com: Early Screening for Diabetes Cost-effective ○ ○
http://www1.allhealth.com/conditions/news/0,4800,2_120789,00.html
A Reuters Health report found at this Web address provides highlights of a report in a recent issue of the *Journal of the American Medical Association,* which concluded that early diagnosis and treatment of non-insulin dependent diabetes mellitus (NIDDM)

proves to be cost effective. Research of the Centers for Disease Control and Prevention (CDC) Diabetes Cost-Effectiveness Study calls for widespread screening and its particular effectiveness in preventing serious diabetic complications.

Columbia-Presbyterian Medical Center: Screening for Diabetes Mellitus ✺ ✺

http://cpmcnet.columbia.edu/texts/gcps/gcps0029.html

Diabetes mellitus screening recommendations are provided through this Columbia-Presbyterian Medical Center site. A general recommendation is followed by discussions of incidence, accuracy of screening tests, effectiveness of early detection, recommendations of other groups, and clinical intervention. Reference citations are also provided.

Cost-Effectiveness of Screening for Type 2 Diabetes Mellitus ✺ ✺

http://www.ncpreventionpartners.org/dmdxcare/index.htm

The slides found at this online series outline findings of the Centers for Disease Control and Prevention Cost-Effectiveness Study Group; graph the average age of diagnosis with and without screening strategies; graph the differences in disease complications based on screening protocols; and provide further information that demonstrates the economic and physical benefits of early detection and complication prevention. Preventive care and common interventions are outlined.

Diabetes Care: Screening for Gestational Diabetes Mellitus ✺ ✺ ✺

http://www.diabetes.org/diabetescare/supplement298/B14.htm

A *Diabetes Care* supplement highlights the proceedings of the Fourth International Workshop-Conference on Gestational Diabetes Mellitus at this site. Visitors will find commentary regarding the purposes of screening, a table outlining maternal risk factors in gestational diabetes, and the sensitivity and specificity of the oral glucose challenge and glycated protein screening. Investigations of the utility of home blood glucose monitoring, alternatives to the oral glucose screen, and pros and cons of universal screening are discussed.

Michigan Diabetes Control Program: Community Screening for Diabetes Recommendations ✺

http://www.diabetes-midon.org/scrning.html

The document found at this site discusses recommendations for diabetes screening in community programs, emphasizing issues to consider in providing widespread public screening and maintaining high-quality procedures. Blood glucose criteria used for referral to additional diagnostic testing is provided.

NIDDK: Diabetes Prevention Program ○ ○ ○
http://www.preventdiabetes.com

Details on the NIDDK Diabetes Prevention Program, the first nationwide research study designed to discover whether type 2 diabetes can be prevented through diet and exercise or medication, are presented at the site. Contact information and Web sites of the medical centers nationwide participating in the study may be accessed. Professionals may wish to view the medical description of the Diabetes Prevention Program, which includes study objectives and secondary research questions, or to view recruitment goals at the accessible press release. Consumer health information is available at the *Millennium Newsletter,* and other diabetes organization and resource sites are accessible.

Quick Reference Guide to Diabetes for Healthcare Providers ○ ○
http://www.diabetes-midon.org/Chapters/QuickCh1.htm

Populations to be screened for diabetes, diabetes diagnosis in adults and children, and normal and abnormal values of the three-hour glucose tolerance test for gestational diabetes are reviewed at this physician's checklist for diabetes mellitus screening.

Hypertension

National Institutes of Health (NIH): Screening for Hypertension ○ ○ ○
http://text.nlm.nih.gov/cps/www/cps.9.html

Screening recommendations for both children and adults are discussed at this site, provided by the National Library of Medicine. The accuracy of screening tests, the usefulness of early detection, and recommendations of other prominent organizations are reviewed. The article presents a complete review of the current literature, with overviews of clinical trials and studies of clinical causes.

Oregon Health Sciences University: Screening for Hypertension ○ ○
http://medir.ohsu.edu/~ohsuhtxt/cps/cps019.html

This update, prepared by the United States Preventive Services Task Force, provides recommendations for hypertension screening, with discussion of screening accuracy, effectiveness of early detection, and a review of recommendations from other private groups and government organizations. Links to related recommendations of the task force are provided throughout the text on topics such as alcohol consumption, physical activity, and smoking.

Ray Williams Institute of Paediatric Endocrinology: Age of Screening for Hypertension ⊙ ⊙
http://www.rwi.nch.edu.au/apegbook/diabn114.htm

Blood pressure screening in children with diabetes mellitus is discussed at this site, with information on factors influencing readings and a table outlining hypertension by age group. Recommendations regarding diagnostic evaluation and considerations with regard to pharmacologic therapy are introduced.

Obesity

Columbia-Presbyterian Medical Center: Screening for Obesity ⊙ ⊙
http://cpmcnet.columbia.edu/texts/gcps/gcps0031.html

Provided by the Columbia-Presbyterian Medical Center, this site offers a guide to screening for obesity. A general recommendation is presented, followed by discussions of incidence, accuracy of screening tests, effectiveness of early detection, recommendations of other groups, and clinical intervention.

National Library of Medicine (NLM): Guide to Clinical Preventive Services: Screening for Obesity ⊙ ⊙ ⊙
http://text.nlm.nih.gov/cps/www/cps.27.html

Recommendations for periodic weight and height measurements are made at this site, along with discussion of screening test accuracy, effectiveness of early detection, professional organization recommendations, and other information that favors obesity screening.

Pediatric Screening

American Academy of Pediatrics: Issues in Newborn Screening ⊙ ⊙
http://www.aap.org/policy/04619.html

This policy statement of the American Academy of Pediatrics addresses newborn screening issues related to phenylketonuria (PKU), congenital hypothyroidism, and further recommendations regarding screening of neonates in clinical practice. Elements of a neonatal screening program, recommendations regarding testing of siblings of children previously diagnosed with one of the disorders of the screening panel, and development of newborn screening protocols are discussed.

Emory University: Screening for Metabolic Disorders ⊙ ⊙ ⊙
http://www.emory.edu/WHSC/GENETICSLAB/biochem/screen.htm

The importance of early and accurate diagnosis of inborn errors of metabolism is stressed at this online article, which emphasizes that all too often these disorders go unrecognized. Predominant clinical signs of disease to be aware of are listed, and selective screenings are indicated where the clinical manifestations listed are present. Comprehensive and general screens to order are presented, with possible initial findings mentioned.

Lexi-Comp Clinical Reference Library: Newborn Screening for Phenylketonuria and Congenital Hypothyroidism ○ ○ ○

http://informatics.drake.edu/lth/html/chapter/mono/ch015700.htm#ch015700

The newborn screening for classic PKU and its variants is reviewed, with an abstract of the test's purpose, reference range, possible panic range, and considerations with regard to false negative and false positive results. The Guthrie method and other methodologies are discussed, and additional information on phenylketonuria, related defects, and dietary measures to be taken are reviewed. A connection to screening for neonatal hypothyroidism is found, which also outlines the characteristic serum findings of the disorder, reference range, test limitations, and other screening considerations.

Thyroid Disease

American College of Physicians/American Society of Internal Medicine (ACP-ASIM): Screening for Thyroid Disease ○ ○ ○

http://www.acponline.org/sci-policy/thyralgo.htm

A position paper on screening for thyroid disease is found at this site of the ACP-ASIM, in addition to a related background paper. Recommendations include screening for subclinical thyroid dysfunction, as well as for overt thyroid disease. A guideline summary may be quickly viewed, or visitors may opt to access the entire text. A glossary of clinical terminology is provided at the bottom of the document, and material on algorithm development for clinical guideline production is accessible.

American Thyroid Association: Guidelines for Detection of Thyroid Dysfunction ○ ○ ○

http://archinte.ama-assn.org/issues/v160n11/ffull/isa90012.html

This screening and diagnosis guideline, published in the online *Annals of Internal Medicine,* defines an optimal approach to identification of patients with thyroid dysfunction. Recommendations of the American Thyroid Association for screening processes and the particularly compelling indications for testing in women are reviewed.

Columbia-Presbyterian Medical Center: Screening for Thyroid Disease ○ ○ ○

http://cpmcnet.columbia.edu/texts/gcps/gcps0030.html

The accuracy of screening tests, information on early detection, and other discussion related to screening for thyroid disease are topics found at this site. Noted is the fact that professional organizations do not ordinarily recommend routine screening for thyroid disease, with the exception of congenital hypothyroidism. Certain populations may benefit from thyroid screening, and discussion of these candidates is provided. Monitoring of patients with a history of thyroid dysfunction and information on remaining alert for subtle or nonspecific symptoms of thyroid dysfunction are discussed.

Journal of the American Medical Association: Cost-effectiveness of Thyroid Screening ○ ○ ○

http://www.glandcentral.com/physician_info/jama_article.html

An overview of findings from a study conducted to evaluate the cost-effectiveness of periodic thyroid dysfunction screening is found at this site of Gland Central. A comparison of this practice with other generally accepted medical screenings is made and the routine evaluation of serum TSH is reviewed. Commentary on the level of cost-effectiveness is provided. Visitors may opt to open an audio file discussion by clicking on the RealAudio link.

12.7 Patient Education and Support

American Dietetic Association (ADA) ○ ○ ○

http://www.eatright.org

The American Dietetic Association is a professional organization that offers support, training, and services to members. For professionals, the site offers a catalog of publications, bibliographies, and links to press releases, position papers, and the *Journal of the American Dietetic Association*. For consumers, the site provides daily nutrition tips, a catalog of publications, a reading list, featured articles, nutrition fact sheets, and information on the food guide pyramid. There is a dietitian listing, information on government affairs, and links to related sites.

Center for Current Research ○ ○ (some features fee-based)

http://www.lifestages.com/health/index.html

This valuable service offers patients summaries of recent medical research on specified disease topics, derived from database searches of articles from the leading medical journals. A wide range of disease topics is found at the site. Alternatively, users may request information on an unlisted topic and will be returned thorough disease overviews. A fee is required for these resources, and the site includes ordering details and a description of all features of the service.

Children with Diabetes ⊙ ⊙ ⊙
http://www.childrenwithdiabetes.com

Children with Diabetes is an online community for young diabetic patients and their friends and families, with links to news articles and updates, a team of physicians available to answer questions from users, and archives of past questions and answers. Information about food and diet, a comprehensive listing of diabetes camps, and connections to articles for parents, kids, adults, and friends are offered. Message boards, chat rooms, and advocacy details are included, in addition to links to major diabetes associations. Regional information and support are provided.

Endocrine Society: Fact Sheets ⊙ ⊙ ⊙
http://www.endo-society.org/pubaffai/factshee.htm

From the Endocrine Society, this site offers links to fact sheets on endocrine-related topics. Topics include the following: animal research, benign prostatic hypertrophy, birth defects, breast cancer, congenital adrenal hyperplasia, contraception, Cushing's syndrome, eating disorders and body weight issues, endometriosis, environmental estrogens, female infertility, genetics, hirsutism, hormone rhythms, male infertility, menopause, osteoporosis, premature birth, premenstrual syndrome, prostate cancer, respiratory distress syndrome, short stature, stress-related disease, thyroid disorders, Turner's syndrome, and diabetes mellitus.

EndocrineWeb ⊙ ⊙ ⊙
http://www.endocrineweb.com

EndocrineWeb.com provides a searchable patient education site about endocrine disorders and endocrine surgery. Articles on the specialty of endocrinology, endocrine surgery, thyroid and parathyroid glands, adrenal glands, diabetes, osteoporosis, and endocrine diseases of the pancreas encompass everything from diagnosis to treatment. Each review provides links to information on specific topics and terms within this colorful, illustrated, and user-friendly site.

Family's Guide to Diabetes ⊙ ⊙
http://diabetes.cbyc.com

The Family's Guide to Diabetes offers a frame or non-frame site version, including information about insulin pumps, a chat room, and a bulletin board. Articles on symptoms, dietary management, and other Internet resources are provided. The site is part of the Diabetes Web Ring, and additional sites in the chain may be consecutively accessed.

Hormone Foundation: Treatment Options for Menopause ⊙ ⊙ ⊙
http://www.hormone.org/contents.html

Maintained by the Hormone Foundation, this page offers an index of information related to treatment options for menopause. All information is provided by the foundation. There are more than 20 articles on a variety of topics including urogenital atrophy, depression, osteoporosis, heart disease, breast cancer, designer estrogens, and mammography.

Human Growth Foundation ○ ○ ○
http://www.hgfound.org
The Human Growth Foundation offers education, support, research, and advocacy for patients with growth-related disorders and includes information appropriate for patients about human growth hormone deficiency, Cushing's syndrome, hypothyroidism, nutritional short stature, intrauterine growth retardation, Russell-Silver syndrome, disproportionate short stature, and achondroplasia. Articles on growth hormone treatment and adult hormone therapy are provided, as well as links to support groups, clinical trials, grant programs, and publications.

International Diabetic Athletes Association (IDAA) ○ ○
http://www.diabetes-exercise.org
The International Diabetic Athletes Association supports diabetics who participate in fitness activities. The site offers membership details and information about regional chapters and support groups. A product catalog and a calendar of upcoming events are posted, as well as links to related sites.

Kelly G. Ripken Program ○ ○ ○
http://thyroid-ripken.med.jhu.edu/offers.htm
This Johns Hopkins Resource for Thyroid Education and Patient Care describes the programs services for those diagnosed with serious thyroid illness. Links to general and specialized thyroid information, details on Kelly's program of care, the Kelly screening program, and answers to questions from Johns Hopkins thyroid specialists are offered.

Kidney Pancreas Transplant Group ○ ○
http://www.egroups.com/group/kptx/info.html
Part of eGroups, this site offers a message board for kidney and pancreas transplant recipients. It is intended to provide support and information for patients and other interested readers.

Medicines for People with Diabetes ○ ○
http://www.niddk.nih.gov/health/diabetes/pubs/med/index.htm
From the NIDDK, this site provides a booklet of information on medicine for people with diabetes. A listing of diabetes medications is presented, and discussions provide information on type 1 and type 2 diabetic treatments, low blood sugar, and help with recognizing whether or not prescribed medicines are working.

MEDLINEplus Health Information: Endocrine Overview ◎ ◎
http://medlineplus.adam.com/ency/article/002351.htm

Part of adam.com, this site provides an overview of the endocrine system, with a disorder listing classified by gland. Links to further information on the hypothalamus, testes, myxedema, goiter, thyrotoxicosis, renal calculi, Addison's disease, adrenogenital syndrome, Cushing's syndrome, pheochromocytoma, dwarfism, acromegaly, diabetes, gigantism, diabetes insipidus, diabetes mellitus, and hypoglycemia are provided, courtesy of the National Library of Medicine.

NIDDK: Financial Help for Diabetes Care ◎ ◎
http://www.niddk.nih.gov/health/diabetes/summary/finanass/finanass.htm

Maintained by the NIDDK, this site provides information on financial help for diabetes care. Details pertaining to Medicaid programs, the Department of Veterans Affairs, the Hill-Burton Program, the Bureau of Primary Health Care, and local public health departments are provided, as well as contact information for the Health Care Financing Administration Office of Beneficiary Relations.

Society for Endocrinology ◎ ◎ ◎
http://www.endocrinology.org

The Society for Endocrinology promotes the advancement of public education in endocrinology. Resources available through the site include an overview of the society, a calendar of events, conference details, information on training courses, a member's handbook, information on journals and other publications, and links to related sites. Details of the society's Young Endocrinologists Committee are also provided. The site also offers an abstract search tool for the *Journal of Endocrinology* and the *Journal of Molecular Endocrinology*, as well as full text of articles published in the society's journal *Endocrine-Related Cancer*.

Support-Group.com ◎ ◎ ◎
http://www.support-group.com

Ample bulletin boards and online chat opportunities are found at this site, specifically geared toward patient-support-related information on the Internet. Over 200 disease categories provide access to several thousand Internet links on the respective disorders. Consumer-oriented background information, organizational links, FAQs, and government information sites are all accessible at Support-Group.com. The A-to-Z topic listing includes pages on diabetes, Graves' disease, hypothyroidism, Klinefelter's syndrome, and a host of additional endocrine-related disorders.

ThyCa: Thyroid Cancer Survivors' Association ◎ ◎ ◎
http://www.thyca.org

This site facilitates patient education, for a better understanding of thyroid cancer; online forums, so that others may learn from personal experieneces; and opportunities for communication among healthcare professionals and patients. News, current research, merchandise, and support group links are provided at this award-winning site.

Thyroid Foundation of America ○ ○ ○
http://www.tsh.org

Provided by the Thyroid Foundation of America, this site contains a patient's guide to thyroid disease. Links to articles on hypothyroidism, Graves' disease, depression and thyroid illness, and management of a thyroid nodule are available. A glossary of terms, answers to Frequently Asked Questions, and updates on the latest in thyroid research are also provided by the Foundation. Links to additional patient and physician information pages on the Internet are offered.

Thyroid Society for Education and Research ○ ○ ○
http://www.the-thyroid-society.org

he Thyroid Society for Education and Research features an illustrated explanation of thyroid disease. There are answers to Frequently Asked Questions, a calendar of hot topics, and links to educational resources. Information is provided about research programs and stipends for medical students. An extensive list of thyroid-related documents is available for download, and there are links to featured articles from professional journals, as well as to other related resources.

13. SUBSPECIALTY TOPICS

13.1 Andropause

Andropause.com: Impact of Low Bioavailable Testosterone ◎ ◎
http://www.andropause.com/impact.html

Typical responses to low bioavailable testosterone are listed at this Web reference, including decreased libido, muscle mass, and strength. Information on testosterone's sexual as well as metabolic functions and a discussion of the andropause literature are offered.

MidLife Passages: Andropause or Viropause ◎ ◎
http://www.midlife-passages.com/hormone.htm

An interesting presentation of the andropause syndrome, associated with lack or absence of testosterone, is introduced at the site, with a review of symptoms and the gradual progression of testicular function decline contrasted with the female menopause. A number of causes of acute testicular failure, diagnosis of andropause, and a table outlining normal androgen values are shown. Complete management is detailed, and in-depth discussion of the various forms of testosterone replacement available is offered.

13.2 Drug Abuse, Endocrinologic and Metabolic Effects

About.com: Alcoholism: Alcohol Metabolism ◎ ◎
http://alcoholism.about.com/health/alcoholism/library/blnaa35.htm?iam=mt&terms=+metabolism

About.com offers this resource on alcohol metabolism from the National Institute on Alcohol Abuse and Alcoholism (NIAAA). Text and graphs describe the metabolic process of alcohol, factors influencing alcohol absorption and metabolism, and the effects of alcohol metabolism on body systems. Commentary by an NIAAA director concludes the article, and references are included.

emedicine: Alcoholic Ketoacidosis ⊙ ⊙ ⊙
http://www.emedicine.com/EMERG/topic21.htm

This continuing medical education publication offers an overview of alcoholic ketoacidosis (AKA). An introduction to AKA includes a general background discussion, accompanied by summaries of pathophysiology and frequency. Typical clinical history and physical presentation is described, followed by summaries of differential diagnoses, typical laboratory work-up, and treatment details. Medications typically prescribed for AKA are summarized in table form, including drug name, contraindications, drug interactions, pregnancy category, and precautions. Follow-up care guidelines and CME review questions conclude the article. A bibliography of references is also available.

emedicine: Cocaine Toxicity ⊙ ⊙
http://emedicine.com/EMERG/topic102.htm

This continuing medical education article reviews the clinical aspects of cocaine toxicity. An extensive introduction includes a history of use and abuse, the drug and its pharmacology, drug interactions, and pathophysiology. Specific system effects are d

Health Aspects of Cannabis ⊙ ⊙
http://users.lycaeum.org/~painter/ENDWAR/marij1.html

This article from *Pharmacologic Reviews* offers a thorough overview of scientific studies documenting the acute and chronic effects of cannabis, possible adverse health effects, and therapeutic uses of the drug. Endocrine and metabolic effects of the drug are discussed, including possible changes in male sex hormone, female reproductive effects, and investigations into possible hypoglycemic effects.

13.3 Genetics

American College of Medical Genetics (ACMG) ⊙ ⊙
http://www.faseb.org/genetics/acmg/index.html

The ACMG is an organization of biochemical, clinical, cytogenic, medical, and molecular geneticists and genetic counselors providing education, resources, and a voice for the medical genetics profession. This site offers ACMG policy statements, standards, and guidelines for clinical genetics laboratories as well as assessment, counseling, and testing guidelines for genetic susceptibility to breast and ovarian cancer. Also provided is information on the college's annual meeting and official journal titled *Genetics in Medicine*, focus group updates, links to related sites including the ACMG Foundation, and comprehensive organizational and membership information.

American Society of Human Genetics (ASHG)
http://www.faseb.org/genetics/ashg/ashgmenu.htm

The ASHG home page provides society policy statements, reports, and publications; an online newsletter; information about the *American Journal of Human Genetics;* and details concerning the ASHG annual meeting. Also included is educational information for those interested in careers in genetics, an application for the ASHG American Association for the Advancement of Science Congressional Fellowship Program, a history of human genetics organizations, and organizational and membership information.

Centers for Disease Control and Prevention (CDC): Office of Genetics and Disease Prevention
http://www.cdc.gov/genetics

Part of the Centers for Disease Control and Prevention, the Office of Genetics and Disease Prevention offers current information to public health professionals, including genetics in the news, recent scientific literature, and upcoming events. Information about the organization and training opportunities is also provided, as well as links to related resources on the Internet.

Endocrine Society: Endocrinology and Birth Defects
http://www.endo-society.org/pubaffai/factshee/birthdef.htm

Created by the Endocrine Society, this fact sheet provides information about endocrinology and birth defects. An overview of birth defects and causes, as well as a discussion of cures for birth defects and the role of endocrinology in advancing cures, is found.

Genetic Alliance
http://www.geneticalliance.org

The Genetic Alliance is an international group composed of individuals, healthcare professionals, and genetic support organizations. Their site offers connections to support groups listed by genetic condition, organization name, and services offered. Useful resources on bioethics, careers in genetics, educational resources, ethnocultural issues, and genetics are found.

Human Biological Data Interchange
http://www.hbdi.org

The Human Biological Data Interchange is a resource for genetic research in diabetes, thyroid disease, and autism. The organization recruits families to answer medical questionnaires and submit blood samples that are analyzed by researchers around the world in genetic and other studies. Information for researchers at the site includes scientific references, researcher applications, and family catalogs. The site also contains details for families wishing to participate.

National Center for Biotechnology Information: Online Mendelian Inheritance in Man (OMIM) ◉ ◉ ◉

http://www3.ncbi.nlm.nih.gov/Omim

Researchers at Johns Hopkins have authored this database of human genes and genetic disorders, developed for the World Wide Web by the National Center for Biotechnology Information. Clinical overviews and detailed literature coverage of recognized genetic diseases are offered, as well as links to the Entrez database of MEDLINE articles and sequence information. Visitors can search the OMIM Database, OMIM Gene Map, and OMIM Morbid Map (a catalog of cytogenetic map locations organized by disease) from the site. Information on the OMIM numbering system, details on creating links to OMIM, site updates, OMIM statistics, information on citing OMIM in literature, and the OMIM gene list are all found at the site. Connections are available to allied resources, and the complete text of OMIM and gene maps can be downloaded from the site.

13.4 Geriatric Endocrinology

American Diabetes Association (ADA): Endocrinology of Aging in the Time of Prometheus ◉

http://www.diabetes.org/pg99/Sessions/morley.asp

This session summary offers an interesting briefing on hormonal secretion decline as one ages; the possibility of its appropriateness as a physiologic response to an aging organism; and other statements regarding the state of the art of the endocrinology of aging.

International Society of Andrology: Endocrinology of Aging in Males ◉

http://www.upmc.edu/isa/97Sep/huhtaniemi.htm

The endocrinology of aging in males is discussed at this page of the International Society of Andrology. Data on testicular endocrinology and Leydig cell failure and discussion of the current knowledge of age-related androgen deficiency in men are presented. The need for further clinical study to determine the significance of age-related hypogonadism is noted.

Mount Rogers/Mount Rainier Clinics: Endocrinology of Aging ◐ ◐
http://www.drcranton.com/endocrinology_of_aging.htm

Lecture notes from an international conference on aging offer information on the use of human growth hormone replacement in reversal of symptoms of aging, as well as discussions of increasing cell resistance to insulin and other peptide hormones in the aging population. Other topics of discussion include the relationship of deep sleep and human growth hormone production, telomeres on chromosomes, other theories on decreasing HGH levels, circadian rhythms, and menopause. Information on additional hormones, their benefits, and generally declining or increasing levels with age are discussed.

Netherlands Institute of Gerontology: Endocrine System and Disorders Poster Sessions ◐ ◐
http://www.nig.nl/congres/3rdeuropeancongress1995/sessions/ses-p25.html

Session abstracts from the Third European Congress of Gerontology are accessible at this address and include clinical review of various subjects in the field of geriatrics and endocrinology. Reference hormone test values in the elderly, aging and diabetes, endocrinopathy in older males, and autoimmune hypothyroidism in the very old are some of the topics addressed.

13.5 Menopause

Menopause and Beyond ◐ ◐ ◐
http://www.oxford.net/~tishy/beyond.html

This site offers information about the physical and psychosocial aspects of menopause and discusses perimenopausal issues, such as heavy bleeding. Ongoing concerns include cardiovascular disease, osteoporosis, breast concerns, pelvic organ disease, vaginal dryness, incontinence, and hot flashes. The site includes information on the pap smear, mammogram, and bone density screening tests, as well as discussion of hysterectomy and colposcopy. A variety of treatments are reviewed, including ovarian hormone replacement, nutritional therapy, herbals, and acupuncture. Discussion boards, self-help book suggestions, and links to related sites make this Web address a comprehensive resource for patients.

North American Menopause Society ◐ ◐ ◐
http://www.menopause.org

The North American Menopause Society is an authoritative source devoted to improving the understanding of menopause through professional education and scientific meetings. Links to professional journals, abstracts, and subscription information are found, and consumers have access to basic information on menopause, as well as answers to frequently asked questions, statistical information, and an article about

Women's Health Clinical Management: Menopause Management for the Millennium ⊙ ⊙ ⊙
http://www.cfs.inform.dk/Sex/menopausecm00.html

This continuing medical education opportunity, courtesy of *Women's Health Clinical Management,* offers clinicians an in-depth article on the menopausal transition. The physiology of menopause and the effects of estrogen deficiency on various systems are reviewed, as is a comprehensive overview of the most current clinical information, opinions, and therapeutic strategies behind management of the medical consequences of menopause. Hormone replacement therapy benefits and risks, current progestin regimens, and new treatments for osteoporosis in the drug pipeline are discussed.

13.6 Osteoporosis in Men

National Osteoporosis Foundation: Men and Osteoporosis ⊙ ⊙
http://www.nof.org/men

Although the disease affects fewer men than women, this fact sheet, provided as a service of the National Osteoporosis Foundation, outlines the special risk factors associated with osteoporosis in men, effective prevention, and treatment. The use of bisphosphonates is discussed, and the *Cutting Edge Report* on the FDA approval of alendronate is accessible. Testosterone replacement therapy, calcitonin, and medications under investigation for use in men are concisely reviewed. The publication, *Strategy on Osteoporosis,* from the National Osteoporosis Foundation's quarterly newsletter, reviews disorders and conditions specific to men that may cause osteoporosis and its gender-specific evaluation.

Osteoporosis Online: Men and Osteoporosis: Not Just a Woman's Disease ⊙ ⊙
http://www.osteoporosis.ca/OSTEO/D01-05.html

This fact sheet offers details on why men are likely to develop osteoporosis and treatment information for males. Personal concerns of men dealing with the disease are presented.

13.7 Pediatric Endocrinology

American Academy of Pediatrics: Endocrinology and Growth ⊙
http://www.aap.org/bpi/Endocrinology.html

Internet endocrinology pages specifically related to endocrinology and growth are included at this listing, with reviews on Web sites included. Children with Diabetes and the Juvenile Diabetes Foundation International are two of the sites reviewed by American Academy of Pediatrics fellows.

Anthropometric Desk Reference ⊙ ⊙ ⊙
http://www.odc.com/anthro/deskref/desktoc.html

The Anthropometric Desk Reference is a resource for professionals and academics studying anthropometric issues. The table of contents includes an anthropometric tutorial, anthropometric reference standards, a section on the validity of international reference standards, and reference data in table, graph, and spreadsheet format. Connections to reference material on the appropriate use of anthropometric indices in children is available in a downloadable format, and databases, such as the World Health Organization's Global Database on Child Growth, are provided.

International Society for Pediatric and Adolescent Diabetes ⊙ ⊙ ⊙
http://www.ispad.org

The International Society for Pediatric and Adolescent Diabetes is a professional organization of doctors and scientists in the field providing information about scientific meetings, membership, and educational activities of the society. Consensus guidelines for managing insulin-dependent patients, abstracts from annual meetings, and links to articles authored by society members may be viewed. Topical coverage of ketoacidosis and the significance of glycosylated hemoglobin values is found at this searchable site.

Juvenile Diabetes Foundation (JDF) International ⊙ ⊙
http://www.jdf.org

Providing diabetes research support, patient education, and advocacy, the JDF maintains a Web site with extensive resources for the diabetes community. A news section with article summaries as well as the full-text articles, a section providing clinical trial information, features devoted to daily care and living with diabetes, questions and answers on important topics, and new book summaries are all available at the site. Links are provided to other resources within the JDF and from government agencies as well as research and treatment centers. Useful reports and abstracts on research topics are accessed through the research section.

Lawson Wilkins Pediatric Endocrine Society (LWPES) ◎ ◎ (some features fee-based)

http://www.lwpes.org

The mission of LWPES is to promote the acquisition and dissemination of knowledge of endocrine and metabolic disorders from conception to adolescence. This Web site contains information of use to both healthcare professionals and patients, including information on grants, awards, and fellowships available through the organization; a state-by-state listing of available positions for pediatric endocrinologists; links to other diabetes-related sites; and a section listing upcoming meetings and conferences. In addition, there is a pediatric endocrinology LISTSERV to which both patients and physicians can subscribe, a members-only section, and other organizational information.

Major Aspects of Growth In Children (MAGIC) Foundation for Children's Growth ◎ ◎

http://www.magicfoundation.org/default.htm

Established by five families of children with growth disorders, the MAGIC (Major Aspects of Growth in Children) Foundation provides support and education regarding growth disorders in children and related adult disorders. The site offers informational brochures on a variety of growth disorders and related topics, the foundation's online newsletter, and information on the annual convention. In addition, there is a LISTSERV, a section for kids, a list of the foundation's services and divisions, and a summary of the history of MAGIC.

University of Michigan Health System: Pediatric Endocrinology Links ◎

http://www.ped.med.umich.edu/RESOURCES/endocrinology.htm

Resources from the University of Michigan are found relating to pediatric endocrinology at this site and include On-line Diabetes Resources and the MAGIC Foundation.

13.8 Reproductive Endocrinology

American Society for Reproductive Medicine ◎ ◎ ◎

http://www.asrm.org

The American Society for Reproductive Medicine exists to advance the study of reproductive medicine and biology. Their Web site offers illustrated audio files of presentations from their annual meeting. Physicians may earn CME credit by viewing the presentations or view details regarding upcoming conferences. Services offered to health professionals include membership, specialty societies, journal articles on fertility and sterility, exam preparation, society news, and information about grants and position placement. Services for patients include answers to frequently asked questions, fact sheets, booklets, and information on current clinical trials. There are links to other professional societies and organizations.

Endocrinology of the Menstrual Cycle ○ ○
http://plpk04.plpk.uq.edu.au/GMC/Physiology/Menstrual_Cycle/index.htm

This slide presentation, written by Simon Manley, explains the endocrinology of the menstrual cycle. Twenty-six slides address a variety of topics, including estrogen and progestin actions, compartments of the ovary, gonadotrophin, hormones of the menstrual cycle, ovarian and uterine phases, abnormalities, menarche, anovulatory cycles, and hypothalamic amenorrhea.

Fertilitext: Overview of Currently Available Drugs ○ ○
http://www.fertilitext.org/p3_pharmacy/medication_overview.html

Tables outlining administration, side effects, actions, considerations, and dosage for selective estrogen receptor modulators, gonadotropins, gonadotropin-releasing hormone agonists and antagonists, and progesterone are found. Generic and trade names, as well as manufacturer contacts, are provided.

Fertilitext: Prescription Medication ○ ○
http://www.fertilitext.org/p3_pharmacy/medication.html

A fertility information page provides a concise review of oral medications used in treatment, a listing of injectable therapies, and details on progesterone and GnRH agonists. Lengthy information on protocols of administrations and an overview of gonadotropins are also provided.

Reproductive Endocrinology Journals ○ ○
http://www.il-st-acad-sci.org/health/oblink2b.html

Maintained by the Illinois State Academy of Science, this site provides links to reproductive endocrinology journals, including *Advances in Contraception*, the *European Journal of Contraception and Reproductive Health Care*, *Gynecological Endocrinology*, and eight others.

Society for the Study of Fertility (SSF) ○ ○
http://www.ssf.org.uk

Members of the SSF promote the study of the biological and medical components of fertility. The site offers a calendar and notices of upcoming events, an employment listing, newsletters, discussion forums, biographies of prominent SSF members, a membership directory, links to related sites, a site search engine, and member registration details. A link is also available to the home page of the *Journal of Reproduction and Fertility,* offering current subscribers access to a free online version.

Society for the Study of Reproduction ✪ ✪
http://www.ssr.org

The Society for the Study of Reproduction provides access to their online journal, *Biology of Reproduction,* at their Web site. There is also information about annual meetings, events, membership, newsletters, and projects, as well as links to other sites of interest.

St. Thomas' Hospital: Endocrines and Reproduction ✪ ✪
http://www.umds.ac.uk/physiology/banks/endorep.html

Written by a doctor of physiology at St. Thomas' Hospital, this tutorial describes reproductive endocrinology. An introduction to hormones is followed by discussions of the pituitary and hypothalamic axis, the thyroid and adrenal glands, sex hormones and reproduction, and the menstrual cycle and pregnancy.

University of Utah: Human Reproduction: Clinical, Pathological and Pharmacologic Correlations ✪ ✪ ✪
http://medstat.med.utah.edu/kw/human_reprod

From the Division of Reproductive Endocrinology and Infertility at the University of Utah, this site offers lecture outlines for a variety of topics, including prolactin, pubertal and midlife changes, male reproductive function, and others. Online seminars, an index of slides and moving images, a glossary, and a section devoted to case studies are provided. The site also provides answers to frequently asked questions, a list of upcoming events, a chat room, and links to related sites.

14. OTHER TOPICAL RESOURCES

14.1 Databases

Glucocorticoid Receptor Resource (GRR) ○ ○ ○
http://nrr.georgetown.edu/GRR/GRR.html

A component of the Nuclear Receptor Resource (NRR), a collection of individual databases on members of the steroid and thyroid hormone receptor superfamily, the Glucocorticoid Receptor Resource is a collection of facts on glucocorticoid receptors (GR), sources for clones and antibodies, maps of GR expression vectors, and phenotypes of mutations. Links are provided to employment information, information on funding for research on nuclear hormone receptors, online journals, related databases, a graphics library, an overview of steroid structures and activities, and a directory of prominent investigators in the field of receptor research.

Illinois State Academy of Science: Andrology Databases ○ ○
http://www.il-st-acad-sci.org/data3.html

Maintained by the Illinois State Academy of Science, this site provides andrology databases of normal laboratory ranges in animals and humans. Human databases describe normal ranges of spermatic vein plasma steroids, seminal plasma IGF-I and IGFBP, semen analysis, and spermatozoa steroids. Links are also available to additional biomedical databases and the American Society of Andrology.

Illinois State Academy of Science: Endocrinology Databases ○ ○
http://www.il-st-acad-sci.org/data2.html

Databases available at this site offer normal ranges of pituitary hormones, steroid hormones, thyroid hormones, insulin-like growth factors, and other hormones present in both humans and animals. Conversion tables for hormones and concentration units, a table outlining steroid nomenclature, and links to other databases are also available.

Kyoto Encyclopedia of Genes and Genomes (KEGG)
http://www.genome.ad.jp/kegg

A project of the Institute for Chemical Research at Kyoto University in Japan, KEGG represents an effort to warehouse current knowledge of molecular and cellular biology. The "Search and Compute" section offers pathway maps, genome maps, prediction tools, and sequence similarity tools. Links are also available to pathway databases, nomenclature and classification databases, and complete genomes and analysis tools.

National Center for Biotechnology Information: Online Mendelian Inheritance in Man (OMIM)
http://www3.ncbi.nlm.nih.gov/Omim

This database of human genes and genetic disorders was developed primarily for use by physicians, researchers, and advanced students concerned with genetic diseases. Reference information, individual disease profiles, texts, and images are found throughout the site, as well as links to the Entrez database of MEDLINE articles and sequence information. Visitors can search the OMIM Database, OMIM Gene Map, and OMIM Morbid Map (a catalog of cytogenetic map locations organized by disease) from the site. Information on the OMIM numbering system, details on creating links to OMIM, site updates, OMIM statistics, information on citing OMIM in literature, and the OMIM gene list are all found at the site. Connections are provided to allied resources, and the complete text of OMIM and gene maps can be downloaded from the site.

National Institutes of Health (NIH): Mammary Genome Anatomy Project (MGAP)
http://mammary.nih.gov/mgap/index.html

Funded by the National Institutes of Health, the Mammary Genome Anatomy Project was initiated to understand the genes and signaling pathways involved in both normal breast development and neoplastic transformations of the breast. An introduction to the project is available, as well as access to cDNA libraries prepared from mammary tissues, detailed molecular information on specific genes expressed in the mammary gland, a microarray database used to profile gene expression patterns in mammary tissue, and links to information on transgenic models used to study breast cancer. Project collaborators are listed at the site.

Prosite Database of Protein Families and Domains
http://www.expasy.ch/prosite

Prosite is a database of protein families and domains. Entries are accessible by descriptions, entry name, author, citation, or by full-text search. The site provides a user manual, list of abbreviations, list of experts, and other professional tools.

Signaling Pathway Database
http://www.grt.kyushu-u.ac.jp/spad

The Signaling Pathway Database contains genetic information and signal transduction systems. The database may be accessed by keyword or by extracellular signal molecules.

Swiss Institute of Bioinformatics (SIB) Expert Protein Analysis System (ExPASy): Enzyme Nomenclature Database (ENZYME)
http://www.expasy.ch/enzyme

Based on recommendations from the Nomenclature Committee of the International Union of Biochemistry and Molecular Biology (IUBMB), ENZYME is a database of information related to the nomenclature of enzymes. Users may access the database by EC number, by enzyme class, by description or alternative name, by chemical compound, by cofactor, or by searching the database. The site also provides an ENZYME user manual and access to other databases and tools.

Weizmann Institute of Science Genome and Bioinformatics: Molecular Biology Databases
http://bioinformatics.weizmann.ac.il/mb/db/enzymes.html

Maintained by the Weizmann Institute of Science Genome and Bioinformatics, this site contains links to 15 databases, including enzyme, metabolic, and signaling pathways databases. Links are also available to information sources on biological pathways, including genetics resources and an annotated bibliography on computational metabolism.

14.2 Ethics

Anabolic Steroid Abuse

National Institute on Drug Abuse (NIDA): Anabolic Steroid Abuse
http://www.steroidabuse.org

The National Institute on Drug Abuse offers resources on anabolic steroid abuse at this address, including a community drug alert bulletin on the use of these drugs, research reports on anabolic steroids, and a NIDA Infofax on anabolic steroid use. A links section offers an index of resources available at this address, as well as links to additional NIDA publications, newsletter articles, and news releases.

National Institute on Drug Abuse
Research Report Series: Anabolic Steroid Abuse ◉ ◉
http://165.112.78.61/ResearchReports/Steroids/AnabolicSteroids.html

Providing an aid to risk recognition, this site answers commonly asked questions regarding anabolic steroid abuse pertaining to health consequences, addiction, and prevention. Topics include steroidal supplements, the scope of steroid abuse in the United States, behavioral effects of anabolic steroids, and treatments for anabolic steroid abuse. The site includes a glossary of terms, links to sources for additional information, and references.

Bioethics

Bioethics, Medical Humanities, and Related Resources ◉ ◉ ◉
http://wings.buffalo.edu/faculty/research/bioethics/other.html

Plentiful material regarding medicine and ethics may be accessed from this one-stop resource, courtesy of the Center for Clinical Ethics and Humanities in Healthcare at the University of Buffalo. More than 60 bioethics centers and organizations, greater than 40 academic medical ethics departments, online databases, and a separate listing of new additions to the site are included for a comprehensive collection of literature, program information, online educational opportunities, and research in the field. Bioethics and classical philosophy, end-of-life issues, philosophy and genetics, and other bioethics topics for physicians are presented.

Georgetown University:
National Reference Center for Bioethics Literature ◉ ◉ ◉
http://www.georgetown.edu/research/nrcbl

The National Reference Center for Bioethics Literature is a collection of books, journals, legal materials, regulations, newspaper articles, and other documents related to issues in biomedical ethics. The site contains a link to BIOETHICSLINE, a bibliographic database supported by the National Library of Medicine and the National Human Genome Research Institute. Connections to educational and teaching resources, bibliographic resources, and library resources are also available through the site. The site also offers links to additional Internet resources related to bioethics.

14.3 Informatics and Software

Diabetes Care: Optimization through Information Technology ◉
http://www.doit-easd.org

The Study Group of the European Association for the Study of Diabetes (EASD) offers this site on the group's past and future meetings and links to resources related to information technology projects in diabetes care. A listing of publications from past meetings and workshops is provided.

Metamedix.com ○ ○
http://www.medilife.com

MetaMedix, a developer of diabetes and health management software, provides opportunities to download its software directly from the site's pages. Mellitus Manager connects glucose meters to personal computers, providing healthcare providers with precise details on blood sugar management. Demo software downloads are available. Information on purchasing glucose meter and insulin pump cables for downloading data directly to the computer is also found. A free diabetes faxable logbook is downloadable in word processing or PDF format.

On-line Diabetes Resources: Software ○ ○ ○
http://www.mendosa.com/software.htm

This site provides links to Web pages dealing with software for diabetes management. Web-based applications include electronic logbooks to keep track of daily blood glucose readings, and access to commercial software programs is, additionally, offered. Disease management programs, medical information organization tools, and a listing of shareware and freeware software programs are included at this extensive compilation.

UMDS Department of Endocrinology, Diabetes, and Metabolic Medicine: Medical Informatics Pages ○ ○
http://www.umds.ac.uk/medicine/endocrinology/mi_info

The United Medical and Dental Schools of Guy's and St. Thomas' Hospitals (UMDS) offer an assortment of medical informatics Web sites related to the specialty of endocrinology and to general practice. Information technology developments for diabetes care, a site dedicated to institutions involved with medical informatics research, and developments in electronic patient record systems are retrievable. A link to medical informatics associations and journals is found.

15. ORGANIZATIONS AND INSTITUTIONS

15.1 Associations and Societies

Below are profiles of more than 50 associations and societies in the fields of endocrinology and metabolism. Those organizations that have a specific focus appear a second time in this volume under particular diseases and disorders or under an appropriate topical heading.

Acid Maltase Deficiency Association (AMDA) ◎ ◎ ◎
http://www.amda-pompe.org

The AMDA was created to support research and public awareness of the disorder, also known as Pompe disease. The site provides a summary of the disorder, including discussions of symptoms, types, and treatment. A section dedicated to respiratory care options, excerpts from an article originally published by the Muscular Dystrophy Association, and information on improving respiration are found, in addition to research developments, clinical trials, and related sites of interest.

American Association of Clinical Endocrinologists (AACE) ◎ ◎ (some features fee-based)
http://www.aace.com/indexjava.htm

The AACE is a professional medical organization with the mission to enhance the practice of clinical endocrinology. The AACE Web site, primarily designed for physicians, contains an extensive amount of information including educational opportunities such as meetings and conferences, publications including journals and newsletters, AACE Clinical Practice Guidelines, and online services available from AACE such as AACE.com text search, a locator for endocrinologists, employment opportunities, and an AACE self-assessment profile. Additional sections include a "Fellows Clinical Corner," a members' area and bulletin board, and an index for this large Web site.

American Association of Diabetes Educators ◐ ◐
http://www.aadenet.org

The American Association of Diabetes Educators is a multidisciplinary organization composed of healthcare professionals who care for and educate diabetes patients. Their site provides information about diabetes legislation and advocacy issues, with details regarding CME meetings and conferences provided. Products available for purchase at the site include professional education resources, patient education materials, and patient products. A list of participating educators and contact information are found.

American Association of Tissue Banks ◐ ◐
http://www.aatb.org

The American Association of Tissue Banks was founded to aid the availability of transplantable human tissues. Its site offers information about the organization, a fact page on organ and tissue donations, and answers to frequently asked questions. Information is provided about accreditation, personnel certification, training courses, and annual meetings. A list of accredited tissue banks is also available.

American Autoimmune Related Diseases Association (AARDA) ◐ ◐ ◐
http://www.aarda.org

Providing both patient and professional resources, the Web site of AARDA offers brief descriptions of more than 50 autoimmune diseases. A discussion of the higher incidence of autoimmune disease in women and a selection of research reports, legislative and advocacy information, a calendar of forthcoming meetings and events, and full-text newsletter articles are also available. In addition, the site includes a link section to other organizations and associations, providing further resources on autoimmune diseases.

American Autoimmune Related Diseases Association (AARDA): Endocrine Autoimmunity ◐ ◐
http://www.aarda.org/endocrine_art2.html

The *InFocus Newsletter* of the American Autoimmune Related Diseases Association provides this online reprint of an article that discusses common autoimmune endocrinology disorders and the risk factors associated with endocrine autoimmunity. General disease features, specific disorders and their diagnosis, and recent advances in endocrine autoimmunity are described. A link found at the bottom of the document brings visitors to an entire collection of related *InFocus* articles, including "Hormones and Autoimmunity" and "Autoimmunity, The Common Thread." Other interesting sites include conference news and promising advances in therapy for autoimmune diseases.

American Diabetes Association (ADA) ◐ ◐ ◐
http://www.diabetes.org

The American Diabetes Association provides research, information, and advocacy in an effort to improve the lives of diabetic patients. The site features diabetes in the news and current association headlines, in addition to advocacy and detailed disorders reviews. Facts and figures, special information for the newly diagnosed patient, and educational material for teachers and healthcare providers are accessible. Links to MEDLINE searches, as well as the association's professional journal, are found.

American Dietetic Association (ADA) ○ ○ ○
http://www.eatright.org

The American Dietetic Association is a professional organization that offers support, training, and services to members. For professionals, the site offers a catalog of publications, bibliographies, and links to press releases, position papers, and the *Journal of the American Dietetic Association*. For consumers, the site provides daily nutrition tips, a catalog of publications, a reading list, featured articles, nutrition fact sheets, and information on the food guide pyramid. Also available are a dietitian listing, information on government affairs, and links to related sites.

American Obesity Association (AOA) ○ ○
http://www.obesity.org

The American Obesity Association is dedicated to education, research, and community action to treat and prevent obesity. The AOA site offers information about the group's mission and membership, facts and statistics about obesity, publications discussing health insurance and treatment for adult obesity, and contact details. Discussions of health conditions associated with obesity and an interactive Weight Wellness Profile are also available.

American Peptide Society ○ ○
http://www.chem.umn.edu/orgs/ampepsoc/apshome.html

The American Peptide Society works to advance knowledge in the chemistry and biology of peptides and proteins. This site provides links to upcoming events and conferences. There are also links to membership applications, awards information, member directories, and employment opportunities. Connections are available to a newsgroup, an online journal, and other related sites.

American Prostate Society ○ ○
http://www.ameripros.org

The American Prostate Society seeks to reduce suffering and death from prostate diseases, with overviews of prostate cancer, prostate enlargement, and prostatitis. Prostate cancer review includes diagnostic and staging information, and articles on second and third opinions, spousal and familial relationships, and prevention are offered. Answers to frequently asked questions, professional article abstracts, and access to archived and current newsletters are provided.

American Society for Reproductive Medicine ◐ ◐ ◐

http://www.asrm.org

The American Society for Reproductive Medicine exists to advance the study of reproductive medicine and biology. Its Web site offers illustrated audio files of presentations from the organization's annual meeting. Physicians may earn CME credit by viewing the presentations or view details regarding upcoming conferences. Services offered to health professionals include membership, specialty societies, journal articles on fertility and sterility, exam preparation, society news, and information about grants and position placement. Services for patients include answers to frequently asked questions, fact sheets, booklets, and information on current clinical trials. There are links to other professional societies and organizations.

American Society of Bariatric Physicians (ASBP) ◐ ◐

http://www.asbp.org

The ASBP is a society composed of professionals who specialize in the treatment of obesity. Professional resources available from the site include a summary of continuing medical education opportunities and calendar, ASBP membership details, and bariatric practice guidelines. Various statements describing bariatric medicine, obesity, and side effects of appetite suppressant medications are also available, as well as contact details for an automated referral service.

American Society of Human Genetics (ASHG) ◐ ◐

http://www.faseb.org/genetics/ashg/ashgmenu.htm

The ASHG home page provides society policy statements, reports, and publications; an online newsletter; information about the *American Journal of Human Genetics;* and information about the ASHG annual meeting. Also included are educational details for those interested in careers in genetics, an application for the American Society of Human Genetics AAAS Congressional Fellowship, a history of human genetics organizations, and other organizational and membership information.

American Society of Transplant Physicians (ASTP) ◐

http://www.a-s-t.org/index.htm

This professional society serves physicians and scientists and promotes research, patient care, advocacy, and education. Information concerning bylaws, CME, meetings, ethics, officers, membership, job postings, publications, and certification is provided. A restricted section for members provides committee reports, slide lectures, a newsletter, CME transcripts, and a member directory. Preregistration for meetings is also possible via the site.

American Society of Transplant Surgeons (ASTS) ◐ ◐

http://www.asts.org

The American Society of Transplant Surgeons exists to promote education and research related to organ and tissue transplantation. This site contains the bylaws of the organization and information on membership, training programs, annual meetings, awards, and fellowships. Sections describing public policy activities and ethics are also available.

American Thyroid Association ○ ○ ○
http://www.thyroid.org

The American Thyroid Association is a professional organization dedicated to increasing scientific and public understanding of the thyroid gland and the management of its diseases. Practice guidelines for physicians, as well as information on thyroid research and Wilson's syndrome, are found. Users may also access journal articles, the association newsletter, conference details, and grant information.

Association of Program Directors in Endocrinology and Metabolism (APDEM) ○ ○ (some features fee-based)
http://www.apdem.org

Members of the APDEM are the directors of training programs that prepare fellows, residents and medical students for clinical research careers in endocrinology and metabolism. The site offers information on fellowships including a "Training Program Finder" where the user can choose a variety of criteria such as preferred discipline, faculty interest, and location to find a desired program. There is also a news and information section which includes job listings, legislative updates, meetings and events, and links to related sites. Also offered are information about the association and a section restricted to members by password.

Canadian Diabetes Association ○ ○
http://www.diabetes.ca

Promoting health through diabetes research, education, and advocacy, the Canadian Diabetes Association offers information for consumers and professionals alike, with general information about diabetes, prevalence statistics, and current research initiatives. A clinical and scientific section of the site offers information for clinicians, and a diabetes educator section is found. Links to publications; information about conferences, events, and awards; and the clinical practice guidelines of the association are found.

Canadian Society for Mucopolysaccharide (MPS) and Related Diseases ○ ○
http://www.mpssociety.ca

The Canadian MPS Society was created to support patients and families affected by lysosomal storage diseases. The site offers information about mucopolysaccharide (MPS) and related diseases. By accessing the "Diseases" link, visitors are taken to discussions on the history of the disease, causes and heredity, diagnosis, symptoms, and treatment options. A chart outlining disease classifications is provided, in addition to a resource library, a discussion forum, and resources for further learning.

Diabetes Insipidus Foundation, Inc. ○ ○ ○
http://diabetesinsipidus.maxinter.net

The Web site of the Diabetes Insipidus Foundation, Inc., with pages available in English, Spanish, or French, contains several articles, facts sheets, and brochures on the symptoms, diagnostic tests, and medications for effective treatment of this disorder.

Endocrine Fellows Foundation (EFF) ○ ○
http://www.endocrinefellows.org

The EFF was established to provide a support system for endocrine fellows. Its Web site provides an array of information of interest to the fellow and professional endocrinologist. Sections include EFF in the news, education and grants, scientific forums, a career center, publications, events, corporate sponsors, and case studies. Links to related sites are also available.

Endocrine Society ○ ○ ○
http://www.endo-society.org/index.htm

The Endocrine Society is devoted to the research, study and clinical practice of endocrinology. This comprehensive site offers a variety of information including fact sheets on many endocrine-related topics, information on publications and Endocrine Society journals, a calendar of scientific meetings, and a placement service for those seeking and trying to fill positions in the field of endocrinology. Other features of this site include an ethics section with several ethics scenarios and a diversity section with information on minority affairs. In addition, the site offers information on awards and grants provided by the society, articles and press releases relevant to the society, information for fellows/students and women in endocrinology, links to related sites, and organizational and membership information.

European Federation of Endocrine Societies (EFES) ○
http://www.unige.ch/efes

The EFES is a nonprofit organization that serves to provide better methods of communication between those interested in endocrinology and to advance research and education in this subject. The site provides information on upcoming events and member organizations from over 30 different countries. The site also contains information regarding EFES's official journal, *European Journal of Endocrinology,* and links to related organizations and societies.

Gauchers Association ○ ○ ○
http://wisebuy.users.netlink.co.uk/gaucher/contents.htm

This comprehensive site provides links to over 200 different patient and professional Internet resources on Gaucher disease, including new sites and an alphabetical listing of the remainder. Articles and references are offered on such topics as enzyme replacement therapy, genetic therapeutics, home infusions, new and investigative treatments, obstetric and gynecological aspects, pain management, and diagnostic testing.

Hormone Foundation

http://www.hormone.org

The Hormone Foundation is the public education affiliate of the Endocrine Society, dedicated to the prevention, diagnosis, and treatment of human diseases influenced by the endocrine system. The site offers an overview of the foundation's mission and leadership, notices of upcoming events, downloadable publications on menopause and ordering details for materials on other endocrine topics, and links to related sites.

Human Growth Foundation (HGF)

http://www.hgfound.org

Through education, research, support and advocacy, the HGF helps individuals with growth-related disorders, as well as their families and healthcare professionals. This Web site provides information on a variety of growth disorders, growth hormone treatment, and adult hormone therapy, as well as a list of related studies and clinical trials. The site also includes a list of publications available from the HGF, information on the foundation's Small Grants Program, and a section on activities and events. For individuals looking to join a mailing list, there is one specifically for adult patients and another specifically for parents of pediatric patients. A children's section of the site provides a question and answer section along with stories from children living with growth disorders.

Hypoglycemia Association, Inc.

http://www.silver-bayou.com/hai/index.htm

The Hypoglycemia Association Inc. offers information and support for hypoglycemia patients, with background information on the disorder and discussions of causes, diagnosis, and treatment. By contacting the organization, users may receive a packet that includes literature lists and useful educational materials. There are links to related sites.

Insulin-Free World Foundation

http://www.insulinfree.org

A nonprofit organization, the Insulin-Free World Foundation provides a forum for information exchange on diabetes through correspondence with leading researchers and collection of research articles and other materials for consumer and professional use. The site offers an overview of the organization, membership information, contact details, a catalog of publications, an online newsletter, and a section devoted to politics and economic issues. Discussions of pancreas transplantation, islet cell replacement, immunology, and future mechanical solutions to diabetes are available, as well as articles describing type I diabetes, type II diabetes, diabetes facts and statistics, and current prevention projects.

International Bone and Mineral Society
http://www.ibmsonline.org

The International Bone and Mineral Society promotes basic and clinical research of the skeleton and mineral metabolism. Information provided at the site includes a society history, current news items, awards, and affiliated societies.

International Diabetic Athletes Association (IDAA)
http://www.diabetes-exercise.org

The International Diabetic Athletes Association supports diabetics who participate in fitness activities. The site offers membership details and information about regional chapters and support groups. A product catalog and a calendar of upcoming events are posted, as well as links to related sites.

International Neuroendocrine Federation
http://www.isneuro.org

Details on the federation's upcoming International Congress of Neuroendocrinology and membership details are found at this organization Web page. A listing of additional upcoming events is provided and includes a pituitary disease workshop and an international meeting on steroids and the nervous system. "The Incredible Walking Brain" link outlines the future status and objectives of the International Neuroendocrine Federation.

International Pancreas and Islet Transplant Association (IPITA)
http://www.jr2.ox.ac.uk/ipita

The IPITA is dedicated to encouraging research, providing a forum for the exchange of relevant information, and promoting contacts between researchers. The site provides information about the association, upcoming meetings, officers, constitution, and bylaws. Other resources include a discussion board, e-mail list, and links to related sites.

International Pompe Association
http://www.pompe.org.uk

This site offers links to information about Pompe's disease produced by the Association for Glycogen Storage Disease (AGSD), Pompe's information elsewhere on the Internet, and background information. From the AGSD, there is a guide for families, information about Pompe's Project, a pamphlet on caring for a child with Pompe's, and current issues of the association's newsletter. Connections to other sites include the Children's Pompe Foundation and the Acid Maltase Deficiency Association. Background information is provided on cell biology and proteolysis.

International Society for Pediatric and Adolescent Diabetes ◎ ◎ ◎
http://www.ispad.org

The International Society for Pediatric and Adolescent Diabetes is a professional organization of doctors and scientists in the field providing information about scientific meetings, membership, and educational activities of the society. Consensus guidelines for managing insulin-dependent patients, abstracts from annual meetings, and links to articles authored by society members may be viewed. Topical coverage of ketoacidosis and the significance of glycosylated hemoglobin values is found at this searchable site.

International Society of Psychoneuroendocrinology (ISPNE) ◎
http://www.ispne.org

Maintained by the International Society of Psychoneuroendocrinology, this site offers information about the organization, including its membership, officers, announcements, conferences, and bylaws.

Lawson Wilkins Pediatric Endocrine Society (LWPES) ◎ ◎ (some features fee-based)
http://www.lwpes.org

The mission of the LWPES is to promote the acquisition and dissemination of knowledge of endocrine and metabolic disorders from conception to adolescence. This Web site contains information of use to both healthcare professionals and patients, including information on grants, awards and fellowships available through the organization; a state-by-state listing of available positions for pediatric endocrinologists; links to other diabetes-related sites; and a section listing upcoming meetings and conferences. In addition, there is a pediatric endocrinology LISTSERV to which both patients and physicians can subscribe, a members-only section, and other organizational information.

National Kidney Foundation (NKF) ◎ ◎ ◎
http://www.kidney.org

The National Kidney Foundation is dedicated to improving life for kidney disease patients. For healthcare professionals, the site offers information on the Council of Nephrology Nurses and Technicians, the Council of Nephrology Social Workers, and the Council on Renal Nutrition. There is also information about research programs, publications, and government relations. For patients, the site offers news, information about programs, publications and periodicals, resources, and membership details. The site also provides educational material concerning organ and tissue donation.

National Mucopolysaccharidoses (MPS) Society ◎ ◎
http://www.mpssociety.org

A chart outlining disease types and links to further information on causes and inheritance are found at the National MPS Society page. Accessing the reference center provides visitors with a listing of publications that may be ordered, and MPS news offers information on upcoming events and legislative updates. By following links to the Online Mendelian Inheritance in Man (OMIM) database site and additional links, visitors gain access to detailed genetic and research information. Information on related diseases, including the oligosaccharidoses, the glycosphingolipidoses, and the mucolipidoses, is provided at the site.

National Ovarian Cancer Association ◐ ◐

http://www.ovariancanada.org

Ovarian cancer information, the organization's ongoing activities, and the association's research page provide a comprehensive Internet source of support and treatment information. Over 2,500 electronic documents are available for rapid viewing and include research summaries on gene therapy, immunotherapy, and anti-angiogenesis. Visitors may search the entire database or access an assortment of clinical trials, treatment agents, and biological approaches to care. Conference reports of the American Society of Clinical Oncology and the American Association for Cancer Research can be accessed.

National Tay-Sachs and Allied Diseases Association, Inc. ◐ ◐

http://www.ntsad.org

The National Tay-Sachs and Allied Diseases Association offers this International Resource Center, structured to provide a comprehensive Web reference on Tay-Sachs and related disease profiles, the basis of genetics, programs sponsored by the organization, and further sources of information, such as recommended reading. The latest events, an online genetic testing center directory, and an assortment of educational materials appropriate for both professionals and the general public may be obtained.

North American Menopause Society ◐ ◐ ◐

http://www.menopause.org

The North American Menopause Society is an authoritative source devoted to improving the understanding of menopause through professional education and scientific meetings. Links to professional journals, abstracts, and subscription information are found, and consumers have access to basic information on menopause, as well as answers to frequently asked questions, statistical information, and an article about natural products. Ordering information for consumer education products and links to other Web resources are provided.

North American Society for the Study of Obesity (NASSO) ◐ ◐

http://www.naaso.org

NAASO was founded to increase and disseminate knowledge related to obesity. The site provides links to press releases, news, and society announcements. A calendar of upcoming events, membership information, funding information, and position announcements are provided, as well as links to the society's online journal, a discussion group, a mailing list, and related sites on obesity management.

Pituitary Tumor Network Association ◎ ◎ ◎
http://www.pituitary.com

The Pituitary Network Association encourages research on pituitary tumors and related pituitary disorders. Information at the site includes articles on emotional aspects of related disorders, general issues, inspiration, insurance issues, patient perspectives, and treatment. There are also articles related to specific disorders, including craniopharyngioma, acromegaly, Addison's disease, Cushing's disease, and prolactinoma. Other information at the site includes clinical trials, medical advances, questions and answers, and physician and hospital referrals. There is a bulletin board and information on publications. There are also links to related sites.

Prader-Willi Association (USA) ◎ ◎ ◎
http://www.pwsausa.org

Downloadable conference registration forms, answers to FAQs, and important medical alerts are available at this searchable organization Web site, dedicated to providing an international network of support and information on Prader-Willi syndrome. Genetic testing details, diagnostic criteria, and position statements on Prader-Willi syndrome are accessible. The organization publishes additional material, such as *The Gathered View* national newsletter, brochures, information kits, and a disease management textbook. A sample copy of the newsletter may be downloaded from the site.

Purine Research Society ◎ ◎
http://www2.dgsys.com/~purine

The secretion of excess uric acid in purine metabolic disease and current progress in research of these disorders is the focus of the Purine Research Society. A simple explanation of metabolic processes, genetic enzyme production, information on purine compounds, and the importance of recognition of purine metabolic diseases are discussed. Concise descriptions of several of these enzyme defects and the future of purine research are reviewed.

Society for Behavioral Neuroendocrinology ◎ ◎
http://www.sbne.org

Connections to society meeting and membership information and a link to the organization's official, professional journal are found at this site of the Society for Behavioral Neuroendocrinology. The organization's mission of providing an investigative forum for the advancement of the understanding of the relationship between behavior and neuroendocrine function is presented. Visitors are encouraged to visit related neuroendocrine Web sites or access related journals at this NeuroRing Web site.

Society for Endocrinology ⊙ ⊙ ⊙
http://www.endocrinology.org

The Society for Endocrinology promotes the advancement of public education in endocrinology. Resources available through the site include an overview of the society, a calendar of events, conference details, information on training courses, a member's handbook, information on journals and other publications, and links to related sites. Details of the society's Young Endocrinologists Committee are also provided. In addition, the site offers an abstract search tool for the *Journal of Endocrinology* and the *Journal of Molecular Endocrinology,* as well as full text of articles published in the society's journal *Endocrine-Related Cancer.*

Society for the Study of Fertility (SSF) ⊙ ⊙
http://www.ssf.org.uk

Members of the SSF promote the study of the biological and medical components of fertility. The site offers a calendar and notices of upcoming events, an employment listing, newsletters, discussion forums, biographies of prominent SSF members, a membership directory, links to related sites, a site search engine, and member registration details. A link is also available to the home page of the *Journal of Reproduction and Fertility,* offering current subscribers access to a free online version.

Society for the Study of Inborn Errors of Metabolism ⊙ ⊙
http://www.ssiem.org.uk

The Society for the Study of Inborn Errors of Metabolism fosters research of inherited disorders of endocrinology and metabolism through scientific meetings and publications. The site provides information about the history, goals, membership, and activities of the organization. Links to publications, training information, and affiliated organizations are offered, as are connections to journals and publishers, societies, diagnostic centers, databases, and other resources.

Society for the Study of Reproduction ⊙ ⊙
http://www.ssr.org

The Society for the Study of Reproduction provides access to their online journal, *Biology of Reproduction,* at their Web site. There is also information about annual meetings, events, membership, newsletters, and projects, as well as links to other sites of interest.

Thyroid Society for Education and Research ⊙ ⊙
http://www.the-thyroid-society.org

The Thyroid Society for Education and Research features an illustrated explanation of thyroid disease. There are answers to frequently asked questions, a calendar of hot topics, and links to educational resources. Information is also provided about research programs and stipends for medical students. An extensive list of thyroid-related documents is available for download, and there are links to featured articles from professional journals as well as other related resources.

Turner's Syndrome Society of the United States ○ ○ ○
http://www.turner-syndrome-us.org

The Turner's Syndrome Society of the United States exists to increase public awareness of the disease and provide information and support for patients. Information about recent and upcoming conferences is found along with a listing of local chapters and contacts. Support features include a chat room and links to related organizations worldwide. Recent research conducted on the disorder and articles discussing early intervention for children are found.

Women in Endocrinology (WE) ○
http://www.women-in-endo.org

WE is an organization devoted to promoting and facilitating the professional development and advancement of women in the field of endocrinology. The site contains a list of activities conducted by WE, such as meetings and awards. The organization's online newsletter, links to related sites, organizational details, and membership details are also provided.

15.2 Foundations and Grant Support

Hundreds of major foundations offer financial support for research in medicine. Below are Web sites that provide access to foundation grants, grant organizations, areas of focus, eligibility, and other relevant data. In addition, several major sources of government research funding are provided, as well as Web sites for grants that are cataloged by specialized organizations and clearinghouses. Major associations and societies that appear in the "Associations and Societies" section frequently include information on research grants, and many offer annual awards for research and study.

Community of Science ○ ○ ○ (free registration)
http://www.cos.com

Community of Science, Inc. (COS) is one of the leading Web networks for professionals in research and development, offering access to information on over 19,000 available research grants, a subscriber-customized Funding Alert, and membership-based abilities to track information on funding and awards at leading national and international research facilities. Related science news and discussion forums are available with the site's free membership.

Foundation Center ○ ○ ○
http://fdncenter.org

The Foundation Center provides direct links to thousands of grant-making organizations, including foundations, corporations, and public charities, along with a search engine to enable the user to locate sources of funding in specific fields. In addition, the site provides listings of the largest private foundations, corporate grant makers, and community foundations. There is also information on funding trends, a newsletter, and grant-seeker orientation material. More than 900 grant-making organizations are accessible through this useful site.

National Institutes of Health (NIH): Funding Opportunities ○ ○ ○
http://grants.nih.gov/grants

Funding opportunities for research, scholarship, and training are extensive within the federal government. At this site for the National Institutes of Health, information is provided on NIH grants and fellowship programs, on research contracts including requests for proposals (RFPs), on research training opportunities in biomedical areas, and on the NIH Guide for Grants and Contracts. The latter is the official document for announcing the availability of NIH funds for biomedical and behavioral research and research training policies. Links are provided to major divisions of the NIH that have additional information on specialized grant opportunities.

Polaris Grants Central ○ ○
http://polarisgrantscentral.net

For the grant seeker, this site provides resources that are available from numerous organizations pertaining to grant identification and application. There are books and publications on grant sources, descriptions of grant information providers, clearinghouses for grant information, federal contacts, grant training materials, and resources on disk or CD-ROM. Within the site, useful sections provide tips and hints on writing grant proposals, grants news from different government agencies and other organizations, information on scholarships and grants for individuals, and information on grant workshops.

Society of Research Administrators (SRA) GrantsWeb ○ ○ ○
http://www.srainternational.org/cws/sra/resource.htm

The Society of Research Administrators has created an extremely useful grant information site, with extensive links to government resources, general resources, private funding, and policy/regulation sites. The site section devoted to U.S., Canadian, and other international resources provides links to government agency funding sources, the commerce business daily, the Catalog of Federal Domestic Assistance, scientific agencies, research councils, and resources in individual fields, such as health and education. Grant-application procedures, regulations, and guidelines are provided throughout the site, and extensive legal information is provided through links to patent, intellectual property, and copyright offices. Associations providing funding and grant information are also listed, with direct links.

15.3 Selected Medical School Departments of Endocrinology and Metabolism

Albert Einstein College of Medicine: Division of Reproductive Endocrinology Infertility ◎ ◎
http://www.aecom.yu.edu/obgyn/divdep/endocrin.html

This site provides information about the Division of Reproductive Endocrinology and Infertility, as well as Montefiore's Fertility and Hormone Center, the Westchester Fertility Network, and the Hartsdale Fertility and Fetal Medicine Institute. Brief descriptions of methods of assisted reproductive technology are provided, including in vitro fertilization, intracytoplasmic sperm injection, assisted hatching, donor eggs, sperm, laboratory services, and surgical treatment of infertility. In addition, there is information available about menopause research and treatment within the division, as well as about the Women's Health Initiative. A list of division staff and links to the Department of Obstetrics and Gynecology, which include access to a newsletter and educational programs for medical students, residents, fellows, and CME for physicians, are also available.

Baylor College of Medicine: Department of Pediatrics, Endocrine and Metabolism Section ◎ ◎
http://www.bcm.tmc.edu/pedi/endo

Provided at this site are a list of faculty and fellows, information about the section's research and academic activities, and a list of current grants providing funding to the section. Also offered are a list of publications authored by faculty members and a section describing faculty awards, appointments and other honors.

Boston Medical Center: Pediatric Endocrinology Services ◎
http://www.bostonchildhealth.org/PediatricsDept/Endocrinology/index.html

The Pediatric Endocrinology Section at Boston Medical Center provides evaluation and care of children and adolescents with endocrine and metabolic disorders. The site provides a brief overview of the section including its mission statement, clinical services, collaborative clinical relationships with Pediatric Primary Care, Adolescent Medicine and Adult Endocrinology, areas of expertise, and contact information. In addition, there are links to other sites within the Boston Medical Center.

Boston University
Department of Medicine: Endocrinology Section ◉

http://medicine.bu.edu/endo.htm

The home page of the Endocrinology Section at Boston University provides a history and description of the section, its various units, and the faculty and their research interests. A list of selected recent publications from the section is also available.

Case Western Reserve University
Department of Medicine: Division of Endocrinology ◉ ◉

http://www.cwru.edu/CWRU/Med/medicine/divcline.htm

The purpose of this site is to provide information about the clinical and molecular endocrinology programs at Case Western Reserve University, University Hospitals of Cleveland, and the Cleveland Veterans Affairs Medical Center. Sections include faculty, current research, clinical activities, fellowship program, contact information, and clinical and molecular endocrinology links. The site also offers multiple links to sites within the Department of Medicine and within the university.

Children's Hospital, Denver: Endocrinology ◉

http://www.childrenshospitalden.org/clinicalindex.html

Affiliated with the University of Colorado Health Sciences Center, this site outlines endocrinology services provided at the Children's Hospital, Denver. Included are a list of problems that are diagnosed and treated at the hospital, information for referral sources, a description of services available, and a list of key contacts. Also available are links to related sites within the hospital.

Children's Memorial Hospital in Chicago
Department of Pediatrics: Division of Endocrinology ◉ ◉

http://www.childmmc.edu/depts/endocrinology/default.asp

Sections at the site of the Division of Pediatric Endocrinology offer information on research projects within the division, a list of staff and their research interests, common endocrinology questions and answers, and links to related sites.

Cincinnati Children's Hospital
Medical Center, Division of Endocrinology ◉ ◉

http://www.chmcc.org/departments/19/index.asp

This site offers an overview of the Division of Endocrinology at Cincinnati Children's Hospital Medical Center, including its mission, faculty and staff, strengths, fellowships available, and a list of conditions treated. Also available are contact information and links to related sites within the Medical Center.

Columbia-Presbyterian Medical Center:
Department of Pediatrics: Division of Pediatric Endocrinology ◎

http://cpmcnet.columbia.edu/dept/pediatrics/pedsend.htm

The pediatric endocrine division provides care to children undergoing evaluation and treatment for endocrine disorders and conducts research in the field. This brief site offers a description of the division, its research activities, and members of the division with their titles and educational background.

Columbia-Presbyterian Medical Center: Presbyterian Hospital
Department of Medicine: Division of Endocrinology ◎

http://cpmcnet.columbia.edu/dept/medicine/endocrinmen.html

The home page of the Division of Endocrinology at the Columbia-Presbyterian Center of New York Presbyterian Hospital provides a description of the division and a list of faculty, clinical programs, and research activities.

Duke University Medical Center:
Division of Endocrinology: Metabolism and Nutrition ◎ ◎ ◎

http://medicine.mc.duke.edu/endro.nsf?Open

The home page of the Division of Endocrinology, Metabolism and Nutrition at Duke University Medical Center provides a description of the division's services, accomplishments, goals, and faculty. The site also lists the types and numbers of procedures and consultations performed through the division. Other resources include profiles of outreach activities, areas of clinical and basic research, special programs, and educational and training activities of the division.

Emory University School of Medicine:
Department of Pediatrics: Division of Endocrinology and Diabetes ◎ ◎

http://wwwph1.cc.emory.edu/PEDS/ENDO

Information provided at this site includes a list of division members and their research interests, references, and biographical data; a description of the division's research activities; a list of clinical facilities; and a description of the fellowship program, including an online application. In addition, there is a section on the division's international adoption research.

Emory University School of Medicine:
Division of Endocrinology and Metabolism ◎ ◎

http://www.emory.edu/ENDOCRINOLOGY

The Division of Endocrinology and Metabolism at Emory University is composed of clinical and basic research faculty with interests in all aspects of endocrinology. The site offers information on the faculty; clinical, research, and teaching activities of the division; and fellowship training programs available. A fellowship application can be downloaded at this site.

Indiana University:
Department of Medicine: Endocrinology Division ◎ ◎

http://medicine.iupui.edu/endo

This site offers a variety of resources for visitors, including descriptions of the following clinical endocrine programs: Indiana Diabetes Center, Thyroid Center, Osteoporosis Center, Hypertension Center, Weight Management Center, and Lipid Control Program. Also provided is information on endocrine laboratory services, division faculty, and fellowship programs. Contact information is available. The site also includes a section describing the Indiana Endocrine Society.

Johns Hopkins School of
Medicine: Division of Endocrinology and Metabolism ◎ ◎

http://www.endocrinology.jhu.edu

Resources for both patients and physicians are available at this new divisional Web site of Johns Hopkins University. Conference and CME updates, faculty research interests and connections, program information and downloadable fellowship applications, and recommended links are provided.

Johns Hopkins School of Medicine:
Division of Pediatric Endocrinology ◎ ◎ ◎

http://www.med.jhu.edu/pedendo/index.html

This site provides information on the Division of Pediatric Endocrinology at the Johns Hopkins University School of Medicine. Sections include training opportunities, research within the division, clinical services, faculty, patient resources, and links to related pediatric sites within and outside of Johns Hopkins. Clinical and research fellowships are available at the division, and applications can be downloaded online. Patient resources available at this site include guides on syndromes of abnormal sex differentiation and congenital adrenal hyperplasia due to 21 hydroxylase deficiency.

Keck School of Medicine
University of Southern California, Department of Pediatrics:
Division of Endocrinology and Metabolism ◎

http://www.usc.edu/schools/medicine

The Division of Endocrinology and Metabolism specializes in the diagnosis and management of children with hormone disorders, diabetes, and other rare and complex carbohydrate conditions such as galactosemia and glycogen storage disease. This site, reached by choosing "Academic Departments" and then "Endocrinology, Diabetes and Metabolism", offers an overview of the division, a description of teaching and research activities, contact information of the division head, and links to other sites within the School of Medicine.

Keck School of Medicine
University of Southern California: Endocrinology Division ◎ ◎
http://www.usc.edu/schools/medicine

The site of the Endocrinology Division of the Keck School of Medicine, reached by choosing "Academic Departments" and then "Endocrinology, Diabetes and Metabolism", includes general information about the division, fellowships, residencies, CME programs, patient care and research activities, and contact information. Multiple links to sites within the university and the school of medicine are also found at the site.

Mayo Clinic:
Endocrinology, Metabolism, Diabetes and Nutrition Division ◎ ◎
http://www.mayo.edu/endocrine/endo-main.htm

This comprehensive site offers information on the Endocrinology, Metabolism, Diabetes and Nutrition Division, including patient information, clinical services available, provider and appointment information, and sections on professional education and research programs offered through the division. A staff directory is available, as well as links to related sites within the Mayo Clinic Rochester.

Mount Sinai School of Medicine, Department of
Medicine: Division of Endocrinology and Metabolism ◎ ◎ ◎
http://www.mssm.edu/medicine/endocrinology/home-page.html

This comprehensive site offers information on the Division of Endocrinology and Metabolism, a directory of physicians, descriptions of research activities and clinical trials, and an education section providing information on courses, clinical fellowships, grand rounds, and training programs. Additional resources include patient information, news and announcements, a site map, and links to related sites.

Mount Sinai School of Medicine, Department of
Pediatrics: Division of Pediatric Endocrinology and Metabolism ◎ ◎
http://www.mssm.edu/peds/endocrin.html

This site describes the services of the Division of Pediatric Endocrinology and Metabolism, including its fellowship training program and faculty. Some basic information on diabetes and a description of the Carole and Michael Friedman and Family Diabetes Unit are also provided.

New York Hospital-Cornell Medical Center: Division of
Endocrinology, Diabetes, and Metabolism/Clinical Research Center ◎
http://www.nycornell.org/medicine/edm/index.html

Offered at this site are a directory of faculty members, a site search engine, and contact information. Links to the home pages of the New York and Presbyterian Hospital, Cornell University Medical College, and the Graduate School of Medical Sciences are also provided.

New York-Presbyterian Hospital Weill Cornell Medical College, Department of Pediatrics: Center for the Study of Endocrine and Metabolic Diseases of Children

http://pedsendo.med.cornell.edu/index.html

This site provides information on the Center for the Study of Endocrine and Metabolic Diseases of Children, including a list of faculty and sections describing the Cornell Juvenile Diabetes Program, the Laboratory of Molecular Endocrinology, congenital adrenal hyperplasia (CAH), and the fellowship program. Included in the section on CAH is information on prenatal diagnosis and genetic testing.

Northwestern University: Division of Endocrinology, Metabolism and Molecular Medicine

http://www.endocrine.northwestern.edu

This site offers information about the Division of Endocrinology, Metabolism, and Molecular Medicine, including faculty research interests, fellowship programs, educational symposia, and seminars. A calendar of events for the Department of Medicine and links to related sites and online journals are also provided.

Ohio State University, Department of Internal Medicine: Division of Endocrinology, Diabetes and Metabolism

http://www.intmed.med.ohio-state.edu/Endo/endocrin_homepage.htm

Resources provided by this home page include an overview of the division, a description of the fellowship training program, a list of publications by members of the division, clinic locations and phone numbers, and a physician directory. In addition, visitors can access links to other divisions within the Department of Internal Medicine.

Oregon Health Sciences University Department of Medicine: Division of Endocrinology, Diabetes and Nutrition

http://www.ohsu.edu/som-Medicine/divisions/endo/index.html

Comprehensive information about the Endocrine Training Program can be found at this site, including program information, profiles of training faculty, application instructions and an application form, and a listing of endocrinology fellows. Other resources include links to sites within the Oregon Health Sciences University and a search engine.

Stanford University School of Medicine Department of Pediatrics: Division of Endocrinology and Diabetes

http://www.med.stanford.edu/school/pediatrics/endocrinology.html

This home page of the Division of Endocrinology and Diabetes within the Department of Pediatrics provides an overview of research activities of the division, including active clinical studies, and a list of faculty with their position, research interests, publications, and contact information. Also provided are the location and hours of the division's clinic as well as links to related sites within the university.

Thomas Jefferson University Hospital:
Division of Endocrinology, Diabetes and Metabolic Diseases ◐ ◐
http://www.jeffersonhealth.org/tjuh/depts/endo/index.html

The Division of Endocrinology, Diabetes and Metabolic Diseases at Thomas Jefferson University Hospital provides comprehensive care for patients with diabetes mellitus, obesity, thyroid nodules, and goiters; other hormonal and glandular disorders involving the thyroid, pituitary, parathyroid, and adrenal glands; and osteoporosis and other bone, cholesterol, and triglyceride metabolism disorders. The site provides descriptions of the division and its services provided through the Endocrinology/Diabetes Clinical Center, the Center for Diabetic Kidney Disease, the Kidney Transplant Program, the Jefferson Thyroid Treatment Center, and the Pancreas Program. Also included at this site are links to Thomas Jefferson University Hospital and its departments, centers, and programs.

University of Alabama at Birmingham Department of Medicine:
Division of Endocrinology and Metabolism ◐ ◐
http://info.dom.uab.edu/endo/index.htm

The Division of Endocrinology and Metabolism provides in-patient and out-patient services, as well as strong clinical and research activities. Information offered at the Web site includes descriptions of clinical activities, research, and fellowship programs available at the division, as well as a list of faculty.

University of Chicago, Department of
Pediatrics: Section of Pediatric Endocrinology ◐
http://www.ucch.org/sections/endo/index.html

Resources provided by this home page of the Section of Pediatric Endocrinology at the University of Chicago include a brief description of programs offered and conditions treated, a list of staff and their research interests and publications, and research studies conducted through the section. Also offered are links to other sites, primarily within the university.

University of Chicago: Section of Endocrinology ◐ ◐ ◐
http://endocrinology.uchicago.edu/index.html

This home page provides a list of faculty and their research interests, clinical research studies conducted through the section, information for prospective fellows, and related links. Visitors can also access the Thyroid Disease Manager, which provides a complete and current analysis of all aspects of human thyroid physiology and thyroid disease; the Center for Polycystic Ovary Syndrome (PCOS), which provides a resource for up-to-date information about PCOS, its diagnosis, treatment, and associated health risks; the Bone Disease Program; and the Section of Pediatric Endocrinology at the University of

Chicago. A faculty and staff e-mail directory and a directory for the Diabetes Prevention Program are also available.

University of Cincinnati College of Medicine: Division of Endocrinology and Metabolism ○

http://www.med.uc.edu/departments/displaydivisionshell.cfm?divisionid=21

The mission of the Division of Endocrinology and Metabolism at the University of Cincinnati is to provide excellence in clinical care, education, and research of patients with diseases of the endocrine system. The division also sponsors an ACGME-accredited training program for subspecialty fellows. This site offers a description of the division, contact information, and links to related sites within the College of Medicine.

University of Iowa College of Medicine Department of Internal Medicine: Division of Endocrinology and Metabolism ○ ○

http://www.int-med.uiowa.edu/Divisions/Endocrine

This page lists patient care, educational, research, and outreach activities of the Division of Endocrinology and Metabolism at the University of Iowa College of Medicine. Additionally, the site offers a list of faculty, fellows, and staff; a site search engine; links to the Virtual Hospital, a digital health sciences library; and links to other sites within the University of Iowa.

University of Iowa College of Medicine Department of Pediatrics: Division of Endocrinology ○

http://www.uihealthcare.com/DeptsClinical
Services/Peds/Divisions/Endocrinology.html

The Division of Endocrinology provides outpatient and inpatient consultation and services for children with endocrine disorders. This site lists the faculty with their educational background and clinical and research interests, an online patient self-referral form, contact information, and links to related sites within the University of Iowa Health Care system.

University of Maryland Department of Medicine: Division of Endocrinology and Metabolism ○

http://www.umm.edu/endo

The Division of Endocrinology and Metabolism at the University of Maryland offers inpatient and private consultations for the evaluation and treatment of patients with endocrine disorders, including obstetric patients. The site lists commonly treated conditions, evaluations, treatments, research activities, and special programs offered through the division. Also offered are links to related sites within the University of Maryland, specialty services available, and recent news releases.

University of Maryland Medical Center
Department of Pediatrics: Division of Pediatric Endocrinology
http://www.mdkids.umaryland.edu/peds/divisions.htm

The Division of Pediatric Endocrinology seeks to make available the latest advances in pediatric research and offers a range of specialized services to support physicians' efforts to evaluate and manage patients with endocrine disorders. The site offers a list of disease specialties, evaluations, treatments, research activities, and special programs available through the division. Contact information and links to other sites within the Department of Pediatrics are provided.

University of Michigan Medical Center:
Division of Endocrinology and Metabolism
http://www.med.umich.edu/intmed/endocrinology

Information provided at this site includes a list of faculty and fellows; resources from the division's fellowship program, including a description of the curriculum and an application available in PDF format; and patient information, including contact numbers, directions, and maps. Also provided are detailed information on the division, clinic and conference schedules, staff listings, grant and financial information, and links to related sites.

University of Minnesota, Department
of Medicine: Endocrinology and Diabetes
http://www.dept.med.umn.edu/medicine/Clinical_services/DEM_Clinic/dem_clinic.html

This site describes endocrinology and diabetes services provided through the Department of Medicine at the University of Minnesota. The site lists phone numbers for appointments and areas for which services are provided, including obesity, thyroid disease and function, pancreas and islet transplantation, treatment methods for diabetes mellitus, and general endocrinology.

University of North Carolina,
Chapel Hill: Division of Endocrinology
http://www.med.unc.edu/wrkunits/2depts/medicine/endocrin

The Division of Endocrinology at the University of North Carolina at Chapel Hill is composed of a full-service clinical component, clinical investigation and research programs, an education program for medical students at the university, a training program for clinical fellows, and basic research in several laboratories. The Web site provides a description of the division, research programs, faculty and staff, clinical services, and postgraduate research and training.

University of Pennsylvania Health System: Department of Medicine: Endocrinology, Diabetes and Metabolism Division ◎ ◎

http://www.med.upenn.edu/health/ms_files/services/me_edm.html

The Endocrinology, Diabetes and Metabolism Division offers diagnostic and therapeutic services for all endocrinologic conditions, including diabetes; disorders of the thyroid, parathyroid, adrenal, and pituitary glands; calcium metabolism; and disorders of the testes and ovaries. This site offers a list of staff with their positions and specialties, clinical services available, and links to related sites. Additionally, there are links to sites within the University of Pennsylvania Health System.

University of Rochester Medical Center, Department of Pediatrics: Division of Endocrinology ◎

http://www.urmc.rochester.edu/Peds/div/endo.htm

At this site visitors will find a brief description of the services and research projects of the Division of Endocrinology, as well as a list of faculty with backgrounds and research interests. The site also offers contact information and links to other divisions within the Department of Pediatrics and the University of Rochester Medical Center.

University of Texas Southwestern Medical Center, Department of Internal Medicine: Division of Endocrinology and Metabolism ◎ ◎

http://www.swmed.edu/home_pages/endocrine/index.shtml

Information provided by this site of the Division of Endocrinology and Metabolism includes a list of faculty and their areas of expertise, descriptions of training opportunities, and links to related sites at the University of Texas (UT) Southwestern and elsewhere. There is also a schedule of Endocrine Grand Rounds at the UT Southwestern Medical Center.

University of Utah, Department of Internal Medicine: Division of Endocrinology ◎

http://int.med.utah.edu:591/Divisions/FMPro?-db=divisions&-format=record%5fdetail.htm&-la

This brief site lists contact information for the Division of Endocrinology and describes research interests and activities.

University of Utah School of Medicine, Department of Pediatrics: Division of Endocrinology and Metabolism ◎

http://www.ped.med.utah.edu/Divisions/Endocrine/index.cfm

Information provided by this division home page includes a listing of consultation and diabetes clinic schedules, contact details for faculty, and a link to the Department of Pediatrics site.

University of Virginia Health System: Division of Endocrinology and Metabolism ✪ ✪ ✪
http://www.med.virginia.edu/internal/endocrine

The Division of Endocrinology and Metabolism at the University of Virginia conducts research and provides state-of-the-art care for patients with a variety of hormonal and metabolic disorders. The division also sponsors a fellowship training program in the field of endocrinology and metabolism. This informative Web site provides information about a variety of centers within the division, including the Virginia Center for Diabetes Professional Education, the Center for Biological Timing, the Center for Research in Reproduction, and the General Clinical Research Center. In addition, there are a list of faculty and staff and their research and educational interests, information about the fellowship training program, a section titled "This Week in Endocrinology," a schedule of seminars and special events, and links to endocrine sites within the University of Virginia Health System.

University of Washington School of Medicine, Department of Medicine: Division of Metabolism, Endocrinology and Nutrition ✪ ✪
http://depts.washington.edu/metab/index.htm

This site provides an overview of the Division of Metabolism, Endocrinology and Nutrition at the University of Washington School of Medicine, and includes a list of faculty, staff, research activities, programs, and centers. The site also offers information about the division's fellowship training program and a list of relevant clinics.

University of Wisconsin, Department of Medicine: Section of Endocrinology ✪
http://www.medicine.wisc.edu/sections/endo

The Section of Endocrinology provides endocrine, metabolic, and nutritional services for outpatients and inpatients; provides fellowship training; and conducts research in areas such as the mechanism of action for production of somatomedins, diabetes and control of insulin secretion, adrenal disease, fertility regulation and regulation of gonadotropin secretion, and other areas. This site includes contact information for the section and its related clinics.

Washington University School of Medicine: Division of Endocrinology, Diabetes, and Metabolism ✪
http://internalmed.wustl.edu/divisions/endo_diab_metab/aplab/map2.htm

The site of the Division of Endocrinology, Diabetes, and Metabolism at Washington University School of Medicine provides a profile of the division's laboratory. The site offers a description of research projects, a list of laboratory staff and publications, and links to related sites.

Washington University School of Medicine: Division of Pediatric Endocrinology and Metabolism ○ ○ ○
http://peds.wustl.edu/div/endometab

This site offers a history and description of the Division of Pediatric Endocrinology and Metabolism at Washington University, a mission statement for the division, contact information and a personnel directory. Also provided are information about the fellowship training program, a fellowship application form, a description of investigational and clinical activities at the division, faculty profiles, and links to related sites. A section for parents includes referral numbers, maps and directions, and an overview of what to expect during a child's treatment.

Yale University School of Medicine Department of Pediatrics: Section of Pediatric Endocrinology ○ ○
http://www.med.yale.edu/yfp/pedguide/endocrin.html

The Section of Pediatric Endocrinology at Yale University is a multidisciplinary unit that conducts research and provides care to patients with endocrine and metabolic diseases. The site offers a description of the section, including its research and clinical activities, and a list of faculty.

Yale University School of Medicine: Section of Endocrinology ○ ○
http://info.med.yale.edu/intmed/endocrin

The Section of Endocrinology is a research-intensive division within the Department of Internal Medicine and focuses on carbohydrate metabolism, mineral metabolism, and developmental biology. The site provides a description of the section, a faculty list with areas of expertise, clinical information, overviews of research and training programs, and notices of seminars. Also available are links to various pages within Yale University.

15.4 Research Organizations

Directories of Research Centers

CenterWatch: Profiles of Industry Providers ○ ○ ○
http://www.centerwatch.com/provider/provlist.htm

CenterWatch has cataloged an extensive listing of preclinical and clinical research, laboratory, monitoring, project management, trial design, patient recruitment, post-marketing services, and regulatory services providers in the United States, organized topically and geographically. For each industry provider, CenterWatch has prepared an in-depth profile, listing services, facilities, and contact information.

Individual Research Centers

Aoki Diabetes Research Institute (ADRI)
http://www.adri.org
The Aoki Diabetes Research Institute is devoted to the study of diabetes and metabolism. This home page offers information on chronic intermittent intravenous insulin therapy (CIIIT), which is the current focus of the center's research, as well as patient stories and annual reports.

Case Western Reserve University Center for Inherited Disorders of Energy Metabolism
http://www.cwru.edu/med/CIDEM/cidem.htm
The Center for Inherited Disorders of Energy Metabolism at Case Western Reserve University provides general information about the institute at this Web site. Resources include a list of relevant publications authored by the center's staff; information about tests offered at the center, including specimen requirements and prices; and contact details.

Center for Research on Reproduction and Women's Health
http://www.med.upenn.edu/~crrwh
From the University of Pennsylvania Health System, this site provides information on the Center for Research on Reproduction and Women's Health. Details are provided on research activities, training, seminar series, and related departments. Other tools offered at the site include e-mail and phone directories, computer information, grant information, and links to related resources.

Cutaneous Biology Research Center
http://cbrc-a12.mgh.harvard.edu
The MGH/Harvard Cutaneous Biology Research Center was established in 1989. The site offers information about the center, faculty, and governance. Topics covered include employment and fellowship opportunities, principal investigators, grants and funding, policies and standards, tutorials, conferences, and symposia. The site also offers links to other resources, including journals.

Diabetes Action Research and Education Foundation
http://www.daref.org
The Diabetes Action Research and Education Foundation is devoted to improving life for those affected by diabetes and its complications. The site offers financial information about the foundation; information about education and program services, including a Native American program, an international program, public service, a diabetes camp for children, and a diabetes university program; and information about

research projects and upcoming events. A recipe and tip of the week and links to related sites are available.

Diabetes and Endocrinology Research Center ○ ○ ○
http://uiderc.icva.gov

From the University of Iowa, this site describes the Diabetes and Endocrinology Research Center. An overview of goals and resources of the center and a description of core facilities are provided, as well as information about core directors and research personnel, research investigators, areas of research, and the center's enrichment pilot project programs. Visitors will also find contact information and links to other diabetes research sites.

Diabetes Institutes Foundation ○ ○
http://www.dif.org

The Diabetes Institutes Foundation supports research at the Leonard R. Strelitz Diabetes Institutes of Eastern Virginia Medical School. The site provides information about the foundation, their supporters, and the patients they have treated. Links to diabetes and nutrition topics, special event details, and related sites are offered.

Diabetes Research and Wellness Foundation ○ ○
http://www.diabeteswellness.net

The Diabetes Research and Wellness Foundation was organized to find a cure for diabetes and provide self-management skills for people with diabetes. There is information on research grants and wellness programs sponsored by the foundation, as well as articles on weight loss, aspirin, and the importance of exercise.

Diabetes Research Institute ○ ○ ○
http://www.drinet.org/html/the_diabetes_research_institut.htm

The Diabetes Research Institute, located at the University of Miami School of Medicine, is devoted entirely to the cure and treatment of diabetes. The site provides patient articles on the following topics: islet cell transplantation, encapsulation, genetic engineering, xenotransplantation, immuno genetics, molecular biology, research lipids, and cardiovascular research. Information about clinical trials, news related to the institute, and a section for kids are also available.

Genetics and In Vitro Fertilization Institute ○ ○
http://www.givf.com

The Genetics and In Vitro Fertilization Institute provides infertility treatment and genetics services in Virginia and Maryland. There are feature articles on such topics as in vitro fertilization, gender selection, preserving reproductive function prior to cancer treatment, cytoplasm transfer, ovary cryopreservation, breast and ovarian cancer risk in Jewish women, preimplantation genetic testing for Huntington's disease, and a colon cancer gene mutation test for Ashkenazi Jews. Sections describing various treatments and services available at the institute are also found at the site.

Joslin Diabetes Center ◉ ◉ ◉
http://www.joslin.harvard.edu

An affiliate of Harvard Medical School, the Joslin Diabetes Center offers news, information, and education related to the disorder. There is information specific to the Boston facilities, including programs for patients, physician profiles, and research volunteers, as well as information about nationwide affiliates. Links to press releases, the latest news, and legislation affecting diabetics are also posted. Research information includes research profiles and links to other research sites. Additional resources include a diabetes library; catalog of books, videotapes, and other educational materials; and a list of continuing medical education courses. Also provided are descriptions of many programs available and links to articles on diabetes, monitoring, insulin, oral medications, nutrition, exercise, and complications.

Neuroendocrine Clinical Center and Pituitary Tumor Center ◉ ◉
http://neurosurgery.mgh.harvard.edu/nendo-hp.htm

Part of Massachusetts General Hospital, this site offers information about the Neuroendocrine Clinical Center and Pituitary Tumor Center. An introduction is followed by information on the attending staff, scheduling, outpatient services, inpatient consultation service, and special expertise. There is also information on stereotactic proton radiosurgery, neuroendocrine clinical conferences, and neuroendocrine lecture series.

Sansum Medical Research Institute ◉ ◉ ◉
http://www.sansum.org

The Sansum Medical Research Institute was founded in 1920 to facilitate research in the treatment of diabetes. Resources provided by this home page include an overview of research conducted at the institute; information about immunology, pathology, and clinical trials; a discussion of pregnancy and diabetes; and a section on nutrition, which includes recipes and helpful hints. Visitors will also find contact information and access to recent newsletters.

University of Maryland Center for Studies in Reproduction ◉ ◉
http://csr.umaryland.edu

This multidisciplinary center is composed of investigators studying developmental endocrinology, ovarian physiology, perinatal endocrinology, uteroplacental physiology, cardiovascular physiology, reproductive behavior, neuroendocrinology, cancer, and mechanisms of hormone action. Resources provided by the center's home page include an overview of the center, a research mission statement, faculty profiles, a description of the center's seminars program, details of training opportunities through the center, and contact information.

University of Minnesota Diabetes Institute for Immunology and Transplantation ◉ ◉ ◉
http://www.diabetesinstitute.org

The Diabetes Institute for Immunology and Transplantation at the University of Minnesota is devoted to finding solutions for diabetics. Information about diabetes at the site includes an overview of the disease, a discussion of the social impact of diabetes, and links to related sites. Other resources include a medical glossary, information about the institute's pancreas and islet programs, a directory of articles on the Internet, a bibliography of other articles, and information about community events and training opportunities. There is also a section devoted to basic and current research.

University of Washington Diabetes Endocrinology Research Center ◉ ◉
http://depts.washington.edu/diabetes

The University of Washington Diabetes Endocrinology Research Center offers an overview of the center's activities at this address, as well as information about affiliates, seminars, directors, and grant programs. Links to other resources are also available.

Vanderbilt University Diabetes Center: Diabetes and Research Training Center ◉ ◉
http://www.mc.vanderbilt.edu/vumc/centers/drtc

One of a network of Core Centers established by the NIDDK, this organization conducts research and training in diabetes mellitus and related endocrine and metabolic disorders. A description of the multidisciplinary program, its core facilities and services, and postdoctoral training details are provided.

Whittier Institute for Diabetes ◉ ◉
http://www.whittier.org

The Whittier Institute for Diabetes is the research and patient care arm of Scripps Health in San Diego, California. This site offers information about ongoing research at the institute; links to diabetes conferences and other related sites; and links to e-mail lists, chat rooms, and personal stories.

15.5 Selected Hospital Endocrinology and Metabolism Departments

Baylor Health Care System: Diabetes Services ◉ ◉
http://www.baylorhealth.com/BaylorsBest/default.asp?Page=service.mid.asp

This site offers information on diabetes services available at Baylor, including program descriptions, contact details, and a list of office locations. Links are available to information on the Diabetes Self-Management Training Program, the Ruth Collins Diabetes Center, the Howard Center, the Gestational Diabetes Management Program, and support groups offered by Baylor and other institutions. Resources on professional programs are also available, including program descriptions, registration forms, and notices of upcoming programs.

Research	The Howard Center at Baylor Medical Center at Irving conducts clinical research into the efficacy of new therapies, and also offers advanced treatment and prevention services for osteoporosis.
Patient Resources	Links to information on patient support groups are available from the site, as well as a list of Baylor Diabetes Center locations.
Location	Dallas, TX

Brigham and Women's Hospital (BWH): Division of Endocrinology-Hypertension ○ ○

http://www.partners.org/pw-cgi/dbml.exe?template=/pweb-view/dept/about/about.dbml&dept_id=34&rso_abbrev=BWH

The George Thorn Center for Endocrinology Disorders in the Division of Endocrinology-Hypertension provides clinical services for patient suffering from hypoglycemia, pituitary diseases, thyroid diseases, adrenal dysfunction, menstrual disorders, gonadal diseases, hirsutism, disorders of calcium metabolism, obesity, osteoporosis, diabetes, hypertension, and sleep disorders. This site offers staff profiles with research interests, referral information, a history of the division, patient resources, information on the division's fellowship and training programs, and discussions of current research projects.

Research	Research in the division is conducted in the areas of diabetes and metabolism, pregnancy-related endocrinology and hypertension, skeletal health and osteoporosis, sleep disorders, hypertension, and thyroid disorders. The research section of this site offers summaries of current research projects related to hypertension, diabetes, calcium disorder and osteoporosis, and sleep disorders.
Patient Resources	Through the "Patient Resources" link, visitors will find descriptions of clinical services and information resources for physicians. Contact details for the patient referral service, the physician referral service, and emergencies are also provided.
Location	Boston, MA

Cleveland Clinic: Department of Endocrinology ○ ○

http://www.clevelandclinic.org/endo

Cleveland Clinic's Department of Endocrinology home page cites the Department's specializations and interests as diabetes mellitus, obesity, osteoporosis, and hypoglycemia; and pituitary, thyroid, parathyroids, adrenals, ovaries, and testes glandular dysfunctions. Also accessible from this home page are links to information for prospective patient participants on research projects, profiles of faculty members, and details on making an appointment.

Research	Information on current clinical research studies, including contact details for patient enrollment, is available through the "Endocrinology Research Projects" link at the home page. A link to staff profiles with research interests is also provided.
Patient Resources	Patient information on diabetes from the department's Data Transfer Project includes an overview of diabetes warning signs, reviews of several commercial blood glucose meters, diabetes management software reviews, diabetes news, and contact details. Additional patient resources include links to important diabetes sites, contact details for enrollment in current clinical studies, and information on making an appointment with the department.
Location	Cleveland, OH

Duke University Medical Center: Division of Endocrinology, Metabolism, and Nutrition ◎ ◎

http://medicine.mc.duke.edu/endro.nsf?Open

This home page of the Division of Endocrinology, Metabolism, and Nutrition offers a description of the division and overview in terms of the number of current faculty and fellows, outpatient visits, inpatient procedures, and inpatient and outpatient consultations. The site also lists specialty procedures, outreach activities, clinical and basic research interests, special programs, and educational activities. Links are also available to a summary of current division goals, information on basic and clinical research training programs, and faculty profiles.

Research	Endocrinology research projects are listed in the areas of osteoporosis, metabolic bone disease, diabetes mellitus, lipid abnormalities, andrologic disorders, pathophysiology, genetics and mitogenic signal transduction.
Patient Resources	Endocrinology-based patient programs at Duke include the Adult Diabetes Education Programs, Inpatient Diabetes Management Programs, and Multidisciplinary Osteoporosis Programs. Faculty profiles with research interests and contact details are also available.
Location	Durham, NC

Johns Hopkins Medical Institutions: Endocrine Surgery ◎ ◎

http://hopkins.med.jhu.edu

Information on endocrine surgery at Johns Hopkins is available from this site, including an overview of endocrine surgery for patients, descriptions of current clinical and basic research interests, faculty profiles with publication bibliographies, and contact information and other resources for appointments and consultations.

Research	Clinical and basic research projects are currently listed in the areas of follicular carcinoma of the thyroid, medullary carcinoma, imaging strategies for parathyroid localization, and gene therapy for metastatic thyroid carcinoma.
Patient Resources	Patients will find an overview of thyroid, parathyroid, adrenal, islet cell tumor, and carcinoid tumor surgery at Johns Hopkins, including clinical details of conditions requiring surgery. Information on services for international patients, the Marburg Pavillion for patients requesting additional comfort and privacy, and patient preparation for admission is provided, as well as contact details for appointments and consultations.
Location	Baltimore, MD

Loyola University: Stritch School of Medicine

http://www.meddean.luc.edu

This address lists specialty imaging and diagnostic services, areas of specialty, and a Diabetes Care Center available through the division. Contact details for physician consultation and referral services and appointment scheduling are also provided. The site also offers links to information on patient services, education programs, research activities, events calendars, and other departments available through LUMC.

Research	Research and clinical services are provided for the treatment of hyperthyroidism in pregnancy, Cushing's syndrome, multiple endocrine neoplasia, hyperthyroidism, hypogonadism, metabolic bone disease, diabetes mellitus, pituitary dysfunction, and neuroendocrinology.
Patient Resources	Information provided through the "Patient Services" link includes a directory of specialty programs and services, primary and specialty physician search engines, and notices of upcoming free health lectures.
Location	Maywood, IL

Massachusetts General Hospital/Harvard Medical School: Neuroendocrine Clinical Center and Pituitary Tumor Center

http://neurosurgery.mgh.harvard.edu/nendo-hp.htm

The Neuroendocrine Clinical Center and Pituitary Tumor Center are comprised of endocrinologists, neurologists, and neurosurgeons serving patients with pituitary and hypothalamic disorders. Visitors will find a directory of attending staff, a newsletter, information on scheduling and referrals, an overview of outpatient and inpatient services, a list of specialty services, information on stereotactic proton radiosurgery for the treatment of pituitary lesions, contact details, and links to suggested sites for patients with pituitary tumors. Details of the neuroendocrine speakers bureau for outside symposia and other events, clinical conferences, and lecture series are also provided.

Research	Information on current hospital research studies available includes evaluation of medical treatments for acromegaly and menstrual dysfunction, as well as new hormonal therapies for the treatment of hormonal deficiencies and HIV positive patients with fat redistribution. The effects of growth hormone on bone and muscle strength in healthy subjects is also being evaluated by the department.
Patient Resources	Resources for patients include details of scheduling and referrals, a list of outpatient services, an overview of proton beam radiosurgery for pituitary lesions, and a list of clinical studies currently open to patient enrollment. Contact details for enrollment are also provided.
Location	Boston, MA

Mayo Clinic: Endocrinology, Metabolism, Diabetes, and Nutrition Division ○ ○ ○

http://www.mayo.edu/endocrine/endo-main.htm

The home page for the Endocrinology, Metabolism, Diabetes and Nutrition Division describes the endocrine system and offers patient information, information for providers on patient referral and care, an overview of clinical services, information on education programs, research summaries, and staff profiles.

Research	Among the Mayo Clinic endocrinology research projects are: metabolic bone disease and osteoporosis; thyroid diseases and thyroid cancer; diabetes mellitus pathophysiology, etiology, complications, and management; diagnosis and management of lipid disorders, obesity, and other nutrition problems; and diagnosis and treatments for pituitary, adrenal and gonadal diseases. Information on the Endocrinology Outcomes and Efficiency Project and molecular and epidemiological endocrinology research is available from the site.
Patient Resources	Patient information available from the site includes details on making an appointment, an overview of the consulting staff in endocrinology at Mayo Clinic, profiles of special support and service programs, and tips for an upcoming visit to the clinic.
Location	Rochester, MN

New England Medical Center (NEMC): Division of Endocrinology, Diabetes, Metabolism, and Molecular Medicine ○ ○

http://www.nemc.org/home/departments/adult/endocrin.htm

This division of the New England Medical Center specializes in the treatment of thyroid disorders, pituitary disorders, adrenal diseases, diabetes, lipid disorders, diseases of calcium regulation, and osteoporosis and other metabolic bone diseases. This site offers an overview of the division and descriptions of specific clinics, including those specializing in bone metabolism, lipid disorders, neuroendocrinology, thyroid diseases, diabetes, and general endocrine disorders. Contact details and information on clinical sessions are also available.

Patient Resources	Patients will find general resources through the "Information" link at this site, including address and telephone contacts, maps and directions, and a searchable database of NEMC physicians.
Location	Boston, MA

New York Presbyterian Hospital ○ ○ ○

http://cpmcnet.cpmc.columbia.edu/dept/medicine/endocrinmen.html

A description of the Division of Endocrinology's strengths in the areas of patient care, teaching and research is available at this address, with clinical programs cited in the areas of metabolic bone diseases, neuroendocrinology thyroid disorders, and diabetes. Visitors will also find listings of endocrinology and affiliated faculty, contact details, and details of special clinical programs and research activities.

Research	Diseases researched through special clinical programs and research activities include metabolic bone diseases, neuroendocrinology, thyroid disorders, and diabetes. A link is available to the Naomi Berrie Diabetes Center home page, offering information on patient care programs, center news and events notices, research highlights, answers to frequently asked questions, and contact details.
Patient Resources	The Berrie Diabetes Center offers support to patients and families with online descriptions of education programs, forums for children and adults, patient perspectives on the disease, clinical trials, and a discussion encouraging family involvement in disease treatment. Visitors will also find an online video presentation of the center, and a section for children.
Location	New York, NY

Northwestern Memorial Hospital: Division of Endocrinology ○ ○

http://www.nmh.org/services/endocrinology.html

The Division of Endocrinology treats and diagnoses pituitary, thyroid, parathyroid and adrenal gland cancers and diseases. Specialized services for diabetes are also provided. This site offers a summary of the division and contact details, as well as resources for Northwestern Memorial Hospital, including a physician directory, news and publications, links to other clinical programs, employment opportunities, contact details, health information for physicians and consumers, and a list of affiliated managed care plans.

Research	The division participates in several research trials sponsored by NIH, including a multicenter trial on diabetes prevention and research into the management of gestational diabetes. Two faculty investigators of the division are also members of the NIH-sponsored National Center for Infertility Research.
Patient Resources	Patients will find health information, a profile of the hospital's Wellness Institute, contact details, an overview of the hospital, and

answers to frequently asked questions on hospital location and other logistical issues.

Location — Chicago, IL

Penn State Milton S. Hershey Medical Center: Endocrinology, Diabetes, and Metabolism Division ◐ ◐

http://www.hmc.psu.edu/medservices/medicine/endo.htm

Members of the division staff specialize in the treatment of growth disorders, hirsutism, metabolic problems, osteoporosis, and diabetes, as well as thyroid, parathyroid, pancreatic, gonadal, pituitary, and adrenal diseases. This site provides a summary of the division and links to general resources from the medical center, including information for patients and visitors, details of academic programs, and information on research facilities and specialty centers.

Research — The center operates a Core Endocrine Laboratory (CEL), offering comprehensive hormone analysis of blood, urine, tissues, and culture media from both humans and experimental animals. The home page of the laboratory is located at http://www.hmc.psu.edu/endo, offering visitors a description of the facility, a profile of the director, a mission statement, detailed information on services provided by the laboratory, a test menu and schedule of fees, a list of previous and current projects and contracts, accreditation details, citations of selected publications, case studies, and links to related endocrinology sites.

Patient Resources — Resources provided for use by patients and health consumers include links to descriptions of medical services, health information on common conditions and other issues, a physician directory, a list of participating insurance plans, news articles and events notices, research profiles, maps and directions, and information on special education programs and support groups for patients and caregivers.

Location — Hershey, PA

Rush-Presbyterian-St. Luke's Medical Center: Department of Internal Medicine ◐

http://www.rpslmc.edu/patients/internal/endocrine.html

An overview of the center's Department of Internal Medicine is available from this site, including links to clinical sections, contact details, information on training programs, clinical trials resources, and related sites of interest. Information on patient services, a medical encyclopedia, and a physician directory are also available. Through the "Clinical Sections" link, visitors will find a brief summary of the Section of Endocrinology's services, include endocrine testing, thyroid biopsy, and diabetes education, as well as contact details for the section.

Research — Research at Rush focuses on diabetes, lipid metabolism, and bone disorders.

Patient Resources	Patient resources include contact details, a directory of physicians, and a medical encyclopedia. Visitors can search the medical encyclopedia by symptom, alphabetically, or by age group. First aid and preventive health information and a multimedia gallery of common health issues are also available.
Location	Chicago, IL

Temple University Hospital: Metabolism, Diabetes and Endocrinology ○

http://www.health.temple.edu/tuh/Health_Care_Information/metabolism.html

The Temple University Hospital home page provides visitors with links to information on clinical programs, academic departments, residency and fellowship programs, medical staff, and a searchable directory of physicians for referrals and appointments. Recent hospital news articles are also available. Visitors can follow the "Academic Departments" link to a listing of links to profiles of departments, including the Metabolism, Diabetes and Endocrinology section within the Department of Medicine. Information on this section includes a description of the department and contact details for appointments.

Research	The Section of Metabolism, Diabetes, and Endocrinology conducts research in several areas, including diabetes and the metabolic aspects of obesity.
Patient Resources	Information for patients is found under the "General Information" link at the home page, and includes contact numbers, directions and parking information, and visiting hours. Special instructions and information for inpatients and day surgery patients are also provided.
Location	Philadelphia, PA

University of Alabama Health System: Division of Endocrinology and Metabolism ○ ○

http://info.dom.uab.edu/endo/index.htm

The Division of Endocrinology and Metabolism home page offers a description of clinical activities and consultation services, a division conference calendar, a faculty directory, a description of the fellowship program, and an overview of research interests in the division.

Research	Basic and clinical research interests currently focus on the molecular basis of diabetic complications, mechanisms of hormonal control of growth and growth factor production, mechanisms of growth hormone action, control of gene transcription, regulation of gene expression by glucose, the cost effectiveness of various insulin initiation schemes, and HLA typing in the identification of susceptibility to diabetes and other endocrine disorders.

Patient Resources   The site provides information on consultation services from the division. Additional information for patients is available from the University of Alabama Health System home page, located at http://www.health.uab.edu, including general health information, news articles, contact details, maps and directions, and information on additional services available to patients and families.

Location   Birmingham, AL

University of California Los Angeles: Medical Center: Division of Endocrinology, Diabetes, and Hypertension ○

http://www.handbook.healthcare.ucla.edu/div.asp?version=5619&div=235

Specializations of this Division of Endocrinology, Diabetes and Hypertension include pituitary disorders, thyroid disorders, disorders of mineral metabolism, adrenal disorders, endocrine pancreas conditions, ovarian conditions, testicular conditions, and hyperlipidemias. This home page includes contact details for information and referral, a link to the division's Diabetes Program, and a listing of faculty members.

Research   Profiles of research at UCLA and its medical center can found through a site search engine. Endocrinology research includes projects investigating insulin-like growth factors (IGFs), pediatric endocrinology, and the effects of estrogen replacement therapy on mood and cognition in postmenopausal women.

Patient Resources   This site offers a list of disorders in which division faculty offer specialized management. Clinical services available through the UCLA Diabetes Program are also listed, as well as contact details.

Location   Los Angeles, CA

University of Chicago Hospitals and Health System ○ ○

http://endocrinology.uchicago.edu

From this introductory page readers can connect to descriptions of research projects, as well as to specialized areas such as the Center for Polycystic Overay Syndrome, the Bone Disease Program, pediatric endocrinology, the Thyroid Disease Manager, and the Diabetes Prevention Program Directory. An e-mail directory, faculty research interests, information on current clinical research studies for patients and physicians, a list of current fellows, information for prospective fellows, links to related sites, and general contact details are also provided.

Research   Clinical studies here include examination of the connection between heredity and Polycystic Ovary Syndrome (PCOS), and specific studies titled Treatment with Troglitazone (Rezulin) for Newly Diagnosed Type 2 Diabetes, Genetics of Type 2 Diabetes in Sibling Pairs, Genetics of Insulin Secretion and Action in PCOS, Pathogenesis and Therapy of PCOS, Study of Families Who Have a History of Type 2 Diabetes Mellitus, Study for Prevention of Type 2 Diabetes, and Study of

Obese Patients With or Without Risk Factors for Type 2 Diabetes. Faculty research interests include molecular genetics of diabetes, type 2 diabetes, gestational diabetes, thyroid autoimmunity and cancer, polycystic ovary syndrome, beta cell function, ion channels, thyroid hormone resistance, iodine transport, and biological rhythms.

Patient Resources — Resources valuable to patients include information on clinical studies open to enrollment, links to the Center for Polycystic Ovary Syndrome and other specialty groups, and a faculty directory with research interests.

Location — Chicago, IL

University of Illinois: Chicago
Medical Center: Division of Andrology ◐ ◑
http://godot.urol.uic.edu

Medical services offered by the Department of Andrology are summarized at the site, including evaluation of male endocrine dysfunction. Connections to the full andrological laboratory services and home pages of the faculty are found.

Research — Research interests of the Andrology Laboratory director focus on basic and applied studies in male reproductive function, including hormonal control of prostatic development, growth, and function. Clinical research interests involve fertility analysis, improvement, and predictability in males with fertility problems.

Patient Resources — Patient resources include consumer-oriented discussions of male infertility testing services, the Patient Sperm Banking Program, and the Donor Sperm Program. Fee schedules, maps and directions, and a catalog of donor sperm samples are also provided.

Location — Chicago, IL

University of Maryland Medicine: Joslin Diabetes Center ◐ ◑
http://www.umm.edu/joslindiabetes

An affiliate of the Joslin Diabetes Center in Boston, this center offers comprehensive health resources for children and adults with diabetes, including clinical services, education and self-care programs, and research. Resources provided by this site include contact information, overviews of services provided to both adults and children, staff profiles, research news, contact details and descriptions for education and self-care programs, facts about diabetes, and information on making an appointment.

Research — The "Research News" section of the site offers descriptions of selected research projects, including those investigating diabetes control and reduction of complications, new technology for the diagnosis of eye complications, cell communication, the impact of lifestyle changes and medications on the delay or prevention of type 2 diabetes, a new chemical for the prevention of blood vessel complications,

	and the prevention of type 1 diabetes in high-risk individuals through small amounts of insulin therapy. Clinical studies seeking volunteers are also listed at the site.
Patient Resources	Services for both adults and the pediatric population are outlined at their respective pages and include screening programs, medical care and complications treatment, a weight and nutrition management program, and access to information on patient participation in clinical trials. An online screening test for diabetes, diabetes fact sheets, and Joslin Center team profiles are available.
Location	Baltimore, MD

University of Michigan Medical Center: Division of Endocrinology and Metabolism ○

http://www.med.umich.edu/intmed/endocrinology

The division's homepage offers faculty and fellow profiles, contact details, fellowship program information, general information for patients, descriptions of current clinical trials, clinic and conference schedules, and links to several related sites.

Research	The clinical study currently listed at this site is titled "Fatty Acids as a Determinant of Blood Pressure."
Patient Resources	Patient information includes an overview of the division, maps and directions, contact details, and descriptions and contact numbers of nursing staff.
Location	Ann Arbor, MI

University of North Carolina, Chapel Hill: Endocrinology Division ○ ○

http://www.med.unc.edu/wrkunits/2depts/medicine/endocrin

Information on research, faculty and staff, clinical services, and postgraduate research and training programs is available through this endocrinology home page. The site also offers an overview of the field of endocrinology, a link to the Diabetes Care Center, and contact details.

Research	Clinical trials pertaining to diabetes are described at the Diabetes Care Center. Other endocrinology research projects are described in the faculty profiles postgraduate training sections of the site.
Patient Resources	Patient can follow a link to the Diabetes Care Center for information on healthcare services, clinical research, and current clinical trials. Patient education resources provided by the center include recipes, a newsletter, details of upcoming events, and links to related sites.
Location	Chapel Hill, NC

University of Pennsylvania Health System: Endocrinology, Diabetes, and Metabolism Division ⊙ ⊙

http://www.med.upenn.edu/health/ms_files/services/me_edm.html

This division specializes in the medical management of diabetes and related complications, male reproductive endocrinology, pituitary diseases, thyroid disorders, and osteoporosis and other metabolic bone diseases. The site offers staff profiles; descriptions of services offered in endocrinology, diabetes, and metabolism; and contact details for appointments.

Research	Research is conducted at the Cox Institute for Diabetes Research in the areas of diabetic retinopathy, nephropathy, and diabetic dermatologic complications. New research technologies used in the diagnosis and management of metabolic bone diseases include dual photon absorptiometry, quantitative computed tomographic scanning, and biopsy of tetracycline labelled bone.
Patient Resources	Patient information includes faculty profiles and contact numbers for appointments. Additional resources are found through connections at the top of the page, including the "Your Health" link, with discussions of nutrition, general health topics, management of chronic conditions, and articles; the "Visitor Information" link, including comprehensive information for each hospital of the UPHS system; and the "Health Plans" link, which lists accepted health plans.
Location	Philadelphia, PA

University of Pittsburgh Medical Center: Division of Endocrinology and Metabolism ⊙ ⊙

http://www.upmc.edu/endodocs/index.html

The Division of Endocrinology and Metabolism's Web site connects readers to a list of clinical services, contact details, information on patient services, annual reports, faculty profiles, descriptions of research projects and clinical facilities, information on the division's fellowship program, and a chart summarizing appropriate treatment of diabetic acidosis. The site also offers a summary of common screening tests for endocrine disorders and a list of normal values of common endocrine tests.

Research	Division research interests include oxytocin and gonadal steroids, regulation of gonadotropin secretion, thyroid physiology, diabetic nephropathy, insulin receptor physiology, glucose and free fatty acid metabolism in diabetic muscle, insulin resistance, steroid-induced osteoporosis, pancreas transplantation, male reproduction, and vasopressin physiology.
Patient Resources	Patients will find descriptions of clinical facilities, a list of clinical services provided by the division, and details for appointments.
Location	Pittsburgh, PA

University of Virginia Health System: Division of Endocrinology and Metabolism ◐ ◐

http://www.med.virginia.edu/internal/endocrine

Resources provided by this home page include descriptions of research and clinical activities, directories of faculty and staff, notices of upcoming events and seminars, information on faculty research and education programs, descriptions of clinical activities and facilities, and an overview of the fellowship training program. The site also offers links to specialty centers devoted to diabetes, biological timing, research in reproduction, and general clinical research, as well as the Endocrine Surgery Service at the University of Virginia.

Research	Numerous research projects are conducted within four specialized centers of the division, including those devoted to diabetes, biological timing, reproduction, and general clinical research.
Patient Resources	The home page offers maps and directions to the University of Virginia. A link to the Diabetes Community Network offers information on upcoming patient education classes, descriptions of services, a description of upcoming Consumer Network Groups, and information on Primary Prevention Programs.
Location	Charlottesville, VA

Vanderbilt University Medical Center: Division of Endocrinology, Diabetes, and Metabolism ◐ ◐

http://medicine.mc.vanderbilt.edu/divisions/endocrin

This site offers an overview of the division, profiles of clinical and research faculty, a downloadable fellowship application form, a bibliography of recent publications, and links to related sites. Information on training, clinical, and research programs is also available.

Research	Research information is provided through profiles of clinical and research faculty members. The Clinical Program offers profiles and links to several specialty groups, including the Diabetes Improvement Program, the Pituitary Center at Vanderbilt, and the Vanderbilt Thyroid and Surgical Endocrinology Clinic. Clinical faculty research interests are also listed. Information on clinical trials is also available.
Patient Resources	Information for patient use includes details of current clinical trials and a link to the Vanderbilt Center for Diabetes Care (VCDC). Resources provided by the VCDC include staff profiles, information on patient education programs, and links to related diabetes sites for patient use. VCDC patients can also access forms for home blood glucose monitoring, which allow users to e-mail home blood glucose results and receive recommendations from their diabetes health care provider.
Location	Nashville, TN

PART FOUR

DISORDERS OF ENDOCRINOLOGY & METABOLISM

Alphabetical Listing of Diseases and Disorders

Abetalipoproteinemia 383
Acquired Hyperlipidemia 379
Acromegaly 268
Acute Intermittent Porphyria 408
Addison's Disease 293
Adrenal Glands 291
Adrenal Hemorrhage 294
Adrenal Hormone Overproduction 295
Adrenal Insufficiency 292
Adrenal Tumors 298
Adrenoleukodystrophy (ALD) 294
Alcaptonuria 393
Aldosterone-Producing
Adrenal Adenoma (Conn's Syndrome) 299
Amenorrhea 307
Amino Acid Metabolism 393
Amyloidosis 417
Androgen Abnormalities 315
Androgen Insensitivity Syndrome
(Male Pseudohermaphroditism) 331
Autoimmune Polyendocrinopathy 415
Benign Prostatic Hyperplasia (BPH) 321
Bone and Mineral Metabolism 335

Bone Mineralization Disorders 338
Calcium Metabolism Disorders, General .. 335
Calcium, Phosphorus, and Vitamin D 335
Carbohydrate Metabolism 387
Carbohydrate-Deficient
Glycoprotein Syndromes 405
Carcinoid Tumors
and Carcinoid Syndrome 411
Carcinoma of the Pancreas 304
Cerebrotendinous Xanthomatosis 399
Collagen Disorders 341
Congenital Adrenal Hyperplasia 332
Congenital Adrenal Hyperplasia (CAH) ... 295
Congenital Erythropoietic Porphyria 408
Congenital Hypothyroidism 275
Coronary Complications 364
Craniopharyngiomas 271
Cryptorchidism 319
Cushing's Disease 269
Dermatologic Manifestations of Diabetes . 365
Development and Sexual Differentiation .. 327
Diabetes Insipidus 263
Diabetes Mellitus 359

Diabetic Foot Ulcers and Disease 365
Disorders of Endocrinology
and Metabolism, General Resources 261
Disturbances of Acid-Base Metabolism 356
Empty Sella Syndrome 265
Energy Metabolism 373
Erectile Dysfunction 316
Essential Fructosuria 387
Fabry's Disease 399
Familial Lecithin
Cholesterol Acyltransferase Deficiency 379
Fatty Acid Oxidation and Carnitine 397
Female Endocrinology 307
Female Pseudohermaphroditism 332
Fluid, Electrolyte, and
Acid-Base Metabolism 353
Fructose-1,6-Bisphosphatase Deficiency 387
Galactokinase Deficiency 388
Galactosemia 388
Galactosylceramide
Lipidosis (Krabbe's Disease) 400
Gastrinoma
(Zollinger-Ellison Syndrome) 302
Gastrointestinal Tract 301
Gastroparesis 366
Gaucher Disease 400
Generalized Gangliosidosis 402
Genetic Syndromes
of Developmental Disorders 327
Gestational Diabetes 362
Glucagonoma 303
Glycogen Storage Diseases: General 389
Glycogen Storage Diseases: Pompe
Disease (Acid Maltase Deficiency) 389
Goiter 283
Graves' Disease 279
Growth and Stature 346
Growth Hormone Deficiency 266
Gynecomastia 317
Hashimoto's Thyroiditis 277
Hereditary Coproporphyria 409
Hereditary Fructose Intolerance 390
Hermaphroditism, General 332
Hirsutism 308
HIV 418
Homocystinuria 394
Hyperaldosteronism 297
Hypercalcemia 335
Hypercortisolism: Cushing's Syndrome 297
Hyperglycemia,
Hyperosmolar, Nonketotic State 370
Hyperkalemia 354
Hyperlipidemia 377
Hypernatremia 355
Hyperparathyroidism: Adenoma 345
Hyperparathyroidism: Carcinoma 345
Hyperparathyroidism: General 344
Hyperphosphatemia 337
Hyperprolactinemia and Galactorrhea 269
Hyperthyroidism 287
Hypobetalipoproteinemia 383
Hypocalcemia 337
Hypoglycemia 370
Hypokalemia 354
Hypolipidemia 382
Hyponatremia 355
Hypoparathyroidism 346
Hypophosphatemia 337
Hypopituitarism 265
Hypothalamic-Pituitary Axis Dysfunction. 263
Hypothyroidism 287
Hypothyroidism, General 274
Infertility 308
Infertility 318
Insulin Resistance 363
Insulinoma 303
Ketoacidosis 366
Klinefelter's Syndrome 327,333
Lipoprotein and
Cholesterol Metabolism 377
Lysosomal Disorders 398
Lysosomal Storage Diseases, General 398
Macrosomia 372
Magnesium Metabolism Disorders 353
Male Endocrinology 315
Male Gonadal Disorders 319
Malignancy 419
Malnutrition 375
Maple Syrup Urine Disease 394
Medullary Thyroid Carcinoma 412
Menstrual
Exacerbations of Medical Problems 309
Metabolic Acidosis 356
Metabolic Alkalosis 357
Metabolism, Inborn Errors 385
Metachromatic Leukodystrophy 402
Mucopolysaccharidoses
(MPS) and Related Diseases 391

Multiple Endocrine Neoplasia	412	Prostate Disorders	321
Myxedema Coma	277	Prostatitis	325
Neoplasms of the Pancreas	302	Pseudohypoparathyroidism	346
Nephropathy	367	Purine and Pyrimidine Metabolic Disorders	398
Neuroendocrine System	263	Pyruvate Carboxylase Deficiency	392
Neurofibromatosis (Recklinghausen's Disease)	413	Pyruvate Dehydrogenase Complex Deficiency	392
Neuropathy	368	Rarer Porphyrias	410
Niemann-Pick Disease	403	Refsum's Disease	403
Non-Functioning Adrenal Incidentaloma	299	Reidel's Thyroiditis	278
Nonthyroidal Illness	288	Renal Osteodystrophy	339
Noonan's Syndrome	328	Retinopathy	369
Obesity	373	Rickets	340
Organ Damage	372	Secondary Hypogonadism: Kallman Syndrome	320
Osteogenesis Imperfecta	341	Sexual Differentiation	331
Osteomalacia	338	Sheehan's Syndrome	268
Osteoporosis	342	Short Stature: General	348
Ovarian Cancer	309	Short Stature: Psychosocial Dwarfism	349
Paget's Disease of the Bone	339	Short Stature: Russell-Silver Syndrome	350
Paraendocrine and Neoplastic Syndromes	411	Skeletal Dysplasias	340
Parathyroid Gland	343	Smith-Lemli-Opitz Syndrome	406
Peroxisomal Disorders	405	Sodium and Water Metabolism Disorders	355
Phenylketonuria (PKU)	395	Subacute or deQuervain's Thyroiditis	280
Pheochromocytoma	300	Subclinical Hypothyroidism	278
Pheochromocytoma Syndromes	413	Subclinical Thyroid Dysfunction	281
Pineal Gland Disorders	271	Syndrome of Inappropriate ADH Secretion	264
Pituitary Apoplexy	267	Systemic Diseases: Endocrine Manifestations	417
Pituitary Disorders: Conditions of Decreased Pituitary Functioning	265	Tall Stature	350
Pituitary Disorders: Conditions of Hormone-Secreting Pituitary Adenomas	268	Tangier Disease	384
Pituitary Disorders: Pituitary Tumors	270	Tay-Sachs Disease	404
Polycystic Ovary Syndrome	311	Testicular Cancer	326
Polyendocrine Disorders	415	Thyroid Gland	273
Porphyria Cutanea Tarda	409	Thyroid Hormone Deficiency	274
Porphyrias	406	Thyroid Hormone Excess	279
Postpartum Thyroid Disease	288	Thyroid Malignancy	284
Potassium Metabolism Disorders	354	Thyroid Storm	280
Prader-Willi Syndrome	328	Thyrotoxicosis Factitia	282
Precocious Puberty and Pubertal Delay	329	Toxic Nodular Goiter (Plummer's Disease)	282
Pregnancy and Thyroid Disorders	286	Turner's Syndrome	333
Premenstrual Syndrome	312	Type 1 Diabetes Mellitus	360
Primary Hypogonadism: Adult Leydig Cell Failure	320	Type 2 Diabetes Mellitus	361
Primary Hypogonadism: General Resources	319	Type I Hyperlipoproteinemia	380
Prostate Cancer	322	Type II Hyperlipoproteinemia	380

Type III Hyperlipoproteinemia 381
Type IV Hyperlipoproteinemia 381
Type V Hyperlipoproteinemia 382
UDPgalactose4-Epimerase Deficiency 391
Urea Cycle Disorders................................395
Uterine Bleeding Disorders 313
Variant Forms
of Hyperphenylalaninemia........................396

Variegate Porphyria..................................410
Vasoactive
Intestinal Peptide Tumor (VIPoma) 304
Vitamin and Trace Mineral Deficiencies ...351
Vitamin D Metabolism Disorders 338
Von Hippel Lindau Disease 414
Wolman's Disease.....................................404

16. GENERAL RESOURCES

16.1 General Resources

**American Autoimmune
Related Diseases Association (AARDA): Endocrine Autoimmunity**
http://www.aarda.org/endocrine_art2.html

The *InFocus Newsletter* of the American Autoimmune Related Diseases Association provides this online reprint of an article which discusses common autoimmune endocrinology disorders and the risk factors associated with endocrine autoimmunity. General disease features, specific disorders and their diagnosis, and recent advances in endocrine autoimmunity are described. A link found at the bottom of the document brings visitors to an entire collection of related *InFocus* articles, including *Hormones and Autoimmunity* and *Autoimmunity, The Common Thread*. Other interesting sites include conference news and promising advances in therapy for autoimmune diseases.

**National Institutes of Health (NIH):
Autoimmunity and Endocrine Disease**
http://grants.nih.gov/grants/guide/pa-files/PA-93-114.html

A guide from the National Institutes of Health offers information on investigator-initiated research grant applications specifically geared toward studying the etiology, diagnosis, and treatment of autoimmune endocrine diseases. Background on autoimmune thyroid disorders, insulin dependent diabetes mellitus, and Addison's disease is provided, as well as details on a recent workshop that identified key research issues in autoimmune endocrinology. Example research topics, study populations, and application procedures are reviewed.

NIDDK: Health Information: Endocrine and Metabolic Diseases ○ ○ ○
http://www.niddk.nih.gov/health/endo/endo.htm

From the NIDDK, this site offers links to publications related to endocrine and metabolic diseases. Patient guides are available on acromegaly, Addison's disease, Cushing's syndrome, cystic fibrosis, familial multiple endocrine neoplasia, Creutzfeldt-Jakob disease, hyperthyroidism, and prolactinoma. This NIH divisional Web site also contains links to research funding opportunities, the NIDDK laboratories, clinical trials, and related health education programs.

OncoLink: Endocrine System Cancers ○ ○ ○
http://cancer.med.upenn.edu/disease/endocrine1

This site of OncoLink, a service of the University of Pennsylvania Cancer Center, offers an excellent starting point for research of the endocrine cancers, with general OncoLink pages offered on adrenal, pancreatic, parathyroid, pituitary, and thyroid cancers. Each resource connection contains regularly updated information on the particular cancer type, with articles from the National Cancer Institute. FAQs related to particular endocrine cancers, CancerLit monthly updates containing current research reports, and a protocol finder for specific cancer trials are available.

Oregon Health Sciences University: Endocrine Gland Neoplasms ○ ○ ○
http://medir.ohsu.edu/cliniweb/C19/C19.344.html

CliniWeb International's resource pages offer an extensive collection of links pertaining to neoplasms of the various endocrine glands. Visitors will find an assortment of clinical articles, pathology information, pre-formatted MEDLINE query links, newsletters, and physician statements of the National Cancer Institute (NCI) for the various ovarian, adrenal, parathyroid, pituitary, testicular, and thyroid neoplasms. Text from major teaching hospitals, such as the Medical College of Wisconsin; advancements in drug treatment; and articles on multiple endocrine neoplasia and neoplastic endocrine-like syndromes are found.

17. NEUROENDOCRINE SYSTEM

17.1 Hypothalamic-Pituitary Axis Dysfunction

Diabetes Insipidus

Diabetes Insipidus Foundation, Inc. ◐ ◐ ◐
http://diabetesinsipidus.maxinter.net
The Web site of the Diabetes Insipidus Foundation, Inc., with pages available in English, Spanish, or French, contains several articles, facts sheets, and brochures on the symptoms, diagnostic tests, and medications for effective treatment of this disorder.

Family Village: Diabetes Insipidus ◐ ◐ ◐
http://www.familyvillage.wisc.edu/lib_di.htm
The Diabetes Insipidus and Related Disorders Network (DIARD), along with other major organizations dedicated to disease research, a medical message board, and the "Never Ending Water Chat Room" provide ample opportunity for both professionals and patients to further research this disorder of insufficient vasopressin secretion. Several fact sheets, from the American Academy of Family Physicians, major diabetes insipidus organizations, and other reputable associations, may be accessed.

Histiocytosis Association Online Library: The Facts About Diabetes Insipidus ◐ ◐
http://www.histio.org/us/lib/diabetes.html
General information on diabetes insipidus may be found at this online fact sheet, provided as a service of the Histiocytosis Association Online Library. Basics on the purpose of vasopressin; the symptoms of polyuria and polydipsia; the diagnostic evaluation, based on intake and output of fluids, urinary measurement of vasopressin,

or magnetic resonance imaging (MRI); further details on synthetic vasopressin administration; and the role of emerging therapies are provided.

Journal of the American Society of Nephrology: Presentation and Follow-up of 30 Patients with Congenital Nephrogenic Diabetes Insipidus ○ ○ ○
http://lww.com/JASN/1046-66739-99p1958.html

Long-term follow-up of patients with congenital nephrogenic diabetes insipidus is presented at this site via a retrospective analysis of clinical data. A description of the initial symptomatology, including failure to thrive, is presented. The hereditary defect of arginine vasopressin signal transduction is reviewed, and the growth retardation in infants, thought to result from inadequate food consumption due to uncontrolled polydipsia, general poor health, and hypernatremia, is detailed. Tables outline symptoms and signs at first referral and gene mutations and laboratory data.

Nephrogenic Diabetes Insipidus Foundation ○ ○
http://www.ndif.org

The Nephrogenic Diabetes Insipidus Foundation supports research, education, and treatment for nephrogenic diabetes insipidus. The site provides information and statistics about the disease, nutrition guidelines, answers to frequently asked questions, terminology review, and journal articles. Conference information, foundation activities, current researchers, and government contacts are listed.

Syndrome of Inappropriate ADH Secretion

emedicine: Syndrome of Inappropriate Antidiuretic Hormone Secretion ○ ○ ○
http://emedicine.com/cgi-bin/foxweb.exe/showsection@d:/em/ga?book=emerg&topicid=784

Emedicine reviews the pathophysiology, specific diagnostic criteria, physical presentation, and multiple causes of this disorder, including CNS disorders, malignancies, and endocrine disorders. Diagnostic differential connections are provided by emedicine so that visitors may easily compare and contrast disease profiles. Laboratory studies and other workup information are reviewed, and treatment in the hospital and emergency department are summarized.

Georgetown University: SIADH (Syndrome of Inappropriate ADH) ○ ○
http://gucfm.georgetown.edu/welchjj/netscut/endocrinology/siadh.html

A table found at this Georgetown University page outlines the multiple etiologies of inappropriate ADH secretion, the most common cause of euvolemic hyponatremia. A link to an algorithm for hyponatremia, more information on plasma osmalality, and emergency treatment measures are provided.

17.2 Pituitary Disorders: Conditions of Decreased Pituitary Functioning

Empty Sella Syndrome

Jefferson Health System: Empty Sella Syndrome ○ ○
http://www.jeffersonhealth.org/diseases/endo/sella.htm
Jefferson Health System provides this online information sheet on empty sella syndrome, its symptoms, and diagnostic testing procedures. A discussion regarding treatment, although treatment is not usually necessary, is found.

Pituitary Tumor Network Association: Empty Sella Syndrome ○
http://www.pituitary.com/FirstAid/Disorders/SymptomsOfEmptySellaSyndrome.htm
The Pituitary Tumor Network Association offers this fact sheet on the most common cause of empty sella syndrome. The syndrome's range of symptomatology and its rare coexistence with pituitary tumors or other disease processes are explained.

Hypopituitarism

emedicine: Hypopituitarism ○ ○ ○
http://www.emedicine.com/EMERG/topic277.htm
The pituitary's role in the endocrine system, details regarding the hormones it secretes, signs of anterior and posterior insufficiencies, and signs and symptoms of a variety of acute and insidious examples of hormone depletion are clinically described. Diagnostic differential links are provided, including the vast array of primary endocrine gland dysfunctions. Laboratory studies for diagnosis, possible imaging studies, emergency basis treatment, and agent profiles for hormone replacement therapy are reviewed in terms of their safety, administration, and contraindications.

Jefferson Health System: Hypopituitarism ○ ○
http://www.jeffersonhealth.org/diseases/endo/hypopit.htm
The endocrinology department of Jefferson Health System offers this online fact sheet pertaining to the variable presentations of hypopituitarism, outlined in table format. Insufficient gonadotropins, growth hormone, thyroid-stimulating hormone, corticotrophic production, and prolactin production and their respective symptoms are

reviewed. Causes of hypopituitarism directly affecting the pituitary gland, such as tumors and infections, and causes of secondary hypopituitarism, as a result of hypothalamic dysfunction, are enumerated. The diagnostic tests necessary and treatment goals are discussed.

Postgraduate Medicine: How to Diagnose Hypopituitarism ◎ ◎ ◎
http://www.postgradmed.com/issues/1998/07_98/schmidt.htm

The features of a variety of secondary hormonal deficiencies, caused by hypopituitarism, are explored in this *Postgraduate Medicine* article. With an emphasis on the correct diagnosis of hypopituitarism, the authors present an illustrative case report of abnormal thyroid function values and possible causes. A variety of abnormalities of or trauma to the pituitary apoplexy, postpartum pituitary necrosis, infiltrative disease, lymphocytic hypophysitis, and other causes, are explored. Clinical features and recognition of hormonal deficiencies in secondary hypothyroidism, adrenal insufficiency, and hypogonadism are reviewed, with T4 levels, serum cortisol levels, low sex hormone levels, and other diagnostic tests and values explained. Hormone replacement therapy, other management considerations, and the long-term outlook for patient and other similarly presenting cases are discussed.

Growth Hormone Deficiency

Hole's Essentials of Human Anatomy and Physiology: Growth Hormone and Growth Disorders ◎ ◎
http://mhhe.com/biosci/ap/holeessentials/student/olc/e-reading2.html

The Online Learning Center of McGraw Hill offers visitors the opportunity to learn more about several pathological conditions associated with abnormal growth hormone (GH) secretion. Chronic hypersecretion in infants and children, genetic determinants of GH structure, the results of chronic hypersecretion, and adults with chronically elevated GH levels are discussed.

Human Growth Foundation: Growth Hormone Deficiency ◎ ◎
http://www.hgfound.org/growth.html

An online booklet is found at this site, which contains information on the hormones responsible for growth regulation, causes of growth hormone deficiency, diagnosis of the disorder, and a treatment option overview. Sources of human growth hormone, the psychosocial aspects of short stature, and the possibility of substitutions for biosynthetic growth hormone varieties as research continues are introduced.

Major Aspects of Growth In Children (MAGIC) Foundation for Children's Growth: Adults Who Live with Growth Hormone Deficiency ◉

http://www.magicfoundation.org/adultlwghd.html

A discussion found at this page includes the effect which growth hormone deficiency may have on mood and emotions, as well as a comparison of growth hormone deficiency in adulthood versus childhood.

Option Care Pediatric Overview: Growth Hormone Therapy ◉

http://www.optioncare.com/growthhormone/pedover.htm

Administration of biosynthetic growth hormone, patient selection following extensive testing, and information on growth failure caused by endocrine disease, systemic disease, and congenital conditions are discussed at this online fact sheet.

United Medical and Dental Schools: Adult Growth Hormone Deficiency ◉ ◉

http://www.umds.ac.uk/medicine/endocrinology/reviews/aghd_rev.htm

Growth hormones regulation of body composition, plasma lipid concentrations, and major quality of life influences are discussed at this page of Guy's and St. Thomas' Hospitals. Discussion of recent clinical trials of GH replacement therapy and resulting benefits in exercise capacity and lipid profiles, as well as improved psychological well-being, is presented.

Vanderbilt University Medical Center: Growth Hormone Deficiency ◉ ◉

http://www.mc.vanderbilt.edu/peds/pidl/endocr/grohorm.htm

Vanderbilt University Medical Center offers a fact sheet that discusses the incidence of growth hormone deficiency, idiopathic hypopituitarism, and a variety of associated defects. The presentation of infants with intrauterine hypopituitarism, a discussion of the delay in skeletal maturation, and further information on the evaluation of children for short stature are offered.

Pituitary Apoplexy

emedicine: Pituitary Apoplexy ◉ ◉ ◉

http://emedicine.com/oph/topic471.htm

Acute hemorrhage or infarction of the pituitary may cause a variety of symptoms, which are reviewed at this site of the emedicine online textbook. The presence of an already existing pituitary adenoma or occasional nonadenomatous gland is reviewed, with the pathophysiology and various theories behind pituitary apoplexy discussed. Headache, vomiting, and other presenting symptoms are reviewed, as well as a variety of causes. Elements of medical management, consisting of high-dose corticosteroids, hormone replacement therapies, and stabilization of the patient, are listed.

University of Virginia: Pituitary Apoplexy ◎ ◎ ◎
http://hsc.virginia.edu/medicine/clinical/internal/conf/chiefs/hypopit.htm

The epidemiology of pituitary apoplexy, associated risk factors, and the pathophysiology of these mechanisms are reviewed. The full clinical syndrome is described, with sudden headache and visual disturbance noted. Endocrine abnormalities and panhypopituitarism, shock, and other findings are discussed, with each problem explained in terms of its relation to its specific endocrine deficiency. Upward enlargement of adenomatous tissue and hypothalamic damage are discussed, in addition to lateral enlargement and downward enlargement of a pituitary adenoma. Other potential complications, such as subarachnoid hemorrhage, and diagnostic tests are reviewed. High-dose steroid replacement, aggressive monitoring of electrolytes and fluids, and additional stabilization and management information is provided.

Sheehan's Syndrome

MDMultimedia: Sheehan's Syndrome ◎
http://www.mdmultimedia.com/a/griffith/gr831.htm

This form of pituitary apoplexy, resulting from postpartum or intrapartum hemorrhage or postpartum infection, is briefly described at the site. The ICD-9 code for the disorder is provided, in addition to synonyms for the disorder.

17.3 Pituitary Disorders: Conditions of Hormone-Secreting Pituitary Adenomas

Acromegaly

Clinical and Investigative Medicine: Diagnosis and Management of Acromegaly ◎ ◎ ◎
http://www.cma.ca/cim/vol-19/0259.htm

This scientific article begins by covering the prevalence, etiology, morphology, and clinical presentation of the disease. Related diagnostic studies, treatment objectives, and therapeutic monitoring are discussed, as are treatment options, such as surgery, drug therapies, and radiotherapy. Various tables and references are included.

HealthCentral: Pediatric Health Encyclopedia: Acromegaly ◉ ◉
http://www.healthcentral.com/peds/top/000321.cfm

From HealthCentral, this site offers patient information on acromegaly. The site provides a list of alternative names, a definition, and discussions of causes, incidence, risk factors, prevention, symptoms, signs and tests, treatment, prognosis, and complications.

Medstudents: Acromegaly and Gigantism ◉ ◉
http://www.medstudents.com.br/endoc/endoc8.htm

Discussions of classical clinical disease features, etiology, and pathology, as well as a chart outlining pituitary tumor types, are found at this online article. The effects of chronic growth hormone (GH) exposure and diagnosis by oral glucose tolerance testing and other laboratory values are explained. An MRI and radiograph of tumor localization are depicted, and goals of medical, surgical, and radiation therapies are reviewed.

NIDDK: Acromegaly ◉ ◉
http://www.niddk.nih.gov/health/endo/pubs/acro/acro.htm

This fact sheet, provided by the NIDDK, offers information about acromegaly, with an overview of the disease and discussions of causes, incidence, diagnosis, and treatment. Treatment options discussed include surgery, drug therapy, and radiation therapy. A list of suggested readings and additional resources is also provided.

Cushing's Disease

Pituitary Tumor Network Association: Cushing's Syndrome ◉
http://www.pituitary.org/FirstAid/Disorders/SymptomsOfCushings.htm

From the Pituitary Tumor Network Association, this site provides information about Cushing's syndrome. An overview, symptom review, and links to a fact sheet and personal account of the disease are offered. Information pertaining to NIH-supported research is discussed, and contact information for physicians interested in referring a patient is accessible.

Hyperprolactinemia and Galactorrhea

Human Reproduction: Prolactin: Physiologic and Pathologic Associations ◉ ◉
http://medstat.med.utah.edu/kw/human_reprod/lectures/prolactin

A detailed overview of prolactin production, lactation, and disorders relating to prolactin secretion is available from this online tutorial. The tutorial lists objectives and definitions of important terms, followed by a presentation of material in outline form.

The outline offers information on prolactin and its role in lactation, the mechanism of the mammary gland as a target of prolactin action, breast changes during physiological hormonal fluctuations influencing the actions of prolactin, prolactin actions, and prolactinomas. Specific subtopics include etiologies and physical findings associated with galactorrhea and imaging techniques of the pituitary gland.

MDMultimedia: Hyperprolactinemia

http://www.mdmultimedia.com/a/griffith/gr437.htm

A basic review of hyperprolactinemia and the elevation of serum prolactin levels is provided at this site, with signs and symptoms and the various causes outlined. Laboratory values and general treatment measures, based on primary cause, are discussed. Pharmacologic intervention, required for tumor regression, is presented, and related disorders and synonyms are listed.

University of Arkansas for Medical Sciences: Hyperprolactinemia

http://physicianlink.uams.edu/CSHyper.htm

The most common clinical scenario surrounding hyperprolactinemia and its symptoms is reviewed at this site, along with the disorder's other causes. Information on pituitary adenomas, a number of different causative pharmacologic agents, and a discussion regarding the various etiologies are found.

17.4 Pituitary Disorders: Pituitary Tumors

General Resources

OncoLink: Pituitary Cancer

http://cancer.med.upenn.edu/disease/pituitary

Pituitary cancer information for both patients and professionals is offered at the connections of this OncoLink clinical Web site. Symptom management and psychosocial support of the cancer patient, as well as month-by-month CancerLit database additions, are found. CancerLit articles include those on manifestations of pituitary tumors, guidelines for treatment, surgical techniques, and case reports of pituitary metastases. Consumer-oriented and physician-directed guidelines on pituitary cancer are found, covering all aspects of pituitary carcinoma. "Pituitary Irradiation Technical Procedures" provides a review of the 3-field vertex procedure.

Pituitary Tumor Network Association ✪ ✪ ✪
http://www.pituitary.com

The Pituitary Tumor Network Association encourages research on pituitary tumors and related pituitary disorders. Information at the site includes articles on emotional aspects of related disorders, general issues, inspiration, insurance issues, patient perspectives, and treatment. There are also articles related to specific disorders, including craniopharyngioma, acromegaly, Addison's disease, Cushing's disease, FMENI, and prolactinoma. Other information at the site includes clinical trials, information on medical advances, questions and answers, and physician and hospital referrals. A bulletin board and information on publications are available, and links to related sites are provided.

Craniopharyngiomas

Pituitary Tumor Network Association: Craniopharyngiomas ✪
http://www.pituitary.org/FirstAid/Disorders/SymptomsOfCraniopharyngiomas.htm

Part of the Pituitary Tumor Network Association, this site offers an overview of craniopharyngioma and a list of symptoms associated with the disorder. Links include a related article and a message board.

17.5 Pineal Gland Disorders

Brain Surgery Information Center: Pineal Region Tumors ✪ ✪
http://www.brain-surgery.com/pineal.html

The pineal gland and its unique functions are described at this site, which includes descriptions of a variety of pineal tumors, diagnostic modalities, and treatment options, including radiation, chemotherapy, and surgical removal.

Chicago Institute of Neurosurgery and Neuroresearch: Pineal Tumors ✪ ✪
http://www.cinn.org/conditions/pinealtumors.html

Information on particular types of pineal tumors may be accessed from this neurological disorders site, including details regarding oligodendroglioma, meningioma, pineal cysts, germinoma, and teratoma. For each indicated tumor type, a fact sheet containing symptoms, diagnosis, and treatment review is found. Within individual fact sheets, further links to diagnostic and treatment modality review are provided.

Epidermoid Cyst of the Pineal Gland

http://www.pinealcyst.freeserve.co.uk

The epidermoid cyst of the pineal gland Web site was created by a patient with the condition. The site provides an overview of the pineal gland and an epidermoid cyst of the pineal gland. Articles are found on symptoms, treatment options, treatment outcomes, and long-term prognosis. Support contact information and links to additional resources are provided, as well as illustrative images.

North Carolina Baptist Hospital: Neoplasms of the Pineal Region

http://www.sma.org/smj/96nov11.htm

Five case reports of pineal region tumors, taken from pathology files of the Pathology Department of North Carolina Baptist Hospital, are offered in this electronic article, including germinoma, pinealoblastoma, pinealoma, astrocytoma, and meningioma. The differential diagnosis of this tumor type and the importance of varying histological, prognostic, and therapeutic approaches to each are defined. Physical exam findings, microscopic tumor examination, and results of treatment are outlined.

18. THYROID GLAND

18.1 General Resources

American Foundation of Thyroid Patients ○ ○
http://www.thyroidfoundation.org

The American Foundation of Thyroid Patients was founded by thyroid patients and provides access to the group's newsletter, a graphic depiction of thyroid disease symptoms, and ordering information for recommended publications. A message board and links to thyroid-related sites are provided.

American Thyroid Association ○ ○ ○
http://www.thyroid.org

The American Thyroid Association is a professional organization dedicated to increasing scientific and public understanding of the thyroid gland and the management of its diseases. Practice guidelines for physicians include links to thyroid disease detection, use of laboratory tests in diagnosis, and hyperthyroidism and hypothyroidism management, as reprinted from several indexed journals. Users may also access the Association newsletter, conference details, and grant information.

Gland Central ○ ○ ○
http://www.glandcentral.com

Gland Central is a comprehensive resource for information about thyroid health, providing a wide variety of facts and statistics about thyroid-related disorders. For physicians, links to articles from the *Journal of the American Medical Association* and recommendations from various thyroid-related organizations are retrievable. Information about the thyroid includes a general overview and discussions of thyroid hormone effects on the body. Further information about hypothyroidism, mild thyroid failure, hyperthyroidism, signs and symptoms, Graves' disease, nodules, and cancer is accessible. Thyroid testing details and answers to frequently asked questions may be found, as well as an online thyroid library containing numerous downloadable documents.

Merck ThyroLink ⊙ ⊙

http://www.thyrolink.com

Professional information at ThyroLink includes conference and symposia updates, descriptions of products, and awards listings. Links to publications, professional societies, and sites specific to iodine deficiency disorders are provided. Patient information is available in English, German, French, and other languages, and connections to interesting thyroid-related Web guides may be accessed.

Thyroid Center ⊙ ⊙ ⊙

http://cait.columbia.edu:88/dept/thyroid

Part of the Columbia-Presbyterian Medical Center, the Thyroid Center is dedicated to the identification and treatment of thyroid disorders. Links are provided to information on such thyroid conditions as hyperthyroidism, hypothyroidism, thyroid eye disease, thyroid nodules, thyroid diseases and women, and hyperparathyroidism. Information on thyroid surgery, parathyroid surgery, postoperative procedures, and radioactive iodine scanning is found, in addition to other resources for thyroid disorders, including the Thyroid Foundation of America and the Thyroid Society.

Thyroid Disease Manager ⊙ ⊙ ⊙

http://www.thyroidmanager.org

Developed by Endocrine Education, Inc., this site offers authoritative, comprehensive information to physicians and medical students on thyroid physiology and thyroid disease. A complete online version of *The Thyroid and its Diseases,* accessible by chapter, is provided, as well as clinical management algorithms. Sections on philosophy, news, CME, and evaluating thyroid function and structure are offered. The site is fully searchable, and a skill-testing "Case of the Month" provides an interesting practice opportunity, as a service of the Knoll Pharmaceutical Company.

18.2 Thyroid Hormone Deficiency

Hypothyroidism, General

American Thyroid Association: Hypothyroidism: The Underactive Thyroid ⊙

http://www.thyroid.org/patient/brochur5.htm

A straightforward information sheet on hypothyroidism, its symptoms, treatment, and a discussion of medication adjustment are found at the site. The differences between the synthetic and desiccated supplements are highlighted.

EndocrineWeb: Hypothyroidism: Too Little Thyroid Hormone ◎ ◎

http://www.endocrineweb.com/hypo1.html

An overview of hypothyroidism, its symptoms, and the potential dangers of the disorder, as well as links to information on diagnosis and treatment, thyroid gland function, diagnostic testing, and goiter formation, are all found at this EndocrineWeb subsite.

Hospital Practice: Recognizing the Faces of Hypothyroidism ◎ ◎ ◎

http://www.hosppract.com/issues/1999/03/dmmmazz.htm

Diverging from the stereotypical picture of hypothyroidism, the author of this article offers four case examples with strikingly diverse clinical pictures. For each study, details regarding the physical exam and laboratory tests are discussed, in conjunction with the author's individually tailored diagnostic algorithms. A middle-aged person with hypercholesterolemia, a young girl with normal thyroid function tests, and an elderly woman presenting with a grand mal seizure are all diagnosed as hypothyroid. Details regarding the physician's conclusions, information on thyroid function testing and several other useful criteria, and a table outlining the common signs and symptoms of mild and severe disease are presented.

Hypothyroidism: Causes, Mechanisms, Clinical Presentation, Diagnosis, and Treatment ◎ ◎ ◎

http://osiris.sunderland.ac.uk/autism/thyroid.htm

The mechanisms that may impair normal thyroid function and general disease classifications are outlined in table format at the site. Differentiation is made between congenital and acquired hypothyroidism, as well as primary and secondary hypothyroidism of

Congenital Hypothyroidism

Columbia University: Screening for Congenital Hypothyroidism ◎ ◎

http://cpmcnet.columbia.edu/texts/gcps/gcps0055.html

The online *Guide to Clinical Preventive Services* provides recommendations regarding the early screening and detection of congenital hypothyroidism. A description of the radioimmunoassay of serum thyroxine (T4) and thyroid-stimulating hormone (TSH) is provided, and the advantages of early intervention are discussed.

Journal of Endocrinology: Thyroid Hormone Actions on Cartilage and Bone ◉ ◉ ◉
http://journals.endocrinology.org/joe/157/joe1570391.htm

The Molecular Endocrinology Group of the Imperial College School of Medicine offers a free downloadable review article providing a discussion of normal linear growth and its crucial genetic, nutritional, and endocrine components. A complete text, courtesy of the *Journal of Endocrinology,* reviews abnormalities in systemic hormone regulation.

Thyroid Society for Education and Research: Congenital Hypothyroidism ◉ ◉
http://www.the-thyroid-society.org/med_letter2.html

The article found at this site, a review on congenital hypothyroidism, provides information on the various malformations or malfunctions of the thyroid gland in the developing fetus. Three categories of permanent congenital hypothyroidism are defined, including abnormalities of thyroid gland formation and growth, abnormalities of enzymatic reaction involved in thyroid hormone release, and malfunction or malformation of the hypothalamus and/or pituitary (central hypothyroidism). Widespread screening and thorough evaluation of positive results are recommended.

Thyroid Society for Education and Research: Congenital Hypothyroidism ◉ ◉
http://www.the-thyroid-society.org/med_letter2.html

A member of the Thyroid Society's Medical Advisory Board is the author of this article on congenital hypothyroidism. The embryonic development of the thyroid, concurrent hypothalamic and pituitary development, and the complex mechanisms that regulate their hormonal interactions are described. Formation and functional failures and the necessity of prompt intervention are discussed. Three categories of permanent congenital hypothyroidism, as well as transient varieties, are reviewed.

Tyler for Life Foundation: Congenital Hypothyroidism ◉ ◉
http://tylerforlife.com/hypothyroidism.htm

The underactivity of the thyroid gland, its estimated incidence, clinical signs, and additional details surrounding treatment are presented at this fact sheet. A state-by-state listing of newborn screening procedures is accessible, as well as other sites of reference for hypothyroidism. Connections include the American Academy of Pediatrics Policy Statement for screening of congenital hypothyroidism, in addition to the MAGIC Foundation.

Hashimoto's Thyroiditis

Adam.com: Chronic Thyroiditis (Hashimoto's Disease)
http://www.adam.com/ency/article/000371.htm

Adam.com's Web-based encyclopedic reference offers an overview of Hashimoto's thyroiditis at the site, with its causes, incidence, and risk factors outlined and its relation to other autoimmune endocrine disorders cited. A scintiscan of an enlarged thyroid may be viewed, and links to further information on symptoms and treatment are found. Diagnostic test preparations and purposes are fully described at the related links.

Thyroid Disease Manager: Hashimoto's Thyroiditis
http://www.thyroidmanager.org/Chapter8/8-contents.htm

Chapter eight of the Thyroid Disease Manager presents a historical review, pathogenesis, disease course, and diagnostic information for Hashimoto's thyroiditis. The autoimmune nature of the condition, goiter description and microscopic findings, and a link to Chapter seven, which provides review of the putative causes of the disease, are found. The disease's incidence and distribution and a table outlining the presentations of Hashimoto's thyroiditis are offered. A discussion surrounding several unusual syndromes believed to be related to or a part of the clinical spectrum of the disorder are cited. A special review of the disease presentation in children is found.

Myxedema Coma

emedicine: Hypothyroidism and Myxedema Coma
http://emedicine.com/cgi-bin/foxweb.exe/showsection@d:/em/ga?book=emerg&topicid=280

The American Academy of Emergency Physicians and emedicine offer visitors this clinical overview of the rare, yet life threatening, myxedema coma. Pathophysiology, demographic details, symptoms and physical presentation, and primary and secondary causes are reviewed. Five diagnostic differential links are provided, with opportunities for comparison of myxedema coma with hypothermia, depression, and septic shock. Electrolytes, arterial blood gases, and secondary studies are enumerated, as well as other testing procedures and a hospital care summary. Thyroid hormone replacement, the mainstay of therapy, is discussed.

Virtual Hospital: Hematologic, Electrolyte, and Disorders of Endocrinology and Metabolism: Myxedema Coma
http://www.vh.org/Providers/ClinRef/FPHandbook/Chapter05/15-5.html

The online University of Iowa *Family Practice Handbook* brings visitors this overview of myxedema coma, which concisely outlines its etiology and treatment.

Reidel's Thyroiditis

DoctorGeorge.com: ⚙
http://www.doctorgeorge.com/clinic/reidels_thyroiditis.htm

Details surrounding the most uncommon form of thyroiditis are found at this online fact sheet. Answers to questions regarding symptoms and signs, laboratory findings, and alternative disease titles are provided, as well as concise treatment and prognosis information.

Thyroid Disease Manager: Reidel's Thyroiditis ⚙ ⚙
http://www.thyroidmanager.org/Chapter19/ch_19__riedels.htm

Information on this rare disorder of thyroid function is presented at this chapter of *The Thyroid and its Diseases*. Demographic details, pathologic exam findings, and a discussion of disease progression are offered. Additional information is provided at this site regarding thyroid manifestations of systemic disease, such as sarcoidosis and amyloidosis, and connections to these related chapters may be accessed.

Subclinical Hypothyroidism

Annals of Internal Medicine: Subclinical Thyroid Disease: A Clinician's Perspective ⚙ ⚙
http://www.acponline.org/journals/annals/15jul98/thyroid.htm

Guidelines at this site of the online *Annals of Internal Medicine* provide unique physician recommendations on dealing with subclinical thyroid disease. Patient symptoms, evidence of organ system involvement, and the cost-benefit analysis are the pivotal topics that this author presents, with earlier physician reviews on the subject questioned and diagnosis warranted where progression to overt disease is not yet discovered.

Health News: A Thyroid Dilemma ⚙ ⚙
http://www.onhealth.com/ch1/in-depth/item/item,14736_1_1.asp

HealthNews, from the publishers of the New England Journal of Medicine, offers this discussion on the asymptomatic hypothyroid patient, with the most common cause discussed and the issue as to whether or not to treat debated. A physician's perspective discusses the biochemical diagnosis, in addition to the main arguments for and against treatment.

18.3 Thyroid Hormone Excess

Graves' Disease

Leicester Royal Infirmary NHS Trust: Thyrotoxicosis
http://www.lri.org.uk/diabetes/end/thy.htm

A basic information sheet on thyrotoxicosis lists symptoms and provides details on the autoimmune nature of the condition, courtesy of the Leicester Royal Infirmary NHS Trust. The next page of this diabetes and endocrinology division also offers details regarding the four classes of commonly used drugs for treatment of thyrotoxicosis. Beta-blocker agents for reduction of hormone effects, carbimazole for hormone reduction, 'block and replace' treatment, surgical gland removal, and radioactive therapy are included. Information on pharmacologic side effects is also provided.

Medical Pathology Course: Graves' Disease
http://www.mcl.tulane.edu/classware/pathology/medical_pathology/thyroid/06Graves.html

This online medical pathology course offers clinical information about Graves' disease, including a three-part definition, example case study, and final diagnosis. Hyperlinks in the text provide supplemental information about key topics.

National Graves' Disease Foundation
http://www.ngdf.org

The National Graves' Disease Foundation is a volunteer effort to provide education and support for Graves' patients. The site provides a bulletin board, contact list, and links to support groups. There are references for recommended readings, product recall notifications, and links to related sites.

Postgraduate Medicine: The Many 'Faces' of Graves' Disease
http://www.postgradmed.com/issues/1999/10_01_99/felz.htm

Important clues to diagnosis of Graves' disease are reviewed at this site of the *Postgraduate Medicine* publication. An analysis of these clinical manifestations, updated information on sensitive thyrotropin assays and additional tests, and clarification regarding the merits and side effects of antithyroid pharmacologic regimens are presented. Part two of the series is accessible from the site and focuses on practical diagnostic testing and management.

Thyroid Disease Manager: Graves' Disease and the Manifestations of Thyrotoxicosis ○ ○ ○
http://www.thyroidmanager.org/Chapter10/10-text.htm

Background information on Graves' disease, Graves' disease as a disorder of thyroid autoimmunity, and a table outlining antibodies in Graves' disease are provided at this site of *The Thyroid and its Diseases*. Theories on the immunological etiology of Graves' disease, incidence and disease distribution, and a complete presentation of the clinical picture and course of the disease are offered. Special details regarding ocular signs and symptoms, as well as related manifestations in other systems of the body, are provided, making this reference a comprehensive presentation of the current literature.

Thyroid Storm

Thyroid Disease Manager: Thyroid Storm ○ ○ ○
http://www.thyroidmanager.org/Chapter12/12-text.htm#THYROID STORM

Thyroid storm, a life-threatening form of thyrotoxicosis, is reviewed in terms of its usual signs and symptoms, with differentiation made between the traditional thyroid crisis and the apathetic storm. Decompensation of various organ systems, including extreme cardiac symptomatology and liver damage, is reviewed. The association of thyroid storm with Graves' disease or toxic nodular goiter is cited, and information on prompt, aggressive intervention is presented. Thyroid storm due to thyroidectomy, postsurgical treatments, and acute infection are discussed. A table reviewing management strategies is found, and an in-depth discussion of the cited methods follows.

Virtual Hospital: Hematologic, Electrolyte, and Disorders of Endocrinology and Metabolism: Thyroid Storm ○ ○
http://www.vh.org/Providers/ClinRef/FPHandbook/Chapter05/13-5.html

Thyroid storm, a life-threatening form of hyperthyroidism, is outlined at this site of the Virtual Hospital from the University of Iowa's *Family Practice Handbook*. The cause, clinical signs, and immediate treatment delivery recommendations are provided.

Subacute or deQuervain's Thyroiditis

PEDBASE: Thyroiditis ○ ○
http://www.icondata.com/health/pedbase/files/THYROIDI.HTM

The epidemiology and pathogenesis of chronic thyroiditis and subacute varieties are presented at this general outline of thyroiditis. Clinical features of Hashimoto's thyroiditis, granulomatous disease, and the lymphocytic subtype are reviewed. Thyroid function tests, antibody detection specific to each, imaging studies, and a medical management summary are provided.

Subacute Thyroiditis ◎ ◎
http://sanantonio360.adam.com/ency/article/000375.htm

Adam.com's online health reviews offer this Web site describing the causes, incidence, and risk factors for subacute thyroiditis, otherwise known as De Quervain's thyroiditis. Enlargeable diagrams of the endocrine system, a link to a symptom listing, laboratory testing procedures, and treatment targeting reduction of pain and inflammation are described.

Thyroid Disease Manager: Subacute Thyroiditis ◎ ◎ ◎
http://www.thyroidmanager.org/Chapter19/ch_19__subacute.htm

This chapter of *The Thyroid and its Diseases* discusses the etiology, pathology, and clinical manifestations of subacute thyroiditis, sometimes referred to as De Quervain's thyroiditis. Differential diagnosis discussion, tables, and figures, symptom relief, and information on spontaneous recovery are presented.

Thyroid Foundation of Canada: Thyroiditis ◎ ◎
http://home.ican.net/~thyroid/Guides/HG05.html

The most common cause of thyroiditis is reviewed at this subsite of the Thyroid Foundation of Canada. Confirmatory biopsy of the thyroid gland and treatment of Hashimoto's thyroiditis by hormone supplementation are summarized. Subacute thyroiditis causing hyperthyroidism as a result of a possible viral infection is of importance, with its distinct clinical features and laboratory tests explained. Treatment for mild to severe forms of subacute thyroiditis is discussed. Also reviewed are silent thyroiditis, with Graves'-like symptoms, and postpartum thyroiditis.

Thyroiditis:
Acute, Subacute, Silent, Chronic Lymphocytic, Riedel's ◎ ◎
http://www.mamc.amedd.army.mil/williams/
NucMed/Endocrine/Thyroid/Thyroiditis/Thyroiditis.html

Acute thyroiditis, a life-threatening thyroid gland infection; subacute thyroiditis; silent thyroiditis; and chronic lymphocytic thyroiditis are reviewed at this site in terms of their pathophysiology and clinical findings. Reidel's thyroiditis, a rare condition also known as invasive fibrous thyroiditis, is mentioned.

Subclinical Thyroid Dysfunction

Subclinical Hyperthyroidism: Just a Low
Serum Thyrotropin Concentration, or Something More? ◎ ◎
http://www.nejm.org/content/1994/0331/0019/1302.asp

An editorial article, courtesy of the *New England Journal of Medicine,* reviews the increased risk of atrial fibrillation and other problems that may be caused by subclinical hyperthyroidism. Noted is the idea that measurement of low thyrotropin concentration may amount to much more than merely a serum value. The concept that careful consideration of antithyroid therapy risks and benefits warrant careful follow-up rather than intervention is described at the site.

Thyrotoxicosis Factitia

Thyroid Disease Manager: Thyrotoxicosis Factitia ○ ○ ○
http://thyroidmanager.bsd.uchicago.edu/Chapter13/Ch-13-3.htm

The online *Thyroid and its Disease* textbook offers a chapter on thyrotoxicosis factitia at this site, explaining the term "factitious" and describing its association with excessive ingestion of thyroid hormone. TSH suppression, thyroid shrinkage, and additional findings are summarized. A table at the site outlines the results of thyroid-function tests in patients with thyrotoxicosis factitia.

Toxic Nodular Goiter (Plummer's Disease)

Case Western Reserve University: Nuclear and Spect Teaching Files: Toxic Nodular Goiter ○ ○
http://www.uhrad.com/spectarc/nucs011.htm

A case example of toxic nodular goiter is shown at this site, with enlargeable images, a clinical history, and a concise discussion of hyperfunctioning thyroid nodules. The differences between toxic nodular goiter and Graves' disease are noted, and therapy specific to toxic nodules is explained, courtesy of Case Western Reserve University.

MEDLINEplus Health Information: Toxic Nodular Goiter ○ ○
http://medlineplus.adam.com/ency/article/000317.htm

General information on toxic nodular goiter, otherwise known as Plummer's disease, is offered at this division of the adam.com Web database. The overview provides causes, incidence, and risk factors, and connections at the top of the document allow interested viewers to recognize abnormal thyroid enlargement via scintiscan. A symptom summary, with specific links found for each; physical examination information and diagnostic tests; and an overview of treatment and complications are offered.

Thyroid Disease Manager: Therapy for Toxic Nodular Goiter ○ ○
http://www.thyroidmanager.org/Chapter17/17_toxic.htm

The Thyroid Disease Manager offers these pages on toxic nodular goiter and reinforces the often severe nature of the condition, due to late diagnosis. Outlined are alternatives necessary for therapy after the multinodular goiter develops further growth and toxicity.

18.4 Goiter

Adam.com: Goiter ○ ○ ○
http://www.adam.com/ency/article/001178.htm

Adam.com's encyclopedic Web reference contains a review of simple goiter and its clinical implications at this Web address. Goiter classifications, endemic information relating to iodine consumption, and hereditary factors are mentioned. Links to pharmacologic leaflets on levothyroxine and liothyronine supplements are accessible from the site, as well as an image of the thyroid on scintiscan. Symptoms, treatment reviews, and diagnostic test listings may also be found.

EndocrineWeb: Thyroid Goiter: Enlargement of the Thyroid ○ ○
http://www.endocrineweb.com/goiter.html

EndocrineWeb's coverage of euthyroid goiter depicts a typical external goiter image and describes a number of factors contributing to the condition. Thyroid hormone supplementation, other treatment modalities where necessary, the possibility of malignancy, and cosmetic considerations of thyroid goiter are discussed.

Thyroid Disease Manager: Multinodular Goiter ○ ○ ○
http://thyroidmanager.bsd.uchicago.edu/Chapter17/17-text.htm

The incidence, etiological theory, and factors involved in the evolution of a multinodular goiter are reviewed at this comprehensive clinical guideline at Chapter 17 of *The Thyroid and Its Disease* textbook. Primary and secondary factors of multinodular origin; a case example of a multinodular goiter caused by a congenital metabolic defect; and additional thyroid stimulating factors, such as epidermal growth and insulin-like growth factors are discussed. By continuing to the article's next page, visitors find discussion on the pathology, natural disease history, and complication of thyrotoxicosis and carcinoma. Diagnostic techniques are summarized, as well as differential diagnosis.

University of Connecticut: Multinodular Goiter ○ ○ ○
http://esynopsis.uchc.edu/S431.htm

The table provided at this Internet address contains a quick review of the etiology, pathogenesis, epidemiology, and general gross description of a multinodular thyroid. Enlargeable thumbnail images of cross-sections are viewable, and microscopic descriptions and examples are available. Additional information and consequences of multinodular goiter are mentioned.

18.5 Thyroid Malignancy

Adam.com: Medullary Carcinoma of Thyroid ⊙ ⊙

http://accessarizona.adam.com/ency/article/000374.htm

The adam.com Web reference provides this page on medullary thyroid carcinoma, with information on the causes and incidence, as well as links to symptom and treatment information. Enlargeable images include a thyroid gland diagram and computed tomography (CT) scan.

CA: A Cancer Journal for Clinicians: Changing Concepts in the Pathogenesis and Management of Thyroid Carcinoma ⊙ ⊙ ⊙

http://www.ca-journal.org/articles/46/5/261-283/46_261-283.html

CA: A Cancer Journal For Clinicians describes the recent advances in the understanding and management of thyroid cancers, from classification and diagnosis with new technologies to insights into the molecular pathophysiology of follicular and parafollicular epithelium tumor development. The prognosis and treatment differences of the thyroid carcinoma categories and the tumor-node-metastasis (TNM) system are summarized. Another formula, based on age at diagnosis, histological tumor grade, disease extent, and size, yields an additional prognostic score. Other recent advances in staging schemes, factors that increase the risk of thyroid carcinoma, molecular events in pathogenesis, and diagnostic criteria are presented. Goals of surgical intervention are reviewed, and accessible figures throughout the text are found, depicting the impact of recurrence, survival rates, and molecular abnormalities.

Cancer Medicine: Medullary Carcinoma of the Thyroid ⊙ ⊙

http://intouch.cancernetwork.com/CanMed/Ch100/100-10.htm

The distinctive diagnosis by needle aspiration cytology, the significance of a single diagnosis in discovering a possible familial disease cluster, and the clinical disease presentation of thyroid medullary carcinoma are reviewed at this chapter of *Cancer Medicine*. The importance of extensive family screening is emphasized, as are facts regarding therapeutic management.

CancerNet: Thyroid Cancer ⊙ ⊙ ⊙

http://cancernet.nci.nih.gov/Cancer_Types/Thyroid_Cancer.shtml

Thyroid cancer introductory overviews, statistics, clinical trials, and additional professionally-oriented information are available at this one-stop resource for thyroid cancer coverage. As a service of the National Cancer Institute, visitors may select from among dozens of documents on genetics, testing, treatment, and coping resources. Sections for both patients and professionals are offered, with complete clinical guidelines and consumer-oriented brochures presented for all aspects of disease and disease management.

EndocrineWeb: Thyroid Nodules ◎ ◎ ◎
http://www.endocrineweb.com/nodule.html

Basic facts about thyroid nodules are reviewed at this site of the EndocrineWeb.com database, with a listing of three questions that should be answered after an appropriate work-up. The use of fine needle aspiration biopsy (FNA), ultrasound examination, and patient complaints and symptoms associated with a thyroid nodule are presented. Links to a nodule exam and biopsy page are found, as well as reassuring information pertaining to radiation exposure and other frequently asked questions regarding diagnosis and treatment.

Frontiers in Bioscience: Images of Thyroid Gland Neoplasms ◎ ◎
http://www.bioscience.org/atlases/tumpath/endo/thyroid/thyroid.htm

Cross-sections and external views of multinodular goiter, follicular adenocarcinoma, lymphoma, and medullary carcinomas of the thyroid gland are viewable at this Frontiers in Bioscience Web site. Each image is accompanied by a brief clinical summary; operative procedure, if applicable; and tumor characteristic listings. A link to microscopic images, with low-, mid-, and high-power magnification, is also available.

North Memorial Health Care Library:
Fine Needle Aspirations of Thyroid Nodules ◎ ◎
http://www.nmmc.com/nmhc/library/htm/thyroid.htm

Common and uncommon etiologies of the prevalent thyroid nodule are reviewed at this site of the North Memorial Health Care Library. The use of fine needle aspiration for differentiation of benign and malignant thyroid growth is discussed, with evaluation protocol and characteristic findings of benign and cancerous nodules outlined. Additional diagnostic procedures such as thyroid scans and ultrasound, for determination of gland volume and cold, warm, and hot nodular growths, are summarized. A listing of thyroid malignancies that may be diagnosed via fine needle aspiration, the prevalence of suspicious cytology, and recommendations regarding the safe and cost-effective fine needle biopsy are discussed.

OncoLink: Cancer of the Thyroid ◎ ◎ ◎
http://cancer.med.upenn.edu/disease/thyroid

Plentiful information on cancers of the thyroid is contained at this OncoLink Web location, as a service of the University of Pennsylvania Cancer Center. An introduction to cancer of the thyroid is found, along with FAQs answering inquiries regarding treatment options for thyroid cancer, radioiodine treatment precautions, and the thyroglobulin assay test. The "Cancer of the Thyroid Menu" also contains a link to automatically subscribe to THYROID-ONC, an online, unmoderated discussion group, as well as a connection to an OncoLink book review pertaining to radiation and thyroid cancer. Articles on medullary carcinoma, thyroid papillary carcinoma, treatment reviews, and a personal account of the illness are provided. CancerLit monthly updates offer extensive article listings on a wide variety of thyroid cancer management topics, and clinical review and guidelines for both patients and professionals are found, courtesy of the National Cancer Institute (NCI).

The Continuing Education Network (TCEN): Management of the Thyroid Nodule ○ ○ ○

http://www.tcen.com/mtn.htm

Text and audio files are provided at this site and allow individual navigation of a thyroid nodule management presentation. The prevalence of thyroid nodules and additional background information on deciding what protocol is required are explained. As visitors advance through the audio presentation, the clinical subgroups of afflicted individuals, differential diagnosis of nodules, history of surgical management, cancer categories, and risk stratification outlines are presented with a slide series, accompanied by a RealPlayer lecture recording.

Thyroid-Cancer.net ○ ○ ○

http://www.thyroid-cancer.net

Provided as a service of the Johns Hopkins Thyroid Tumor Center, this page contains access to surgical treatment information for thyroid nodules and cancer, and topical coverage of diagnosis, treatment, medications, and innovations in thyroid tumor cancer management. Specific clinical situations are addressed in terms of surgical outcome, and plenty of answers to Frequently Asked Questions.

18.6 Pregnancy and Thyroid Disorders

General Resources

Thyroid Foundation of Canada: Thyroid Disorders and Pregnancy ○ ○ ○

http://home.ican.net/~thyroid/Articles/EngE11A.html

Professors from the University of Western Ontario and the University of California at San Diego offer this online review of the spectrum of thyroid disease in pregnancy. The autoimmune nature of some thyroid disorders in pregnancy and postpartum thyroiditis are discussed, in addition to the issues of thyroid disease and fertility and pregnancy planning for women with thyroid disease. A pregnant woman's thyroid gland function, as well as that of the fetus is reviewed, and hypothyroidism, hyperthyroidism, solitary thyroid nodule, and fetal thyroid disease presentations are found.

Hyperthyroidism

Memorial Health System: Hyperthyroidism in Pregnancy ○ ○
http://www.qualityoflife.org/fprp/noontopics/020798.htm

This informative basic introduction to hyperthyroidism in pregnancy reviews the natural course of Graves' disease and also lists nine other possible causes of hyperthyroidism during gestation. Complications, both maternal and fetal, are reviewed, in addition to therapeutic goals.

Thyroid Disease Manager: Thyrotoxicosis ○ ○
http://thyroidmanager.bsd.uchicago.edu/Chapter14/Ch-14-4.htm

The management of hyperthyroidism in the pregnant patient is reviewed at this clinical article, with the classical causes and causes specific to the pregnancy outlined. The courses of the conditions, the fetal risks associated with them, and the separate management considerations are reviewed. Clinical features suggestive of Graves' in the pregnant patient are outlined in a table summary, and additional information charts on fetal outcome and treatment guidelines are found. Further discussion with regard to gestational transient thyrotoxicosis and nodular thyroid disease in pregnancy may be found.

Hypothyroidism

Endocrine Society:
Recommendations in Response to Major Hypothyroidism Study ○ ○
http://www.endo-society.org/maternalthyroiddeficiency

An Endocrine Society press release, a position paper related to the assessment and treatment of maternal thyroid hormone deficiency during pregnancy, and common questions and answers related to hypothyroidism are available from this address. The position paper provides background information on recent research and resulting Endocrine Society recommendations.

National Institutes of Health News Release:
Hypothyroidism during Pregnancy Linked to Lower IQ for Child ○ ○
http://www.nih.gov/news/pr/aug99/nichd-18.htm

The National Institutes of Health press release at this address offers an overview of recent research suggesting a link between untreated maternal hypothyroidism and lower IQ test scores in offspring. The article explains the research study and resulting data and also offers a chart outlining average IQ test scores and percentage of test scores below 85 in children with healthy mothers, hypothyroid mothers treated during pregnancy, and hypothyroid mothers untreated during pregnancy.

Thyroid Disease Manager: Primary Hypothyroidism ◎ ◎ ◎
http://www.thyroidmanager.org/Chapter14/Ch-14-3.htm

This article offers a technical discussion of primary hypothyroidism and its clinical importance in pregnancy. Topics include the prevalence of reduced thyroid function in apparently healthy pregnant women, as well as pregnant women previously diagnosed with hypothyroidism, the effects of hypothyroidism on pregnancy outcome, screening and diagnosis of hypothyroidism during pregnancy, and therapeutic considerations. Tables outline the prevalence of abnormally elevated thyroid-stimulating hormone (TSH) in 2,000 consecutive women at 15 and 18 weeks gestation, and thyroxine dosage for maintaining normal serum TSH concentration before and during pregnancy in patients with primary hypothyroidism.

Postpartum Thyroid Disease

Thyroid International: Postpartum Thyroiditis ◎ ◎ ◎
http://www.thyrolink.com/data/HTML/THYINT/JOURNAL/5-96INT.HTM

Postpartum thyroiditis (PPT) or hypothyroidism is the subject of the *Thyroid International* Web location. The variable incidence, significant clinical features, and clinical spectrum of disease are summarized, with special attention to the transient nature of the condition and its association with depression. PPT's relation to exacerbation of underlying thyroid disease and immune rebound are discussed. Figures accessible throughout the text illustrate changes in hormone level and abnormal thyroid ultrasound, and a graph depicting the course of postpartum thyroid function may be viewed.

University of Palermo: Postpartum Thyroiditis ◎ ◎
http://mbox.unipa.it/~radpa/p7/ppt.html

The pathology of postpartum thyroiditis (PPT) is reviewed at this site, with a case example presentation and specific patient findings outlined. Echographic examination, hormonal values, cytological exam, and therapeutic results are summarized. A description of this autoimmune thyroid condition and special considerations with regard to diagnosis are presented.

18.7 Nonthyroidal Illness

Postgraduate Medicine: Sick Euthyroid Syndrome ◎ ◎ ◎
http://www.postgradmed.com/issues/1999/04_99/camacho.htm

The online edition of *Postgraduate Medicine,* offers an article on sick euthyroid syndrome, which discusses thyroid physiology, types of abnormalities, etiology of abnormalities, clinical significance, diagnosis, and treatment. The article, provides a thorough explanation of abnormal thyroid function patterns in acutely ill patients.

University of Alabama:
Sick Euthyroid Syndrome Clinical Resources ✪ ✪ ✪ (some features fee-based)
http://www.slis.ua.edu/cdlp/uab/clinical/endocrinology/thyroid/ses.htm

Professional clinical resources specific to sick euthyroid syndrome are found at the site, which offers relevant documents that range from online texts and tutorials to clinical guidelines of major endocrinology associations and the National Guidelines Clearinghouse. Miscellaneous resources, such as WebMedLit in endocrinology and a link to similar resource pages that are suitable for patients and families, are accessible. Some sites require registration and subscription, while others may be visited on a free trial basis, such as the *MDConsult Reference Books*.

19. ADRENAL GLANDS

19.1 General Resources

Addison and Cushing International Federation
http://www.spin.nl/nvap0302.htm
Background information on Addison's disease, Cushing's syndrome, and acromegaly is found at this site, with details on current treatment research for professional reference. Links to member organizations, various support groups, and a connection to a useful table, which outlines the strength of various forms of glucocorticoids, are found.

CliniWeb International: Adrenal Gland Diseases
http://www.ohsu.edu/cliniweb/C19/C19.53.html
From CliniWeb International, this site offers links to resources on adrenal gland diseases, including diseases of the adrenal cortex, adrenal gland hyperfunction, adrenal gland neoplasms, adrenal hyperplasia, and Waterhouse-Friderichsen syndrome. Sources of information include the Medical College of Wisconsin, Oncolink, and the University of Utah, with the option to instantly access preformatted PubMed query links provided.

National Adrenal Diseases Foundation
http://www.medhelp.org/nadf
The National Adrenal Diseases Foundation provides education and support to individuals affected by adrenal diseases and offers an overview of Addison's disease, including symptoms and prognosis. Publications of the organization include fact sheets on Addison's disease, Cushing's syndrome, congenital adrenal hyperplasia, and hyperaldosteronism. Links to news, answers to frequently asked questions, a book list, international support groups, and current research related to the genetic basis of Addison's disease and its treatment are provided.

Temple University School of Medicine: Hormonal Hypertension ◐ ◐
http://blue.vm.temple.edu/~pathphys/endocrine/hypertension.html

Primary aldosteronism, pheochromocytoma, and Cushing's syndrome are all discussed in this Internet outline regarding their relationship to hypertension of hormonal origin. The pathogenetic subtypes of mineralocorticoid hypertension, manifestations, laboratory abnormalities and diagnostics, and other mineralocorticoid excess syndromes are listed. Diagnosis of pheochromocytoma, biochemical measurements, and precipitating events are recognized. A general discussion of Cushing's syndrome and manifestations of steroid excess are found.

University of Pennsylvania: Adrenal Diseases ◐ ◐
http://www.health.upenn.edu/surgery/clin/gi/adrenal.html

From the University of Pennsylvania Health Systems, this site discusses surgically correctable diseases related to the adrenal gland, including Cushing's syndrome, Conn's disease, and pheochromocytoma. Facility and contact information is provided.

19.2 Adrenal Insufficiency

General Resources

emedicine: Adrenal Insufficiency and Adrenal Crisis ◐ ◐ ◐
http://www.emedicine.com/emerg/topic16.htm

Adrenocortical hypofunction and severe, acute adrenocortical hypofunction are the subjects of this emedicine review, which describes the physiological effects of glucocorticoids, aldosterone, idiopathic primary adrenal insufficiency, and secondary insufficiency due to hypothalamic-pituitary disease and other causes. Rapidly progressing adrenal crisis; clinical and physical findings; a multitude of causes, diagnostic differentials, and their emedicine links; and diagnostic evaluative procedures are presented. Aggressive emergency care and profiles of corticosteroid drugs are included.

Merck Manual of Diagnosis and Therapy: Adrenal Cortical Hypofunction ◐ ◐
http://www.merck.com/pubs/mmanual/section2/chapter9/9b.htm

Information related to adrenal cortical hypofunction disorders, including Addison's disease and secondary adrenal insufficiency, is available through this fact sheet. Topics related to Addison's disease include etiology and incidence, pathophysiology, symptoms and signs, laboratory findings, diagnosis, prognosis, and treatment. The article also lists symptoms and signs; diagnosis; and treatments available for secondary adrenal insufficiency. Links are available to similar resources on adrenal cortical hyperfunction, pheochromocytoma, and nonfunctional adrenal masses.

University of Alabama:
Hypofunction of the Adrenal Cortex Clinical Resources ○ ○ ○

http://www.slis.ua.edu/cdlp/WebDLCore/clinical/endocrinology/adrenal/hypo.html

The clinical resources accessible from this site provide encyclopedic review, clinical guidelines, and a host of miscellaneous documents pertinent to hypofunction of the adrenal cortex. Practice guidelines include those of the National Guidelines Clearinghouse and the National Institute of Diabetes and Digestive and Kidney Diseases (NIDDK). A related patient and family resource page may be connected to directly from the site.

Addison's Disease

Australian Addison's Disease Association ○ ○ ○

http://addisons.org.au

The site of the Australian Addison's Disease Association, a rapidly growing organization, provides extensive information about Addison's disease. The topics covered concerning this disease, include causes, symptoms, diagnosis, and treatment. Information on the adrenocorticotropic hormone (ACTH) stimulation test and the insulin-induced hypoglycemia test is found, as well as medical articles, case studies, and support and coping resources. Newsletters, information about the association, answers to frequently asked questions, and links to related sites are found.

emedicine: Addison's Disease ○ ○ ○

http://emedicine.com/cgi-bin/foxweb.exe/
showsection@d:/em/ga?book=med&topicid=42

emedicine's guide to primary adrenocortical insufficiency is reviewed at this site, with sections included on the background, pathophysiology, and presentation of chronic disease. Causes, differentials links, laboratory studies and, other diagnostic workup tests are reviewed. Imaging findings, histologic findings, medical management, and drug profiles are also included in this comprehensive disorder review.

NIDDK: Office of Health Research Reports: Addison's Disease ○ ○ ○

http://www.mystical-www.co.uk/adison.htm

Information about primary and secondary adrenal insufficiency and coverage of symptoms, diagnosis, and treatment options are offered at this publication of the National Institutes of Health. Specific tests for diagnosis; special problems, such as surgery and pregnancy in an Addison's patient; patient education material; and suggested reading are provided.

Adrenal Hemorrhage

Definitive Adrenal Insufficiency Due to Bilateral Adrenal Hemorrhage and Primary Antiphospholipid Syndrome ○ ○

http://jcem.endojournals.org/cgi/content/full/83/5/1437?&searchid=976570205097_8092

Adrenal manifestations of antiphospholipid syndrome are reviewed at this article abstract, courtesy of the *Journal of Clinical Endocrinology and Metabolism*. Spontaneous bilateral adrenal hemorrhage leading to acute adrenal insufficiency is described, and a case example of a woman with primary antiphospholipid syndrome is presented, with abdominal computed tomography (CT) images shown. The laboratory findings and principal features of occult hemorrhage are reviewed, as well as confirmatory diagnostic tests and a rapid treatment response.

Adrenoleukodystrophy (ALD)

Kennedy Krieger Institute and Academic Medical Center: Mutation Database for X-Linked Adrenoleukodystrophy ○ ○

http://www.x-ald.nl/index.htm

This database for X-linked adrenoleukodystrophy offers an information source of mutations and polymorphisms in the X-ALD (ABCD1) gene and provides various pages on mutation, frame shift, deletions, polymorphisms, and other mutations and error types. An additional page lists all mutations sorted by amino acid position, and the clinical manifestations of several different phenotypes are described.

National Institute of Neurological Disorders and Stroke (NINDS): Adrenoleukodystrophy ○ ○

http://www.ninds.nih.gov/health_and_medical/disorders/adrenolu_doc.htm

The National Institutes of Health (NIH) provides this fact sheet on adrenoleukodystrophy, courtesy of NINDS. This genetic, progressive dysfunction of the adrenal gland and the resulting damage to the myelin sheath are reviewed, with several disease features listed. Treatment, prognosis, and references to journal articles and additional in-depth information on the illness are offered.

19.3 Adrenal Hormone Overproduction

General Resources

Merck Manual of Diagnosis and Therapy: Adrenal Cortical Hyperfunction ◐ ◐
http://www.merck.com/pubs/mmanual/section2/chapter9/9c.htm

The *Merck Manual* offers a thorough discussion of adrenal cortical hyperfunction through this online review. Specific subtopics include adrenal virilism, Cushing's syndrome, and hyperaldosteronism. Symptoms, signs, diagnosis, and treatment details are typically provided for each subtopic. Links are also available to similar resources devoted to adrenal cortical hypofunction, pheochromocytoma, and nonfunctional adrenal masses.

Congenital Adrenal Hyperplasia (CAH)

American Family Physician: Congenital Adrenal Hyperplasia: Not Really a Zebra ◐ ◐ ◐
http://www.aafp.org/afp/990301ap/1190.html

American Family Physician presents an in-depth article on congenital adrenal hyperplasia, its elusive diagnosis, and carefully monitored treatment regimens. The deficiency in cortisol synthesis in mild to severe disease forms, the inadequacy of glucocorticoid production, and the electrolyte disturbances and related symptomatology of insufficient mineralocorticoid synthesis are reviewed. A table presents the enzymatic pathway for cortisol and aldosterone biosynthesis, and the results of 21-hydroxylase deficiency are noted. Signs and symptoms in children and adults, specifically women, are outlined. Differences in clinical manifestations and recognition of the classical and mild types are discussed, with a clinical algorithm presented. Prenatal diagnosis and therapy in afflicted families are recommended.

Congenital Adrenal Hyperplasia ◐ ◐
http://www.rwi.nch.edu.au/endcond/endcond6.htm#E9E4

The key enzymes of adrenal steroid biosynthesis are listed at this Web site, which fully reviews congenital adrenal hyperplasia. In addition, visitors may access pages that describe the physiological basis of the disorder, differentiate between the severe classical form and the non-classical form, provide information on genetics and prenatal testing, and present features of the salt-losing CAH. Case histories, biochemical disease features, and causes of adrenal insufficiency other than congenital adrenal hyperplasia are reviewed.

Congenital Adrenal Hyperplasia Support Group ◐ ◐
http://www.rch.unimelb.edu.au/CAH

The Australian Congenital Adrenal Hyperplasia Support Group provides fact sheets on CAH excerpted from *Your Child with Congenital Adrenal Hyperplasia*. The lack of cortisol and aldosterone and the abundance of androgen, the disease implications in fetal development, the diagnosis in both girls and boys, and differentiation between CAH with and without aldosterone absence are presented. *CAH: A Guide For Young Women* offers information on fertility, pregnancy, and polycystic ovary disease in girls with poorly controlled CAH. Related publications, videos, and Internet links are found at the site.

Endocrine Society:
Endocrinology and Congenital Adrenal Hyperplasia ◐ ◐
http://www.endo-society.org/pubaffai/factshee/cah.htm

Severe and mild forms of CAH are reviewed at this fact sheet, offered as a service of the Endocrine Society. The prevalence of the condition in specific populations, steroid treatment, prenatal diagnosis and management, newborn blood screening, and current research into the precise amino acid defects of the genes are mentioned.

Family Village: Adrenal Hyperplasia ◐ ◐ ◐
http://www.familyvillage.wisc.edu/lib_adrh.htm

Family Village's collection of resources on adrenal hyperplasia include the MAGIC Foundation for Children's Growth, the National Adrenal Diseases Foundation (NADF), and links to the Online Mendelian Inheritance in Man (OMIM) summaries on adrenal hyperplasia types I-V. Message boards and additional Web sites on congenital adrenal hyperplasia are accessible, such as the Late Onset (Non-Classic) Congenital Adrenal Hyperplasia home page.

New York Weill Cornell Center: Congenital Adrenal Hyperplasia ◐ ◐
http://pedsendo.med.cornell.edu/cah

The New York Weill Cornell Centers Division of Pediatric Endocrinology addresses CAH, with mild disease forms and the less common classical CAH reviewed. Prenatal diagnosis for 21-hydroxylase deficiency via DNA analysis is discussed, and a link to the *CAH Genetics Testing Fact Sheet* provides answers to the most frequent inquiries regarding CAH and genetic testing.

Hyperaldosteronism

E-note for Adult Medicine: Hyperaldosteronism
http://enotes.tripod.com/hyperaldosteronism.htm
Presented as a service of Massachusetts General Hospital, this E-note offers clinicians a quick reference to the differential diagnosis and treatment for the various causes of hyperaldosteronism. Offering concise information for clinicians, the page describes components of both primary and secondary disease.

Family Practice Notebook.com: Aldosteronism
http://fpnotebook.com/END3.htm
This chapter of the Family Practice Notebook offers an outline of aldosteronism, including epidemiology, causes, signs and symptoms, and laboratory diagnostics. Links to further details on laboratory tests, the motor examination, headache, hypertension, and adrenal adenomas are found.

Hyperaldosteronism: The Facts You Need to Know
http://www.medhelp.org/www/nadf9.htm
Excess production of aldosterone is reviewed at the site, with the hormone's purpose and symptoms of its excess and deficiency explained. Adrenal hyperplasia or benign tumors are the causes discussed, and tests that search for excess hormone in the blood and urine, as well as tests that may differentiate between hyperplasia and tumor, are summarized. Treatment, depending on the cause, is outlined. Aldosterone blocking, antihypertensives, and surgical tumor removal in the case of Conn's syndrome are discussed.

Hypercortisolism: Cushing's Syndrome

Centre for Neuroendocrinology: Cushing's Syndrome
http://www.studentbmj.com/back_issues/0400/education/100.html
This portion of an endocrinology series on Cushing's syndrome explains the physiology of glucocorticoid secretion, the disease etiology, and concise reviews of both ACTH independent and dependant causes. Psuedo Cushing's syndrome, clinical features, and complete workup information involved are summarized. Biochemical disease confirmation, problems in diagnosis, differential diagnosis, and treatment regimens for various clinical pictures are presented.

Cushing's Support and Research Foundation
http://world.std.com/~csrf
Founded in 1995, the Cushing's Support and Research Foundation is a resource for patients and healthcare professionals alike. The site provides a fact sheet on Cushing's

syndrome, which includes a general overview of the disorder and articles on causes, incidence, symptoms, diagnosis, treatment, current research, and current studies of the National Institutes of Health. Suggested readings, information about the foundation, current news and events, and contact information are provided.

EndocrineWeb:
Diseases of the Adrenal Cortex: Cushing's Syndrome ⊙ ⊙ ⊙

http://www.endocrineweb.com/obesity.html

A core description of Cushing's syndrome and a thorough and illustrated guide to the disease are found at this interesting, online presentation. Common causes of excess steroids, tests for Cushing's syndrome, and treatment details are provided. Several links throughout the page lead readers to further basic and clinical information on adrenal imaging, operations for adrenal tumors, laparoscopic adrenalectomy, and adrenal carcinoma.

MedNets: Cushing's Disease ⊙ ⊙

http://www.mednets.org/cushings.htm

MedNets consumer information offers a thorough introduction to Cushing's syndrome, its causes, symptoms, and diagnosis. Details on research currently being conducted by the National Institutes of Health is presented. Readers will find answers to most basic questions regarding adrenal tumors, ectopic ACTH syndrome, pituitary adenomas, and testing procedures.

National Institute of Neurological Disorders
and Stroke (NINDS): Cushing's Syndrome Information Page ⊙ ⊙

http://www.ninds.nih.gov/health_and_medical/disorders/cushings_doc.htm

Offered as a service of the National Institute of Neurological Disorders and Stroke, this fact sheet contains basic information on Cushing's syndrome, with treatment, prognosis, and current research of NINDS summarized. Selected references and related Web site listings complete this governmental resource.

19.4 Adrenal Tumors

General Resources

OncoLink: Adrenal Cancer ⊙ ⊙ ⊙

http://cancer.med.upenn.edu/disease/adrenal

The latest listing of adrenal cancer trials of the University of Pennsylvania and related oncological medical groups is found at the "OncoLink's UPCC Protocol Finder" on this Web page. The site also offers answers to frequently asked questions about adrenal cancer as well as monthly updates of related CancerLit citations. Specific patient and physician guidelines are provided for both pheochromocytoma and adrenocortical cancers that offer cellular and staging classifications, as well as treatment option overviews.

OncoLink: Adrenal Neoplasms ◐ ◐

http://pathcuric1.swmed.edu/ScribeService/Resources/
path/objectives/Endocrine/endocrine-Adrenal-2.html

This site offers a general review of adrenal neoplasms, comparing and contrasting the histological findings of both adrenal cortical adenomas and adrenocortical carcinoma. Also provided is demographic and clinical information on pheochromocytoma.

University of Alabama: Adrenal Neoplasms Clinical Resources ◐ ◐ ◐

http://www.slis.ua.edu/cdlp/WebDLCore/clinical/oncology/endocrine/adrenal.html

Clinical resources for adrenal neoplasms are listed and accessible directly from this site, with supplementary resource directories for patients and families also available. References include the *Merck Manual* chapter on adrenal disorders, the British Columbia Cancer Agency Information for Health Care Providers, clinical guidelines from CancerNet and the National Guidelines Clearinghouse, and miscellaneous resources from notable medical Internet databases.

Aldosterone-Producing Adrenal Adenoma (Conn's Syndrome)

Conn's Syndrome ◐ ◐

http://www.mcevoy.demon.co.uk/Medicine/
Pathology/GenPath/Endocrine/Adrenal/Conns.html

This rare syndrome of primary aldosteronism is differentiated from hyperaldosteronism with bilateral nodular hyperplasia. The presence of a single, benign secretory adenoma; the effects of hypersecretion of aldosterone; and the clinical features of the syndrome are listed.

Non-Functioning Adrenal Incidentaloma

Adrenal Adenoma, Non-hyperfunctioning ◐ ◐

http://www.mamc.amedd.army.mil/williams/
GU/Adrenal/Benign/Adenoma/Adenoma.htm

The clinical presentation of adrenal adenoma is offered at this text-only site. Descriptions of computed tomography, magnetic resonance, positron emission tomography, and scintigraphic findings are provided.

Family Practice Notebook.com: Adrenal Adenoma

http://www.fpnotebook.com/END2.htm

Family Practice Notebook offers outlines of the pathophysiology of a variety of diseases, including this page of its adrenal diseases chapter. Six points related to aldosterone excess and links to further information on hypertension and hypokalemia are provided.

Pheochromocytoma

Lycos: Pheochromocytoma Support Site

http://www.angelfire.com/hi/Pheochromocytoma/index.html

The index of pheochromocytoma Web sites offered at this support page contains tributes to members who established the support group and information on physicians at the National Institutes of Health who are currently studying pheochromocytoma and multiple endocrine neoplasia. An article addressing the biochemical diagnosis of pheochromocytoma, instructions for blood sampling and shipping of specimens, and a compilation of personal Internet pages are found.

National Cancer Institute: MedNews: Pheochromocytoma

http://www.meb.uni-bonn.de/cancernet/102494.html

From MedNews and the National Cancer Institute, this site offers professional information about pheochromocytoma, with articles related to cellular classification, stage information, treatment options, and localized benign, regional, metastatic, and recurrent pheochromocytoma.

20. GASTROINTESTINAL TRACT

20.1 General Resources

National Pancreas Foundation ○ ○ ○
http://www.pancreasfoundation.org

The National Pancreas Foundation supports research of disease related to the pancreas and provides information and services to people affected by these illnesses. Their site provides information about the pancreas, pancreatic cancer, and pancreatitis. Nutritional information, answers to FAQs, and links to pancreatic disease-related material on the Internet may be accessed.

Pancreas.org ○ ○ ○
http://www.pancreas.org

Pancreas.org was created to provide information for patients, physicians, and research on pancreatic disorders. Computed tomography images, a glossary of terms, and links to pancreatic cancer resources are offered. Research study reviews, disorder introductions and treatment details, and links to the National Pancreas Foundation, the Pancreatic Cancer Action Network, and the Midwest Multicenter Pancreatic Study Group are found.

20.2 Neoplasms of the Pancreas

General Resources

Cancer Medicine:
Neoplasms of the Gastroenteropancreatic Endocrine System ◎ ◎ ◎
http://intouch.cancernetwork.com/CanMed/Ch103/103-0.htm

Carcinoid tumors, glucagonoma, insulinomas, and other neoplasms classified according to their secretory products are discussed at this online chapter of *Cancer Medicine*. Growth factors and receptors expressed in gastroenteropancreatic tumors, neuroendocrine characteristics, anatomic distribution, and information on accurate diagnosis are presented. Effective treatment agents for pancreatic islet cell carcinomas are, additionally, reviewed.

Johns Hopkins Medical Institutions:
Islet Cell/Endocrine Tumors of the Pancreas ◎ ◎ ◎
http://162.129.103.69/MCGI/SEND%5EWEBUTLTY(704)/787106207

This subsite of Johns Hopkins Medical Institutions highlights the histological characteristics of endocrine neoplasms of the pancreas and describes the general principles applicable to the management of these functional tumors. The clinical syndromes for insulinoma, gastrinoma, VIPoma, and glucagonoma are summarized, and radioimmunoassay (RIA) for insulin, gastrin, VIP, and glucagon hormonal measurement is described. Tumor staging and imaging techniques for localization and other diagnostic techniques are reviewed, as well as surgical treatment and chemotherapeutic intervention. Nonfunctional tumors, as well as the rare somatostatinoma, are discussed.

Gastrinoma (Zollinger-Ellison Syndrome)

Cancer Control Journal: Gastrinoma: State of the Art ◎ ◎ ◎
http://www.hlmcc.org/cancjrnl/v4n1/article4.html

The article found at this Web site reviews the literature and developments in the diagnosis, imaging, operative and nonoperative management, and follow-up of gastrinoma patients since the identification of Zollinger-Ellison syndrome in 1955. Recent advance in H2-blockers and the use of omeprazole for greater control of acid production are discussed, in addition to improved imaging methods of tumor localization. Summaries of diagnosis and management, including two algorithmic reviews, and recognition of hypercalcemia and other endocrine abnormalities seen in multiple endocrine neoplasia syndrome type 1 (MEN 1) are presented. Computed tomography (CT), magnetic resonance imaging (MRI), ultrasonography, and selective angiography modalities for diagnosis of primary and metastatic disease are discussed.

Neoplastic Endocrine-Like Syndromes ◐ ◑
http://www.niddk.nih.gov/health/digest/summary/zolling/zolling.htm

The National Digestive Diseases Information Clearinghouse offers this informational brochure on Zollinger-Ellison syndrome, a potentially fatal disorder in which pancreatic, often cancerous, tumors secrete excess gastrin. The symptoms, diagnosis, and treatment of the disorder are outlined. The clearinghouse encourages free copy and distribution of the publication.

Zollinger-Ellison Syndrome ◐ ◑
http://www.5mcc.com/SUMMARY/1012.html

A concise description of Zollinger-Ellison syndrome, including its related tumors, synonyms, and causes, may be found at the site, with reference to the disorder's ICD-9 code and additional Web connections.

Glucagonoma

Adam.com: Glucagonoma ◐ ◑
http://accesswaco.adam.com/ency/article/000326.htm

This fact sheet describes clinical aspects of glucagonoma, a tumor of the pancreas resulting in excess glucagon production. The overview includes a summary of causes, incidence, and risk factors; symptoms; and treatment. A diagram of the endocrine system is available, and links are provided to explanations of unfamiliar terms.

emedicine: Glucagonoma Syndrome ◐ ◑ ◒
http://www.emedicine.com/DERM/topic168.htm

Professionals will find an informative overview of glucagonoma and pseudoglucagonoma syndromes at this address. An introduction to these syndromes includes a detailed discussion of pathophysiology and demographics. Clinical topics include typical patient presentations, physical findings, possible causes, differentials, laboratory analysis, and treatments. Representative images of erythema associated with the syndromes are available, and a bibliography of references is also provided. CME review questions are offered in conclusion.

Insulinoma

MEDLINEplus Health Information: Insulinoma ◐ ◑
http://medlineplus.adam.com/ency/article/000387.htm

From the adam.com Web database comes this overview of insulinoma, also known as islet cells adenoma or insuloma. The causes, incidence, and risk factors of this usually benign tumor of the endocrine pancreas are reviewed at the site, and links to symptoms, treatment, and prevention information are provided.

Vasoactive Intestinal Peptide Tumor (VIPoma)

**Cancer Medicine:
Vasoactive Intestinal Peptide Tumor (VIPoma)** ◐ ◐

http://intouch.cancernetwork.com/CanMed/Ch103/103-9.htm

Vasoactive intestinal peptide tumor (VIPoma), a rare, noninsulin-secreting tumor of the pancreatic islets, is described in this article. A historical overview of the disease is followed by a thorough discussion of distinguishing features. Specific topics include sites of tumors secreting vasoactive intestinal peptide, biochemical diagnosis and experience, and appropriate treatments. Reference citations are available.

**Washington University
School of Medicine: VIPoma Metastatic to Liver** ◐ ◐

http://gamma.wustl.edu/ot001te173.html

A diagnosis of a VIPoma metastatic to the liver is made at this example review, based on patient history, octreotide scintigraphy, SPECT imaging, and angiographic computed tomography (CT). Abnormal liver findings representing metastatic spread are discussed.

20.3 Carcinoma of the Pancreas

Ask NOAH About: Islet Cell Carcinoma ◐ ◐ ◐

http://noah.cuny.edu/cancer/nci/cancernet/100790.html

The distinct cancers of the islet cells of the pancreas, their unique metabolic and clinical manifestations, and surgical and chemotherapeutic management are reviewed within this New York Online Access to Health (NOAH) Web document. Cellular classifications of secreted agents, tumor types, and their respective illnesses are presented. Diagnostic tests for each syndrome are reviewed, and treatment option overviews for gastrinoma, insulinoma, and miscellaneous islet cell tumors are presented.

CancerNet: Islet Cell Carcinoma ◐ ◐ ◐

http://cancernet.nci.nih.gov/Cancer_Types/Islet_Cell_Carcinoma.shtml

A service of the National Cancer Institute, CancerNet offers comprehensive resources on a wide variety of topics important to cancer patients and health professionals. General resources include an overview of support sources, complementary and alternative medicine, genetic causes and risk factors, prevention, clinical trials, and statistics. Physician Data Query (PDQ) resources on the topic of islet cell carcinoma are available for both patients and healthcare professionals. The professional PDQ treatment overview includes an introduction to cancer of the endocrine pancreas, cellular classification details, disease staging guidelines, and treatment options relevant to gastrinoma, insulinoma, miscellaneous islet cell carcinoma, and recurrent islet cell carcinoma. Reference citations are provided throughout the document.

Lustgarten Foundation for Pancreatic Cancer Research ☼ ☼ ☼
http://www.lustgartenfoundation.org

The Lustgarten Foundation for Pancreatic Cancer Research offers information for foundation supporters, medical researchers, and patient advocates at their site. For medical researchers, the site offers the latest news in pancreatic cancer research with links to relevant journal articles. For patients, the site offers a pancreatic cancer patient resource guide, including sections on clinical trials, managing pain, and coping with fatigue. A glossary of terms and links to additional resources are found, as is organizational and membership information.

OncoLink: Pancreatic Cancer ☼ ☼ ☼
http://cancer.med.upenn.edu/disease/pancreas

OncoLink's resource collection on pancreatic cancer includes general information, courtesy of the National Cancer Institute (NCI), as well as monthly CancerLit additions for islet cell carcinoma regarding treatments, trials, surgical procedures, diagnostics, and case studies. Useful external links include scintigraphy teaching files and the pancreas cancer home page of Johns Hopkins Medical Institutions.

Pancreas Cancer Home Page ☼ ☼ ☼
http://www.path.jhu.edu/pancreas

Provided by Johns Hopkins Medical Institutions, this site provides articles on such topics as pancreatic surgery and medical treatment, genetic research, and other scientific endeavors. Information regarding discoveries made at the institute, its new laboratory for research, and its clinicians and investigators is provided. Answers to FAQs, a bibliography on pancreatic cancer, and information on genetic testing are also offered.

Pancreatic Cancer Action Network ☼ ☼
http://www.pancan.org

The Pancreatic Cancer Action Network is dedicated to raising awareness of the disorder and the urgent need for research programs. The site provides information about events, programs, and campaigns. An e-mail list, a suggested reading list, and links to press releases are found, as are facts from the National Cancer Institute and links to pancreatic cancer practice guidelines.

Pancreatic Cancer Online

http://www.healthyfoundations.com/pancreatic

Pancreatic Cancer Online offers self-help ideas and alternative treatment options for pancreatic cancer. The self-help section provides information on diet and nutrition, supplements, exercise, medication, and stress reduction. Alternative treatment options discussed include the Gerson program, the Gonzales program, bovine and shark cartilage, dietary intervention, hydrazine sulfate, designer chemotherapy, Rubitecan, and direct injection of high-dosage radiation. A list of surgeons who perform the Whipple procedure and a listing of message boards, links to resources, and links to other sites of interest are found.

Ronald S. Hirshberg
Memorial Foundation for Pancreatic Cancer Research

http://www.pancreatic.org/main.htm

The Ronald S. Hirshberg Memorial Foundation for Pancreatic Cancer Research is dedicated to promoting research and providing information and advocacy to patients and their families. Information about pancreatic cancer at the site includes a definition of the disorder and statistical facts. There are also sections on diagnosis, prognosis, treatment, and research. Links to related sources of information include Johns Hopkins and OncoLink.

21. FEMALE ENDOCRINOLOGY

21.1 General Resources

Human Reproduction:
Menstrual Disorders and Other Common Gynecology Problems ◯ ◯
http://medstat.med.utah.edu/kw/human_reprod/lectures/gyn_disorders
This online tutorial provides an overview of menstrual disorders and other common gynecology problems, including dysmenorrhea, abnormal uterine bleeding, and premenstrual syndrome. Definitions of terms are presented, followed by a presentation of material in outline form. Causes, diagnosis, and management considerations are reviewed, with a flow diagram for treatment of premenstrual syndrome included.

21.2 Amenorrhea

American Academy of Pediatrics:
Amenorrhea in Adolescent Athletes ◯ ◯
http://www.aap.org/policy/02626.html
This article from the American Academy of Pediatrics Committee on Sports Medicine offers a discussion of amenorrhea in adolescent athletes and resulting health problems. The article offers an overview of possible mechanisms of amenorrhea, as well as recommendations for amenorrhea management and prevention. Reference citations are provided.

Vanderbilt University Medical Center: Secondary Amenorrhea ◐ ◐
http://www.mc.vanderbilt.edu/peds/pidl/adolesc/ammenorh.htm

Secondary amenorrhea in adolescents is described in this fact sheet. The article discusses appropriate clinical investigations, clinical assessment, and possible causes. Reference citations are provided.

21.3 Hirsutism

Adam.com: Excessive Hair on Females ◐ ◐
http://www.adam.com/ency/article/003148.htm

This patient fact sheet offers an overview of hirsutism, including alternative clinical names, clinical considerations, and possible coexisting medical symptoms. Common causes are outlined, and treatment details are reviewed. A summary of routine medical tests during an initial evaluation of hirsutism is provided, as well as links to specific causative disease entities.

Advanced Fertility Center of Chicago: Hirsutism and Hyperandrogenism in Women ◐
http://www.advancedfertility.com/hirsute.htm

Diagnostic classifications of hyperandrogenism, causes of hirsutism in women, and evaluations of hirsute women are reviewed. Initial testing, information on testosterone levels, tumor workup, and treatment with oral contraceptives, spironolactone, and flutamide are outlined.

21.4 Infertility

Advanced Reproductive Care: Hormonal Therapy ◐ ◐
http://www.fertilityusa.com/hormonetherapy.html

Ovulation and hormonal therapy used in the treatment of infertility are discussed in this detailed article. A table of hormonal therapy medications includes generic and brand names, type of administration, and mechanisms of action. Hormonal therapies listed and discussed include GnRH agonists, human menopausal gonadotropins, follicle stimulating hormone, clomiphene citrate, human chorionic gonadotropin, progesterone, and bromocriptine, with other therapeutic considerations available. The article includes graphic representations of hormonal fluctuations throughout the menstrual cycle and in-vitro fertilization occurring throughout the menstrual cycle. Visitors will also find an overview of infertility, including prevention, evaluation, diagnosis, and treatment, in addition to a glossary of terms.

Finch University of Health Sciences/Chicago Medical School: Antibodies to Hormones and Neurotransmitters ◐ ◐

http://repro-med.net/papers/antibod.html

This site of the Chicago Medical School offers information about antibodies to hormones and neurotransmitters. The introduction describes five categories of immune problems that cause difficulties in fertility and pregnancy. There is a section describing treatments and a section devoted to outcomes.

Recurrent Pregnancy Loss: Hormonal Causes ◐ ◐ ◐

http://www.drdaiter.com/preg6.html

A board-certified physician in reproductive endocrinology and infertility presents this article describing hormonal causes for pregnancy loss. The article discusses the coordination of ovulation and embryo implantation in pregnancy and hormonal effects on this mechanism resulting in infertility and pregnancy loss. Three potential classes of luteal phase defects are described, including inadequate luteal phase production of progesterone, inadequate progesterone production after luteal rescue by the placental hCG, and inadequate placental production of progesterone. Other topics include the use of endometrial biopsy as a diagnostic tool and conflicting reports of progesterone teratogenicity.

21.5 Menstrual Exacerbations of Medical Problems

Journal of the American Medical Association Women's Health Info Center: Effects of the Menstrual Cycle on Medical Disorders ◐ ◐

http://www.ama-assn.org/special/womh/library/readroom/arch98/ira70759.htm

This article offers a detailed overview of the menstrual cycle within a larger discussion of medical problems exacerbated by normal hormonal fluctuations in premenopausal women. An overview of the menstrual cycle is followed by discussions of gonadotropin-releasing hormone agonists, menstrual migraines, catamenial epilepsy, asthma, rheumatoid arthritis, irritable bowel syndrome, diabetes, and other miscellaneous disorders in light of the menstrually-related exacerbation of these disorders. The article provides reference citations.

21.6 Ovarian Cancer

Fertility Drugs and Ovarian Cancer: A Review of the Evidence Purporting a Causal Association ◐ ◐

http://www.iaac.ca/articles/fertovar.html

A proposed hypothesis for ovarian cancer pathogenesis is found at this online article, with review of the malignant transformation of the epithelium lining and a multifactorial etiology, including a genetic transmission hypothesis, environmental factors, and additional theories. The link between nulliparity/infertility and ovarian cancer, debate over the causal role of fertility drugs in ovarian cancer, and a review of criteria for establishing a causal association between risk factors and disease are highlighted.

Gilda Radner Familial Ovarian Cancer Registry ◎ ◎
http://rpci.med.buffalo.edu/departments/gynonc/grwp.html
The Gilda Radner Familial Ovarian Cancer Registry is based at the Roswell Park Cancer Institute. The site provides information and statistics about ovarian cancer, with a section on risk factors and answers to frequently asked questions provided. Contact information and details about registering with the service are found.

National Ovarian Cancer Association ◎ ◎
http://www.ovariancanada.org
Ovarian cancer information, the organization's ongoing activities, and the association's research page provide a comprehensive Internet source of support and treatment information. Over 2,500 electronic documents are available for rapid viewing and include research summaries on gene therapy, immunotherapy, and anti-angiogenesis. Visitors may search the entire database or access an assortment of clinical trials, treatment agents, and biological approaches to care. Conference reports of the American Society of Clinical Oncology and the American Association for Cancer Research can be accessed.

National Ovarian Cancer Coalition ◎ ◎
http://www.ovarian.org
A support organization founded by ovarian cancer survivors, the National Ovarian Cancer Coalition promotes education, public awareness, and medical research. Information about the organization, answers to frequently asked questions, reports on the psychological aspects of ovarian cancer, and links to related sites are included, as well as a library of books and products for ovarian cancer patients. Information about upcoming events and programs is found, and news updates are provided.

Ovarian Cancer Alliance Canada ◎ ◎
http://www.ocac.ca
Ovarian Cancer Alliance Canada was organized by ovarian cancer survivors to promote improved diagnosis, treatment, and outcome of the disease. Information about ovarian cancer at the site includes an overview and discussions of risk factors, symptoms, and treatments available. A fact sheet for newly diagnosed women, a quarterly newsletter, and special topic discussions on nonconventional therapies and benign ovarian masses are offered.

Ovarian Cancer National Alliance ○ ○
http://www.ovariancancer.org

The Ovarian Cancer National Alliance seeks to increase public and professional understanding of the disease and encourage research efforts. A fact sheet about ovarian cancer is found, in addition to a downloadable conference brochure, a treatment and clinical trials page, and highlights of the alliance newsletter.

University of Michigan:
Ovarian Cancer and Women's Health Bibliography ○ ○
http://www-personal.umich.edu/~bethany/books.html

This site contains an ovarian cancer and women's health bibliography. Publication topics include ovarian cancer prevention, medical texts, nutrition, and alternative medicine. Books for caregivers, and on such topics as pain control, coping with the terminal phase of illness, and infertility may be found.

21.7 Polycystic Ovary Syndrome

allHealth.com: Stein-Leventhal Syndrome ○ ○
http://www.allhealth.com/ahtools/encyclopedia/article/0,8895,000369,00.html

IVillage and allHealth.com offer provide an overview at this site of Stein-Leventhal syndrome, also know as polycystic ovary syndrome. A description of the abnormal ovarian function, its related symptoms and signs, and theories related to estrogen production and hypothalamic-ovarian feedback are discussed. Test values that may be abnormal are listed at the "Symptoms" link, and pharmacological and surgical management options are described.

Case Studies: Polycystic Ovary Syndrome ○ ○
http://www.cs.umu.se/~medinfo/CaseStudies/256_4.html

A case study of PCOS, otherwise known as Stein-Leventhal disease, provides a description of the clinical syndrome. Late consequences, such as infertility and cardiovascular disease, are reviewed, as well as the characteristics of the current study group and results with regard to the parameters tested. Body mass index and hormonal values are measured.

DotPharmacy: Hirsute Pursuits ○ ○
http://www.dotpharmacy.com/uphirsut.html

An overview of PCOS, with special attention given to recognition of the male-pattern hair growth, is offered at this site. Differentiation between ovarian cysts and the ovaries of PCOS sufferers is made, and the underlying excessive androgen production is reviewed. The full range of symptoms associated with the illness is mentioned and includes diabetes, heart disease, cancer, and chronic fatigue. Oral contraceptive therapy and additional effective treatment modalities for hirsutism are explored.

HealthGate:
Polycystic Ovarian Syndrome (Stein-Leventhal Syndrome) ◐ ◐
http://www.healthgate.com/sym/sym366.shtml

Polycystic ovarian syndrome, also known as Stein-Leventhal disease, is reviewed at Healthgate's Symptoms, Illness, and Surgery information database. The fact sheet found offers a general overview of the disease, signs and symptoms, and the hormonal imbalance involved. Expectations regarding diagnostic testing, appropriate healthcare measures, and a treatment review are provided.

Vanderbilt University Medical Center: Polycystic Ovary Syndrome ◐ ◐
http://www.mc.vanderbilt.edu/peds/pidl/adolesc/polcysov.htm

Polycystic ovary syndrome is described in this clinical article. The article discusses in detail this clinically heterogeneous syndrome, including incidence, symptoms, common clinical features, diagnosis, and treatment. Reference citations are provided, and links are available to other topics, organized by body system.

21.8 Premenstrual Syndrome

Endocrine Society: Endocrinology and Premenstrual Syndrome ◐ ◐
http://www.endo-society.org/pubaffai/factshee/premenstrual.htm

Premenstrual syndrome is described for professionals and consumers in this fact sheet. Common questions are answered, providing information on the clinical importance of premenstrual syndrome, the definition of the syndrome, premenstrual syndrome diagnosis, and the role of endocrine factors in premenstrual syndrome. Visitors can also access Endocrine Society resources through this address, including publications, meeting notices, patient information resources, and links to related sites.

University of Alabama:
Premenstrual Syndrome Clinical Resources ◐ ◐ ◐
http://www.slis.ua.edu/cdlp/WebDLCore/clinical/gynecology/pms.htm

The Clinical Digital Libraries Project of the University of Alabama offers viewers a compilation of easily accessible clinical guidelines, textbook chapters, clinical trials, and news resources on the Internet related to premenstrual syndrome. Additional pages of general gynecology clinical resources and resources on premenstrual syndrome for consumers are accessible from the site.

21.9 Uterine Bleeding Disorders

American Family Physician: Abnormal Uterine Bleeding ◉ ◉ ◉
http://www.aafp.org/afp/991001ap/1371.html

Diagnostic aspects of abnormal uterine bleeding are described in this professional article. Tables summarize terminology used to describe abnormal uterine bleeding, differential diagnosis of abnormal uterine bleeding, characteristics of ovulatory and anovulatory menstrual cycles, and treatment options for dysfunctional uterine bleeding. Flow charts diagram suggested initial approaches to abnormal uterine bleeding in premenopausal, perimenopausal, and postmenopausal women. The article discusses clinical history and physical examinations appropriate to premenopausal, perimenopausal, and postmenopausal women. Reference citations are included.

MedInfoSource:
Practical Management of Dysfunctional Uterine Bleeding ◉ ◉
http://www.cmea.com/resource/c-dysf.html

A technical overview of dysfunctional uterine bleeding is available from this article, including discussions of hormonal and organic etiologies and diagnosis. Treatment strategies are summarized, including medical and surgical therapies. The article also provides reference citations.

22. MALE ENDOCRINOLOGY

22.1 Androgen Abnormalities

Androgen Insensitivity Syndrome ◐ ◐ ◐
http://www.geneclinics.org/profiles/androgen/details.html

Funded by the National Institutes of Health and developed by the University of Washington, this Web page contains a summary of the disease characteristics, diagnosis and testing, and genetic counseling procedures offered for androgen insensitivity syndrome (AIS). Synonyms for the condition, classifications of AIS phenotypes, laboratory findings, and links to tables and literature citing other findings are provided. Testing used in the molecular diagnosis of AIS is reviewed, and clinical descriptions of complete AIS, partial AIS, mild AIS, and Reifenstein syndrome are found. A large portion of the site is devoted to differential diagnosis, management, and related literature and MEDLINE abstracts. A useful resource listing at the end of the document provides contact information and links to national and international support groups.

Complete Androgen Insensitivity Syndrome ◐ ◐
http://www.rch.unimelb.edu.au/publications/CAIS.html

Information on complete androgen insensitivity syndrome is contained at this new 28-page information booklet, published by Dr. Garry Wayne of the Royal Children's Hospital. Visitors may obtain the booklet, free of charge, by contacting the department directly or may download the publication in its entirety directly from the site.

22.2 Erectile Dysfunction

Alberta Medical Association: Laboratory Endocrine Testing Guidelines for Investigation of Impotence and Male Androgen Insufficiency ◉ ◉

http://www.amda.ab.ca/cpg/catalogue/documents/endocrinology/impotence/guideline.html

These guidelines describe appropriate endocrine laboratory tests in the evaluation of impotence, including a summary of recommendations, background discussion, important notes on the applicability of the guidelines, and reference citations.

American Association for Geriatric Psychiatry: Treating Erectile Dysfunction ◉ ◉ ◉

http://macmcm.com/aagp/aagp99-tedepciams.htm

This report reviews topics recently discussed at the American Association for Geriatric Psychiatry meeting relating to the etiology, psychological assessment, and treatment of erectile dysfunction (ED) in late life. Several causes of ED, the physiological requirements for normal sexual functioning, and review of medical and mechanical solutions are discussed. Specific medications that may interfere with proper erectile function and the psychological impact of ED are presented.

American Association of Clinical Endocrinologists (AACE): Clinical Practice Guidelines for the Evaluation and Treatment of Male Sexual Dysfunction ◉ ◉ ◉

http://www.aace.com/clin/guides/sexualdysfunction.html

Clinical practice review offered at this site is provided as a joint venture of the AACE and the American College of Endocrinology. A framework for the evaluation, diagnosis, and management of erectile dysfunction, with an emphasis on cost-effectiveness and relationship issues, is offered. The role of the endocrinologist in the treatment of male sexual dysfunction, erectile physiology and pathophysiology, and medical conditions and drug-related causes of dysfunction are discussed. A comprehensive table outlining sexual side effects of common medications is found, in addition to an algorithm for evaluation of ED. History and examination considerations, laboratory and other assessments, and psychological, medical, and hormonal therapies are reviewed. Several nonspecific therapies are discussed, such as vacuum devices and venous constriction rings.

Ask NOAH About: Impotence (Erectile Dysfunction) ◉ ◉ ◉

http://www.noah.cuny.edu/wellconn/impotence.html

An impotence discussion, provided as a service of the New York Online Access to Health (NOAH) educational Web site, offers information on penile anatomy and disorders frequently associated with impotence, as well as information specific to older men, men with serious medical conditions, and other risk factors. Discussion is provided on the deprivation of oxygen-rich blood supply to the penis, specific medical factors that may interfere with normal functioning, the process of aging, and the relationship of abnormal testosterone levels to impotence. Hypogonadism, other hormonal abnormalities, and several other factors that may contribute to impaired sexual function are reviewed. Symptoms, diagnosis, lifestyle changes, and extensive review of current medical treatment are also presented.

Lahey Clinic Center for Sexual Dysfunction: American Association of Clinical Endocrinologists Clinical Practice Guidelines for Male Sexual Dysfunction ◉ ◉ ◉
http://www.impotence-center.com/clinguide.htm

The focus of these guidelines is the treatment of male erectile dysfunction. However, discussions of all medical, psychological, and behavioral aspects of libido and ejaculatory difficulties are included. The guideline document offers a mission statement, followed by topical discussions of the role of the endocrinologist in the treatment of male sexual dysfunction, types of sexual dysfunction, evaluation of sexual dysfunction, and the clinical management possibilities. Erectile physiology, aging, related erectile changes, and causes of erectile dysfunction are reviewed, and charts and figures accompany the text. Included is a listing of sexual side effects of common prescription medications.

University of Alabama: Erectile Dysfunction Clinical Resources ◉ ◉ ◉
http://www.slis.ua.edu/cdlp/unthsc/clinical/urology/infertility/erectiledysfunction.htm

Clinical resources related to erectile dysfunction are directly accessible from this site of the University of Alabama's Clinical Digital Libraries Project. Several fee-based and free online textbook chapters are available, such as Harrison's Online and the *Merck Manual*. Practitioner guidelines from the American Urological Association, the American Association of Clinical Endocrinologists, MD Consult, and the National Guideline Clearinghouse are also available, providing a review of organic erectile dysfunction, evaluation, and treatment. A listing of miscellaneous resources is found from both Yahoo! and Health Reviews for Primary Care Providers.

22.3 Gynecomastia

American Academy of Family Physicians: Gynecomastia: When Breasts Form in Males ◉ ◉
http://familydoctor.org/handouts/080.html

This consumer-oriented information page provides several paragraphs that review the causes of gynecomastia; laboratory tests needed to diagnose the cause; and treatment details where tenderness, tumors or other diseases, or specific medications are involved.

Pediatric Bulletin: Gynecomastia ◐ ◐

http://home.coqui.net/myrna/gyne.htm

Breast tissue development in males is divided into four types, including pubertal or benign adolescent breast hypertrophy, type II physiological gynecomastia, type III general obesity and type IV pectoral muscle hypertrophy. Idiopathic, familial, and specific diseases causing type II gynecomastia are outlined.

22.4 Infertility

Columbia University College of Physicians and Surgeons: Male Infertility ◐ ◐

http://cpmcnet.columbia.edu/texts/guide/hmg10_0007.html

The "*Health Concerns of Men*" chapter of the Columbia University College of Physicians and Surgeons *Complete Home Medical Guide* offers a discussion of the three major categories of male infertility, causes, diagnosis by semen analysis, and treatment of the underlying cause. The often treatable conditions reviewed at the site include failure to deliver sperm, buildup of sperm antibodies by either the man or woman, undescended testicles, and sperm immobility.

IVF.com: Male Infertility Overview: Assessment, Diagnosis, and Treatment ◐ ◐ ◐

http://www.ivf.com/shaban.html

As its title implies, IVF.com's Web site offers information on the management of male factor infertility, with details provided on myotonic dystrophy, bilateral anorchia, Sertoli-cell-only syndrome, and other causes of male infertility. By beginning at this address, visitors are led through several pages describing male reproductive physiology, various conditions, and additional review of diagnosis and treatment.

Lycos: Health with WebMD: Finding the Cause ◐ ◐ ◐

http://webmd.lycos.com/content/dmk/dmk_summary_account_1499

WebMD provides background information on male infertility, with an overview, treatment and diagnosis details, complementary therapies, and self-care summary. In addition, users may access several related articles of interest in each category directly from the site, including an illustrated anatomy article, an overview of the male reproductive system, and an inclusive report from *FDA Consumer* on overcoming infertility. Articles regarding etiology and treatment are available as a service of the *Fertility Sourcebook,* and more technically oriented material from the *British Medical Journal* and *Patient Care* for investigating and managing infertile patients is found.

22.5 Male Gonadal Disorders

Cryptorchidism

University of Louisville Pediatric Urology: Cryptorchidism
http://louisvillesurgery.com/urology/crypto.htm

This clinical review of cryptorchidism, otherwise known as undescended testes, includes details regarding the incidence, etiology, and pathophysiology of the condition. Diagnosis, associated conditions, and treatment options are reviewed. Images are accessible throughout the text.

Uro.com: Undescended Testicle
http://www.uro.com/undesc.htm

Provided by the Virginia Urology Center, this fact sheet offers viewers a discussion of the undescended testicle, with diagnostic information, treatment details, and possible complications associated with surgical, therapeutic intervention.

Primary Hypogonadism: General Resources

American Association of Clinical Endocrinologists (AACE): Clinical Practice Guidelines for the Evaluation and Treatment of Hypogonadism in Adult Male Patients
http://www.aace.com/clin/guides/hypogonadism.html

This practice guideline, developed by the AACE and the American College of Endocrinology, provides specific recommendations regarding the diagnosis and management of hypoganadism, with several target populations mentioned. Prepubertal and postpubertal general manifestations with either testosterone deficiency or loss of testicular function are outlined, and significant details of the history and physical examination are reviewed. Testosterone level and gonadotropin determinations, dynamic tests, and other studies, such as bone densitometry, are discussed. Specific syndromes of hypergonadotropic hypoganadism and hypogonadotropic hypogonadism are addressed, and therapeutic goals are presented.

Family Practice Notebook.com: Hypogonadism
http://www.fpnotebook.com/URO2.htm

Primary and secondary causes of hypogonadism are outlined at the site, with signs and symptoms specific to prepubertal and postpubertal onset listed. Laboratory findings, testosterone therapy, and links to related sites within the online *Family Practice Notebook* are found.

Merck Manual of Diagnosis and Therapy: Male Hypoganadism ◉ ◉ ◉
http://www.merck.com/pubs/mmanual/section19/chapter269/269g.htm

Classifications of hypogonadism, symptoms and signs (dictated by age of onset), and laboratory measurements of serum testosterone, leutinizing hormone, and follicle-stimulating hormone are discussed. Other testing procedures, treatment directed at correction of the underlying disorder, if applicable, and testosterone replacement therapy are reviewed.

Primary Hypogonadism: Adult Leydig Cell Failure

Wellman Clinic: Hypogonadism ◉ ◉
http://www.weymouthclinic.co.uk/wellman/paper2.html

Testosterone production and hypogonadism are discussed in this informative fact sheet. The article discusses the production of testosterone by the testes and adrenal glands, testosterone circulation, and reduction of testosterone levels with age. Physiological changes associated with testosterone deficiency are listed, including both symptomatic and biological alterations. The article also presents a discussion of the ongoing development of a biochemical definition of hypotestosteronaemia.

Secondary Hypogonadism: Kallman Syndrome

Online Mendelian Inheritance in Man (OMIM): Kallman Syndrome ◉ ◉ ◉
http://www3.ncbi.nlm.nih.gov/htbin-post/Omim/dispmim?308700

Alternative disease titles, a clinical synopsis link, and connections to related databases, such as LocusLink, are found at this site of the OMIM database. Case examples, extensive literature review, and extensive MEDLINE citation links are found throughout the entry. Seven selected examples of allelic variants may be viewed.

University of Utah: Kallman's Syndrome ◉ ◉
http://medstat.med.utah.edu/kw/human_reprod/seminars/seminar1B2.html

The University of Utah offers this seminar chapter on sexual differentiation, explaining this mechanism of gonadotropin deficiency. A graphic representation is enlargeable at the site, and results of this disorder of sexual differentiation are outlined.

22.6 Prostate Disorders

General Resources

American Prostate Society ⊙ ⊙
http://www.ameripros.org

The American Prostate Society seeks to reduce suffering and death from prostate diseases, with overviews of prostate cancer, prostate enlargement, and prostatitis. Prostate cancer review includes diagnostic and staging information; and articles on second and third opinions, spousal and familial relationships, and prevention are offered. Answers to frequently asked questions, professional article abstracts, and access to archived and current newsletters are provided.

Prostate Health ⊙ ⊙ ⊙
http://www.prostatehealth.com

Maintained by a board of academic urologists, private practice urologists, radiologists, and primary care physicians, the Prostate Health Web site provides comprehensive information regarding disorders of the prostate. Prostate anatomy and physiology; an index of articles, reports, and multimedia presentations on prostate-related topics; an interactive symptom index information on early cancer detection; and details regarding symptoms, tests, and treatments for prostatitis are presented.

Benign Prostatic Hyperplasia (BPH)

APIMALL Health Channel: BPH Disease Management ⊙ ⊙
http://apinet.site.yahoo.net/apinet/benproshyp.html

Contemporary management of benign prostatic hyperplasia in North America and Europe, considering the increase in an aging population and healthcare expectations, is reviewed at this site. Accepted first-line pharmacotherapy in North America and basic management protocol of practicing physicians are outlined. Differences in practice across Europe, although not objectively analyzed, occur, with sales of various therapies markedly variable between different countries and a decline in the prostatectomy rate in certain nations noted. Brief reviews of medical treatment trends in Germany, Italy, the United Kingdom, and France are found.

MDMultimedia: Prostatic Hyperplasia, Benign ⊙ ⊙
http://www.mdmultimedia.com/a/griffith/gr736.htm

A description of benign prostatic hyperplasia is offered at this address, accompanied by a lengthy list of signs and symptoms. Possible causes, differential diagnosis information, laboratory tests, pathological findings, and diagnostic procedures are outlined. In addition, visitors will find general and surgical treatment measures, drugs of choice, patient monitoring details, and possible complications listed. The symptom index for BPH, adapted from the American Urological Association, is found.

Merck Manual of Diagnosis and Therapy: Benign Prostatic Hyperplasia ○ ○

http://www.merck.com/pubs/mmanual/section17/chapter218/218a.htm

The pathophysiology and symptomatology of benign prostatic hyperplasia is discussed at this chapter of the online *Merck Manual of Diagnosis and Therapy*. Links are found to additional chapters on urinary stasis and calculus formation, a table outlining the American Urological Association Symptom Score, and information on prostate cancer.

University of Alabama: Benign Prostatic Hyperplasia ○ ○ ○ (some features fee-based)

http://www.slis.ua.edu/cdlp/unthsc/clinical/urology/prostate/bph.htm

Clinical resources pertaining to benign prostatic hyperplasia are found at this site of the Clinical Digital Libraries Project of the University of Alabama. An assortment of textbook entries, pathology images, and clinical guidelines regarding diagnosis and therapeutics for BPH are found at this site, including the full clinical guidelines of the Agency for Healthcare Research and Quality (formerly the Agency for Health Care Policy and Research). Although free reference material is provided, some links may require a user subscription.

Prostate Cancer

Association for the Cure of Cancer of the Prostate (CURE) ○ ○

http://www.capcure.org

CaPCURE is an association dedicated to the cure of cancer of the prostate, with current headlines related to the disorder accessible. Upcoming events, disease discussions, and recent clinical trials are reviewed. Statistical information and an article on living with prostate cancer are found, in addition to reference to additional publications.

Canadian Prostate Cancer Research Foundation (CPCRF) ○ ○

http://www.prostatecancer.on.ca

A Canadian organization solely devoted to eliminating prostate cancer, the CPCRF is committed to raising funds for research into the cause, cure, and prevention of the disease. The site offers related news releases, scientific and funding information, and details related to upcoming events and campaigns.

Doctor's Guide: Prostate Cancer Information and Resources ◎ ◎
http://www.pslgroup.com/PROSTCANCER.HTM

From the Doctor's Guide to the Internet, Prostate Cancer Information and Resources, the site provides links to prostate cancer news and alerts, prostate cancer information, discussion groups, and other related sites.

Education Center for Prostate Cancer Patients ◎ ◎
http://www.ecpcp.org

The ECPCP was organized to improve the quality of life for patients through education, counseling, and research. Information about the ECPCP and articles on diagnosis and treatment options are found. There is a newsletter and information about books, publications, conferences, and contributions.

Massachusetts Prostate Cancer Research Institute ◎ ◎ ◎
http://www.cureprostatecancer.com

Provided by the Massachusetts Prostate Cancer Research Institute, this site offers a guide to the management of prostate cancer, with background information on diagnostic testing and discussions of cryosurgery, radical surgery, seed implants, x-ray therapy, and hormone therapy treatment options. The latest research, publications by members of the faculty, and journal reviews are accessible.

OncoLink: Prostate Cancer ◎ ◎ ◎
http://www.oncolink.upenn.edu/disease/prostate

The University of Pennsylvania Cancer Center provides general cancer information, an overview of prostate cancer, disease FAQs, and recommendations with regard to prostate cancer screening and diagnostics. Additional interesting connections discuss genetics, treatment options, and clinical trials, including an online trial protocol finder. Psychosocial support resources, a collection of useful news items, and special coverage of hormones and their connection to prostate cancer are offered, making this OncoLink site an all-inclusive resource for both patients and healthcare professionals.

Prostate Cancer Dot Com ◎ ◎
http://www.prostatecancer.com

Maintained by the Prostate Cancer Research and Education Foundation, this site serves as a support and educational resource. The site offers review of current research and educational goals, including lifestyle changes investigation, herbs and alternative medicine studies, cryosurgery/immunology study, prostate cancer vaccine research, photo-dynamic laser therapy study, and nutrition cancer prevention study.

Prostate Cancer Research Institute ○ ○ ○
http://www.prostate-cancer.org

The Prostate Cancer Research Institute is devoted to educational and research initiatives into the prevention and management of prostate cancer. A newsletter and a mailing list for clinical question posting are available, as are several PowerPoint presentations. Review includes high-dose ketaconazole and hydrocortisone treatment, cytoxan, estrogens, the challenge of prostate cancer, anemia of androgen deprivation, androgen independent prostate cancer, intermittent hormone blockade, staging, and bone integrity. Links to papers by noted experts in the field are offered, accompanied by data sheets, an acronym listing, and a glossary of related terms.

University of Michigan Comprehensive Cancer Center: Prostate Cancer Program ○ ○
http://www.cancer.med.umich.edu/prostcan/prostcan.html

Maintained by the University of Michigan Comprehensive Cancer Center, this site offers information about the institute's prostate cancer program, as well as connections to current journal articles related to treatment options and clinical trials. Cancer staging information, educational resources for patients and professionals, and links to information about the prostate cancer genetic project are found.

University of Wisconsin Comprehensive Cancer Center: Prostate Cancer Answers ○ ○
http://www.medsch.wisc.edu/pca

Maintained by the University of Wisconsin Comprehensive Cancer Center, this site provides information on cancer research, prevention, detection, diagnosis, and treatment. There is a section on clinical trials, new research results, and answers to frequently asked questions.

WellnessWeb: Prostate Cancer Center ○ ○ ○
http://www.wellweb.com/PROSTATE/prostate.htm

Part of the WellnessWeb, the Prostate Cancer Center provides comprehensive information about the disorder, with a detailed overview, diagnostic screening tools, a discussion regarding the screening controversy, and available disease treatments. Outcomes and prognosis with regard to impotence and incontinence are explored, and an article entitled *What's New in Prostate Cancer?* outlines the results of current research into available hormonal therapies, radiation treatment, and the recent examinations of prognosis and therapeutic side effects.

Prostatitis

General Infirmary at Leeds:
National Guideline for the Management of Prostatitis ○ ○ ○
http://www.agum.org.uk/CEG/S46_prostatitis.html

The etiology, clinical features, diagnosis, and management for both acute and chronic prostatitis are provided at this online review of MEDLINE-based references, authored by physicians of the General Infirmary at Leeds. A description of prostatic massage for treatment of the chronic disease form, investigations and interpretations of results, and recommended antibacterial regimens are discussed.

Prostatis Foundation ○ ○
http://www.prostate.org

The Prostatitis Foundation Web site offers information about the disease, including articles on symptoms, causes, treatments, prostate drainage, and diagnostics. Scientific reports and lists of clinics specializing in prostatitis are found, as well as information about current clinical studies and upcoming workshops.

Prostatitis Foundation: Prostatitis ○ ○ ○
http://prostatitis.org/index.html

Causes, symptoms, and treatments for prostatitis may be accessed at this comprehensive healthcare resource. A symptom index, scientific literature, and a listing of clinics specializing in prostatitis are, additionally, included. Details regarding NIH-sponsored clinical trials and current and previous International Workshops are offered, as is a welcome page for physicians, which reviews "The Feliciano Method," otherwise known as the Philippine cure. Dr. Feliciano's description of how to perform a prostatic drainage, clinical books, and a Stanford University study on a behavioral approach to prostatitis without drugs or surgery are found. This international resource is available for viewing in four languages.

University of Alabama:
Prostatitis Clinical Resources ○ ○ ○ (some features fee-based)
http://www.slis.ua.edu/cdlp/cchs/clinical/urology/prostate/prostatitis.htm

Clinical resources specifically for prostatitis diagnosis and treatment are found at this page of the Clinical Digital Libraries Project of the University of Alabama. Included are links to online textbooks, such as the respective *Merck Manual of Diagnosis and Therapy* chapter; organ system pathology images; government-sponsored clinical trials; and clinical practice guidelines of the National Guidelines Clearinghouse. Most connections are accessible at no charge, although one requires an online subscription to the Health Sciences Library.

22.7 Testicular Cancer

Cancerlinks ◉ ◉ ◉
http://www.cancerlinks.org/testicular.html

Part of Cancerlinks, this site provides links to sites related to testicular cancer general medical information, genetics, online testicular support groups, cell culture drug resistance, high-dose chemotherapy, and pain management. Survivors of testicular cancer tell their stories, and useful information on advocacy and legislation may be accessed. This comprehensive, searchable resource also offers journal sections, information on metastatic stages, and links to current clinical trials.

National Cancer Institute (NCI): Testicular Cancer ◉ ◉ ◉
http://www.graylab.ac.uk/cancernet/201121.html

Provided by the National Cancer Institute, this site provides patient information about testicular cancer, with a detailed disease description, staging information, and an overview of treatment alternatives. Discussion of recurrent testicular cancer is provided, as are contacts for further information.

Orchid Cancer Appeal ◉ ◉
http://www.orchid-cancer.org.uk/testicular_cancer.html

From the Orchid Cancer Appeal, this site provides information about testicular cancer. The site describes warning signs and self-examination procedures, with information about causes and prevention included.

Testicular Cancer Resource Center ◉ ◉ ◉
http://www.acor.org/diseases/TC

Hosted by the Association of Cancer Online Resources, the Testicular Cancer Resource Center offers information and support to patients. Resources include instructions for self-examination, a testicular cancer primer, a glossary of related terms, and an e-mail support group. Links to patient information, physician information, case studies, news, statistics, and personal stories are found, in addition to information on tumor markers, causes of testicular cancer, fertility overview, and chemotherapeutic intervention.

23. DEVELOPMENT AND SEXUAL DIFFERENTIATION

23.1 Genetic Syndromes of Developmental Disorders

Klinefelter's Syndrome

Adam.com: Klinefelter's Syndrome ◎ ◎
http://www.adam.com/ency/article/000382.htm
The failure of development of secondary sexual characteristics in boys and other symptoms of Klinefelter's syndrome are reviewed at this site of the adam.com encyclopedic reference. A link explaining treatment options is provided.

emedicine: Klinefelter's Syndrome ◎ ◎ ◎
http://emedicine.com/cgi-bin/foxweb.exe/showsection@d:/em/ga?book=ped&topicid=1252
Klinefelter's syndrome and its variants are reviewed at this site of the emedicine online textbook. The aberrant genotype and its major consequences are discussed, as well as variable manifestations in growth, the central nervous system, dentition, the circulatory system, and sexual characteristics. Other problems to be considered and diagnostic differentials are reviewed. Cytogenic studies, hormonal tests, imaging procedures, and histologic findings are presented.

Hospital Practice: Diagnosis and Treatment of Klinefelter Syndrome ◎ ◎ ◎
http://www.hosppract.com/issues/1999/0915/cesmyth.htm

A case presentation provides to practitioners and other interested readers an awareness of the prevalence of Klinefelter's syndrome, its most common features, and the impact that the disease has on the physical and social development of its victims. Treatment regimens, related disorders, and a figure demonstrating cases of nondisjunction in meiosis and a mosaic karyotype are found. Clinicians may earn CME credit for the presentation.

Noonan's Syndrome

Family Village: Noonan Syndrome Links ◎ ◎ ◎
http://laran.waisman.wisc.edu/fv/www/lib_noon.htm

Internet organization pages, fact sheets, and an entry from the Online Mendelian Inheritance in Man (OMIM) database are all accessible at this collection of Web links. Specific connections to the Noonan Syndrome Support Group and the Noonan Syndrome Society provide access points for diagnostic, therapeutic, research, and support-oriented information.

PEDBASE: Noonan Syndrome ◎ ◎
http://www.icondata.com/health/pedbase/files/NOONANSY.HTM

The Pediatric Database (PEDBASE) contains this entry on the epidemiology, pathogenesis, and organ malformations associated with Noonan syndrome. Clinical disease features, including endocrine manifestations; karyotyping and other investigations; management details; and a connection to the Noonan Syndrome Information and Resources site are found.

Prader-Willi Syndrome

Prader-Willi Association (UK): Genetics of Prader-Willi Syndrome ◎ ◎
http://www.pwsa-uk.demon.co.uk/genetics.htm

Information about the genetics of Prader-Willi syndrome, photographs of typical appearance, and an outline of four variants of genetic abnormality are shown, including chromosome 15 deletion, maternal disomy, chromosomal translocation, and chromosome imprinting error. This online leaflet includes methods to aid in the initial diagnosis and discussion of research done at the Clinical Genetics Unit of Birmingham Maternity Hospital.

Prader-Willi Association (USA) ○ ○ ○
http://www.pwsausa.org

Downloadable conference registration forms, answers to FAQs, and important medical alerts are available at this searchable organization Web site, dedicated to providing an international network of support and information on Prader-Willi syndrome. Genetic testing details, diagnostic criteria, and position statements on Prader-Willi syndrome are conveniently accessible. The organization publishes additional material, such as *The Gathered View* national newsletter, brochures, information kits, and a disease management textbook. A sample copy of the newsletter may be downloaded from the site.

University of Chicago: Clinical Features of Prader-Willi Syndrome ○ ○
http://genes.uchicago.edu/ucgs/special-diagnostics/PW-AS/PWfeatures.html

Clinical Laboratory Services at the University of Chicago Department of Genetics offers a list of clinical features associated with Prader-Willi syndrome for handy, professional reference. Major and minor criteria, directions for score interpretation, and comments regarding terminology use in criteria are found.

23.2 Precocious Puberty and Pubertal Delay

allHealth.com: Precocious Puberty in Boys ○
http://www1.allhealth.com/childrens/qa/0,4801,6_121328,00.html

allHealth.com offers a description of precocious puberty in boys as a response to a patient question posted at the site. The physician provides answers to the significant event of precocious puberty in boys, defines the body organs, and provides a focus of what practitioners look for in diagnosis.

American Family Physician: Disorders of Puberty ○ ○ ○
http://www.aafp.org/afp/990700ap/209.html

Published by the American Academy of Family Physicians, this online review offers practitioners a discussion of the normal processes of puberty and provides tables outlining pubertal milestones in boys and girls. An approach to the child presenting with premature or atypical puberty is depicted in table format, and assessment for delayed puberty is presented, including patient grouping according to initial assessment. Diagnostic testing approaches, a cost comparison of tests used for evaluation, and a variety of syndromes are discussed, with the goals of medical treatment and methods of accomplishment reviewed. A patient information handout on early and delayed puberty, written by the authors of this article, may be accessed from the site.

Covenant Health: Precocious Puberty in Girls
http://www.covenanthealth.com/features/health/hormonal/HORM4707.htm

The Health Information Library of Covenant Health offers this fact sheet, which outlines normal pubertal milestones, symptoms of precocious puberty, and facts about prevention.

Family Practice Notebook.com: Precocious Puberty
http://www.fpnotebook.com/END112.htm

A chapter on early puberty is offered at this family medicine resource. A definition of premature sexual development in both girls and boys, precocious puberty types and causes, and links to additional topics on abnormal sexual development are provided.

Family Practice Notebook.com: Pubertal Delay
http://www.fpnotebook.com/END111.htm

An online notebook chapter offers an outline regarding pubertal delay, with basic facts on delayed adolescence in both males and females presented. Hypogonadotropic and hypergonadotropic etiology, variants, and defects are concisely reviewed.

HealthlinkUSA: Precocious Puberty
http://healthlinkusa.com/251.html

HealthLinkUSA provides an extensive assortment of Internet links on precocious puberty at this site, including fact sheets, a question and answer page, and information regarding the prevalence of precocious puberty among girls. Prevention, acromegaly, treatment, and precocious puberty in boys are a handful of the topics discussed, with information provided by noteworthy Internet sources and organization Web sites.

Ray Williams Institute of Paediatric Endocrinology: Normal Puberty and Pubertal Disorders
http://www.rwi.nch.edu.au/endcond/endcon20.htm

Several slides accessible from this site describe normal puberty in both boys and girls, abnormalities of puberty, and basic investigations in the diagnosis of pubertal disorders. Therapeutic goals and alternatives are outlined.

Tulane University: Reproductive Endocrine Conference: Delayed Puberty
http://www.tmc.tulane.edu/departments/ob-gyn/reproendo/dpubertylect.html

An outline of the normal sequence of puberty, diagnostic workup, and classification of delayed puberty is provided at this Web page. Hypergonadotropic hypogonadism, hypogonadotropic hypogonadism, and eugonadism are introduced, along with their treatment modalities.

23.3 Sexual Differentiation

General Resources

George Washington University: Abnormal Prenatal Differentiation
http://gwu.edu/~twon/abnormal.html

Five sex chromosome disorders are defined at this site of George Washington University. The fetally androgenized female, androgen insensitivity syndrome, Turner's syndrome, and Klinefelter's syndrome are included.

Johns Hopkins Children's Center: Syndromes of Abnormal Sex Differentiation
http://www.med.jhu.edu/pedendo/intersex

Prepared by physicians at Johns Hopkins Hospital, this site offers a complete, downloadable copy of a guide to syndromes of abnormal sex differentiation. Normal sex differentiation is described in order to assist patients and other interested readers in understanding the problems of ambiguous sex differentiation. Specific syndromes are discussed and accompanied by tables outlining the aberrant development of each disorder. Endocrine, surgical, and psychological treatment modalities are presented, along with a glossary of terms and a useful listing of support groups.

Androgen Insensitivity Syndrome (Male Pseudohermaphroditism)

Androgen Insensitivity Syndrome Support Group
http://www.medhelp.org/www/ais

The Androgen Insensitivity Syndrome Support Group was founded to raise awareness of the disorder, increase availability of information to patients, and support those affected by the disorder. Information about androgen insensitivity syndrome (AIS) includes an overview of the disorder and discussions of severity, as well as information on related conditions, gonadectomy, hormone replacement therapy, and vaginal hypoplasia. An article relating to diagnosis is found, in addition to several personal stories. Links to newsletters, pages in foreign languages, and medical, psychosocial, and gender identification studies and research are provided.

Family Practice Notebook.com: Male Pseudohermaphroditism
http://www.fpnotebook.com/END105.htm

This page of Family Practice Notebook.com contains an outline of the causes and signs of male pseudohermaphroditism. True hermaphroditism and additional related topics may be accessed from the sidebar menu.

Congenital Adrenal Hyperplasia

University of Utah:
Congenital Adrenal Hyperplasia ◉ ◉ (some features fee-based)
http://medstat.med.utah.edu/kw/human_reprod/seminars/seminar1B5.html

The most common form of congenital adrenal hyperplasia, the autosomal recessive inheritance pattern, and additional enzyme defect variants are discussed at this chapter of an online seminar in sex differentiation. An enlargeable image of enzyme pathways and a password-protected photograph of clitoromegaly in congenital adrenal hyperplasia are found.

Female Pseudohermaphroditism

Family Practice Notebook.com: Female Pseudohermaphroditism ◉ ◉
http://www.fpnotebook.com/end104.htm

Family Practice Notebook.com offers a quick reference to the several causes and differential diagnosis of female pseudohermaphroditism. Related pages may be accessed directly from a convenient sidebar menu.

Hermaphroditism, General

Healthwise Knowledgebase: Hermaphroditism, True ◉ ◉ ◉
http://www.healthynetwork.com/kbase/nord/nord772.htm

Brought to viewers by the National Organization for Rare Disorders, Inc., this site contains a related disorders list and connections, a general discussion of hermaphroditism, symptoms of the condition, summary of causes, and review of standard therapies. A reference listing and Internet resources are provided.

Online Mendelian Inheritance in Man (OMIM): Hermaphroditism ◉ ◉
http://www3.ncbi.nlm.nih.gov/htbin-post/Omim/dispmim?235600

The OMIM database offers a clinical synopsis link, as well as reports of true hermaphroditism, as excerpted from the clinical literature. MEDLINE references are provided. Familial cases, mode of inheritance, and discussion of a report of genetic, cytogenic, and histologic findings in an affected family are found.

Klinefelter's Syndrome

Klinefelter Syndrome and Associates, Inc. ⊙ ⊙
http://www.genetic.org/ks
Klinefelter's Syndrome and Associates was organized in an effort to provide information and support for patients with Klinefelter's syndrome, as well as educational material for clinicians. The site provides links to articles and information about sex chromosome variations, with connections to regional news, details about upcoming conferences, and highlights from past meetings. Information about the group's newsletter and access to articles from past issues are found.

Turner Center: Klinefelter's Syndrome: An Orientation ⊙ ⊙
http://www.aaa.dk/turner/engelsk/kline.htm
An orientation to Klinefelter's syndrome, published by the National Society of Turner Contact Groups in Denmark, offers information on the causes of the disorder and a section dedicated to the chromosomal constitution of these patients. The books mentioned in the list of literature at the end of this online booklet provide referral to further information on chromosomal aberrations.

XXY Information ⊙ ⊙ ⊙
http://www.globalwebsol.com/vv/index.htm
This site offers information about Klinefelter's syndrome, with a brief disorder overview and several short discussions on treatment, sexuality and fertility, and chromosomal variations. Professional journal articles, a medical dictionary link, an online book store, and an e-mail list are offered, as well as connections to additional international sites of interest. Special connections for parents relate to behavior management, learning disabilities, and legal assistance.

Turner's Syndrome

Family Practice Notebook.com: Turner's Syndrome ⊙ ⊙
http://www.fpnotebook.com/END110.htm
The signs and symptoms of the gonadal dysgenesis of Turner's syndrome are presented at this site of the Family Practice Notebook.com. Laboratory tests and findings are briefly reviewed.

Rare Disease Clinical Trials ⊙ ⊙
http://rarediseases.info.nih.gov/ord/wwwprot/menu/dx05844.html
This site provides links to clinical trials pertaining to Turner's syndrome, including a controlled study of estrogen's effects on cognitive and social functioning in girls with Turner's syndrome. A link to a phase II randomized study of oxandrolone versus

placebo for growth-hormone-treated girls with Turner's syndrome is also offered. By clicking on a chosen study, visitors are given protocol details, including study objectives, entry criteria, and participating investigator information.

Turner's Syndrome Society of the United States ◎ ◎ ◎
http://www.turner-syndrome-us.org

The Turner's Syndrome Society of the United States exists to increase public awareness of the disease and provide information and support for patients. Information about recent and upcoming conferences is found along with a listing of local chapter information and contacts. Support features include a chat room and links to related organizations worldwide. Recent research conducted on the disorder and articles discussing early intervention for children are found.

Turner's Syndrome Society, Texas ◎ ◎
http://www.onr.com/ts-texas

This site provides definitions, synonyms, and clinical abnormalities associated with Turner's syndrome. Links to frequently asked questions, local societies and chapters, newsgroup discussions, a chat room, and associated Web sites are offered. The site also provides a link to an online medical dictionary.

University of Michigan: Turner's Syndrome: A Case Study ◎ ◎
http://www-personal.umd.umich.edu/~jcthomas/
JCTHOMAS/1997%20Case%20Studies/C.Duda.html

A case study of Turner's syndrome reviews the presentation of a typical female with the disorder, with a focus on chromosomal abnormalities and how they impact the patient with Turner's syndrome. Variation in symptoms is discussed, as is a variety of chromosomal aberrations. The likelihood of spontaneous abortion in Turner conceptions is mentioned.

University of Utah: Gonadal Dysgenesis ◎ ◎ (some features fee-based)
http://medstat.med.utah.edu/kw/human_reprod/seminars/seminar1B3.html

As part of an online seminar on sexual differentiation, this page provides a discussion of gonadal dysgenesis, characterized by Turner's syndrome. A description of problems associated with X chromosome abnormalities, mention of space-form blindness, and additional X chromosome structural abnormalities are presented. An image offered at the site is password protected.

24. BONE AND MINERAL METABOLISM

24.1 Calcium, Phosphorus, and Vitamin D

Calcium Metabolism Disorders, General

Merck Manual of Diagnosis and Therapy: Calcium Metabolism ✪ ✪ ✪
http://www.merck.com/pubs/mmanual/section2/chapter12/12d.htm
From the *Merck Manual of Diagnosis and Therapy,* this site provides extensive information on calcium metabolism, with sections on the normal regulation of calcium metabolism, hypocalcemia, and hypercalcemia. For each disorder, there is a discussion of etiology and pathogenesis, symptoms, diagnosis, and treatment. Specific drugs are discussed in detail.

Hypercalcemia

Hypercalcemia Outline ✪ ✪
http://www.outlinemed.com/demo/nephrol/6740.htm
Mechanisms of calcium regulation, symptoms of the disorder, and evaluation of underlying causes are provided in this concise Web outline. Connections to information on malignancy with bone destruction, paraneoplastic syndrome details, an outline of hyperparathyroidism, and additional links related to the evaluation, diagnosis, and treatment of hypercalcemia are presented.

MDMultimedia: Hypercalcemia Associated with Malignancy ✪ ✪
http://www.mdmultimedia.com/a/griffith/gr430.htm
Differentiation of hypercalcemia associated with malignancy from other, more treatable conditions is reviewed at this Web address. Signs and symptoms of disease,

several causes, a differential diagnosis listing, and laboratory tests are enumerated. Loop diuretics, calcitonin, glucocorticoids, and several additional pharmacotherapeutic interventions are mentioned.

National Cancer Institute: Hypercalcemia ◎ ◎ ◎
http://imsdd.meb.uni-bonn.de/cancernet/304462.html

An overview of this common, yet serious, metabolic disorder is presented at this site of the National Cancer Institute. Normal calcium homeostasis, as well as mechanisms of cancer-associated hypercalcemia, is discussed, and potentiating factors, such as immobility, hormonal therapy, and hematologic malignancy, are reviewed. The article stresses the importance of diagnosis and timely intervention and notes the possibility of withholding therapy in refractory malignancy.

University of Chicago Health Services: Hypercalcemia Annotated Bibliography ◎ ◎
http://uhs.bsd.uchicago.edu/uhs/topics/hypercal.bib.html

This Web address of a University of Chicago medical group offers reference listings for general information regarding hypercalcemia, citations to primary hyperparathyroidism literature, and links to abstracts related to miscellaneous causes of hypercalcemia. References include journal abstracts regarding the determination of disease cause, management of acute symptoms, disease complications, and other guidelines. Each bibliographic entry is followed by a brief description and rating of the material's content.

University of Illinois
Primary Care Template: Hypercalcemia ◎ ◎
http://gopher.uicomp.uic.edu/IntMedRes/template/Hyprcalc.htm

A medical definition of hypercalcemia, three pathophysiologic mechanisms for hypercalcemia, clinical manifestations of disease, and several causes of the disorder are outlined at this site of the University of Illinois College of Medicine at Peoria. Diagnostic criteria, therapeutic measures in acute and long-term management, and a reference listing are provided.

University of Texas M.D. Anderson Cancer Center:
Management of Recurrent Persistent Hyperparathyroidism ◎ ◎ ◎
http://endrcr06.mda.uth.tmc.edu/management/default.html

A discussion of hyperparathyroidism, characterized by the presence of hypercalcemia, is found at this article, with issues surrounding surgical management, a table outlining the conditions associated with hyperparathyroidism, and successful approaches to the imaging and localization of affected parathyroid tissue included.

Hypocalcemia

emedicine: Hypocalcemia
http://www.emedicine.com/emerg/topic271.htm

A profile and clinical guideline for hypocalcemia is offered at this site of the emedicine database. An introduction provides background, pathophysiology, frequency, and mortality rates. Diagnostic review, differential links for contrast and comparison, and discussions of treatment, medication, and follow-up procedures are all provided at this condensed management review.

Hyperphosphatemia

emedicine: Hyperphosphatemia
http://www.emedicine.com/emerg/topic266.htm

This site of the online emedicine database offers background information about the role of phosphorus in the body, with coverage of disease pathophysiology, frequency, and mortality. Patient history, clinical presentation, and disease causes are reviewed, and information is provided about diagnosis, treatment, medications, and follow-up care.

Hypophosphatemia

emedicine: Hypophosphatemia
http://www.emedicine.com/emerg/topic278.htm

This medical teaching file provides background into normal phosphate levels, pathophysiology, and disease prevalence. In outline form, the site also discusses the clinical aspects of analyzing patient histories, performing physical examinations, understanding risk factors, and comprehending laboratory studies in serum phosphate and other electrolyte levels. A treatment section contains information on emergency room care and special medication tables cover drug information on adult and pediatric dosage, contraindications, and precautions. Moreover, the site deals with inpatient care, treatment complications, and appropriate patient education.

Vitamin D Metabolism Disorders

University of California San Francisco: Researchers Clone Gene Vital for Vitamin D Metabolism ○ ○
http://www.ucsf.edu/daybreak/1997/11/1103_met.htm

Daybreak, a news service of the University of California San Francisco, discusses the identification of the elusive enzyme involved in vitamin D metabolism. The impact that this discovery has on vitamin D regulation research and genetic and acquired conditions that may be corrected by normalizing vitamin D metabolism are discussed.

Vitamin D Metabolism and Rickets ○ ○ ○
http://georgia.ncl.ac.uk/VitaminD/vitaminD.html

Information about vitamin D's involvement in bone growth and development, biochemical details, and descriptions of vitamin D-sensitive rickets may be accessed from the site. X-linked hypophosphatemia, familial disease, and additional links to information on vitamin D-resistant rickets are found. An entry from the Online Mendelian Inheritance in Man (OMIM) database provides complete research history, and additional research projects and sites are offered. The clinical picture in adults, inheritance models, and an online teaching file, providing a radiograph of rickets and enlarged detail, are found. An abstract collection offers headings on therapeutic research, dental problems, and disease presentation.

24.2 Bone Mineralization Disorders

Osteomalacia

MDMultimedia: Osteomalacia and Rickets ○ ○
http://www.mdmultimedia.com/a/griffith/gr636.htm

Signs and symptoms, a wide range of causes, differential diagnosis, and pathological findings are reviewed in this Web outline. Treatment of osteomalacia, dependent upon the cause; medications; and other management details are presented.

University of Washington: Osteomalacia ○ ○
http://courses.washington.edu/bonephys/opmal.html

Discussion of the causes of osteomalacia is found at this subsite of the University of Washington Department of Medicine. The clinical diagnosis of rickets, hereditary disease causes, and information on lack of proper bone mineralization are reviewed. A table outlines the causes of osteomalacia, in addition to some of the associated biochemical abnormalities. Bone biopsy photographs show the appearance of normal bone tissue, osteomalacia, and disease specifically caused by vitamin D deficiency. An

X-ray of rickets and a connection to a site about hereditary hypophosphatemia are found.

Paget's Disease of the Bone

Methodist Health Care System: Paget's Disease of the Bone ○ ○
http://methodisthealth.com/bone/pagets.htm

From the Methodist Health Care System, this site provides disease information, with a definition and discussions of causes, symptoms, diagnosis, and treatment. The site provides links to other bone disorders, including fibrous dysplasia, osteogenesis imperfecta, and primary hyperparathyroidism. A listing of bone cancers and a glossary are offered.

National Institutes of Health (NIH): Paget's Disease of Bone ○ ○ ○
http://www.osteo.org/paget.html

From the National Institutes of Health Osteoporosis and Related Bone Diseases National Resource Center, this site provides information on Paget's disease, with a fact sheet offering a definition and discussion of several related topics. Causes, prevalence, symptoms, diagnosis, hearing loss, exercise, medical treatment, and surgical treatments are addressed.

Paget Foundation ○ ○
http://www.paget.org

The Paget Foundation provides information and programs for consumers and physicians on Paget's disease and related disorders. The site sponsors patient information on Paget's disease of the bone, primary hyperparathyroidism, fibrous dysplasia, osteoporosis, and breast cancer metastatic to the bone. Professionals who join the foundation from this site are provided with the latest news on treatment and research. The site also provides a link to the National Institutes of Health Osteoporosis and Related Bone Diseases National Resource Center.

Renal Osteodystrophy

Harvard Medical School: Renal Osteodystrophy ○ ○
http://www.med.harvard.edu/JPNM/BoneTF/Case21/WriteUp21.html

A case presentation of renal osteodystrophy is found at this site, with blood chemistries, findings, and a review of the clinical presentation. Access to the patient's bone scintigram and radiographs is provided, as well as discussion of the major mechanisms of etiology.

Virtual Children's Hospital: Renal Osteodystrophy ◐ ◐

http://www.vh.org/Providers/TeachingFiles/PAP/MSDiseases/RenalOsteodys.html

The Virtual Children's Hospital provides a discussion of the etiology of renal osteodystrophy as a result of chronic renal disease. Radiographic changes of both rickets and secondary hyperparathyroidism are summarized.

Rickets

Rickets: A General Overview ◐ ◐

http://georgia.ncl.ac.uk/VitaminD/ricketsOV.html

Alternative names; causes, incidence, and risk factors; prevention details; and a symptom review are all provided at this online presentation. Musculoskeletal examination and other signs and tests are discussed, as well as treatment goals, expectations, and complications of vitamin D deficiency and rickets.

24.3 Skeletal Dysplasias

Adam.com: McCune-Albright Syndrome ◐ ◐

http://www.adam.com/ency/article/001217.htm

Adam.com provides a concise, yet comprehensive overview of the causes, incidence, and risk factors associated with McCune-Albright syndrome. Answers to questions regarding the long-term prognosis of fibrous dysplasia, precocious puberty, and further details on symptoms, treatment, and prevention are found, as well as complications, alternative disease names, and links to related information.

Family Village: McCune-Albright Syndrome ◐ ◐ ◐

http://laran.waisman.wisc.edu/fv/www/lib_mcas.htm

A collection of links at this page offers visitors general disease reviews, as well as support group Web links, related online chats, and clinical information connections of the Online Mendelian Inheritance in Man (OMIM) database and PedBase.

Greenberg Center for Skeletal Dysplasias ◐ ◐ ◐

http://www.med.jhu.edu/Greenberg.Center/Greenbrg.htm

Located at the Johns Hopkins Hospital Center for Medical Genetics, the Greenberg Center for Skeletal Dysplasias provides a tutorial on genetics that includes reviews of the evaluation and diagnosis of an individual with short stature, in addition to genetics and various modes of inheritance. Clinical summaries of achondroplasia, hypochondroplasia, pseudoachondroplasia, cartilage hair hypoplasia, chondroectodermal dysplasia, and other conditions are found. The site also provides links to articles of interest and related references.

Multiple Epiphyseal Dysplasia Support Page ◐ ◐
http://www.geocities.com/Athens/Ithaca/7000/en_english/index.html

This site offers information about multiple epiphyseal dysplasia (MED) in English, French, German, Italian, Spanish, and Portuguese. A definition of the disorder and sections on symptoms, diagnosis, and treatment are provided. A networking section offers links to organizations and individuals around the world who are working on improving treatment methodologies or who are affected by the disease. There are links to related sites and summaries of interesting, related articles.

Online Mendelian Inheritance in Man (OMIM): Achondroplasia ◐ ◐ ◐
http://www3.ncbi.nlm.nih.gov/htbin-post/Omim/dispmim?100800

Information on the most common form of short-limb dwarfism is found at this site of the OMIM database. OMIM offers visitors several pages of clinical information, patterns of inheritance, molecular genetics, diagnosis, and clinical management for the disorder, as well as a clinical synopsis page and mini review of the disorder and the related indexed literature.

24.4 Collagen Disorders

Osteogenesis Imperfecta

Osteogenesis Imperfecta Foundation ◐ ◐ ◐
http://www.oif.org

The Osteogenesis Imperfecta (OI) Foundation is a health organization created to help people manage problems resulting from the disease. For healthcare professionals, this site offers an information kit with brochure, resource lists, and relevant contact details. Information provided at the site includes a fact sheet and sections on bone densitometry, rodding surgery, and understanding the structure of bone in OI. Discussions of fracture management, genetics, hearing loss, nutrition, osteoporosis, pain management, pregnancy, and psychosocial needs of the family are presented, and a resource center offers current publications and additional educational products. Links to related law and advocacy information, a newsletter, support groups, and related organizations are accessible from the site.

24.5 Osteoporosis

Foundation for Osteoporosis Research and Education ◉ ◉ ◉
http://www.fore.org

The Foundation for Osteoporosis Research and Education seeks to prevent osteoporosis through research and education. Their site provides information about the foundation, a calendar of events, and information about the disorder, including a section on prevention, optimal calcium intake guidelines, and answers to frequently asked questions. The site offers details regarding osteoporosis risk assessment and bone mineral density testing dates and locations. Links are also found to publications, newsletters, and press releases.

International Bone and Mineral Society ◉ ◉
http://www.ibmsonline.org

The International Bone and Mineral Society promotes basic and clinical research of the skeleton and mineral metabolism. Information provided at the site includes a society history, current news items, awards, and affiliated societies.

International Osteoporosis Foundation ◉ ◉
http://www.osteofound.org

The International Osteoporosis Foundation supports national societies to coordinate their efforts and maximize their efficiency. Their site provides information about their mission, as well as disease review, including descriptions of symptoms, risk factors, prevention, and member societies. Special projects, meetings, and press releases may also be found at this searchable site.

National Institutes of Health (NIH): Osteoporosis and Related Bone Diseases/National Resource Center ◉ ◉ ◉
http://www.osteo.org

Part of the National Institutes of Health, the Osteoporosis and Related Bone Diseases National Resource Center provides information to patients, professionals, and the general public. Bone health information at the site includes sections on osteoporosis, Paget's disease, osteogenesis imperfecta, and related disorders. This searchable site also provides access to newsletters, bibliographies, and related Web pages.

National Osteoporosis Foundation ◉ ◉ ◉
http://www.nof.org

The National Osteoporosis Foundation features informative books for consumers and physicians at their Web site. News at the site includes statistics and press releases, reports on current research, legislative news, and patient news and information. Information about the disorder includes disease facts and sections on bone health, bone density, and men and osteoporosis. Information for professionals includes clinical guidelines, research grants, professional partners networks, clinical symposia, and legislation. There is information on prevention, including discussions of risk factors, calcium, exercise, and medications. Patient information connections include medication fact sheets, links to support groups, patient news, regional offices, and tips on preventing falls.

Osteoporosis Medical News and Alerts ◎ ◎
http://www.pslgroup.com/OSTEOPOROSIS.HTM

Medical news and alerts at this page are continuously updated and include current review of the latest in osteoporosis treatment information. Article links include calcium supplementation, testosterone therapy for men, bisphosphonates, hormone replacement therapy, and the relation of corticosteroid treatment and osteoporosis risk. Treatments on the horizon, such as parathyroid hormone, and further developments in management are retrievable. The Pharmacists Caring for Osteoporosis link and a multitude of additional connections related to disease management are provided.

24.6 Parathyroid Gland

General Resources

University of Alabama:
Parathyroid Diseases Clinical Resources ◎ ◎ ◎ (some features fee-based)
http://www.slis.ua.edu/cdlp/WebDLCore/clinical/endocrinology/parathyroid/index.htm

Provided as a service of the Clinical Digital Libraries Project, this site offers access to parathyroid disease clinical resources by subtopic, as well as clinical resources related to parathyroid evaluation and diagnosis. By connecting to any chosen subtopic, visitors gain access to an extensive collection of authoritative textbook chapters, pathology resources, news, clinical guidelines, and trials related to the particular disease or management method. Patients and families will find a related consumer-oriented listing of sites. Some textbook chapters require a user subscription, although most resources are free of charge.

Your Parathyroid.com ◎ ◎
http://www.parathyroid.com

Every aspect of parathyroid function and disease is summarized at this parathyroid information source. By clicking on any of the parathyroid topic pages, visitors will be led to further text on parathyroid adenomas, hyperplasia, symptoms, osteoporosis, calcium metabolism, and diagnostic testing procedures. Parathyroid surgical techniques, parathyroid cancer, and related subjects are offered within the more than 70 Web pages and 65 detailed illustrations. By clicking on the disorder and treatment button, visitors will find a listing of 10 topical links to get started with their searches.

Hyperparathyroidism: General

American Academy of Family Physicians: Hyperparathyroidism ❂ ❂ ❂
http://www.aafp.org/afp/980415ap/allerhei.html

From *American Family Physician,* this site offers an informative article on hyperparathyroidism. Sections of the article include pathophysiology, diagnosis, differential diagnosis, effects of hyperparathyroidism on body systems, asymptomatic effects, nonsurgical management, surgical management, and recommendations of the National Institutes of Health. Diagrams and illustrations are included, and a link to a patient information handout on the disorder is provided.

Baylor College of Medicine
Grand Rounds Archive: Primary Hyperparathyroidism ❂ ❂ ❂
http://www.bcm.tmc.edu/oto/grand/12094.html

Hyperparathyroidism (HPT), its various presentations, historical information with regard to the glands' discovery, and distinctions between primary, secondary, and tertiary HPT are offered. Methods for discovery of the underlying pathology are discussed, and details surrounding the debates as to the disorder's true etiology are found. Treatment alternatives and questions as to preoperative localization are introduced, and varying schools of thought regarding surgical approaches are summarized, with the advantages of each considered. Convenient treatment algorithms following surgery are provided, and surgical pitfalls that may interfere with appropriate intervention are examined.

National Institutes of Health (NIH): Diagnosis and
Management of Asymptomatic Primary Hyperparathyroidism ❂ ❂ ❂
http://text.nlm.nih.gov/nih/cdc/www/82txt.html

The full text of a consensus panel statement regarding hyperparathyroidism management is provided at this site, as a service of the NIH. Established are definitive diagnostic criteria, current and appropriate management, and the conclusion that not all cases of hyperparathyroidism warrant surgical intervention. A discussion regarding the most cost-efficient and accurate methods of diagnosis, demonstrated by persistently elevated levels of serum calcium and parathyroid hormone (PTH) is presented. Elaboration on the monitoring of asymptomatic individuals, detected incidentally, is provided, offering both nonsurgical and surgical alternatives. Additionally, monitoring procedures and lifestyle recommendations are examined. Gland localization imaging technologies and information on further research regarding the effects of asymptomatic hyperparathyroidism are included.

NIDDK: Hyperparathyroidism ◐ ◐
http://www.niddk.nih.gov/health/endo/pubs/hyper/hyper.htm

Hyperparathyroidism, its symptoms, and diagnosis are reviewed at this informational brochure, as a service of the NIDDK. A sketch of the glands' location is provided, and their distinct hormones and function, the calcium-phosphorus balance, rare familial causes, and diagnosis through serum hormone and calcium level measurements are explained.

Hyperparathyroidism: Adenoma

Harvard Medical School: Hyperparathyroidism: Clinical Case ◐ ◐
http://www.med.harvard.edu/JPNM/TF93_94/May3/CaseMay3.html

A case example of hypercalcemia caused by a localized parathyroid adenoma is reviewed at this site, with a diagnostic description and online image demonstrating diseased tissue in the right lower pole of the right thyroid lobe. By accessing the full case report, a discussion regarding improvement of parathyroid scintigraphy is found.

Hyperparathyroidism: Carcinoma

National Cancer Institute (NCI): Parathyroid Cancer ◐ ◐
http://www.medhelp.org/lib/cancernet/200541.HTM

The article found at this site, courtesy of the National Cancer Institute, examines cancerous conditions of the parathyroid glands, with localized, metastatic, and recurrent disease stages defined. Surgery, radiation, and chemotherapeutic treatment, according to cancer stage, are reviewed, and sources of further reading and information are offered.

OncoLink: Parathyroid Cancers ◐ ◐ ◐
http://cancer.med.upenn.edu/disease/parathyroid

Information from the National Cancer Institute (NCI) on parathyroid cancers includes monthly CancerLit citations regarding new trials, treatments, and current research. OncoLink's physician and patient information statements on parathyroid cancer are available from the site and review general information, cellular classifications and staging, treatment option overviews, and localized, metastatic, and recurrent carcinoma management. The "OncoLink Protocol Finder" database offers a search engine for finding open clinical trials available through the University of Pennsylvania and other cooperative oncology groups.

Hypoparathyroidism

EndocrineWeb: Hypoparathyroidism: Too Little Parathyroid Hormone Production ◎ ◎
http://www.endocrineweb.com/hypopara.html

EndocrineWeb.com presents a colorful brochure at the site, reviewing insufficient parathyroid hormone (PTH). Three disease categories, their etiologies, and treatment with vitamin D and calcium supplementation are discussed. Congenital, idiopathic, and postsurgical causes of deficient parathyroid secretion are defined, as well as secretion of biologically inactive hormone and the rare occurrence of parathyroid hormone resistance (pseudo-hypoparathyroidism).

Pseudohypoparathyroidism

Nephrogenic Diabetes Insipidus Foundation: Pseudohypoparathyroidism ◎
http://www.ndif.org/Terms/pseudohypoparathyroidism.html

Pseudohypoparathyroidism is described at this entry of the Nephrogenic Diabetes Insipidus Foundation. The major disease cause and characteristic findings are briefly reviewed.

Wheeless' Textbook of Orthopedics: Pseudohypoparathyroidism ◎ ◎
http://www.medmedia.com/05/311.htm

The lack of responsiveness to parathyroid hormone, a clinical picture resembling hypoparathyroidism, and other characteristics of the disorder are reviewed. Links are found to more details about hypoparathyroidism, the actions of parathyroid hormone, and the hypocalcemia and hyperphosphatemia that often result.

24.7 Growth and Stature

General Resources

Family Village: Growth Disorders ◎ ◎ ◎
http://www.familyvillage.wisc.edu/lib_grow.htm

This Family Village resource page offers several references to specific growth disorder Web sites, including those on Russel-Silver syndrome, adrenal hyperplasia, McCune-Albright syndrome, and Turner syndrome. Sites specific to pituitary dwarfism and the above-mentioned diseases as well as listings that include such organizations as the

MAGIC Foundation for Children's Growth may be accessed. Two Internet mailing lists, courtesy of the Human Growth Foundation, are offered. Major association missions and aims are described.

Human Growth Foundation: Growth and Growth-Related Disorders ◉ ◉
http://www.hgfound.org/disordersframe.html

This fact sheet, accompanied by a sidebar table of contents, outlines eight growth disorders as well as growth-related diseases caused by poor nutrition, systemic diseases, or bone disorders. Deficiency of human growth hormone, intrauterine growth retardation, and several other conditions are described. The home page of the foundation, accessible from this site, provides an index containing access to growth hormone treatment, Internet support listings, studies and clinical trials, and publication links.

Major Aspects of Growth In Children (MAGIC) Foundation for Children's Growth: Underlying Conditions of Growth Abnormalities ◉ ◉ (some features fee-based)
http://www.magicfoundation.org/default.htm

Underlying conditions of growth abnormalities are the focus of the MAGIC foundation, with information provided at its site regarding hereditary, hormonal, nutritional, and psychosocial causes of poor growth. Causes of excessive or rapid growth are discussed, and links to disease and informational brochures, fundraisers, and convention details are provided. The *MAGIC Touch* and *MAGIC Star* quarterly newsletters are available online to members, and a networking system for families affected by growth disorders is offered.

MEDLINEPlus Health Information: Growth Disorders ◉ ◉ ◉
http://medlineplus.nlm.nih.gov/medlineplus/growthdisorders.html

MEDLINEPlus offers an assortment of government and other resources by category at this site, including general overviews, clinical trials, symptoms, organizations, specific conditions, and treatment considerations of growth disorders. Access to the respective National Institutes of Health research division; government and industry-sponsored clinical trials on achondroplasia and growth hormone deficiencies and abnormalities; a growth chart, courtesy of the Turner's Syndrome Society of the United States; and a link to the Growth Hormone Forum of MedicineNet are found.

Short Stature: General

American Academy of Pediatrics: Causes of Growth Retardation
http://www.aap.org/policy/re9701t1.htm

Intrinsic short stature due to genetic or intrauterine growth retardation, constitutional delay in growth, and systemic disorders causing short stature are outlined at this American Academy of Pediatrics Web site.

Endocrine Society: Endocrinology and Short Stature
http://www.endo-society.org/pubaffai/factshee/shrtstat.htm

An Endocrine Society fact sheet offers visitors the opportunity to learn more about this descriptive and statistical term, with a discussion of the influences of stature, medical conditions causing short stature, and other variations in normal growth. The role of basic and clinical research in endocrinology, in order to better understand the mechanisms of underlying growth abnormalities, is outlined.

Genentech: Growth Failure Caused by Hormones
http://outcast.gene.com/Medicines/Endocrine/parents/growth/endodisease.html

Excess cortisol, growth hormone deficiency, and adult growth hormone deficiency are reviewed at this online fact sheet, as a service of Genentech Endocrinology. A variety of causes for each syndrome is presented.

HealthlinkUSA: Dwarfism
http://www.healthlinkusa.com/95.html

HealthlinkUSA provides four pages of connections to Web pages related to dwarfism, including achondroplasia references, prenatal diagnosis, genetic information, and answers to frequently asked questions. Clinical problems associated with dwarfism, dwarfism type listings, support organizations, and dwarfism genetic research pages can be accessed, with three pages and more than twenty informative connections in all.

Human Genome Database: Types of Dwarfism
http://www.dwarfism.org/medical/types.phtml

Information on over 800 types of dwarfism and dysplasia is provided at this database, courtesy of dwarfism.org. Visitors may select from an alphabetical listing of disorders and access the respective Online Mendelian Inheritance in Man (OMIM) entry, which includes a clinical synopsis and text with MEDLINE citation links.

Little People of America
Dwarfism Resources: Dwarfism Types and Definitions ⊙ ⊙ ⊙
http://www.lpaonline.org/resources_dwarftypes.html

This page provides a centralized resource for dwarfism types and definitions, as a service of Little People of America. The most common of over 200 estimated types of dwarfism are reviewed at the page, including achondroplasia, congenital adrenal hyperplasia, osteogenesis imperfecta, and growth hormone (GH) deficiency. Further descriptions and clinical summaries may be accessed throughout the page for each individual disorder and are provided by major teaching institutions and research foundations.

Manbir Online: Short Stature ⊙
http://www.manbir-online.com/htm3/gh.1.htm

A percentile breakdown of diseases associated with short stature is presented at this colorful site, with constitutional growth delay comprising 98% of cases of short stature. Important causes of short stature, syndromes of short stature, and tests involved in establishing a definitive diagnosis regarding the causes are listed.

Ray Williams Institute of
Paediatric Endocrinology: Growth and Disorders of Growth ⊙ ⊙
http://www.rwi.nch.edu.au/endcond/endcon33.htm

The slides available from this Web address outline disorders of growth, with details regarding prenatal and postnatal growth, the growth axis, growth hormone stimulation tests, and causes of short stature. Information on the assessment and treatment of short stature is also provided.

Short Stature: Psychosocial Dwarfism

emedicine: Child Abuse and Neglect: Psychosocial Dwarfism ⊙ ⊙ ⊙
http://emedicine.com/cgi-bin/foxweb.exe/
showsection@d:/em/ga?book=ped&topicid=566

Psychosocial dwarfism, known by a variety of other names, is reviewed at this site of the emedicine Web reference. The growth failure associated with emotional deprivation or a pathological psychosocial environment is discussed, with three distinct subtypes described. Historical factors important in making the diagnosis, significant aspects of the physical exam, and the transient growth hormone deficiency not related to inadequate nutritional intake are discussed. Diagnostic differential links may be accessed directly from the site for convenient comparison with dwarfism, growth failure, and classic growth hormone deficiency. Baseline screening for failure to thrive and additional laboratory diagnostics are outlined, as well as imaging studies and a medical care review.

Short Stature: Russell-Silver Syndrome

Family Village: Russell-Silver Syndrome ○ ○ ○
http://www.familyvillage.wisc.edu/lib_rss.htm

Family Village has compiled a useful and varied list of references at this subsite, including links to the Association for Children with Russell-Silver Syndrome, a dwarfism LISTSERV, and connections to fact sheets on the disease, courtesy of the Online Mendelian Inheritance in Man (OMIM) database.

Major Aspects of Growth In Children (MAGIC) Foundation for Children's Growth: Russell-Silver Syndrome ○ ○
http://www.magicfoundation.org/rss.html

Interesting and unsettling aspects of the syndrome, common characteristics, and rarer traits of diagnosed patients are outlined. Information for consumers interested in taking an active part in their own care is found, its a listing of potential therapies. The long-term effects of Russell-Silver syndrome and its effect on quality of life are discussed.

Tall Stature

Family Practice Notebook.com: Tall Stature ○ ○
http://www.fpnotebook.com/END19.htm

This site of the Family Practice Notebook provides a concise outline of the various causes of tall stature and the evaluation involved in diagnosis. Connections to specific conditions associated with tall stature, such as Klinefelter's syndrome and precocious puberty, are found, and further diagnostic testing procedure detail may be accessed.

Genentech: Familial Tall Stature and Causes of Abnormal Tall Stature ○
http://outcast.gene.com/Medicines/Endocrine/parents/growth/tall_stature.html

This fact sheet on familial tall stature also outlines several endocrine causes of abnormal tall stature, such as early puberty and growth hormone excess.

25. VITAMIN AND TRACE MINERAL DEFICIENCIES

25.1 General Resources

American Society for Nutritional Sciences: Nutrient Information ○ ○
http://www.nutrition.org/nutinfo

Valuable nutrient information is available through this directory, including food sources, diet recommendations, symptoms and health problems caused by deficiencies, symptoms of acute and chronic toxicity, clinical uses, and summaries of recent research. Reference citations are also listed for further reading. Forty-three nutrient topics are listed, including vitamins, minerals, trace elements, lipids, energy, and fiber.

Arbor Nutrition Guide ○ ○ ○
http://arborcom.com

By clicking on the clinical link of the Arbor Nutrition Guide visitors will be taken to a complete guide to nutritional deficiency information and nutrition-related diseases. Individual nutrients and deficiencies are found at the nutrients and vitamins/minerals link, and the nutrition assessment page offers practice guidelines and nutritional assessment tools. Nutritional assessment guidelines, research papers on nutritional status assessment, and isotopic tools for evaluating nutrition are provided. Other topical headings include surgical nutrition support, iron status disorders, and at-risk groups for disease.

Summary of Diseases Associated with Mineral/Vitamin Deficiencies ○ ○
http://www.b-c-g.com/diseases.htm

A summary of diseases associated with mineral/vitamin deficiencies are listed at this online table, which includes disorders resulting from biotin, calcium, chromium, folic acid, essential fatty acids, iron, magnesium, vitamin D and C, and a host of additional trace minerals and nutrients.

26. FLUID, ELECTROLYTE, AND ACID-BASE METABOLISM

26.1 Magnesium Metabolism Disorders

emedicine: Hypermagnesemia ○ ○ ○
http://www.emedicine.com/emerg/topic262.htm

A concise medical resource is offered by emedicine at this Web address, covering the role of magnesium in various metabolic pathways. Featured are sections regarding patient history, physical manifestations, and causes of the disease. This all-inclusive reference provides detailed review of necessary laboratory studies, treatment, medication options, and follow-up care.

emedicine: Hypomagnesemia ○ ○ ○
http://www.emedicine.com/emerg/topic274.htm

This professional health resource provides an introduction to general magnesium metabolism and disorder pathophysiology and frequency. The site includes a clinical section that provides information on interpreting patient history, examining physical manifestations, and understanding disorder causes. Sections devoted to laboratory tests, treatment procedures, medications, and follow-up care are provided.

26.2 Potassium Metabolism Disorders

Hyperkalemia

emedicine: Hyperkalemia ◉ ◉ ◉
http://www.emedicine.com/emerg/topic261.htm

This technical guide of the emedicine electronic textbook provides a short background into the disorder, along with pathophysiology, prevalence, and mortality information. The site offers a useful guide to analyzing patient history, physical signs, and causes and assists in interpreting laboratory studies, ECG tests, and cortisol and aldosterone values. A treatment section includes information on emergency room care and consultations, and a medication profiles section offers details on calcium gluconate and chloride, insulin, sodium bicarbonate, beta agonists, diuretics, and binding resins therapies. Additionally, the site deals with follow-up care, complications, prognosis, and patient education. Examples of ECG tests are posted, and a comprehensive bibliography is included.

Hypokalemia

emedicine: Hypokalemia ◉ ◉ ◉
http://www.emedicine.com/emerg/topic273.htm

This guide provides background information on potassium balance in humans and covers pathophysiology and prevalence details. In an outline form, the site includes beneficial information on patient histories, physical manifestations of the disease, and causes. A review of interpreting laboratory, imaging, and electrocardiogram tests and treatment sections dealing with prehospital care, emergency care, and consultations are found. Moreover, the site offers information on medication, follow-up care, complications, prognosis, patient education, and other special concerns. Included are an image of an ECG test and an extensive bibliography.

University of Alabama: Hypokalemia ◉ ◉ ◉ (some features fee-based)
http://www.slis.ua.edu/cdlp/uab/clinical/nephrology/electrolyte/potassium/hypokalemia.htm

Provided by the University of Alabama, this site offers an assortment of professional, clinical resources related to hypokalemia. Online textbooks, clinical guidelines, clinical trials listings, and miscellaneous resources are provided. Many materials are free, although some may require an online subscription.

26.3 Sodium and Water Metabolism Disorders

General Resources

Merck Manual of Diagnosis and Therapy: Water and Sodium Metabolism ○ ○ ○
http://www.merck.com/pubs/mmanual/section2/chapter12/12b.htm
This tutorial from the *Merck Manual of Diagnosis and Therapy* offers comprehensive information about water and sodium metabolism and disorders of water and sodium metabolism. Disorders discussed include extracellular fluid volume contraction, extracellular fluid volume expansion, hyponatremia, and hypernatremia. For each disorder, a discussion of etiology, pathology, diagnosis, and treatment is provided.

Hypernatremia

emedicine: Hypernatremia ○ ○ ○
http://www.emedicine.com/emerg/topic263.htm
This site offers an overview of hypernatremia, with background information and sections on pathophysiology, frequency, and mortality. Clinical information at the site includes discussions of patient history, physical findings, and causes. There are also sections on diagnostic workup, treatment, medication, and follow-up care.

University of Medicine and Dentistry of New Jersey (UMDNJ): Management of Hypernatremia ○ ○
http://www4.umdnj.edu/rwjcweb/hypern/index.html
This site offers clinical information about hypernatremia, discussing the etiology of several types of hypernatremia, including isovolemic hypernatremia, hypovolemic hyponatremia, and hypervolemic hypernatremia. A diagnostic approach is presented, and there is information on treatment of the three types of the disorder.

Hyponatremia

emedicine: Hyponatremia ○ ○ ○
http://www.emedicine.com/EMERG/topic275.htm
This site provides a comprehensive clinical guide to hyponatremia. An introduction offers background material, pathophysiology, frequency, and mortality figures. Clinical information includes patient history, physical manifestations, and causes. Sections on diagnosis, treatment, medication, and follow-up care are provided.

HealthCentral: Dilutional Hyponatremia ◎ ◎
http://www.healthcentral.com/peds/top/000394.cfm

From HealthCentral, this site offers information about dilutional hyponatremia, with alternative names, a definition, and a discussion of causes, incidence, and risk factors provided. Information on prevention, symptoms, tests, treatment, prognosis, and complications is introduced.

University of Alabama: Hyponatremia ◎ ◎ ◎ (some features fee-based)
http://www.slis.ua.edu/cdlp/WebDLCore/clinical/
nephrology/electrolyte/sodium/hyponatremia.htm

This site provides links to clinical resources related to hyponatremia, provided as a service of the Clinical Digital Libraries Project. Documents related to etiology, clinical features, diagnosis, clinical approach, and treatment of the disease are found, as well as clinical guidelines, drug trials, and miscellaneous clinical resources. Online textbook chapters and material specific to pediatrics are provided. Visitors will find most connections to be freely accessible, although some may require an online library subscription.

26.4 Disturbances of Acid-Base Metabolism

Metabolic Acidosis

emedicine: Metabolic Acidosis ◎ ◎ ◎
http://www.emedicine.com/EMERG/topic312.htm

This clinical teaching file includes an introduction to metabolic acidosis with background disease information, pathophysiology, and mortality figures. Clinical review includes patient history, physical findings, and causes. Sections are provided on diagnosis, treatment, medication, and follow-up care.

Metabolic Acidosis ◎ ◎
http://www.aacb.asn.au/educ/noel/bgas/tsld022.htm

This site offers a reference summary of metabolic acidosis. The site includes information about pathophysiology and diagnosis, as well as causes of various disease varieties.

Temple University School of Medicine: Metabolic Acidosis ◎ ◎ ◎
http://blue.temple.edu/~pathphys/renal/metabolic_acidosis.html

This site offers a tutorial on metabolic acidosis, with definitions, formulae, and a section on the anion gap. The site outlines the pathogenesis, secondary response, and symptoms and signs associated with acidosis. Discussions of specific syndromes, including elevated anion gap acidosis and normal anion gap acidosis, are provided.

Metabolic Alkalosis

HealthCentral: Pediatric Health Encyclopedia: Alkalosis
http://www.healthcentral.com/peds/top/001183.cfm

From HealthCentral, this site offers a profile of alkalosis, including alternative names, a definition, and a discussion of causes, incidence, and risk factors. Information about prevention, symptoms, signs and tests, treatment, prognosis, and complications is provided.

Temple University School of Medicine: Metabolic Alkalosis
http://blue.temple.edu/~pathphys/renal/metabolic_alkalosis.html

This outline of metabolic alkalosis includes a discussion of the primary process and its effects. Information about compensatory responses to metabolic alkalosis and discussions of generation versus maintenance, saline-sensitive versus saline-resistant metabolic alkalosis, and disorder diagnosis are found.

27. DIABETES MELLITUS

27.1 General Resources

Ask NOAH About: Diabetes ○ ○ ○
http://www.noah.cuny.edu/diabetes/diabetes.html

From Ask NOAH, this site offers a well-organized menu of links to diabetes-related information, with an assortment of fact sheets, clinical articles, patient information, and glossaries related to etiological factors, diagnosis, age-specific and gender-specific issues, exercise, medications, monitoring, nutrition, prevention, trials, statistics, news, and research in the field.

Centers for Disease Control and Prevention (CDC): Diabetes and Public Health Resource ○ ○
http://www.cdc.gov/nccdphp/ddt

Part of the National Center for Chronic Disease Prevention and Health Promotion, the Division of Diabetes Translation maintains this Web site. In addition to conference and program information, the site offers answers to frequently asked questions about diabetes and links to statistics, special projects, and related publications.

Medscout: Diabetes Mellitus ○ ○ ○
http://medscout.com/diseases/endocrine/diabetes/index.htm

From Medscout, this site offers links to association information, news, guidelines and consensus statements, training material, a diabetes chat, diabetes among different nationalities and other statistical information, diabetes in pregnancy, clinical trial review, current research, and treatment. Special attention to cardiac, foot, and dermatologic complications is provided, as well as discussion relating to diabetes and genetics.

On-line Diabetes Resources ◐ ◓ ◑

http://www.mendosa.com/faq.htm

This site indexes diabetes-related resources on the Internet, categorized as organizations and charities, universities, hospitals, physicians, and research. Additional topical headings include companies, publications, diabetes medications, diabetes software, blood glucose meters, and diabetic neuropathy, with brief site descriptions provided for the entries.

27.2 Type 1 Diabetes Mellitus

American Family Physician: Educational Guidelines for Achieving Tight Control and Minimizing Complications of Type 1 Diabetes ◐ ◓ ◑

http://www.aafp.org/afp/991101ap/1985.html

An article authored by a professor at the University of Maryland School of Medicine provides a clinical opinion for achieving maximum control of type 1 diabetes through regular blood glucose testing. The goals of the American Diabetes Association for glucose control are set forth, as are the onset, peak, and duration of action of various insulins. Several additional recommendations for tight blood sugar control are provided, and a related patient information handout summarizes the author's discussion.

American Family Physician: Type 1 Diabetes Mellitus and Use of Flexible Insulin Regimens ◐ ◓ ◑

http://www.aafp.org/afp/991115ap/2343.html

This article, published by the American Academy of Family Physicians, was authored by a professor of medicine in the endocrinology and nutrition division of the University of Washington School of Medicine. The text provides background information on the pharmacology of insulins, pharmacokinetic parameters and pitfalls, general recommendations regarding treatment strategies, and discussion of flexible insulin dosing regimens. Review of the landmark Diabetes Control and Complications Trial, stressing frequent self-monitoring for a successful program, is emphasized.

Insulin-Free World Foundation: General Articles ◐ ◓ ◑

http://www.insulinfree.org/articgen.htm

Provided by the Insulin-Free World Foundation, this site offers links to over 25 professionally oriented articles on type 1 diabetes, including discussions of genetics, diet, prevalence, heart disease, eye diseases, nervous system impairment, diabetic retinopathy, hypoglycemia, and mortality.

27.3 Type 2 Diabetes Mellitus

General Resources

American Academy of Family Physicians: Benefits and Risks of Controlling Blood Glucose Levels in Patients with Type 2 Diabetes Mellitus ☉ ☉ ☉
http://www.aafp.org/clinical/diabetes/allofit.html

This review of the evidence and recommendations of the American Academy of Family Physicians and the American Diabetes Association includes an executive summary on the magnitude of benefits of tight glycemic control. Methodology of the literature review is explained, and an overview of clinical trial designs is set forth. Microvascular and macrovascular outcomes, derived from observational studies and evidence from clinical trials, are summarized, and all-cause mortality and a summary of the application of these studies are found. The potential harms of intensive glycemic control are introduced, and outcomes estimates and determining the probability of benefits and harms, are reviewed and accompanied by a discussion of example mathematical models.

American Diabetes Association (ADA): Screening for Type 2 Diabetes ☉ ☉ ☉
http://journal.diabetes.org/FullText/Supplements/DiabetesCare/Supplement100/s20.htm

This *Diabetes Care* supplement offers a position statement, courtesy of the American Diabetes Association, on the early detection and prompt intervention necessary to reduce disease complications and decrease risk for serious coronary episodes. Diabetes prevalence and risk factors, symptoms, and general recommendations for screening by physicians are reviewed. Screening testing procedures, general recommendations for community screening programs, and references to other *Diabetes Care* abstracts are found.

American Family Physician: Oral Pharmacologic Management of Type 2 Diabetes ☉ ☉ ☉
http://www.aafp.org/afp/991201ap/2613.html

The American Academy of Family Physicians provides an in-depth article at this Web address, discussing the epidemiological and interventional studies regarding oral pharmacologic diabetes management. Recommendations of the American Diabetes Association, review of pharmacologic agents, and comparison of clinical effects of oral antihyperglycemic drugs are provided. Discussions on treatment initiation, oral agent combinations, and principles of blood glucose monitoring are presented. Additional information on the social and economic benefits of various treatments is reviewed based on the current literature.

Insulin-Free World Foundation: General Articles ◎ ◎
http://www.insulinfree.org/artictype2.htm

Provided by the Insulin-Free World Foundation, this site provides links to articles about type 2 diabetes that discuss glycemic control, the prevalence of type 2 diabetes among minorities, and oral medications.

Gestational Diabetes

Diabetes Care:
Position Statement: Gestational Diabetes Mellitus ◎ ◎ ◎
http://journal.diabetes.org/FullText/Supplements/DiabetesCare/Supplement100/s77.htm

The position of the American Diabetes Association regarding the management of gestational diabetes mellitus is found at this site and includes the latest approaches to detection and diagnosis, obstetric and prenatal considerations, and therapeutic strategies during pregnancy regarding monitoring and management. A table outlines long-term therapeutic considerations.

Michigan Diabetes Outreach Network:
Quick Reference Guide to Diabetes: Gestational Diabetes ◎ ◎
http://www.diabetes-midon.org/Chapters/QuickCh12.htm

A quick reference guide chapter found at this site offers testing criteria, nutritional intervention, and monitoring guidelines for gestational diabetes mellitus. Blood glucose goals, insulin administration, and facts about activity and pregnancy, breast feeding, and diabetes after delivery are provided.

University of Texas Medical Branch at Galveston (UTMB):
Gestational Diabetes Mellitus: An Update and Review ◎ ◎ ◎
http://www.pajournal.com/pajournal/cme/pa903a.htm

Continuing medical education is provided at this online series chapter, which allows readers to complete an online test for credit after reading. Pathogenesis, risk factors, screening and diagnosis, and fetal complications associated with gestational diabetes mellitus are reviewed, as well as maternal complications and medical and nonpharmacologic management. Viewers will be provided with information to assist in the identification of gestational diabetes mellitus, in addition to details on the pathophysiological defects and basic management involved.

Insulin Resistance

Dr. Gale's Web Pages on Insulin Resistance ○ ○ ○
http://people.enternet.com.au/~agale

A diagram of the action of insulin and an article on the physiological actions of insulin and insulin resistance (IR) are found at this physician's Web site, in addition to cases of type 2 diabetes diagnosis and other discussions of IR causes. Cancer and IR, publications on IR, and dietary recommendation discussions are provided. Case reports of IR, details on a Consensus Development Conference on Insulin Resistance, and a host of additional interesting resources on IR's pathophysiology and diagnosis are found.

Insulin Resistance Information ○ ○
http://commodore.perry.pps.pgh.pa.us/~odonnell/ir1.html

The Insulin Resistance Information page offers links and information related to the disorder, including symptoms, effects of high blood insulin, conditions stemming from the disorder, diagnosis, and progression of the disease. Links to related sites are offered.

27.4 Complications

General Resources

American Academy of Family Physicians: Guidelines on the Care of Diabetic Nephropathy, Retinopathy, and Foot Disease ○ ○ ○
http://www.aafp.org/afp/971115ap/zoorob.html

Strategies for facilitating patient compliance with recommended glycemic control, recommendations with regard to diabetic complications, and discussion of the use of angiotensin-converting enzyme inhibitors in diabetics with proteinuria or hypertension are reviewed at this address of the American Academy of Family Physicians. Practice parameters for nephropathy, retinopathy, and foot care are outlined, and a patient information handout on diabetes care may be accessed from the site.

Barbara Davis Center for Childhood Diabetes: Long-Term Complications of Diabetes ○ ○
http://www.uchsc.edu/misc/diabetes/chap21.html

Created by the Barbara Davis Center for Childhood Diabetes, this site contains a chapter on the long-term complications of diabetes. Links are available to information about eye problems, retinopathy, kidney disease, neuropathy, joint contractures, and birth defects. Related information about macrovascular problems, foot problems, thyroid disorders, adrenal disorders, and discovered connections between diabetes and celiac disease, skin problems, and sexual function are reviewed.

Centers for Disease Control and Prevention (CDC): Prevention and Treatment of Complications of Diabetes Mellitus ◎ ◎ ◎
http://aepo-xdv-www.epo.cdc.gov/wonder/prevguid/p0000063/p0000063.htm

The United States Department of Health and Human Services, the Centers for Disease Control and Prevention, and the National Center for Chronic Disease Prevention and Health Promotion have collaborated to bring visitors this online practice guideline regarding the prevention and treatment of complications of diabetes mellitus. Categorized by complication types and organ system, the guideline provides management review of acute glycemic complications, adverse outcomes of pregnancy, eye disease, kidney disease, cardiovascular illness, diabetic neuropathy, and foot disorders. Charts found at the site depict the natural history of diabetic nephropathy in persons with insulin-dependent diabetes as well as clinical manifestations of diabetes-related eye disease. For each section, prevention, detection, treatment, and reference information is provided.

Postgraduate Medicine: Symposium on Complications of Diabetes ◎ ◎ ◎
http://www.postgradmed.com/issues/1999/02_99/symp_int.htm

This *Postgraduate Medicine* issue is a four full-text symposium on diabetes complication management, including articles on coronary artery disease and diabetes, diabetic nephropathy, limited joint mobility, and avoiding emergencies away from home. A number of studies that validate the role of antilipemic agents in diabetic patients with coronary artery disease are provided, and additional secondary prevention measures are stressed.

Coronary Complications

British Medical Journal: Risk Factors for Coronary Artery Disease in Non-Insulin Dependent Diabetes Mellitus ◎ ◎
http://www.bmj.com/cgi/content/full/316/7134/823

This article from the *British Medical Journal* describes a United Kingdom study of risk factors for coronary artery disease in non-insulin dependent diabetes mellitus. The full article is available, including a concluding discussion of major risk factors for coronary artery disease in the general diabetic population and patients with type 2 diabetes mellitus. Acknowledgements and reference citations are listed, and data tables accompany the article.

CNN.com: Diabetes Joins List of Heart Disease Risk Factors ◎
http://207.25.71.12/HEALTH/heart/9909/02/diabetes.heart/index.html

CNN posted this article in September of 1999, introducing the decision of the American Heart Association to add diabetes to the list of controllable risk factors for heart disease and stroke. Reference to a study of the National Heart, Lung, and Blood Institute to study hyperglycemia and related risks of heart disease is found.

Dalhousie University Cardiac Prevention Research Centre (CPRC): Diabetes and Coronary Heart Disease ◎
http://www.chebucto.ns.ca/Health/CPRC/diabetes.html

Created as an educational resource for health consumers, this article offers a discussion of coronary heart disease associated with diabetes. The site presents an overview of type 1 and type 2 diabetes, coronary heart disease and other risk factors, and treatments. Information on high blood cholesterol levels, high blood pressure, smoking, nutrition, obesity, and exercise is provided through links at the site.

Postgraduate Medicine: Coronary Artery Disease and Diabetes ◎ ◎ ◎
http://www.postgradmed.com/issues/1999/02_99/bohannon.htm

Attention to secondary prevention is the focus of this *Postgraduate Medicine* article, which details the prevalence of large-vessel coronary artery disease in the diabetic population. Coronary risk factors, a table outlining the effect of diabetes on lipid values, and the benefits of antilipemic therapy are reviewed. Additional interventions and preventative measures are set forth.

Dermatologic Manifestations of Diabetes

Dermatology Online Journal: Diabetes Mellitus ◎ ◎
http://matrix.ucdavis.edu/DOJvol1num2/diabetes/dmreview.html

From *Dermatology Online Journal*, this site contains an article on skin manifestations of diabetes mellitus, with an overview and sections on cutaneous infection in diabetes mellitus, dermal manifestations of diabetes mellitus, vascular manifestations of diabetes mellitus, and other skin markers of disease. Review of diabetic neuropathy and the skin is offered.

Diabetic Foot Ulcers and Disease

Amputation Prevention Global Resource Center ◎ ◎ ◎
http://www.diabetesresource.com/html/educ.htm

Dedicated to helping prevent amputations in people with diabetes, this site provides information for healthcare professionals and patients. Training materials include guidelines for foot ulcer prevention for persons with diabetes and for healthcare professionals. Guidelines for grading wound severity in diabetic neuropathic foot ulcers, a list of audiovisual materials available for purchase, publications, and a searchable bibliography are provided.

Diabetic Foot Disease: An Interactive Guide ❂ ❂ ❂
http://www.diabetes.usyd.edu.au/foot/Main.html

Supported by a peer-reviewed grant of the Regional Diabetes Support Scheme, this site offers chapters on diabetic foot infection, neuropathic ulcers, peripheral vascular disease, Charcot's arthropathy, and painful neuropathy. Foot examination and care, illustrations, and images make this guide a useful tool for professional review or patient education.

Wound Management:
The Complexities of Wound Management in the Diabetic Foot ❂ ❂ ❂
http://www.jcn.co.uk/2_2_6.htm

Wound management in diabetic foot ulceration is reviewed at the site, with background information on this common diabetes complication and a table that distinguishes neuropathy from neuro-ischaemia found. A discussion of a case example is offered, with details of the examination and indications for referral stated. Wound management and many options for ultimate healing are set forth, as are principles that should be applied to the choice of dressings. A general discussion about impediments to wound healing in the diabetic is included.

Gastroparesis

NIDDK: Gastroparesis and Diabetes ❂ ❂
http://www.niddk.nih.gov/health/digest/pubs/gastro/gastro.htm

Created by the National Institute of Diabetes and Digestive and Kidney Diseases, this site offers a patient discussion of gastroparesis. An overview of the condition is followed by discussions of symptoms, complications, causes, diagnosis, and treatment.

Ketoacidosis

Clinical Pediatrics: Diabetic Ketoacidosis Treatment Guidelines ❂ ❂
http://www.ispad.org/clin-2.htm

These guidelines describe the treatment of diabetic ketoacidosis (DKA), representing a consensus by the International Society for Pediatric and Adolescent Diabetes (ISPAD). The article discusses the cause, definition, clinical presentation, and treatment of the condition. Treatment guidelines include considerations of fluid therapy, insulin, monitoring, and transition therapy, as well as management of possible complications.

Tables outline the monitoring of DKA treatment and clinical signs of intracerebral crisis during management. Reference citations are available.

emedicine: Diabetic Ketoacidosis ✪ ✪ ✪
http://www.emedicine.com/EMERG/topic135.htm

Diabetic ketoacidosis is described in detail through this continuing medical education article. An introduction to the disease, including demographics, is followed by a detailed clinical overview. Typical clinical history, causes, differentials, laboratory diagnostics, and treatments are listed. Detailed tables of corresponding medications include drug name, dosage information, contraindications, drug interactions, pregnancy risks, and important precautions. The article also discusses follow-up inpatient and outpatient care, possible complications, prognosis, and important patient education issues. Review questions are available, and a bibliography of references is also listed.

Georgetown University Community and Family Medicine Web Server: Diabetic Ketoacidosis ✪ ✪
http://gucfm.georgetown.edu/welchjj/netscut/endocrinology/diabetic_ketoacidosis.html

Visitors to this address will find a detailed overview of the symptoms and appropriate treatment related to diabetic ketoacidosis. Treatment topics include vascular repletion, electrolyte correction, insulin administration, monitoring, and emergency management.

Nephropathy

Diabetes Insight: Diabetes and Nephropathy ✪ ✪
http://www.diabetic.org.uk/guides/complic/nephpthy.htm

The online *Diabetes Insight* offers this page on kidney disease and diabetes, with general information regarding prevalence and additional demographic details. Three major risk factors for nephropathy and additional educational information for complication prevention are presented at this fact sheet.

NIDDK: Kidney Disease of Diabetes ✪ ✪
http://www.niddk.nih.gov/health/diabetes/pubs/kdd/kdd.htm

Maintained by the NIDDK, this site offers information about kidney disease resulting from diabetes. There are sections on the course of kidney disease, preventing and slowing kidney disease, dialysis and transplantation, management, and future research and management directions. References are provided.

University of Alabama:
Diabetic Nephropathy Clinical Resources ◎ ◎ ◎ (some features fee-based)
http://www.slis.ua.edu/cdlp/uab/clinical/
nephrology/glomerulonephritis/multisystem/diabetic.htm

The Clinical Digital Libraries Project of the University of Alabama offers a listing of online textbook chapters, clinical guidelines related to diabetic nephropathy, and additional nephropathy clinical resources. Direct access to pages of the online *Merck Manual* and the Family Practice Handbook are offered, as well as targeted PubMed searches, courtesy of Oregon Health Sciences University. Although most material is free, some services are fee based and require an online subscription. Complete consumer-oriented information is also accessible at the glomerular disease patient resource link.

Neuropathy

Centers for Disease Control and Prevention (CDC): Neuropathy ◎ ◎
http://aepo-xdv-www.epo.cdc.gov/wonder/prevguid/p0000063/body0010.htm

Background on persons with diabetes who develop neuropathy, three major types of diabetic neuropathy, and three overlapping clinical syndromes are discussed at this online fact sheet, courtesy of the Centers for Disease Control and Prevention. Complications that may occur with autonomic neuropathy are outlined in table format. Possible prevention with glycemic control is discussed, and detection with patient interview techniques, physical examination, distal temperature sensation, and other methods is reviewed. The differential diagnoses and reasons for exclusion of other possible causes of neuropathy are listed.

NIDDK: Diabetic Neuropathy ◎ ◎
http://www.niddk.nih.gov/health/diabetes/pubs/neuro/neuro.htm

This subsite of the NIDDK offers consumers information on diabetic neuropathy, with an introduction to the condition followed by discussions of incidence, causes, symptoms, major types, diagnosis, treatment, foot care, and experimental treatments. A list of organizations providing additional resources and a suggested reading list are provided.

On-line Diabetes Resources: Diabetic Neuropathy ◎ ◎
http://www.cruzio.com/~mendosa/neuro.htm

This site contains a list of more than 30 Web resources for diabetic neuropathy. For each resource, a link and review are included.

Retinopathy

American Diabetes Association (ADA): Screening for Diabetic Retinopathy ◎ ◎ ◎
http://diabetes.org/diabetescare/Supplement/s20.htm

This American Diabetes Association position statement details the natural history of diabetic retinopathy, the efficacy of laser photocoagulation surgery, and its latest stance with regard to management of patients with diabetes. A method for preventing vision loss by following a step-by-step list of guidelines is presented.

Diabetic Retinopathy Foundation ◎ ◎ ◎
http://www.retinopathy.org/index.html

The Diabetic Retinopathy Foundation supports research and awareness of diabetic retinopathy, a major cause of blindness. The site provides consumer information in such areas as eye functioning, early and advanced stages of retinopathy, treatment in all stages, and important points of prevention. Links are provided to related sites of interest, including the Juvenile Diabetes Foundation and the American Academy of Ophthalmology.

National Eye Institute: Diabetic Eye Disease ◎ ◎
http://www.nei.nih.gov/publications/diabeye.htm

From the National Eye Institute, this site provides information about diabetic eye disease, with an overview of various conditions, including diabetic retinopathy, cataract, and glaucoma. There are also discussions of incidence, risk factors, symptoms, diagnosis, treatment, prevention, and current research. A subsite, maintained by the National Eye Institute's National Eye Health Education Program, offers program materials discussing diabetic eye disease for patients and consumers. Fact sheets, brochures, public service announcements, and press releases are available, as well as information about National Diabetes Month activities.

New York Eye and Ear Infirmary: Diabetic Retinopathy Clinical Overview ◎ ◎ ◎
http://www.nyee.edu/diglib/diabetic/text/part1.htm

As a service of the Department of Ophthalmology at the New York Eye and Ear Infirmary, this site charts the effects of hyperglycemia on retinal circulation, vascular changes in the diabetic, and the three major types of retinopathy. A definition of clinically significant macular edema is illustrated, and a presentation of a fluorescein angiogram for evaluation of areas of retinal leakage or non-perfusion is found. Several other graphics at the site demonstrate laser treatment and treatment stages.

Hyperglycemia, Hyperosmolar, Nonketotic State

emedicine: Hyperosmolar Hyperglycemia Nonketotic Coma ○ ○ ○
http://www.emedicine.com/emerg/topic264.htm

The similarity between diabetic ketoacidosis and hyperosmolar hyperglycemic nonketotic coma (HHNC) is discussed, with the pathophysiology and clinical presentation of the disease presented. The cascade of metabolic changes and resulting neurological deficits are listed, with expected vital signs, skin findings, and other physical exam symptoms noted. The most frequent causes and major illnesses that may initiate the syndrome are presented, and 17 diseases that may mimic HHNC have accessible links for convenient disease comparisons. Standard laboratory studies, imaging studies, and emergency and hospital care are outlined. Insulin, electrolytes, and other drug categories are reviewed, with specific medication profiles presented.

Merck Manual of Diagnosis and Therapy: Nonketotic Hyperglycemic-Hyperosmolar Coma ○ ○
http://www.merck.com/pubs/mmanual/section2/chapter13/13d.htm

This complication of type II diabetes mellitus is discussed in terms of its symptoms, signs, and diagnosis, as well as immediate aims of treatment. Links to information on additional diabetes complications are offered.

Hypoglycemia

emedicine: Hypoglycemia ○ ○ ○
http://emedicine.com/cgi-bin/foxweb.exe/showsection@d:/em/ga?book=emerg&topicid=272

An emedicine textbook chapter offers an all-inclusive review and management guide to hypoglycemia, with symptoms, examination findings, causes, and differentials included. Visitors may access several differential links for convenient comparisons or browse the information on laboratory testing, patient care, and pharmacology. Complete glucose supplement and glucose elevating agent profiles are found.

Home Health Care Consultant: Management of Hypoglycemia in Diabetes in the Home Care Setting ○ ○ ○
http://www.mmhc.com/hhcc/articles/HHCC9911/kauloish.html

An article from a home health care publication reviews the experiences of patients treated with either insulin or sulfonylureas, with an overview of hypoglycemia, insights into its recognition, and comprehensive steps for effective prevention and management. A table outlines normal hypoglycemic counterregulation, symptoms of hypoglycemia, and medication-related considerations for avoidance. Special information on the elderly and drugs that may induce hypoglycemia are presented.

Hypoglycemia Association, Inc.
http://www.silver-bayou.com/hai/index.htm

The Hypoglycemia Association offers information and support for hypoglycemia patients, with background information on the disorder and discussions of causes, diagnosis, and treatment. By contacting the organization, users may receive a packet of information with literature lists and useful information. There are links to related sites.

Hypoglycemia Homepage Holland: Clinical Causes of Hypoglycemia
http://lightning.prohosting.com/~hypoglyc/causes.htm

A clinical definition of hypoglycemia; postprandial hypoglycemia and its causes; fasting hypoglycemia resulting from decreased gluconeogenesis, endocrine gland insufficiency, or excessive insulin; and diseases that can lead to hypoglycemia are discussed.

International Diabetes Monitor: Hypoglycemia: Think Drugs, Diabetes
http://www.medforum.nl/idm/hypoglycemia_think_drugs,_diabetes.htm

A summary and discussion of an original article entitled *Causes, Management, and Morbidity of Acute Hypoglycaemia in Adults Requiring Hospital Admission* are found at this site. The authors discuss the high incidence of neurological manifestations this patient group typically exhibits and the populations's high-risk status and generally poor prognosis. The differential diagnosis of drug-induced hypoglycemia and its associated risk factors are presented.

Ray Williams Institute of Paediatric Endocrinology: Hypoglycemia in Diabetes
http://www.rwi.nch.edu.au/apegbook/diabne58.htm#E9E58

The acute complication of hypoglycemia in diabetic patients is reviewed at the site, with value definition, neurogenic and neuroglycopenic symptoms, and symptoms of hypoglycemia in diabetic children. Recommendations for its correction and grading of hypoglycemia severity are found. Possible adverse consequences of hypoglycemia on the brain and other occurrences are outlined. Counter-regulatory responses to hypoglycemia are reviewed, including endogenous insulin secretion suppression, rapid release of counter-regulatory hormones, and stimulation of glucogenesis in prolonged hypoglycemia. Growth hormone and cortisol responses and permanent or reversible effects of adrenaline responses are enumerated.

Macrosomia

Diabetes Care:
Growth Factors and the Regulation of Fetal Growth ○ ○ ○
http://www.diabetes.org/diabetescare/supplement298/B60.htm

This illustrated supplement to *Diabetes Care* contains an overview of the proceedings of the Fourth International Workshop-Conference on Gestational Diabetes Mellitus. The usefulness of fibroblast growth factor in determining fetal development and assessing maternal pathology in pregnancies complicated by diabetes is discussed, and the contribution of both insulin and insulin growth factors and the macrosemia associated with poorly controlled diabetes are reviewed. The article is accompanied by an extensive reference listing that provides direct access to related literature abstracts.

emedicine: Infant of Diabetic Mother ○ ○ ○
http://emedicine.com/cgi-bin/foxweb.exe/
showsection@d:/em/ga?book=ped&topicid=845

Abnormal glucose control in pregnancy or gestational diabetes mellitus is reviewed, with emedicine authors discussing the multiple problems infants born to mothers with glucose intolerance face. The etiology of associated complications, including growth problems; medical history; and complete review of diagnostic studies are provided. Procedures necessary to reduce respiratory distress, hypoglycemic management, electrolyte management, and profiles of minerals for hypocalcemia treatment are presented. The concern that these infants will manifest weight problems as they age is discussed.

Organ Damage

Diabetes Mall: Organ Damage in Diabetes ○ ○
http://diabetesnet.com/orgdmg.html

The Diabetes Mall features an informative article on diabetes and organ damage. Links are provided to control tips, Internet resources, alternative therapies, complications, and information on the latest technology. Additional resources found through the site highlight current diabetes research and news, new medication information, clinical trials, and research tools for diabetics.

28. ENERGY METABOLISM

28.1 Obesity

American Obesity Association (AOA)
http://www.obesity.org

The American Obesity Association (AOA) is dedicated to education, research, and community action to treat and prevent obesity. The AOA site offers information about the group's mission and membership, facts and statistics about obesity, publications discussing health insurance and treatment for adult obesity, and contact details. Discussions of health conditions associated with obesity and an interactive Weight Wellness Profile are also available.

American Society of Bariatric Physicians (ASBP)
http://www.asbp.org

ASBP is a society comprised of professionals who specialize in the treatment of obesity. Professional resources available from the site include a summary of continuing medical education opportunities and calendar, ASBP membership details, and bariatric practice guidelines. Various statements describing bariatric medicine, obesity, and side effects of appetite suppressant medications are also available, as well as contact details for an automated referral service.

Human Obesity Gene Map
http://www.loop.com/~bkrentzman/obesity/gen-mol.biol/200obesitygenes.html

An abstract of an article related to the published results of the human obesity gene map is found at this site, with a full-text article accessible exploring human obesity genetics and links to further information in genetics and molecular biology.

Merck Manual of Diagnosis and Therapy: Obesity ◎ ◎ ◎
http://www.merck.com/pubs/mmanual/section1/chapter5/5a.htm

The epidemiology, etiology, and signs of overweight and obesity are reviewed at this text of the online *Merck* reference. Diagnosis, complications, prognosis and treatment, and details on surgical and behavioral intervention are provided. Etiological breakdown includes genetic determinants, environmental factors, and regulatory determinants, such as drugs and endocrine factors.

National Heart, Lung, and Blood Institute (NHLBI): Clinical Guidelines on the Identification, Evaluation, and Treatment of Overweight and Obesity in Adults ◎ ◎ ◎
http://whi.nih.gov/guidelines/obesity/ob_home.htm

Assessment of the obese and overweight, as well as management by reduction of excess weight and institution of measures to control accompanying risk factors, are reviewed at the summary of this guideline of the NHLBI. Weight classifications by body mass i

National Library of Medicine (NLM): Screening for Obesity ◎ ◎ ◎
http://text.nlm.nih.gov/cps/www/cps.27.html

Literature review discussing the prevalence of overweight and obesity, risk factors, and observational study data establishing a clear association between overweight and hypercholesterolemia are presented. Associated clinical risks; clinical methods for detecting obesity, including tables of desirable weights; anthropometric methods of detection; and the effectiveness of early identification and intervention are summarized. Recommendations of the American Academy of Family Physicians, the American Heart Association, the American Medical Association, and other reputable sources are presented.

North American Society for the Study of Obesity (NASSO) ◎ ◎
http://www.naaso.org

NAASO was founded to increase and disseminate knowledge related to obesity. The site provides links to press releases, news, and society announcements. A calendar of upcoming events, membership information, funding information, and position announcements are provided, as well as links to the society's online journal, a discussion group, a mailing list, and related links on obesity management.

University of Alabama: Obesity Clinical Resources ◎ ◎ ◎ (some features fee-based)
http://www.slis.ua.edu/cdlp/cchs/clinical/endocrinology/obesity.html

Clinical guidelines, including free and professional, fee-based services on obesity are accessible from this site of the Clinical Digital Libraries Project of the University of Alabama. Textbook chapters include those of the online *Merck Manual* and professional material of the American Academy of Family Physicians, the American Association of Clinical Endocrinologists, and the National Institute of Diabetes and Digestive and Kidney Diseases (NIDDK). Direct links to the National Guidelines Clearinghouse and nutritional and metabolic disease trials of ClinicalTrials.gov are provided.

University of Alabama: Obesity Patient/Family Resources ○ ○ ○
http://www.slis.ua.edu/cdlp/cchs/patientinfo/endocrinology/obesity.html

The University of Alabama's Clinical Digital Libraries Project offers this page of patient-and consumer-oriented Web links on obesity. Visitors may access the encyclopedic adam.com or OnHealth Web databases directly from the site, as well as find a chapter from the *Complete Home Medical Guide* entitled "Basics of Good Nutrition." For information on personal health management, the site offers several easy-to-understand documents regarding the effects of obesity and tools for its successful management.

28.2 Malnutrition

Drug Base: Protein-Energy Malnutrition ○ ○
http://www.drugbase.co.za/data/med_info/pem.htm

Conditions resulting from a diet with excessive nonprotein calories or severe inadequacy of both energy and nutrients are reviewed at this DrugBase Web site. The epidemiology of both marasmus and kwashiorkor, pathophysiology, diagnosis, treatment, and prognosis are succinctly reviewed.

MDMultimedia: Malnutrition, Protein-Calorie ○ ○
http://www.mdmultimedia.com/a/griffith/gr550.htm

The conditions associated with protein-calorie malnutrition and the impairment in normal physiological processes are outlined at the site, with distinctions among first, second, and third degree forms of disease. Signs and symptoms, risk factors, differential diagnosis, and laboratory tests are enumerated. Pathological findings of both marasmus and kwashiorkor, other tests and diagnostic procedures, and general treatment measures are reviewed. Follow-up as well as expected course and prognosis are presented.

29. LIPOPROTEIN AND CHOLESTEROL METABOLISM

29.1 Hyperlipidemia

General Resources

American Heart Association (AHA): Hyperlipidemia ○ ○
http://www.americanheart.org/Heart_and_Stroke_A_Z_Guide/hyp.html
From the Heart and Stroke Guide of the AHA, this site provides a patient guide to hyperlipidemia, with a listing of five families of plasma lipoproteins and discussion of various types of hyperlipidemia. Related AHA publications and access to online guides regarding specific syndromes, pharmacotherapeutics, and diets are found.

Detection and Management of Lipid Disorders in Diabetes ○ ○ ○
http://www.diabetes.org/diabetescare/Supplement/s96.htm
This *Diabetes Care* supplement offers a Consensus Statement on the epidemiology, pathophysiology, treatment, and goals of therapy of hyperlipoproteinemias in diabetes mellitus. A list of studies urgently needed to resolve important issues regarding lipid level control in patients with diabetes mellitus is provided.

Hyperlipidemia File ○ ○ ○ (fee-based)
http://www.lifestages.com/health/hyperlip.html
By downloading the files found at this site of the Center for Current Research, compiled from the National Library of Medicine database and the National Institutes of Health, visitors gain access to late-breaking research from renowned experts in the field. Discussions of current findings in lipid metabolism management, courtesy of

well-recognized research centers and institutions, include those of the Baylor Lipid Clinic and the Lipid and Arteriosclerosis Prevention Clinic at the University of Kansas Medical Center. Drug therapies, comparative studies of effectiveness and safety, non-drug management, and dietary therapies for hyperlipidemia are covered in the organized Hyperlipidemia File for a modest fee.

Hyperlipoproteinemia Classifications ◎ ◎
http://webteach.mccs.uky.edu/cls872hazard/biochem/section3.html

The Frederickson classes of hyperlipidemia type I through type V are reviewed at this article, as well as the scheme of classification based on metabolic pathways and related abnormalities. Notable hypoproteinemias, risk factors for coronary artery disease, and additional diseases causing secondary dyslipidemias are summarized.

Stanford University: Management of Common Lipid Disorders ◎ ◎ ◎
http://scrdp.stanford.edu/lipids.html

Authored by a physician at Stanford University Division of General Internal Medicine, this site offers overviews of three categories of common lipid disorders, with example patient cases and in-depth discussions. Management procedures for each are detailed, with drugs of choice, genetics, and gender-specific information provided. Screening recommendations are reviewed, and references on lipid disorder management are cited.

Terre Haute Center for Medical Education: Hyperlipoproteinemias ◎ ◎ ◎
http://www.dentistry.leeds.ac.uk/biochem/thcme/hyperlip.html

A great wealth of information on more than 15 clinical variations of hyperlipoproteinemias may be accessed from this site of the University of Leeds. By clicking on familial hypercholesterolemia, hyperlipoproteinemia types I-V, Wolman disease, or any of the other listed disease variants, visitors will be taken to the respective disorder's Online Mendelian Inheritance in Man (OMIM) entry, provided as a service of the National Library of Medicine and the National Institutes of Health. Descriptions of example cases cited from the literature, allelic variants, a clinical synopsis, and complete reference listing are accessible. Related MEDLINE citations are noted throughout the text, and several additional databases may be accessed directly from the site, including the Human Gene Nomenclature Database, LocusLink, and Coriell Cell Line Repository.

University of Alabama: Hyperlipidemia Clinical Resources ◎ ◎ ◎ (some features fee-based)
http://www.slis.ua.edu/cdlp/uab/clinical/cardiology/cardiovascular/hyperlipidemia.html

This site provides an Internet research starting point, with links to clinical resources for hyperlipidemia. Documents include relevant chapters of the *Merck Manual* and the *Family Practice Handbook,* as well as a connection to the Heart Information Network, CliniWeb professional information, and other authoritative sources. Clinical guidelines from the American Heart Association may be accessed. Several resources at the site require an online subscription.

Acquired Hyperlipidemia

Adam.com: Hyperlipidemia; Acquired ◐ ◐
http://pcs.adam.com/ency/article/000403.htm

High blood cholesterol levels secondary to other disease processes are explained at this page of the adam.com Web database. Descriptions of lipoprotein types are provided, accompanied by links to further details on lipid forms. Secondary causes of hyperlipidemia are reviewed, including disease risk factors, such as diabetes mellitus. Drug risk factors, saturated fat intake, and additional variables are listed. Information on lipoprotein analysis and therapeutic goals may be accessed.

Merck Manual of Diagnosis and Therapy: Secondary Hypertriglyceridemia ◐
http://www.merck.no/pubs/mmanual/section2/chapter15/15g.htm

The *Merck Manual of Diagnosis and Therapy* provides an overview at this Web address of secondary triglyceridemia, with an explanation regarding the disorder's appearance secondary to other disease processes. Connections to additional hyperlipidemia topics may be accessed at the page.

Familial Lecithin Cholesterol Acyltransferase Deficiency

Online Mendelian Inheritance in Man (OMIM): Lecithin: Cholesterol Acyltransferase Deficiency (LCAT Deficiency) ◐ ◐ ◐
http://www3.ncbi.nlm.nih.gov/htbin-post/Omim/dispmim?245900

This error of lipid metabolism is reviewed at the site, with noted cases and reports of clinical features. Various authors have examined families with lecithin: cholesterol acyltransferase deficiency (LCAT) and the important role which LCAT plays in lipoprotein metabolism. Selected examples of allelic variants in Italian, Japanese, German, Swedish, Norwegian, Danish, Canadian, and Dutch families are reviewed, with access to all referenced article abstracts provided.

Type I Hyperlipoproteinemia

Online Mendelian Inheritance in Man (OMIM): Hyperlipoproteinemia, Type I
http://www3.ncbi.nlm.nih.gov/htbin-post/Omim/dispmim?238600

Alternative names, a variety of related database links, and discussion of reported occurrences from the literature of type I hyperlipoproteinemia are found at this entry of the Online Mendelian Inheritance in Man (OMIM) database. Closely related MEDLINE citations may be accessed at different points throughout the text. Allelic variants and a variety of related discussions are found, including information on infants found to have lipoprotcin lipase deficiency (LPL), hemolysis in plasma of patients with LPL deficiency, antioxidant therapy, and gender differences.

Type II Hyperlipoproteinemia

Adam.com: Familial Combined Hyperlipidemia
http://www.adam.com/ency/article/000396.htm

Causes, incidence, and risk factors of this inherited hyperlipidemia are reviewed, with a symptom link, information on laboratory testing, treatment goals and therapeutics, and dietary intervention presented.

Online Mendelian Inheritance in Man (OMIM): Hyperlipoproteinemia, Type II
http://www3.ncbi.nlm.nih.gov/htbin-post/Omim/dispmim?144400

Otherwise known as familial hypercholesterolemic xanthomatosis, this disease is reviewed at this OMIM site, with features of the condition and links to related PubMed entries and literature provided.

University of Illinois: Familial Hypercholesterolemia
http://www2.uic.edu/~eburka1/phyb569ppp/index.htm

A tutorial on familial hypercholesterolemia provides background information on this autosomal dominant disease, disorder characteristics, and review of structural and functional abnormalities of the low-density lipoprotein receptor. Genetic variations and suggestions for using the presented information for treatment purposes are presented. A graphic version of this concise review is offered.

Type III Hyperlipoproteinemia

Apo E Genotype Test for Type III Hyperlipoproteinemia ○ ○
http://www.kimballgenetics.com/tests-apo_e.html

The value of apolipoprotein E (apo E) genotyping for patients at risk is discussed at this genetic testing site. Indications for definitive diagnosis, presentation of symptoms, recommended sequence of tests, and a description of testing services available are found.

Online Mendelian Inheritance in Man (OMIM): Apolipoprotein E ○ ○ ○
http://www3.ncbi.nlm.nih.gov/htbin-post/Omim/dispmim?107741

Hyperlipoproteinemia III, known by several alternative titles, is reviewed in depth at this Online Mendelian Inheritance in Man (OMIM) database entry. A description, including early delineation, the molecular basis of polymorphism, and the role of dyslipidemias in cardiovascular disease, Alzheimer's disease, and in other progressive neurological disorders, is presented. Genetic mapping, allele distribution worldwide, and selected examples of allelic variants are presented, with closely related journal citations accessible throughout the discussion. Interested visitors are provided convenient access to the nomenclature, LocusLink, genome, and additional database links.

Type IV Hyperlipoproteinemia

Merck Manual of Diagnosis and Therapy: Type IV Hyperlipoproteinemia ○ ○
http://www.merck.no/pubs/mmanual/section2/chapter15/15e.htm

This common disorder is reviewed at this chapter of the *Merck* online reference. Information found includes symptoms, signs and diagnosis, prognosis, and treatment. The association of this lipidemia with insulin resistance and obesity and suggestions regarding weight reduction and limitation of alcohol consumption are made.

Online Mendelian Inheritance in Man (OMIM): Hyperlipoproteinemia, Type IV: Carbohydrate hyperlipidemia ○ ○ ○
http://www3.ncbi.nlm.nih.gov/htbin-post/Omim/dispmim?144600

A discussion of persistently elevated plasma triglycerides and its clinical manifestations is presented at this Online Mendelian Inheritance in Man (OMIM) entry. Contributing environmental factors, additional conditions causing hyperlipoproteinemia IV, and individual cases of the hyperlipoproteinemia IV phenotype are summarized. Related journal abstracts referencing the association of rheumatic manifestations, glycogen storage disease I, and other conditions are accessible, in addition to a clinical synopsis entry.

Type V Hyperlipoproteinemia

Merck Manual of Diagnosis and Therapy: Type V Hyperlipoproteinemia ⊙ ⊙
http://www.merck.no/pubs/mmanual/section2/chapter15/15f.htm

The appearance of eruptive xanthomas, lipemia retinalis, and additional telltale symptoms of this rather uncommon lipidemia are reviewed at this *Merck* publication chapter. Additional signs, concern over pancreatitis, and recommendations with regard to weight reduction and additional therapeutic measures are outlined.

Online Mendelian Inheritance in Man (OMIM): Hyperlipidemia, Type V ⊙ ⊙
http://www3.ncbi.nlm.nih.gov/htbin-post/Omim/dispmim?238400

A brief review and clinical synopsis of hyperlipidemia type V is found at this database entry, with markedly elevated triglycerides and similarities to type III noted.

29.2 Hypolipidemia

General Resources

Differential Diagnosis of Low HDL-Cholesterol ⊙
http://www.healthyheart.org/Education/hdl/hdl08.htm

A table found at this site of the Healthy Heart Program summarizes an approach to the differential diagnosis of low high-density lipoproteins (HDL). A distinction between primary and secondary disease is shown within this flowchart of lipid disorder identification.

Merck Manual of Diagnosis and Therapy: Hypolipidemia ⊙ ⊙
http://www.merck.com/pubs/mmanual/section2/chapter16/16a.htm

Low levels of plasma lipoproteins as seen in rare familial disorders or secondary to several systemic diseases are reviewed at this site of the online *Merck* reference, offering comprehensive overviews for practitioners and consumers alike. Discussions of raising high-density lipoprotein levels in hypoalphalipoproteinemia, the mutations causing hypobetalipoproteinemia, the rare, congenital abetalipoproteinemia, and Tangier disease are provided at the site. General measures for raising high-density lipoprotein (HDL) levels are reviewed.

Oregon Health Sciences University: Hypolipoproteinemia
http://medir.ohsu.edu/cliniweb/C18/C18.452.648.556.485.html

CliniWeb International pages provide preformatted query links to the National Library of Medicine's PubMed database, including this page on searches for review articles, therapeutic studies, and diagnostic investigations of hypolipoproteinemia. Abetalipoproteinemia, hypobetalipoproteinemia, lecithin acyltransferase deficiency, and Tangier disease literature may be retrieved by clicking on the respective links.

Abetalipoproteinemia

Adam.com: Bassen-Kornzweig Syndrome
http://thirdage.adam.com/ency/article/001666.htm

An encyclopedic entry, provided by the adam.com database, offers background information on this autosomal recessive disorder, as well as links to symptom listings, diagnostic tests, and dietary treatment, which details an increased consumption of medium-chain triglycerides and avoidance of long-chain triglycerides. Information on the fat-soluble vitamins may be accessed and includes links specifying vitamin functions and appropriate food sources.

Terre Haute Center for Medical Education: Abetalipoproteinemia: Kornzweig Syndrome
http://www.dentistry.leeds.ac.uk/biochem/thcme/hypolip.html

By accessing the links specific to hypobetalipoproteinemia, abetalipoproteinemia, or Tangier disease, visitors are directed to the related Online Mendelian Inheritance in Man (OMIM) database entries. Each document provides a review of the literature, citing interesting case examples. MEDLINE references are provided throughout the text, with connections to journal abstracts, a clinical synopsis, and related databases.

Hypobetalipoproteinemia

Online Mendelian Inheritance in Man (OMIM): Apolipoprotein B
http://www3.ncbi.nlm.nih.gov/htbin-post/Omim/dispmim?107730

The two main forms of apolipoprotein B hypolipoproteinemia and their genetic coding are discussed in the text of this Online Mendelian Inheritance in Man (OMIM) entry. The clinical picture of familial hypobetalipoproteinemia is reviewed, with reference to asymptomatic individuals, an array of secondary diseases and symptoms, and causative defects and mutations. Information on genetic frequencies of allelic variants, seventeen selected allelic variant examples, and a clinical synopsis entry are found.

Tangier Disease

National Center for Biotechnology
Information (NCBI): Genes and Disease: Tangier Disease
http://web.ncbi.nlm.nih.gov/disease/tangier.html

The National Center for Biotechnology Information (NCBI) provides a well-presented overview of this genetic disorder of cholesterol transport, named after its location of first identification. An illustration of the mutations causing cholesterol to accumulate within the cell is displayed, and the understanding of the inverse relationship between high-density lipoprotein (HDL) levels and coronary artery disease is discussed, exemplifying how research into rare conditions may offer useful information for more common, familial forms of disease.

Online Mendelian Inheritance in Man (OMIM):
High Density Lipoprotein Deficiency, Tangier Disease
http://www3.ncbi.nlm.nih.gov/htbin-post/Omim/dispmim?205400

Characteristic clinical enlargement of the liver, spleen, and tonsils; locations of affected individuals; neuropathic manifestations; and the possibility of severe visual impairment are reviewed for this high-density lipoprotein (HDL) deficiency. Examples of studied cases consistent with increased risk for premature vascular disease are provided, with related PubMed citations accessible throughout the text.

30. METABOLISM, INBORN ERRORS

30.1 General Resources

Baylor College of Medicine: Metabolic Myopathies ◎ ◎
http://svt.ee.tut.fi/korpinen/emg147.htm
The etiologies, clinical features, and expected abnormal findings are outlined for acid maltase deficiency, the glycogenoses, McArdle's disease, carnitine deficiency, carnitine palmitoyl transferase deficiency, and myadenylate deaminase deficiency at this site of the Baylor College of Medicine. Strategies for diagnosis and EMG procedures are presented.

Case Western Reserve University Center for Inherited Disorders of Energy Metabolism ◎ ◎
http://www.cwru.edu/med/CIDEM/cidem.htm
Part of Case Western Reserve University, the Center for Inherited Disorders of Energy Metabolism is a group of specialized laboratories that focus on disorders of mitochondrial function. Their site provides general information about the center and its staff. There are descriptions of general tests performed at the center including acylcarnitine profile, carnitine screening, fatty acid oxidation, electron transport chain, and many others. Details about each test, including costs, are available. There is also a list of selected publications authored by faculty and staff.

MedWebPlus: Mitochondrial Myopathies ◎ ◎ ◎
http://medwebplus.com/subject/Mitochondrial_Myopathies.html
MedWebPlus provides an assortment of interesting Internet links related to physician management, expert opinion, support, and research of mitochondrial myopathies. The connections provided include the Washington University School of Medicine Neuromuscular Disease Center, the United Mitochondrial Disease Foundation, the "Ask the Experts" about mitochondrial myopathies page of the Muscular Dystrophy Associa-

tion, and a physician's guide to care. The physician's guide, downloadable in Adobe Acrobat format, offers a variety of clinical articles on diagnosis, treatment, and research advances, and an article on carnitine palmitoyl transferase deficiency offers current medical news and a "Food Pharmacy" page with articles from noted specialists and organizations.

National Institute of Neurological Disorders and Stroke (NINDS): Mitochondrial Myopathies Information Sheet ◐ ◐

http://www.ninds.nih.gov/health_and_medical/disorders/mitochon_doc.htm

The informational brochure at this site, presented as a courtesy of the National Institute of Neurological Disorders and Stroke of the National Institutes of Health, offers a discussion of mitochondrial myopathies, including symptoms, treatment options, and prognosis details. A listing of references and organizations that may offer in-depth information is provided.

Presbyterian Hospital of Dallas Neuromuscular Center: Mitochondrial Myopathies ◐ ◐ ◐

http://www.thr.org/nmc/mitochondrial_myopathies.htm

A connection to the Neuromuscular Center of the Presbyterian Hospital of Dallas provides visitors with an overview of mitochondrial defects, including a description of the clinical presentation of these disorders, clarification of their molecular basis, and a discussion of treatment. Potential therapeutic benefits of vitamin C, K3, and riboflavin are examined, as is treatment with antioxidants, glucocorticoids, and ubiquinone. Detailed entries on succinate dehydrogenase, fumarase deficiency, mitochondrial DNA deletion and point mutation, and pyruvate dehydrogenase are accessible. Additional connections review the pathophysiology of disorders of muscle energy metabolism, inheritance patterns, and symptoms.

Society for the Study of Inborn Errors in Metabolism ◐ ◐

http://www.ssiem.org.uk

The Society For the Study of Inborn Errors of Metabolism fosters research of inherited Disorders of Endocrinology and Metabolism through scientific meetings and publications. The site provides information about the history, goals, membership, and activities of the organization. Links to publications, training information, and affiliated organizations are offered, as are connections to journals and publishers, societies, diagnostic centers, databases, and other resources.

United Mitochondrial Disease Foundation ◐ ◐ ◐

http://www.umdf.org

The United Mitochondrial Disease Foundation promotes research for cures and treatments of mitochondrial diseases. Information about mitochondrial diseases includes a glossary of terms, reviews of the literature, other publications, a medical article database and library, and a patient registry. A discussion of mitochondria and disease and descriptions of 42 mitochondrial diseases are provided. This Web page also offers information on current research, news and events, and information about the Foundation. Links to support groups and related sites are included.

30.2 Carbohydrate Metabolism

General Resources

Terre Haute Center for Medical Education: Defects in Fructose, Galactose, and Glycerol Metabolism ○ ○ ○
http://www.dentistry.leeds.ac.uk/biochem/thcme/othrcarb.html

Six specific defects in fructose, galactose, and glycerol metabolism are listed at this page, and information on each error of inborn metabolism is discussed at the related Online Mendelian Inheritance in Man (OMIM) link. Hereditary fructose intolerance, fructosuria, and classic galactosemia, as well as other disorders, are discussed at this collection of OMIM pages, with each providing information on recognized cases, hereditary and mutation facts, and biochemical and biophysical characterization of disease variants. Selected examples of allelic variants, links to MEDLINE listings, and literature references are offered.

Essential Fructosuria

Online Mendelian Inheritance in Man (OMIM): Fructosuria ○ ○
http://www3.ncbi.nlm.nih.gov/htbin-post/Omim/dispmim?229800

Allelic disease variants, a discussion of this benign defect of metabolism, and recognized cases of fructosuria are reviewed at this Online Mendelian Inheritance in Man (OMIM) entry. Related research abstracts are accessible throughout the text, and genetic mapping information is found.

Fructose-1,6-Bisphosphatase Deficiency

Oxford Medical Informatics: Fructose-1,6-Diphosphatase Deficiency ○
http://oxmedinfo.jr2.ox.ac.uk/Pathway/Disease/31087.htm

Physical, neurological, and other disease manifestations are concisely outlined at the site, in addition to treatment and carrier detection. A link connects visitors to an illustration of carbohydrate metabolism.

Galactokinase Deficiency

Online Mendelian Inheritance in Man (OMIM): Galactokinase Deficiency ○ ○ ○
http://www3.ncbi.nlm.nih.gov/htbin-post/Omim/dispmim?230200

The OMIM database presents a review of galactokinase deficiency at this site, which includes previously reported case examples, genetic mapping information, reference listings, and specific PubMed links. A clinical synopsis and cytogenetic map location table are found.

Oxford Medical Informatics: Galactokinase Deficiency ○
http://oxmedinfo.jr2.ox.ac.uk/Pathway/Disease/38544.htm

The physical, neurological, and biochemical characteristics of galactokinase deficiency are listed at the site, and access to an illustration of the metabolic pathway of carbohydrate metabolism is offered, depicting galactokinase deficiency, galctosemia, and galactose epimerase.

Galactosemia

Children's Liver Alliance: Galactosemia Links ○ ○
http://www.livertx.org/galactosemialinks.html

The *Merck Manual,* online newborn screening manuals, and several research and resource pages are available at this collection of galactosemia Web connections. Visitors will find an assortment of educational material at www.galactosemia.org, accessible from the site, which includes information for the newly diagnosed, conferences and newsletters, current research initiatives, and links regarding potential complications. Entries from PEDBASE and the Online Mendelian Inheritance in Man (OMIM) database may be accessed, in addition to articles abstracts specific to cognitive function, a prevalent mutation of galactosemia in African Americans, and the molecular basis for the Duarte and Los Angeles variants.

Nebraska Health and Human Services System: Practitioner's Manual: Galactosemia ○ ○
http://www.hhs.state.ne.us/nsp/pmg.htm

Clinical features of the severe form of the disease and a discussion of a qualitative screening test are found at the site. Confirmatory testing and screening practice considerations are concisely reviewed.

Texas Department of Health: Galactosemia Handbook ◎ ◎ ◎
http://www.tdh.state.tx.us/newborn/handbook.htm
Provided by the Texas Department of Health, this handbook was designed to help parents care for children with galactosemia. A general overview of the disorder, inheritance factors, complications, treatment, and diet information are provided, as well as information about reading labels, specific foods, support group links, and references.

Glycogen Storage Diseases: General

Family Village: Glycogen Storage Disease ◎ ◎
http://www.familyvillage.wisc.edu/lib_gsd.htm
Family Village provides a collection of Internet resources related to glycogen storage diseases, including connections to associations related to specific diseases, a LISTSERV for networking of professionals and patients, and a variety of informational brochures on the various disease types.

Terre Haute Center for Medical Education: Glycogen Storage Diseases Database ◎ ◎ ◎
http://www.dentistry.leeds.ac.uk/biochem/thcme/glycstor.html
This database of the University of Leeds affords direct access to specific pages of the Online Mendelian Inheritance in Man (OMIM) database for types 0 through X glycogen storage diseases. Von Gierke's, Pompe, Cori, Andersen, McArdle, Hers, and Tarui diseases are included in the OMIM collection, with each entry providing a clinical synopsis, allelic variants, text discussion, and references. Visitors have the opportunity to access related MEDLINE document listings from various points throughout the OMIM pages.

Glycogen Storage Diseases: Pompe Disease (Acid Maltase Deficiency)

Acid Maltase Deficiency Association ◎ ◎ ◎
http://www.amda-pompe.org
The Acid Maltase Deficiency Association (AMDA) was created to support research and public awareness of this disorder, also known as Pompe disease. The site provides a summary of the disorder, including discussions of symptoms, types, and treatment. A section dedicated to respiratory care options, excerpts from an article originally published by the Muscular Dystrophy Association, and information on improving respiration are found, in addition to research developments, clinical trials, and related sites of interest.

Children's Pompe Foundation ◐ ◐
http://www.pompe.org

The Children's Pompe Foundation is dedicated to finding a cure for Pompe disease and offers information about the foundation and the disorder, including overviews of the five basic disease forms. Press releases and articles about the foundation, information about upcoming events and recent fundraising efforts, and links to related sites are provided.

International Pompe Association ◐ ◐
http://www.pompe.org.uk

This site offers links to information about Pompe disease produced by the Association for Glycogen Storage Disease (AGSD), Pompe's resources elsewhere on the net, and background information. Available from the AGSD are a guide for families, information about Pompe's Project, a pamphlet on caring for a child with Pompe's, and current issues of the association's newsletter. Connections to other sites include the Children's Pompe Foundation and the Acid Maltase Deficiency Association. Background information is provided on cell biology and proteolysis.

Hereditary Fructose Intolerance

Adam.com: Hereditary Fructose Intolerance ◐ ◐
http://wzzk.adam.com/ency/article/000359.htm

This adam.com Web article discusses the causes and incidence of hereditary fructose intolerance, otherwise known as disaccharide malabsorption or fructosemia. Overviews of symptoms, signs and tests, and disease complications are found, as well as a link regarding genetic testing.

Boston University: Hereditary Fructose Intolerance and Aldolase ◐ ◐
http://www.bu.edu/aldolase

Boston University offers access to information on hereditary fructose intolerance (HFI) diagnosis, treatment, and current research at this Internet page. An aldolase biochemistry, genetics, and molecular biology evolution page link is provided, in addition to information on the university's HFI support group.

Online Mendelian Inheritance in Man (OMIM): Fructose Intolerance, Hereditary ◐ ◐ ◐
http://www3.ncbi.nlm.nih.gov/htbin-post/Omim/dispmim?229600

An Online Mendelian Inheritance in Man (OMIM) entry is found at this Web address, which provides several database links, recognized cases of hereditary fructose intolerance, discussion regarding genetic mutations, and the biochemical and biophysical disease characterizations. Selected examples of allelic variants and links to referenced PubMed listings are found.

Mucopolysaccharidoses (MPS) and Related Diseases

Canadian Society for Mucopolysaccharide (MPS) and Related Diseases

http://www.mpssociety.ca

The Canadian MPS Society was created to support patients and families affected by lysosomal storage diseases. The site offers information about MPS and related diseases. By accessing the diseases link, visitors are taken to discussions on the history of the disease, causes and heredity, diagnosis, symptoms, and treatment options. A chart outlining disease classifications is provided, in addition to a resource library, a discussion forum, and resources for further learning.

National Mucopolysaccharidoses (MPS) Society

http://www.mpssociety.org

A chart outlining disease types and links to further information on causes and inheritance are found at the National MPS Society page. Accessing the reference center provides visitors with a listing of publications that may be ordered, and MPS news offers information on upcoming events and legislative updates. By following links to the Online Mendelian Inheritance in Man (OMIM) database site and additional links, visitors gain access to detailed genetic and research information. Information on related diseases, including the oligosaccharidoses, the glycosphingolipidoses, and the mucolipidoses, is provided at the site.

UDPgalactose 4-Epimerase Deficiency

Oxford Medical Informatics: Galactose 4 Epimerase Deficiency

http://oxmedinfo.jr2.ox.ac.uk/Pathway/Disease/57744.htm

The absence of symptomatology of galactosemia III is concisely reviewed at this site, and a link to an illustration of the metabolic pathway of galactose metabolism is accessible, with galactokinase deficiency, galactosemia, and galactose epimerase detailed.

Pyruvate Carboxylase Deficiency

emedicine: Pyruvate Carboxylase Deficiency ✹ ✹ ✹
http://www.emedicine.com/PED/topic1967.htm

Emedicine's pediatric topics include this in-depth clinical review of pyruvate carboxylase deficiency, also referred to as congenital infantile lactic acidosis or Leigh necrotizing encephalopathy. Malfunction of the citric acid cycle and gluconeogenesis and the resulting metabolic acidosis are summarized, along with pathophysiology, clinical and physical presentation, and diagnostic differential links. Laboratory and imaging studies, as well as profiles of pharmacologic agents used to correct acidosis and to activate the pyruvate dehydrogenase complex, are reviewed.

iBionet: Pyruvate Carboxylase Deficiency: Symptoms, Self-Assessment, and Links ✹ ✹
http://www.ibionet.com/rarediseases/PyruvateCarboxylaseDeficiency.html

A symptom checklist for pyruvate carboxylase deficiency is found at this iBio symptoms and self-assessment search engine. In addition, visitors will discover a listing of links to genetic counseling, genetic testing, and information on research and genetics in the field of endocrinology, courtesy of the Endocrine Society, the University of Kansas Medical Center, and the International Birth Defects Information System.

Pyruvate Dehydrogenase Complex Deficiency

Healthwise Knowledgebase: Pyruvate Dehydrogenase Deficiency ✹ ✹ ✹
http://www.healthynetwork.com/kbase/nord/nord413.htm

The Healthwise Knowledgebase of the National Organization for Rare Disorders, Inc. (NORD) offers a listing of synonyms for the condition, a general discussion and review of symptoms, and genetic cause. Affected populations, related disorders, and standard and investigational therapies are examined. The page also offers references and a list of related Web resources.

National Library of Medicine (NLM): Pyruvate Dehydrogenase Complex Deficiency ✹ ✹
http://wwwils.nlm.nih.gov/mesh/jablonski/syndromes/syndrome548.html

The National Library of Medicine provides information at this site related to the major features of pyruvate dehydrogenase complex deficiency. By accessing the full entry, visitors are able to view historical references and a MEDLINE bibliography.

30.3 Amino Acid Metabolism

General Resources

**Oregon Health Sciences University:
Amino Acid Metabolism, Inborn Errors** ◎ ◎
http://medir.ohsu.edu/cliniweb/C18/C18.452.648.66.html
A variety of clinical reference links are accessible from this page of Oregon Health Sciences University. CliniWeb International provides several direct links to preformatted PubMed literature searches specific to a variety of inborn errors of amino acid metabolism. Also found are fact sheets and in-depth disease reviews, courtesy of the Medical College of Wisconsin and the Online Mendelian Inheritance in Man (OMIM) database.

**Terre Haute Center for Medical Education: Introduction to Amino
Acid Metabolism and Inborn Errors of Amino Acid Metabolism** ◎ ◎
http://web.indstate.edu/thcme/mwking/amino-acid-metabolism.html
Introductions to amino acid metabolism and inborn errors of amino acid metabolism are found at this site of the Terre Haute Center for Medical Education. Detailed reviews of amino acid biosynthesis and amino acid catabolism are provided, as well as connections to specific pages of the Online Mendelian Inheritance in Man (OMIM) database for amino acid defects, urea cycle defects, and defects in amino acid transport.

Alcaptonuria

emedicine: Alkaptonuria ◎ ◎ ◎
http://emedicine.com/cgi-bin/foxweb.exe/
showsection@d:/em/ga?book=ped&topicid=64
Authored by a professor at Virginia Commonwealth University, this emedicine entry details the hallmark of the disease, the inherited biochemical abnormality, and an autosomal recessive mode of inheritance. Disease causes, homogentisate identification and other testing procedures, and medical and dietary treatment of alkaptonuria are outlined in this organized management guideline.

**King Faisal Specialist Hospital and Research Centre:
Alkaptonuria: Case Report and Review of the Literature** ◎ ◎
http://www.kfshrc.edu.sa/annals/185/98-055.html
A description of this rare metabolic disease and a report of a child with presymptomatic alkaptonuria are found at the site. Review of the relevant literature, clinical aspects, and management are discussed.

MEDLINEplus Health Information: Alcaptonuria
http://medlineplus.adam.com/ency/article/001200.htm

MEDLINEPlus Health Information and the adam.com Web encyclopedia present this overview of alcaptonuria, a rare inherited condition. Causes, incidence, and risk factors are provided, as well as pages devoted to symptom recognition and treatment and links to related terminology.

Homocystinuria

Online Mendelian Inheritance in Man (OMIM): Homocystinuria
http://www3.ncbi.nlm.nih.gov/htbin-post/Omim/dispmim?236200

This extensive resource, provided as a service of the OMIM database, offers a review of compiled worldwide data regarding the disease features of various systems, biochemical disease specifications, pathogenesis, and population genetics for homocystinuria. Specific genetic mutations, discussion of worldwide frequency, pharmacologic management, surgical procedures for ophthalmic manifestations, and follow-up information regarding the first known case of homocystinuria are found. Allelic disease variants are referenced.

Tyler for Life Foundation: Homocystinuria
http://tylerforlife.com/homocystinuria.htm

Facts regarding this hereditary error of metabolism, symptoms associated with the illness, and thoughts on the autosomal recessive mode of inheritance are reviewed for homocystinuria. A state-by-state listing of disorders screened for in each state and additional online educational material may be accessed, such as the associated National Organization for Rare Disorders (NORD) entry and a personal homocystinuria Web page.

Maple Syrup Urine Disease

emedicine: Maple Syrup Urine Disease
http://emedicine.com/cgi-bin/foxweb.exe/showsection@d:/em/ga?book=ped&topicid=1368

This completed topic heading of the emedicine encyclopedic reference provides a concise clinical management guide to maple syrup urine disease, otherwise known as MSUD or branched-chain ketonuria. Authored by a physician at Baylor College of Medicine, the article details the branched-chain alpha-keto acid dehydrogenase complex deficiency and the related pathophysiology. Demographic information, distinct clinical phenotypes, laboratory study review, and goals of dietary therapy are reviewed.

Family Village: Maple Syrup Urine Disease ◎ ◎
http://www.familyvillage.wisc.edu/lib_msud.htm

Family Village offers a collection of connections at this site appropriate for both professional and consumer reference. Contact information for support groups, subscription information to a related Web chat, fact sheets on maple syrup urine disease, and a connection the Online Mendelian Inheritance in Man (OMIM) entry for the disorder are easily accessible. A Pediatric Database (PEDBASE) article and a connection to the Maple Syrup Urine Disease Family Support Web site are also offered.

Phenylketonuria (PKU)

National Library of Medicine (NLM): Screening for Phenylketonuria (PKU) ◎ ◎
http://text.nlm.nih.gov/cps/www/cps.50.html

A discussion of this inborn error of metabolism and recommendations regarding genetic screening of newborns by measurement of phenylalanine level are provided at this online article. The accuracy of screening with the Guthrie test, information on false-positive and false-negative results, and the effectiveness of early detection are reviewed. An update on recommendations of several organizations, such as the American Academy of Pediatrics (AAP), regarding screening times and repeat screenings is found.

National PKU News ◎ ◎ ◎
http://205.178.182.34

The National PKU News Home Page offers information about phenylketonuria, including genetics, screening, diet composition, diet maintenance, maternal PKU, and PKU treatment programs. The PKU research link contains papers on alternative treatments for inborn errors of metabolism, the follow-up study to the 1967-1983 National Collaborative Study of Children Treated for PKU, and diet treatment and supplement review. The National PKU news index provides research review, special features, and food and nutrition notes.

Urea Cycle Disorders

National Urea Cycle Disorders Foundation ◎ ◎ ◎
http://www.nucdf.org

The National Urea Cycle Disorders Foundation exists to save children's lives. Information about the foundation includes a news section, medical research and grant information, conference updates, a membership application, and contribution information. Information about this group of disorders includes general overviews and articles on symptoms, types, and treatment options. Details on the organization's family support network and connections to additional Internet resources, including pediatric databases, dietary specialties, genetics sites, and research trials, are provided.

Organic Acidemia Association: Management of Urea Cycle Disorders ○ ○ ○
http://just4u.com/oaa/tuchma1.htm

A professor of pediatric and laboratory medicine at the University of Minnesota Hospital presents this interesting article discussing prevention of the devastating effects of urea cycle disorders. Long-held beliefs regarding traditional management of these disorders are challenged by the author, and ideas and suggestions to stimulate further discussion are presented. Problems associated with obtaining proper plasma ammonia levels, problems with glucose administration related to ammonia levels, the idea of genetically determined glutamine levels, and theory regarding their use as a marker for adequate therapy are presented. Dietary management, the administration of arginine and methods of increasing mitochondrial ornithine concentrations, and additional examples to stimulate progress in urea cycle disorder amelioration are presented.

Vancouver Hospital Health Sciences Center: Urea Cycle Defects ○ ○
http://www.vanhosp.bc.ca/html/wellness_amdc_findout_urea.html

The five varieties of urea cycle defects, according to enzyme type, are defined at this Health and Wellness Web site. By clicking on the links above the introductory text, visitors gain access to the enzyme listing and a colorfully illustrated explanation of the urea cycle. Patterns of inheritance of the various disorders, dietary management and other ammonia reduction therapy, and discussion of the need for balance between meeting body protein requirements while eliminating ammonia are explained. A related Web site and contact information for associated organizations are provided.

Variant Forms of Hyperphenylalaninemia

Mead Johnson: Hereditary Tyrosinemia ○ ○ ○
http://www.meadjohnson.com/metabolics/hereditarytyrosinemia.html

An overview of hypertyrosinemia is found at this Web site and includes information on the diagnosis and dietary management of patients with this disorder. The inborn errors of tyrosine catabolism or secondary disease causes are explained, and an illustration at the site outlines the degradation of phenylalanine and tyrosine. Screening procedures, nondietary management options, and references are provided.

National Dysautonomia Research Foundation (NDRF): Tetrahydrobiopterin Deficiency ⊙

http://www.ndrf.org/tetrahyd.htm

An explanation of this less commonly recognized anomaly in amino acid metabolism is found at this site of the NDRF. Links providing further information are recommended and accessible.

Tetrahydrobiopterin Home Page ⊙ ⊙

http://www.bh4.org

Connections from this page allow interested viewers to learn more about recognized tetrahydrobiopterin deficiencies, their biochemical background, and specific syndrome phenotypes, pathophysiology, treatment, and diagnosis. A patient database, mutations database, and parent support group listing are accessible.

University of Washington: Phenylalanine Hydroxylase Deficiency ⊙ ⊙ ⊙

http://ribosome.geneclinics.org/profiles/pku/details.html

This site, funded by the National Library of Medicine and the National Human Genome Research Institute, details both hyperphenylalaninemia and phenylketonuria. Disease characteristics of the classic and variant disease types are summarized, and diagnosis by newborn screening is examined, with two types of molecular genetic testing discussed. Additional discussion focuses on the reliability of current tests to accurately discern concentrations in newborns, due to time-dependent serum concentrations. Clinical disease descriptions, molecular genetic testing, and genotype-phenotype correlations are examined. Prevalence, a historical perspective, management across a variety of patient populations, and links to references and genomic databases are conveniently provided. Selected organization and clinic contact information and Web sites are listed.

30.4 Fatty Acid Oxidation and Carnitine

Presbyterian Hospital of Dallas: Metabolic Myopathies: Lipid Defects ⊙ ⊙

http://www.thr.org/nmc/lipid_defects.htm

Discussion of carnitine deficiency, carnitine palmitoyl transferase deficiency, and acyl CoA dehydrogenase are accessible from this site of the Neuromuscular Center at the Presbyterian Hospital of Dallas. Each overview offers information on the particular metabolic defect, symptoms, and treatment recommendations.

30.5 Purine and Pyrimidine Metabolic Disorders

Purine Research Society
http://www2.dgsys.com/~purine

The secretion of excess uric acid in purine metabolic disease and current progress in research of these disorders is the focus of the Purine Research Society. A simple explanation of metabolic processes, genetic enzyme production, information on purine compounds, and the importance of recognition of purine metabolic diseases are discussed. Concise descriptions of several of these enzyme defects and the future of purine research are reviewed.

30.6 Lysosomal Disorders

Lysosomal Storage Diseases, General

Medstudents: Lysosomal Storage Diseases
http://www.medstudents.com.br/metdis/metdis6.htm

This Medstudents' page offers concise reviews of three lysosomal storage diseases, including Gaucher's disease, Fabry's disease, and Niemann-Pick disease, with clinical manifestations, diagnosis, and treatment information outlined.

Rare Genetic Diseases in Children: Lysosomal Storage Diseases
http://mcrcr2.med.nyu.edu/murphp01/lysosome/lysosome.htm

Education for those interested in the variety of lysosomal storage diseases is presented at this site, with a guide to cellular processes and lysosomal function, a quick reference guide to disorders, suggestions for further reading and informational links, and a lysosomal lexicon associated with lysosomal diseases. By accessing the reference guide, visitors are presented with a table outlining glycogenosis disorders, glycolipidoses, mucopolysaccharide disorders, oligosaccharides/glycoprotein disorders, and lysosomal enzyme and lysosomal membrane transport diseases. Respective enzyme defects, substances stored, chromosome locations, and Online Mendelian Inheritance in Man (OMIM) database entry links are found.

Cerebrotendinous Xanthomatosis

Bombay Hospital Journal
Case Reports: Cerebrotendinous Xanthomatosis ○ ○
http://www.bhj.org/journal/1997/3901_jan/case_180.htm

This site of the *Bombay Hospital Journal* provides readers with a case report of this rare autosomal recessive disorder, with past history, examination, and images of bilateral fusiform swellings over the tendoachilles. An explanation of the defective synthesis of primary bile acids in the liver and concomitant increases in cholesterol and decreases in cholic and chenodeoxycholic acid is provided. Discussion of the clinical picture and mention of lipid profiles and other, rare autosomal recessive disorders of lipid metabolism are provided.

Fabry's Disease

Fabry Disease Home Page ○
http://www.sci.ccny.cuny.edu/~fabry

From the City College of New York, this page provides clinical and biochemical information about the inborn error of glycolipid metabolism. The mode of inheritance of this enzymatic defect, links to additional sites related to Fabry disease, and an educational disease outline are provided.

Fabry Support and Information Group ○ ○ ○
http://www.cpgnet.com/fsig.nsf

The Fabry Support and Information Group offers information and emotional support to Fabry patients and their families, with detailed background information of the disorder that includes an explanation of metabolic defect, disease inheritance, clinical symptoms, and treatment. Information about membership in the organization and participation in a clinical trial is found, in addition to links to other sites and additional online information. There is also a discussion page with personal biographies.

International Center for Fabry Disease ○ ○ ○
http://www.mssm.edu/crc/Fabry/fabry.html

From the Department of Human Genetics at Mount Sinai School of Medicine, this site offers information and support for Fabry disease patients. An explanation of the disease includes an introduction and sections on the nature of the metabolic defect in Fabry disease, inheritance, clinical symptoms, diagnosis, treatment, specific therapy, and prenatal diagnosis. A research update section, information regarding free diagnostic studies, and Fabry disease references are provided, including clinical publications, biochemical research, and molecular genetic research.

Metabolic Disease and Stroke: Fabry's Disease ○ ○ ○
http://emedicine.com/cgi-bin/foxweb.exe/
showsection@d:/em/ga?book=neuro&topicid=579

Background information on this X-linked lysosomal disorder is presented at this site of the emedicine online textbook. Deficiency of alpha-galactosidase and further pathophysiology, multi-organ system involvement, physical examination findings, and diagnostic differential links are provided. Laboratory diagnostics, medical and surgical interventions, and profiles of antiplatelet agents and anticoagulants are found. In addition, visitors are presented with information on medical and legal pitfalls in management. Referenced Medline abstracts may be directly accessed at emedicine articles.

National Institutes of Health (NIH): Fabry's Disease ○ ○
http://www.ninds.nih.gov/health_and_medical/disorders/fabrys_doc.htm

From the National Institute of Neurological Disorders and Stroke, this patient information booklet provides basic information on Fabry's disease. An overview of the disorder and discussions of treatment, prognosis, and current research of this National Institutes of Health division are found.

Galactosylceramide Lipidosis (Krabbe's Disease)

Globoid Cell Leukodystrophy or Krabbe's Disease ○ ○
http://metro.peacelink.it/appeal/gianmarco/v.html

The clinical features and examination findings in Krabbe's disease are reviewed in this article, along with biochemical features and genetic mapping. Molecular and population genetics, an animal model discussion, and allelic disease variants are presented.

UTHealth.com: Globoid Cell Leukodystrophy (GCL) A.K.A. Krabbe's Disease ○
http://www.uthealth.com/ut/mental/encyc/krabbe.htm

Pharmacology Research Corporation presents a concise, online fact sheet regarding the treatment, prognosis, and current research goals. Reference to in-depth disease information is provided.

Gaucher Disease

Gauchers Association ○ ○ ○
http://wisebuy.users.netlink.co.uk/gaucher/contents.htm

This comprehensive site provides links to over 200 different patient and professional Internet resources on Gaucher disease. New sites and an alphabetical listing of the remainder are provided, with articles and references to enzyme replacement therapy, genetic therapeutics, home infusions, new and investigative treatments, obstetric and gynecological aspects, pain management, and diagnostic testing provided.

Gauchers Association: Living With Gaucher Disease ○ ○ ○
http://www.wisebuy.co.uk/gaucher/living.htm

Offered by the Gauchers Association, this guide is intended for patients, parents, relatives, and friends of those affected with Gaucher disease. The site provides an introduction and history of the disorder, with further discussion of lysosomal storage defects, variations in manifestations, causes, diagnosis, and emotional and social aspects of disease. Current research and treatment information is offered at this comprehensive reference.

National Gaucher Foundation ○ ○ ○
http://www.gaucherdisease.org

Maintained by the Gaucher Disease Foundation, this site offers information on the clinical course of Gaucher disease and a section on prevention and treatment with reference to carrier testing and enzyme replacement therapy. A discussion of prevalence and transmission is provided, as well as links to additional Internet resources, guides for patients and clinicians, e-mail discussion lists, and news updates.

National Gaucher Foundation: Gaucher Disease: Clinical Course ○ ○
http://www.gaucherdisease.org/info/course.htm

This lipid storage disease is described in clinical terms at the site, with the accumulation of glucocerebroside and the loss of mineral in the bones explained. Distinctions between different types of the disorder are mentioned.

Pittsburgh Genetics Institute: Gaucher Disease: A Clinical Trial of Gene Therapy ○ ○ ○
http://neuro-www2.mgh.harvard.edu/gaucher/genetherapy.html

A gene therapy clinical trial as a treatment for Gaucher disease is discussed at this site of the Pittsburgh Genetics Institute. Current management options, such as bone marrow transplantation and enzyme replacement therapy, are explained at the site, and the promising mechanisms of somatic gene therapy as a cure, rather than a treatment, is thoroughly detailed.

Generalized Gangliosidosis

National Library of Medicine (NLM): Gangliosidosis GM1, Type I ⊙ ⊙
http://wwwils.nlm.nih.gov/mesh/jablonski/syndromes/syndrome309.html

A disease synopsis and full record entry for generalized gangliosidosis is offered, courtesy of the National Library of Medicine health information site. Several synonyms, a disorder summary, and major features of various systems are listed. By accessing the full entry option, visitors are able to view historical reference information and a MEDLINE bibliography.

Online Mendelian Inheritance in Man (OMIM): Gangliosidosis, Generalized GM1, Type I ⊙ ⊙ ⊙
http://www3.ncbi.nlm.nih.gov/htbin-post/Omim/dispmim?230500

Generalized gangliosidosis is discussed at this site of the Online Mendelian Inheritance in Man Web database. A listing of allelic variants and descriptions, definitive description of this disease entity, and a complete review of related literature are provided. A clinical synopsis and several database links are found, including the nomenclature, genome, and gene map locus connections.

Metachromatic Leukodystrophy

Medical College of Wisconsin
Health Link: Metachromatic Leukodystrophy ⊙
http://141.106.32.35/article/921440824.html

The Medical College of Wisconsin Physicians and Clinics offers a fact sheet on this genetic enzyme deficiency. Symptoms of the late infantile, juvenile, and adult forms are reviewed, and additional facts, provided as a service of the National Institute of Neurological Disorders and Stroke (NINDS), are stated.

Selected Medical Images: Metachromatic Leukodystrophy ⊙ ⊙
http://matweb.hcuge.ch/matweb/Selected_images/
Developmental_genetic_diseases/metachromatic_leukodystrophy.htm

Online magnifications of metachromatic leukodystrophy of the brain, as well as neuropathological images are available at this site. Sources include Cornell University Medical College and the University of Connecticut Health Center and are provided as a service of MATWEB.

Niemann-Pick Disease

National Institute of Neurological Disorders and Stroke (NINDS): Niemann-Pick Disease
http://www.ninds.nih.gov/health_and_medical/disorders/niemann.doc.htm

A mini-information sheet, courtesy of the National Institute of Neurological Disorders and Stoke (NINDS), is offered at the site, with overviews of treatment, prognosis, and current genetic and therapeutic research. An article listing provides reference to more in-depth information.

National Niemann-Pick Disease Foundation, Inc.
http://www.nnpdf.org

The National Niemann-Pick Disease Foundation supports research, advocacy, and awareness of the disorder and provides an assortment of fact sheets on the disorder that discuss diagnosis, symptoms, transmission, and treatment. Information about the foundation includes a history, membership information, contact information, a newsletter, and descriptions of services, as well as conference details and agenda.

Niemann-Pick Disease Group (UK)
http://www.nnpdf.org/npdg-uk/index.html

The Niemann-Pick Disease Group provides information and support to families and professionals around the world regarding Niemann-Pick disease. The group's current newsletter is available at their site, which offers research and fund-raising updates, membership information, and links to related groups.

Refsum's Disease

Infantile Refsum's Disease
http://home.pacifier.com/~mstephe

A personal page on infantile Refsum's disease offers information on professionals and centers participating in research, general disease overview, and details regarding otology and auditory impairment, deafness and blindness, and ophthalmic concerns. A connection is found to the Infantile Refsum's Disease Web ring.

Westminster Hospital of London: Diet Treatment of Refsum's Disease
http://www.alphalink.com.au/~dijon/index3.htm

As a service of the Westminster Hospital of London, this page provides visitors with information on the phytanic acid level of various food groups and the principles of the dietary restrictions explained. Phytanic acid-free foods, medium-risk foods, and foods known to contain a high content of phytanic acid are reviewed at the table on page two of the Web site.

Tay-Sachs Disease

Ask NOAH About: Pregnancy: Tay-Sachs Disease Public Health Education Information Sheet ◐ ◐
http://www.noah.cuny.edu/pregnancy/march_of_dimes/birth_defects/taysachs.html

New York Online Access to Health offers this Web site, courtesy of the March of Dimes, regarding background and treatment information on Tay-Sachs disease. Portions of the fact sheet address disease inheritance patterns, prenatal diagnosis, carrier screening, and other details pertaining to Tay-Sachs research.

National Tay-Sachs and Allied Diseases Association, Inc. ◐ ◐
http://www.ntsad.org

The National Tay-Sachs and Allied Diseases Association offers this International Resource Center, structured to provide a comprehensive Web reference on Tay-Sachs and related disease profiles, the basis of genetics, programs sponsored by the organization, and further sources of information, such as recommended reading. The latest events, an online genetic testing center directory, and an assortment of educational materials appropriate for both professionals and the general public may be obtained.

Wolman's Disease

King Faisal Specialist Hospital and Research Centre: Wolman's Disease ◐ ◐
http://www.kfshrc.edu.sa/annals/182/97-264.html

This rare, autosomal recessive lysosomal storage disease is reviewed at this site via retrospective clinical, radiological, biochemical, and histopathological findings of diagnosed patients. The necessity of a plain abdominal radiograph to check for the characteristic pattern of adrenal calcification is emphasized.

Online Mendelian Inheritance in Man (OMIM): Wolman Disease ◐ ◐ ◐
http://www3.ncbi.nlm.nih.gov/htbin-post/Omim/dispmim?278000

Alternative disease titles, related database links, and an in-depth discussion of the severe, infantile and the milder, adult-onset cholesterol ester storage disease (CESD) are presented at this site of the Online Mendelian Inheritance in Man (OMIM) database. The large increases in cholesterol of the organs in the acute, infantile form and clinical presentation are described, with several reported cases cited. Interesting review of the molecular basis of CESD, and a phenotypic mouse model of human CESD, which biochemically and histopathologically mimics human Wolman disease, are reviewed. Allelic variants and connections to closely related PubMed abstracts are found.

30.7 Peroxisomal Disorders

Peroxisomal Disorders ○ ○ ○
http://home.pacifier.com/~mstephe/peroxisome.htm

This page of the infantile Refsum's Disease Web page provides general information on the current state of knowledge regarding the nature and functions of the peroxisome, as well as the diseases resulting from peroxisomal dysfunction. An overview of the organelle, biochemical reactions that occur in the cell, and peroxisomal biogenesis are presented. Characterizations of and distinctions among the various disorders are discussed, and links to their respective entries in the Online Mendelian Inheritance in Man (OMIM) database are accessible.

The Peroxisome Website: Peroxisomal Single Enzyme Disorders ○ ○ ○
http://www.peroxisome.org/Scientist/Biochemistry/disorders/1enzymedisorders.html

Nine peroxisomal single enzyme disorders are reviewed at this biochemistry Web site of Johns Hopkins University School of Medicine. Visitors are encouraged to access specific disorders and may learn more about the peroxisomal biochemistry of metabolic pathways of these abnormalities by accessing information at the sidebar frame. Clinical presentation, molecular genetics, common mutations, and summary information on possible treatments are offered, with selected abstract references and Online Mendelian Inheritance in Man (OMIM) entries. By linking to the home page of the Peroxisome Website, created by Stephen J. Gould, visitors are afforded additional access to information geared especially for scientists, physicians, and laypersons.

30.8 Carbohydrate-Deficient Glycoprotein Syndromes

Healthwise Knowledgebase:
Carbohydrate-Deficient Glycoprotein Syndrome Type 1 ○ ○ ○
http://www.healthwise.org/kbase/nord/nord1071.htm#Synonyms

The Healthwise Knowledgebase of the National Organization for Rare Disorders, Inc. (NORD) offers synonyms for the condition, a related disorders listing, a general discussion of its characterization and clinical presentation, and various phases of symptoms in infants through adults. Causes of carbohydrate-deficient glycoprotein syndrome, affected populations, standard therapies, and investigational treatment are reviewed.

30.9 Smith-Lemli-Opitz Syndrome

Smith-Lemli-Opitz Syndrome Advocacy and Exchange ○ ○ ○
http://members.aol.com/slo97

Symptoms and diagnosis of Smith-Lemli-Opitz syndrome are presented here, with a listing of the most common defects associated with the disease shown. The natural history of the disorder and the metabolic impairment associated with the disease are reviewed at the biochemistry section of the page. The autosomal recessive nature of the disease and other genetic details are highlighted, along with major medical obstacles and treatment strategies. A variety of related links and articles are included.

30.10 Porphyrias

General Resources

American Porphyria Foundation ○ ○ ○
http://www.enterprise.net/apf

This American Porphyria Foundation provides pages at its site relating to acute intermittent porphyria, porphyria cutanea tarda, erythropoietic protoporphyria, and additional disease variations. Topical discussions include drugs and porphyria, multiple chemical sensitivity syndrome, and testing for porphyrias. Information on telemedicine consultations and links to other porphyria-related sites are offered.

Canadian Porphyria Foundation, Inc. ○ ○
http://www.cpf-inc.ca

The Canadian Porphyria Foundation exists to improve the quality of life for people with the disorder. The site provides a guide to porphyria with an overview of the disease and discussions of causes, types, symptoms, diagnosis, treatment, surgery, heredity, prognosis, and drugs. Links to current and archived newsletters may be accessed.

MediCAD: The Porphyrias ○ ○
http://www.medicad.com/porphyria.html

MediCAD's multimedia presentations include this page reviewing the mechanisms, etiology, and skin lesion histopathology of the various porphyrias. Attack prevention and treatment specific to the various disorder types are reviewed. A table organizes information on heredity, cutaneous manifestations, and extracutaneous manifestations.

Millennium Meeting on Porphyrins and Porphyrias ◐ ◐
http://perso.wanadoo.fr/porphyries-france/millennium_meeting.htm

Information on the Millennium Meeting on Porphyrins and Porphyrias is presented at the conference Web site, with a listing of abstracts accepted by the millennium meeting's scientific committee for poster or oral presentation and discussion of the provisional program. Additional information is downloadable from the site, and registration details and opportunities are provided. Topics include gene replacement therapy in porphyrias, hemoproteins in relation to disease, and clinical aspects, pathophysiology, and management.

Terre Haute Center for Medical Education: The Porphyrias ◐ ◐ ◐
http://www.dentistry.leeds.ac.uk/biochem/thcme/porphyri.html

The Terre Haute Center for Medical Education provides this subsite of the Inborn Errors of Metabolism Page, containing eight links to information on the various porphyrias. Congenital erythropoietic, acute intermittent, porphyria cutanea tarda, and hereditary coproporphyria pages are but a handful of the Online Mendelian Inheritance in Man (OMIM) database pages accessible from the site. Each OMIM entry offers alternative disease titles, a comprehensive literature review, information on modes of inheritance, and additional governmental database links. A clinical synopsis and mini-OMIM entry are found, offering diagnostic and treatment information. A list of allelic variants is offered for most entries.

University of Queensland Porphyria Research Unit: Porphyria: A Patient's Guide ◐ ◐ ◐
http://www.uq.edu.au/porphyria

This online consumer reference contains a discussion of acute porphyria, a safe and unsafe drug listing grouped by drug classification, diagnostic review, and management strategies. Basic information on porphyrin production and enzyme deficiencies, brief review of the various porphyria types, and the care of the skin in porphyria are discussed. A clinical section addresses the features of an acute attack and reviews the possibility of convulsions, fluid and electrolyte imbalances, and neuropathic features.

University of Texas Houston Medical School: Porphyrias ◐ ◐
http://medic.med.uth.tmc.edu/path/00000884.htm

A table outlining the laboratory diagnosis summary is found at this site, as well as connections to several facts sheets on the various porphyrias. Each connection offers further details regarding laboratory findings and treatment.

Acute Intermittent Porphyria

Brent's Porphyria Page ○ ○
http://members.tripod.com/~theaipforum

This personal page, dedicated solely to porphyria news and treatment, includes "Daily Porphnews!," facts from the American Porphyria Foundation, and an enormous assortment of acute intermittent porphyria Web links, updated weekly. Live Internet chat options, laboratory result interpretation information, and porphyria testing details are all included.

Porphyria Foundation of Canada: Acute Intermittent Porphyria ○ ○
http://www.rural.escape.ca/porphyria/p_aip.htm

The Porphyria Foundation of Canada offers visitors general information on acute intermittent porphyria at the site, with stage one through stage four symptomatology reviewed. Dietary instructions, diagnosis via the "Watsom-Schwartz" test, and additional tests for aminolevulinic acid and porphobilinogen are discussed. The dominant inheritance pattern is described, and access to the foundation's main page is provided.

University of Texas Houston Medical School: Acute Intermittent Porphyria ○
http://medic.med.uth.tmc.edu/path/00000805.htm

A discussion of this autosomal dominant disorder is found at this Web address, with information on estimated prevalence, neurological dysfunction seen in acute attacks, additional manifestations, and laboratory findings. Treatment information is reviewed.

Congenital Erythropoietic Porphyria

Biosynthesis of Haem: Erythropoietic Porphyria (Congenital Erythropoietic Porphyria) ○
http://www.broombio.demon.co.uk/presentations/Porphyria/tsld011.htm

A concise description of erythropoietic porphyria is found at this Web site and includes quick facts relating to inheritance, prevalence, and symptoms.

emedicine: Erythropoietic Porphyria ○ ○ ○
http://emedicine.com/cgi-bin/foxweb.exe/
showsection@d:/em/ga?book=derm&topicid=145

This professional reference offers details on erythropoietic porphyria, also known as congenital erythropoietic porphyria. The pathophysiology of this error of porphyrin-heme synthesis, its multi-system manifestations, diagnostic differential links, and a review of all laboratory and diagnostic tests are presented. Histologic dermatopathologic findings, crucial management strategies, and a drug profile of oral photoprotectant medication are supplied.

University of Texas Houston
Medical School: Congenital Erythropoietic Porphyria ◉
http://medic.med.uth.tmc.edu/path/00000810.htm

Clinical manifestations of the skin and erythron are reviewed at this site, which also provides mention of complications, laboratory findings, and prophylactic skin protection measures.

Hereditary Coproporphyria

Healthwise Knowledgebase: Porphyria, Hereditary Coproporphyria
http://www.healthynetwork.com/kbase/nord/nord323.htm

Related disorders, a general discussion of this rare condition, and reviews of symptoms, causes, and standard therapies are provided at this site, sponsored by the National Organization for Rare Disorders, Inc. Details regarding investigational therapies are, additionally, provided.

Porphyria Foundation of Canada:
Hereditary Coproporphyria (HCP) ◉
http://www.rural.escape.ca/porphyria/g_hcp.htm

This synopsis of hereditary coproporphyria reviews inheritance pattern, clinical symptoms, laboratory findings, and treatment.

Porphyria Cutanea Tarda

Iron Disorders Institute: Porphyria Cutanea Tarda ◉ ◉
http://www.irondisorders.org/disorders/pct/index.htm

Six pages of information are accessible from this site, including discussion of the risk groups, symptoms, detection, and treatment of this inherited metabolic disorder. Visitors may click on the sidebar menu to retrieve specific information or view consecutive pages of this disorder entry. Information is concise and includes references.

Postgraduate Medicine: Porphyria Cutanea Tarda ◉ ◉ ◉
http://www.postgradmed.com/issues/1999/04_99/rich.htm

Background information on acquired and inherited porphyrias is introduced at this online article, courtesy of *Postgraduate Medicine*. Medical histories and discussion of the most prevalent variety of the porphyrias are presented and include disease hallmarks, a listing of drugs that may exacerbate symptoms, laboratory abnormalities, and characteristic clinical findings.

Rarer Porphyrias

Merck Manual of Diagnosis and Therapy: Less Common Porphyrias ○ ○ ○
http://www.merck.no/pubs/mmanual/section2/chapter14/14c.htm

The *Merck Manual of Diagnosis and Therapy* offers information regarding several of the less commonly encountered porphyrias, including delta-aminolevulinic acid dehydratase deficiency, congenital erythropoietic porphyria, hepatoerythropoietic porphyria, and additional disorders. Comparisons of symptoms and signs, considerations in diagnosis, and treatment summaries are presented.

Porphyria Foundation of Canada: Rare Forms of Porphyria ○
http://www.rural.escape.ca/porphyria/g_rare.htm

Four rare forms of porphyria are discussed at this Web site, with symptoms and some diagnostic information presented. Connections to an online guide reviewing porphyria types and to the HEME Biosynthetic Pathway table are found.

Variegate Porphyria

New Scientist: Fit For a King ○ ○
http://www.newscientist.com/ns/19990522/newsstory6.html

The improper synthesis of haem is reviewed at this news article, which describes a wide range of symptoms encountered in variegate porphyria, along with a hereditary account of the disease of the British royal family. *New Scientist* explains current research at Dartmouth Medical School in New Hampshire regarding recently recognized, naturally occurring enzymes that are able to detoxify porphyrins.

Porphyria Foundation of Canada: Variegate Porphyria ○ ○
http://www.rural.escape.ca/porphyria/g_vp.htm

The classic photosensitivity and neurovisceral crises present in variegate porphyria are discussed at this site. Theories regarding precipitating factors, symptoms in an acute attack, and treatment measures are outlined.

University of Virginia: Variegate Porphyria Pedigree ○
http://www.people.virginia.edu/~rjh9u/varpor.html

A pedigree of this autosomal dominant disorder of haem metabolism is shown at this page. A characterization of the disease and occurrence information is presented.

31. PARAENDOCRINE AND NEOPLASTIC SYNDROMES

31.1 Carcinoid Tumors and Carcinoid Syndrome

Ask NOAH About: Gastrointestinal Carcinoid Tumor ◐ ◐
http://www.noah.cuny.edu/cancer/nci/cancernet/201064.html
This site features a patient-friendly resource guide that explains the intricacies of gastrointestinal carcinoid tumor. It provides information on the stages of carcinoid tumors, including localized, regional, metastatic, and recurrent stages. In nonscientific language, the site describes treatment options at each stage of the disease. Additionally, the site provides visitors with the telephone numbers and addresses of institutions that offer more information.

Carcinoid Cancer Foundation, Inc. ◐ ◐
http://www.carcinoid.org
The Carcinoid Cancer Foundation encourages and supports research and education related to carcinoid tumors. Their site provides links to newsworthy items, information about special events, and topics of special interest. Visitors may submit questions to a physician to be answered via e-mail or phone. Links to discussion and support groups, personal Web pages, and other sites of interest are found.

H. Lee Moffit Cancer Center and Research Institute: Cancer Control Journal: Carcinoid Tumors of the Gut ◐ ◐ ◐
http://www.moffitt.usf.edu/cancjrnl/v3ns/article2.html
This scientific article offers many insights into carcinoid tumors, beginning with the history of the disorder and continuing with discussions of the pathology, diagnosis, and biochemical characterization of carcinoid tumors. The article provides details on the surgical management of foregut, midgut, and hindgut carcinoid tumors and

reviews prognosis and survival rates. Histological types of carcinoid tumors, magnified images, and biochemical identification review are provided. The primary features of the carcinoid syndrome, useful diagnostic tests, and current treatment recommendations are outlined.

31.2 Medullary Thyroid Carcinoma

Cancer Medicine: Neoplasms of the Neuroendocrine System: Medullary Thyroid Carcinoma (MTC) ◐ ◐

http://intouch.cancernetwork.com/CanMed/Ch102/102-3.htm

A separate chapter on medullary thyroid carcinoma, courtesy of the *Cancer Medicine* publication, offers information on the epidemiology, pathologic considerations, biologic characteristics, and clinical disease features. The distinguishing biochemical features of medullary thyroid carcinoma, diagnostic tests, and considerations with regard to surgical management and treatment of recurrent or metastatic disease are presented.

31.3 Multiple Endocrine Neoplasia

Cancer Medicine: Multiple Endocrine Neoplasia (MEN) Syndromes ◐ ◐ ◐

http://intouch.cancernetwork.com/CanMed/Ch102/102-5.htm

Multiple endocrine neoplasia type 1 and multiple endocrine neoplasia 2A and 2B are presented at this electronic edition of *Cancer Medicine*. Epidemiology, pathologic characteristics, biologic characteristics, clinical features, diagnostic screening tests, and therapeutic considerations are all presented. Treatment of recurrent or metastatic disease is summarized.

Disease Manifestations: Multiple Endocrine Neoplasia Type 2B ◐ ◐

http://www.iadh.org/multiple.htm

The chromosomal mutation associated with multiple endocrine neoplasia type 2B, the purpose of the gene, and the disease's familial or sporadic occurrence are discussed. The autosomal dominant mode of inheritance, oral mucosal neuromas, and a range of endocrine and nonendocrine abnormalities often present are described. Pheochromocytoma, medullary thyroid carcinomas, and other characteristic neoplasms are reviewed, in addition to diagnostic procedures and prognosis.

Italian Multiple Endocrine Neoplasia Network (MENNET) ◐
http://www.dfc.unifi.it/mennet

This Italian study group offers information at its Web site on multiple endocrine neoplasia types 1 and 2, with aims and interests of the collaboration and contact information for genetic testing.

Massachusetts General Hospital: Familial Multiple Endocrine Neoplasia Type I ◐ ◐
http://neurosurgery.mgh.harvard.edu/men-1.htm

Massachusetts General Hospital offers this Web review of familial multiple endocrine neoplasia type 1 (FMEN1) and the various glands that may be affected. Overactivity of the parathyroids, islet cell tumor development, overproduction of pituitary hormones, and less commonly occurring tumors and complications are explained. Treatment of pancreatic cancer in FMEN1, a discussion regarding the considerable variation in symptom presentation, and the future of abnormal gene identification for diagnosis and additional research are reviewed.

NIDDK: Familial Multiple Endocrine Neoplasia Type I ◐ ◐ ◐
http://www.niddk.nih.gov/health/endo/pubs/fmen1/fmen1.htm

Familial multiple endocrine neoplasia type 1 (FMEN1), a genetic disorder, and its effects on the pancreas, pituitary, and parathyroids are described at this information sheet, courtesy of the NIDDK. Hypercalcemia, prolactinomas, rare complications such as islet cell tumors or carcinoids, and FMEN1 genetic testing discussions are offered. The providers of the text encourage its duplication and distribution.

31.4 Pheochromocytoma Syndromes

Neurofibromatosis (Recklinghausen's Disease)

National Neurofibromatosis Foundation, Inc. ◐ ◐ ◐
http://www.nf.org

Details on the organization's International Consortium and individual sections for both patients and healthcare professionals are accessible from the site. The organization's news reel provides information on the latest developments in disease research, and neurofibromatosis trial details are provided. The scientific link offers professionals a worldwide clinician's forum, for specific case discussion, as well as a compilation of recent publications and details on programs of the Foundation. Diagnostic and management details, clinic listings, and pages in foreign languages are included.

Von Hippel Lindau Disease

Von Hippel Lindau Family Alliance ◐ ◐ ◐
http://www.vhl.org

This Von Hippel Lindau Family Alliance page may be viewed in any of several languages listed at the sidebar menu and includes current and archived issues of an online newsletter, DNA testing information, the organization's online bookstore link, and interactive e-mail discussion groups. The professional information link offers a site on the genetic, clinical, and imaging features of Von Hippel Lindau syndrome, as well as patient handouts, VHL conference details, an overview of VHL from the National Cancer Institute, and current suggestions for screening protocols. Support groups in the United States and abroad are listed, and articles from the press contain news related to current research, genetic discoveries, and personal accounts.

32. POLYENDOCRINE DISORDERS

32.1 Autoimmune Polyendocrinopathy

Irish Medical Journal: Unusual Manifestations of Type I Autoimmune Polyendocrinopathy ◉ ◉
http://imj.ie/issue02/Paper5UnusualManifestations.htm

This electronic article contains information regarding the clinical manifestations of autoimmune polyendocrinopathy, with discussion relating to the possibility of a defect in suppressor T-cells. The recent recognition of three distinct syndromes and the findings most commonly found in each are reviewed. Five case examples are summarized, with premature ovarian failure, ocular abnormalities, dental abnormalities, and characteristic adrenal failure described.

Online Mendelian Inheritance in Man (OMIM): Autoimmune Polyendocrinopathy Syndrome ◉ ◉ ◉
http://www3.ncbi.nlm.nih.gov/htbin-post/Omim/dispmim?240300

The OMIM database offers this clinical synopsis of autoimmune polyendocrinopathy syndrome, type 1, also referred to as polyglandular deficiency syndrome. The presence of moniliasis and hypoparathyroidism, and the subsequent onset of adrenal insufficiency, are described at the site, along with allelic variants of the disease and the spectrum of clinical findings in the three syndrome types. Related Medline abstract links are accessible throughout the text.

Online Mendelian Inheritance in Man (OMIM): Schmidt Syndrome ◉ ◉ ◉
http://www3.ncbi.nlm.nih.gov/htbin-post/Omim/dispmim?269200

Schmidt syndrome, also known as type 2 polyglandular autoimmune syndrome, is the subject of this OMIM Web site. The syndromal associations, possibly linked to aberrations on chromosome 6, are reviewed, along with susceptibility in patients to immunological malfunction of a particular immune-response gene. Addison's disease, insulin-dependent and noninsulin-dependent diabetes mellitus, hypothyroidism and hyperthyroidism, and pernicious anemia are the characteristic features described. The disease's possible affiliation with interstitial myositis is cited, and MEDLINE abstracts are accessible throughout the text.

33. SYSTEMIC DISEASES: ENDOCRINE MANIFESTATIONS

33.1 Amyloidosis

Amyloidosis ◎ ◎
http://www.mdmultimedia.com/a/griffith/gr41.htm
An outline of several types of amyloidosis is found at this site, with information on signs and symptoms, causes, risk factors, diagnosis, and treatment alternatives concisely reviewed. References are provided.

Amyloidosis Support Network ◎ ◎ ◎
http://amyloidosis.org
The Amyloidosis Support Network was created to provide education and resources to patients and the general public. At its Web site the organization offers an overview of the disorder, opportunities for patient and family networking, case histories, potential new treatments, and financial issues. Professional information includes links to published papers, conferences and contact information, and article abstracts. Links to related topics are found.

LifeForce Hospitals: Amyloidosis ◎ ◎
http://czubeck.home.texas.net/newpage1.htm
Provided by LifeForce Hospitals, this site contains an in-depth article about amyloidosis, with general considerations summarized and a detailed classification table distinguishing systemic and localized disease variations. Sections on the pathogenesis of amyloidosis, its pathology, and clinical aspects are found. Components of amyloid deposits and information on standards for diagnosis are reviewed.

Mayo Clinic: Primary Amyloidosis ○ ○
http://www.mayo.edu/mmgrg/rst/aapamph.htm

Provided by the Mayo Clinic Rochester, this site offers patient information on primary amyloidosis, with a general overview of amyloidosis and discussions of its effects on the kidneys, heart, and nerves. Diagnosis, treatment, and infection information is provided, in addition to contact details.

33.2 HIV

AIDS Knowledge Base: Endocrine Abnormalities ○ ○
http://hivinsite.ucsf.edu/akb/1997/05endo

A chapter on endocrine abnormalities associated with the human immunodeficiency virus (HIV) is found at this Web site, with an overview of the topic, as well as specific discussion of adrenal insufficiency, hypogonadism, pituitary dysfunction, pancreatic dysfunction, calcium metabolism, and thyroid function abnormalities in HIV.

Aids Treatment News:
Endocrine Complications of HIV Progression ○ ○ ○
http://www.aegis.org/pubs/atn/1991/ATN14001.html

This article, excerpted from *Aids Treatment News*, offers a look at the particular endocrine system disturbances that may result from HIV progression. Endocrine problems as a direct result of the chronic disease process or as a consequence of secondary opportunistic infections are discussed, with signs of endocrine dysfunction generally reviewed. A transcript of an interview with a specialist in the field of adrenal dysfunction covers examples of decreased dehydroepiandrosterone (DHEA) levels, insufficient secretion of cortisol, and related pituitary involvement in AIDS.

Parkland Pocket Guide to HIV Care:
Endocrine Manifestations of HIV ○ ○ ○
http://www.hivbook.com/endo.html

Endocrine manifestations of HIV infection are reviewed at the site, including hyperthyroidism and hypothyroidism, adrenal insufficiency, gonadal dysfunction, and hypertriglyceridemia. Pharmacologic agents used in AIDS treatment and their potentials for inducing endocrine changes are reviewed, with a table outlining specific drugs and their associated side effects. Treatment of AIDS wasting syndrome using a multitude of agents, including androgenic anabolic steroids and human growth hormone, is discussed.

33.3 Malignancy

Cancer Medicine: Adrenal Dysfunction
http://intouch.cancernetwork.com/canmed/Ch187/187-3.htm

This online chapter offers an overview of adrenal dysfunction associated with cancer, including adrenal metastases and adrenal insufficiency. Evaluation of adrenal metastases is discussed in detail, and reference citations are provided.

Cancer Medicine: Endocrine Complications
http://intouch.cancernetwork.com/canmed/Ch187/187-0.htm

A professional overview of endocrine complications of neoplastic illness is found at this Web address, with a review of individual complications followed by specific discussions of thyroid dysfunction, adrenal dysfunction, and pituitary dysfunction. Reference citations are listed.

34. RARE DISORDERS

34.1 National Organization for Rare Disorders (NORD)

The National Organization for Rare Disorders (NORD) is a unique federation of voluntary health agencies, individuals, and medical professionals dedicated to the identification, treatment, and cure of rare "orphan" diseases. There are more than 6,000 of these serious health conditions, most of which are genetically caused. Each orphan disease affects fewer than 200,000 Americans, but combined, they affect more than 25 million people in the United States.

Researching Rare Disorders

NORD rare disorder profiles are available at http://www.rarediseases.org. Clicking on the rare disorders database and entering a search term will return all related glossary entries. A summary of the rare disorder is provided, and a full report containing additional re-sources is available for a nominal sum. The database contains information on over 1,100 diseases written in layman's terminology, including: General Description (abstract), Synonyms, Symptoms, Causes (etiology), Affected Population (epidemiology), Related Disorders (for differential diagnosis), Standard Treatments, Investigational Treatments, Resources (contacts for further information), and References (bibliography). The database can be searched using the disease name, synonyms, or symptoms.

Other Programs

Organization Database
This database lists approximately 1,200 disease-specific organizations and support groups, registries, clinics, Web sites, umbrella organizations, and service agencies. Information includes addresses, phone and fax numbers, Web addresses, publications, and services available through each agency. Most are American agencies, but Canadian and European rare disease organizations are also listed.

Orphan Drug Designation Database
The FDA has designated almost 1,000 pharmaceuticals as "orphan drugs." This database of approved and investigational orphan products lists officially designated orphan drugs, the indications for which they are approved, and ways in which to contact the manufacturers of these orphan drugs. The database is searchable by the name of the product, manufacturer, or the name of the disease.

Contacting NORD

We invite you to contact NORD through the Web site http://www.rarediseases.org, by phone 203-746-6518 (or recorded Help-Line: 1-800-999-6673), or via mail at: NORD, P.O. Box 8923, New Fairfield, CT 06812.

PART FIVE

GENERAL MEDICAL WEB RESOURCES

35. REFERENCE INFORMATION AND NEWS SOURCES

35.1 Abbreviations and Acronyms

Common Medical Abbreviations ○ ○
http://courses.smsu.edu/jas188f/690/medslpterm.html

Several hundred major medical abbreviations are defined in an alphabetical listing at this educational information site.

National Council for Emergency Medicine Informatics (NCEMI) ○ ○ ○
http://www.ncemi.org

The National Council for Emergency Medicine Informatics provides a searchable database for medical abbreviations and acronyms. By clicking on "Abbreviation Translator" and entering the letters to be identified, single or multiple definitions will be returned.

35.2 Abstract, Citation, and Full-text Search Tools

Doctor Felix's Free MEDLINE Page ○ ○
http://www.beaker.iupui.edu/drfelix/index.html

This site, a useful resource for those interested in performing MEDLINE searches for article citations, offers links to sites providing free MEDLINE access to visitors. More than thirty sites are profiled, with information on database coverage, frequency of updates, registration requirements, usage restrictions, document delivery information, and links to additional information on the site. Miscellaneous sources for full MEDLINE access trial periods are also listed.

Infomine: Scholarly Internet Resources ◉ ◉ ◉
http://infomine.ucr.edu/search/bioagsearch.phtml

Infomine offers searchable biological, agricultural, and medical resource collections. Web sites can be browsed by title of resource, subject and title, subject, and keyword. Recently added sites are stored in a separate section. The site also offers links to additional Internet medical resources.

Internet Grateful Med at the National Library of Medicine (NLM) ◉ ◉ ◉
http://igm.nlm.nih.gov

Internet Grateful Med (IGM) is one of the two NLM-sponsored free MEDLINE search systems. The default MEDLINE search includes articles published from 1966 to the present and includes PreMEDLINE. This version of IGM takes advantage of PubMed's ability to display related articles and links to the full text of participating online journals. Other searchable databases include AIDSLINE, AIDSDRUGS, AIDSTRIALS, BIOETHICSLINE, ChemID, DIRLINE, HealthSTAR, HISTLINE, HSRPROJ, OLDMEDLINE, POPLINE, SDILINE, SPACELINE, and TOXLINE. The site also offers a user's guide and specific information on new features of the site.

MEDLINE/PubMed at the National Library of Medicine (NLM) ◉ ◉ ◉
http://www.ncbi.nlm.nih.gov/PubMed

PubMed is a free MEDLINE search service providing access to 11 million citations with links to the full text of articles of participating journals. Probably the most heavily used and reputable free MEDLINE site, PubMed permits advanced searching by subject, author, journal title, and many other fields. It includes an easy-to-use "citation matcher" for completing and identifying references, and its PreMEDLINE database provides journal citations before they are indexed, making this version of MEDLINE more up-to-date than most.

35.3 General Medical Supersites

American Medical Association (AMA) ◉ ◉ ◉
http://www.ama-assn.org

The AMA develops and promotes standards in medical practice, research, and education; acts as advocate on behalf of patients and physicians; and provides discourse on matters important to public health in America. General information is available at the site about the organization; journals and newsletters; policy, advocacy activities, and ethics; education; and accreditation services. AMA news and consumer health information are also found at the site. Resources for physicians include membership details, information on AMA CPT/RBRVS Electronic Medical Systems, Y2K information and preparation suggestions, AMA Alliance information (a national organization of physicians' spouses), descriptions of additional AMA products and services, a discussion of legal issues for physicians, and information on AMA's global activities. Links are provided to AMA member special interest groups for physicians and students. Information for consumers includes medical news; detailed information on a wide range of conditions; general health topic discussions; family health resources for children, adolescents, men, and women; interactive health calculators; healthy recipes; and general safety tips. Specific pages are devoted to comprehensive resources related to HIV/AIDS, asthma, migraines, and women's health. Healthcare providers and patients will find this site an excellent source for accurate and useful health information.

BioSites ○ ○ ○
http://www.library.ucsf.edu/biosites

BioSites is a comprehensive catalog of selected Internet resources in the Biomedical Sciences. The sites were selected as part of a project by staff members of Resource Libraries within the Pacific Southwest Region of the National Network of Libraries of Medicine. Sites are organized by medical topic or specialty field, and users can also search the site by keyword. Featured Web sites are listed by title, but detailed descriptions are not provided.

CenterWatch ○ ○ ○
http://www.centerwatch.com/main.htm

This clinical trials listing service offers patient resources, including a listing of clinical trials by disease category, links to current NIH trials, listings of new FDA drug therapy approvals, and current research headlines. Background information on clinical research is also available to patients unfamiliar with the clinical trials process. Industry professional resources include research center profiles, industry provider profiles, industry news, and career and educational opportunities. Links to related sites of interest to patients and professionals are available at the site.

Health on the Net (HON) Foundation ○ ○ ○
http://www.hon.ch

The Health on the Net Foundation is a nonprofit organization advancing the development and application of new information technologies, notably in the fields of health and medicine. This site offers an engine that searches the Internet as well as the foundation's database for medical sites, hospitals, and support communities. A media gallery contains a searchable database of medical images and videos from various sources. The site also features a list of online journals, articles and abstracts, and papers from conferences and various other medical sources. The HON MeSH tool allows users to browse Medical Subject Headings (MeSH), a hierarchical structure of medical concepts from the National Library of Medicine (NLM). Users can also select a target group, such as healthcare providers, medical professionals, or patients and other individuals, to receive more tailored search results.

HealthGate ◎ ◎ ◎
http://www.healthgate.com

HealthGate offers information resources and health-related articles for healthcare professionals and the general public. Health professional resources include links to research tools, including online journals, drug information, and medical search engines, continuing medical education (CME) resources, news, and patient education materials. Resources for the general public and patients include articles on current health issues and advances, drug and vitamin information, symptoms and medical tests information, and several Webzines devoted to specific topics, including alternative medicine, fitness, nutrition, mental well-being, parenting, travel health, and sexuality. A joint effort of two medical publishers allows site access to full-text journal articles. Search engines allow users to search the site, MEDLINE, or a medical dictionary for information. The site provides users with a good starting point for medical information.

Medical Matrix ◎ ◎ ◎ (free registration)
http://www.medmatrix.org

Medical Matrix offers a list of directories categorized into specialties, diseases, clinical practice resources, literature, education, healthcare and professional resources, medical computing, Internet and technology, and marketplace resources containing classifieds and employment opportunities. Additional features include a site search engine, access to MEDLINE, clinical searches, and links to symposia on the Web, medical textbook resources, patient education materials, continuing medical education information, news, and online journals. Free registration is necessary to access the site.

MedNets ◎ ◎ ◎
http://www.internets.com/mednets

This site houses a collection of proprietary search engines, searching only medical databases. Users can access search engines by medical specialty or disease topic. Other resources include links to the home pages of associations, journals, hospitals, companies, research, government sites, clinical practice guidelines, medical news, and consumer and patient information. The site also includes a set of medical databases and links to search engines provided on the Internet by medical schools.

Medscape ◎ ◎ ◎ (free registration)
http://www.medscape.com

Medscape offers a searchable directory of specialty Web sites that provide information on a wide range of medical specialties. Registration is free, and users can customize the site's home page from a particular computer by choosing a medical specialty. Information in a personalized home page includes news items, conference summaries and schedules, treatment updates, practice guidelines, and patient resources, all pertaining to the chosen field of specialization. The site also includes clinical feature articles and links to special clinical resources.

Megasite Project: A Metasite Comparing Health Information Megasites and Search Engines ○ ○ ○
http://www.lib.umich.edu/megasite/toc.html

The Megasite Project, created by librarians at Northwestern University, the University of Michigan, and Pennsylvania State University, evaluates and provides links to 26 Internet sites providing health information. Criteria for evaluation and comparison include administration and quality control, content, and design. Users can access results of site evaluations, tips for successful site searches, lists of the best general and health information search engines reviewed, and site comparisons listed by evaluation criteria. A bibliography of articles on Web design and Internet resource evaluation is found at the address, as well as descriptions of other aspects of the project.

National Library of Medicine (NLM) ○ ○ ○
http://www.nlm.nih.gov

The National Library of Medicine, the world's largest medical library, collects materials in all areas of biomedicine and healthcare and works on biomedical aspects of technology, the humanities, and the physical, life, and social sciences. This site contains links to government medical databases, including MEDLINE and MEDLINE plus, information on funding opportunities at the National Library of Medicine and other federal agencies, and details of services, training, and outreach programs offered by NLM. Users can access NLM's catalog of resources (LocatorPlus), as well as NLM publications, including fact sheets, published reports, and staff publications. NLM research programs discussed at the site include topics in Computational Molecular Biology, Medical Informatics, and other related subjects.

The Web site features 15 searchable databases, covering journal searches via MEDLINE, AIDS information via AIDSLINE, AIDSDRUGS, AIDSTRIALS, bioethics via BIOETHICSLINE, and numerous other important topics. The "master search engine," nicknamed Internet Grateful Med (IGM), searches MEDLINE using the retrieval engine called PubMed. It is very user-friendly. There are 9 million citations in MEDLINE and PreMEDLINE and the other related databases. Additionally, the NLM provides sources of health statistics, serials programs, and services maintained through a system called SERHOLD.

WebMD ○ ○ ○ (some features fee-based)
http://www.webmd.com

High-quality consumer health information and resources for healthcare professionals are available at this address. Consumer resources include information on conditions, treatments, and drugs; medical news and articles on specific topics; a medical encyclopedia; drug reference resources; a forum for asking health questions; online chat events with medical experts; transcripts of past chat events; message boards; and articles and expert advice on general health topics. Consumers can also join a "community" for more personalized information and forums. Physicians services are available for a fee of US$29.95 monthly (in a twelve-month contract), and includes access to medical news, online journals, and reference databases; online insurance verification and referrals; e-mail, voice mail, fax, and conference call capabilities; practice management tools; online trading; financial services; and other resources. The site includes a preview tour of the service for interested professionals.

35.4 Government Information Databases

CRISP: Computer Retrieval of Information on Scientific Projects
http://www-commons.cit.nih.gov/crisp

CRISP is a searchable database of federally-funded biomedical research projects conducted at universities, hospitals, and other research institutions. Users, including the public, can use CRISP to search for scientific concepts, emerging trends and techniques, or to identify specific projects and/or investigators. This site provides a direct gateway into the searchable database. The NIH funds the operation of CRISP.

Government Information Locator Service
http://www.access.gpo.gov/su_docs/gils/gils.html

Intended to pool access to government information through one search engine, this federal locator service enables a search by topic in which the search word or phrase is placed in quotation marks. Instructions for searching are located at the site.

Healthfinder
http://healthfinder.gov/moretools/libraries.htm

Healthfinder provides links to national medical libraries, such as the National Library of Medicine and the National Institutes of Health Library, and other medical or health sciences libraries on the Internet. Directories of libraries are also available to find local facilities. Visitors can also use a site search engine to find specific health Web resources.

MEDLINEplus: Health Information Database
http://www.nlm.nih.gov/medlineplus/medlineplus.html

A comprehensive database of health and medical information, MEDLINEplus serves a different purpose from its sister service, MEDLINE, which is a bibliographic search engine to locate citations and abstracts in medical journals and reports. MEDLINEplus offers the ability to search by topic and obtain full information rather than citations. The search engine brings up extensive resources on every possible topic, giving complete information on all aspects of the topic. One can search body systems, disorders and diseases, treatments and therapies, diagnostic procedures, side effects, and numerous other important topics related to personal health and the field of medicine in general.

35.5 Government Organizations

Government Agencies and Offices

Administration for Children and Families (ACF) ◎ ◎ ◎
http://www.acf.dhhs.gov

This site provides descriptions of, resources for, and links to ACF programs and services. These sites detail programs and services that relate to areas such as welfare and family assistance, child support, foster care and adoption, Head Start, and support for Native Americans, refugees, and the developmentally disabled. Updated news and information is provided as well.

Administration on Aging ◎ ◎ ◎
http://www.aoa.dhhs.gov

This site provides resources for seniors, practitioners, and caregivers. Resources include news on aging, links to Web sites on aging, statistics about older people, consumer fact sheets, retirement and financial planning information, and help finding community assistance for seniors.

Agency for Toxic Substances and Disease Registry (ATSDR) ◎ ◎ ◎
http://www.atsdr.cdc.gov/atsdrhome.html

The mission of this agency is "to prevent exposure and adverse human health effects and diminished quality of life associated with exposure to hazardous substances from waste sites, unplanned releases, and other sources of pollution present in the environment." Toward this goal, the site posts national alerts and health advisories. It provides answers to frequently asked questions about hazardous substances and lists the minimal risk levels for each of them. The site has a HazDat database developed to provide access to information on the release of hazardous substances from Superfund sites or from emergency events and on the effects of hazardous substances on the health of human populations. A quarterly Hazardous Substances and Public Health Newsletter is available for viewing on the site, as are additional resources for kids, parents, and teachers.

Center for Nutrition Policy and Promotion (CNPP) ◎ ◎ ◎
http://www.usda.gov/cnpp

The Center for Nutrition Policy and Promotion is "the focal point within USDA where scientific research is linked with the nutritional needs of the American public." It provides statistical information and resources for educators, and contains dietary guidelines for Americans, official USDA food plans, and means to request additional publications and information by mail or phone.

Department of Health and Human Services (HHS) ◉ ◉ ◉
http://www.os.dhhs.gov

This site lists HHS agencies and provides links to the individual agency sites. It offers news, press releases, and information on accessing HHS records and contacting HHS officials. It also provides a search engine for all federal HHS agencies and access to HealthFinder.

Epidemiology Program Office ◉ ◉ ◉
http://www.cdc.gov/epo/index.htm

Information and resources on public health surveillance is available here. Publications and software related to epidemiology are available for download. Updated news, events, and international bulletins are also featured at the site.

Federal Web Locator ◉ ◉ ◉
http://www.infoctr.edu/fwl

This is a useful search engine for links to federal government sites and information on the World Wide Web. Users can search agency names and access a table of contents.

Food and Drug Administration (FDA) ◉ ◉ ◉
http://www.fda.gov

The FDA is one of the oldest consumer protection agencies in the United States, monitoring the manufacture, import, transport, storage, and sale of about $1 trillion worth of products each year. This comprehensive site provides information on the safety of foods, human and animal drugs, blood products, cosmetics, and medical devices. The site also contains details of field operations, current regulations, toxicology research, medical products reporting procedures, and answers to frequently asked questions. Users can search the site by keyword and find specific information targeted to consumers, industry, health professionals, patients, state and local officials, women, and children.

Food and Nutrition Service (FNS) ◉ ◉ ◉
http://www.fns.usda.gov/fns

The Food and Nutrition Service (FNS) "reduces hunger and food insecurity in partnership with cooperating organizations by providing children and needy families access to food, a healthful diet and nutrition education in a manner that supports American agriculture and inspires public confidence." The site provides details of FNS nutrition assistance programs such as Food Stamps, WIC, and Child Nutrition. Research, in the form of published studies and reports, is also made available at the site.

Food Safety and Inspection Service ◉ ◉ ◉
http://www.fsis.usda.gov

The Food Safety and Inspection Service (FSIS) is "the public health agency in the U.S. Department of Agriculture responsible for ensuring that the nation's commercial supply of meat, poultry, and egg products are safe, wholesome, and correctly labeled and packaged." This site offers a description of the FSIS and their activities, and provides news, consumer information, publications, and resources for educators.

Government Printing Office (GPO) Access ◉ ◉ ◉
http://www.access.gpo.gov/su_docs

Formed by the Government Printing Office to facilitate the transition of electronic documents, this site is the central location for accessing documents from all three branches of the federal government. It provides free access to the official government versions of some 140,000 titles in plain text or PDF format. GPO Access also contains links to governmental databases, including the Federal Register, the Code of Federal Regulations, and the Congressional Record.

Healthcare Financing Administration ◉ ◉ ◉
http://www.hcfa.gov

Information on Medicare, Medicaid, and Child Health insurance programs is provided here. Statistical data on enrollment in the various programs as well as analysis of recent trends in healthcare spending, employment, and pricing is also provided. The site offers consumer publications and program forms, which are available for download.

Indian Health Service (IHS) ◉ ◉
http://www.ihs.gov

Indian Health Service (IHS) is an agency "within the U. S. Department of Health and Human Services and is responsible for providing federal health services to American Indians and Alaska Natives." This site offers related news and press releases. It details management resources, medical programs, jobs, scholarships, office locations, and contact information.

National Bioethics Advisory Commission (NBAC) ◉ ◉
http://bioethics.gov/cgi-bin/bioeth_counter.pl

NBAC "provides advice and makes recommendations to the National Science and Technology Council and to other appropriate government entities regarding the appropriateness of departmental, agency, or other governmental programs, policies, assignments, missions, guidelines, and regulations as they relate to bioethical issues arising from research on human biology and behavior." It also advises on the applications, including the clinical applications, of that research. This site lists meeting dates, transcripts of meetings, reports, news, and links to related sites.

National Center for Chronic Disease Prevention and Health Promotion ◎ ◎ ◎

http://www.cdc.gov/nccdphp/nccdhome.htm

This site "defines chronic disease, lists major chronic diseases, and describes the cost burden of treating them as well as the cost-effectiveness of prevention." Risk behaviors that lead to chronic disease are discussed, and comprehensive and disease-specific approaches to prevention of chronic diseases are addressed. The site provides access to selected Center reports, newsletters, brochures, and CD-ROMs. Information on conferences, meetings, and news publications is provided along with links to related sites.

National Center for Environmental Health (NCEH) ◎ ◎ ◎

http://www.cdc.gov/nceh/ncehhome.htm

The NCEH "is working to prevent illness, disability, and death from interactions between people and the environment." Site links and information on programs and activities are provided, and access is available to publications and products including NCEH fact sheets, brochures, books, and articles. The site also offers current employment opportunities and information on training programs. Spanish and young adult versions of the NCEH site are also available.

National Center for Health Statistics (NCHS) ◎ ◎ ◎

http://www.cdc.gov/nchs/default.htm

The National Center for Health Statistics (NCHS) is the foremost federal government agency responsible for gathering, analyzing, and disseminating health statistics on the American population." To accomplish the mission of the Center, the NCHS Web site has a site-based search engine and collections of health related statistics organized alphabetically by topic. frequently asked questions are answered on various statistical topics. Useful resources at the site include contact information for obtaining copies of vital records, related catalogs, publications, and other information products.

National Center for Infectious Diseases ◎ ◎ ◎

http://www.cdc.gov/ncidod/index.htm

The mission of the National Center for Infectious Diseases "is to prevent illness, disability, and death caused by infectious diseases in the United States and around the world." The site contains an online bimonthly journal that tracks trends and analyzes new and reemerging infectious disease issues around the world. Resources include general information on infectious diseases, specific infectious disease discussions and descriptions, and links to organizations, associations, journals, newsletters, and other publications. One section of the site is devoted to resources related to travel health.

National Center for Toxicological Research (NCTR) ○ ○
http://www.fda.gov/nctr/index.html

The mission of NCTR "is to conduct peer-reviewed scientific research that supports and anticipates the FDA's current and future regulatory needs." This research is aimed at understanding critical biological events in the expression of toxicity and at developing methods to improve assessment of human exposure, susceptibility, and risk. The site details the accomplishments, current programs, and future goals of the NCTR.

National Guideline Clearinghouse (NGC) ○ ○ ○
http://www.guidelines.gov/index.asp

The National Guideline Clearinghouse (NGC) is a database of evidence-based clinical practice guidelines and related documents produced by the Agency for Health Care Policy and Research (AHCPR), in partnership with the American Medical Association (AMA) and the American Association of Health Plans (AAHP). Users can search the database by keyword or browse by disease category.

National Institute for Occupational Safety and Health (NIOSH) ○ ○ ○
http://www.cdc.gov/niosh/homepage.html

NIOSH "is part of the Centers for Disease Control and Prevention and is the only federal institute responsible for conducting research and making recommendations for the prevention of work-related illnesses and injuries." The site contains updated news, listings of special events and programs, and information on downloading or ordering related publications. It also provides access to databases such as a pocket guide to hazardous chemicals and a topic index of occupational safety and health information.

National Science Foundation, Directorate for Biological Sciences ○ ○ ○
http://www.nsf.gov/bio/ibn/start.htm

The Division of Integrative Biology and Neuroscience (IBN) supports research aimed at understanding the living organism-plant, animal, microbe-as a unit of biological organization. Current scientific emphases include biotechnology, biomolecular materials, environmental biology, global change, biodiversity, molecular evolution, plant science, microbial biology, and computational biology (including modeling). Research projects generally include support for the education and training of future scientists. IBN also supports doctoral dissertation research, research conferences, workshops, symposia, Undergraduate Mentoring in Environmental Biology (UMEB), and a variety of NSF-wide activities. This site describes in detail the activities and divisions of IBN, and offers a staff directory, award listings, and deadline dates for funding applications.

Office of National Drug Control Policy (ONDCP) ○ ○ ○
http://www.whitehousedrugpolicy.gov

This site states the missions and goals of the ONDCP. It has a clearinghouse of drug policy information with a staff that will respond to the needs of the general public, providing statistical data, topical fact sheets, information packets and more. There is information on related science, medicine, and technology. There are also resources on prevention, education, and treatment programs. Information on the enforcement of the policies is provided for the national, state, and local levels.

Office of Naval Research: Human Systems Department ⊙ ⊙
http://www.onr.navy.mil/sci_tech/personnel/default.htm#biological

This site details Medical Science and Technology, and the Cognitive and Neural Science and Technology programs of the Human Systems Department. Procedures for submitting proposals are also outlined at the site.

Public Health Service (PHS) ⊙ ⊙
http://phs.os.dhhs.gov/phs/phs.html

Links to public health service agencies and program offices, and Health and Human Services vacancy announcements are available at this site. The site is linked to the Office of the Surgeon General, providing transcripts of speeches and reports, a biography of the current Surgeon General, and a history and summary of duties associated with the position.

Substance Abuse and Mental Health Services Administration (SAMHSA) ⊙ ⊙ ⊙
http://www.samhsa.gov

SAMHSA "is the federal agency charged with improving the quality and availability of prevention, treatment, and rehabilitation services in order to reduce illness, death, disability, and cost to society resulting from substance abuse and mental illnesses." The site provides substance abuse and mental health information, including details of programs for prevention and treatment in these areas, updated news and statistics, and notices of grant opportunities.

NIH Institutes and Centers

Center for Information Technology (CIT) ⊙ ⊙ ⊙
http://www.cit.nih.gov/home.asp

The Center for Information Technology incorporates the power of modern computers into the biomedical programs and administrative procedures of the NIH by conducting computational biosciences research, developing computer systems, and providing computer facilities. The site provides information on activities and the organization of the Center, contact information, resources for Macintosh users, and links to many useful Information Technology sites. Users can search the site or the CIT Help Desk Knowledgebase for specific information.

Center for Scientific Review (CSR) ○ ○ ○
http://www.drg.nih.gov

The Center for Scientific Review is the focal point at NIH for the conduct of initial peer review, which is the foundation of the NIH grant and award process. The Center carries out a peer review of the majority of research and research training applications submitted to the NIH. The Center also serves as the central receipt point for all such Public Health Service applications and makes referrals to scientific review groups for scientific and technical merit review of applications and to funding components for potential award. To this end, the Center develops and implements innovative, flexible ways to conduct referral and review for all aspects of science. The site contains contact information, transcripts of public commentary panel discussions, news and events listings, grant applications, peer review notes, and links to additional biomedical and government sites.

Centers for Disease Control and Prevention (CDC) ○ ○ ○
http://www.cdc.gov

The mission of the Centers for Disease Control and Prevention is to promote health and quality of life by preventing and controlling disease, injury, and disability. The site provides users with links to 11 associated Centers, Institutes, and Offices; a Web page devoted to travelers' health; publications; software; and other products, data, and statistics; training and employment opportunities; and subscription registration forms for online CDC publications. Highlighted publications include *Emerging Infectious Disease Journal* and *Morbidity and Mortality Weekly Report,* both of which can be e-mailed on a regular basis by registering on this site. Links are available to additional CDC resources, and state and local agencies concerned with public health issues. CDC offers a comprehensive, alphabetical list of general and specific health topics at the site. Visitors can also search the site by keyword, and read spotlights on current research and information presented by the Web site.

Computer Retrieval of Information on Scientific Projects (CRISP) ○ ○ ○
http://www-commons.cit.nih.gov/crisp

CRISP is a comprehensive compilation of abstracts describing the federally funded research projects of academic, healthcare, and research institutions. The database, maintained by the Office of Extramural Research at the National Institutes of Health, includes projects funded by many of the major government agencies, such as the National Institutes of Health (NIH), the Food and Drug Administration (FDA), and the Centers for Disease Control and Prevention (CDCP). Visitors to the site can use the CRISP search interface to identify emerging research trends and techniques or to locate specific projects and/or investigators. General information about the CRISP database and answers to frequently asked questions about CRISP are also available.

Fogarty International Center (FIC) ⊙ ⊙ ⊙

http://www.nih.gov/fic

The Fogarty International Center for Advanced Study in the Health Sciences leads NIH efforts to advance the health of the American public, and citizens of all nations, through international cooperation on global health threats. Resources at the site include Center publications, regional information on programs and contacts, research and training opportunities, a description of the Center's Multilateral Initiative on Malaria (MIM), details of the NIH Visiting Program for Foreign Scientists, and news and vacancy announcements.

National Cancer Institute (NCI) ⊙ ⊙ ⊙

http://www.nci.nih.gov

The National Cancer Institute leads a national effort to reduce the burden of cancer morbidity and mortality, and ultimately to prevent the disease. Through basic and clinical biomedical research and training, the NCI conducts and supports programs to understand the causes of cancer; prevent, detect, diagnose, treat, and control cancer; and disseminate information to the practitioner, patient, and public. The site provides visitors with many informational resources related to cancer, including CancerTrials for clinical trials resources and CancerNet for information on cancer tailored to the needs of health professionals, patients, and the general public. Additional resources relate to funding opportunities, and events and research at NCI.

National Center for Biotechnology Information (NCBI) ⊙ ⊙ ⊙

http://www.ncbi.nlm.nih.gov

A comprehensive site that provides a wide array of biotechnology resources to the user, the NCBI includes sources such as a genetic sequence database (GenBank); links to related sites, a newsletter, site and genetic sequence search engines; information on programs, activities, and research projects; seminar and exhibit schedules; and database services. Databases available through this site include PubMed (for free MEDLINE searching) and OMIM (Online Mendelian Inheritance in Man) for an extensive catalog of human genes and genetic disorders.

National Center for Complementary and Alternative Medicine (NCCAM) ⊙ ⊙ ⊙

http://nccam.nih.gov

The National Center for Complementary and Alternative Medicine identifies and evaluates unconventional healthcare practices, supports, coordinates, and conducts research and research training on these practices, and disseminates information. The site describes specific program areas; answers common questions about alternative therapies; and offers news, research grants information, and a calendar of events. Information resources at the site include a citation index related to alternative medicine obtained from MEDLINE, a bibliography of publications; the NCCAM clearinghouse of information for the public, media, and healthcare professionals; and a link to the National Women's Health Information Center (NWHIC).

National Center for Research Resources (NCRR) ○ ○
http://www.ncrr.nih.gov

The National Center for Research Resources creates, develops, and provides a comprehensive range of human, animal, technological, and other resources to support biomedical research advances. The Center's areas of concentration are biomedical technology, clinical research, comparative medicine, and research infrastructure. The site offers more specific information on each of these research areas, grants information, news, current events, press releases, publications, research resources, and a search engine for locating information at the site.

National Eye Institute (NEI) ○ ○ ○
http://www.nei.nih.gov:80

The National Eye Institute conducts and supports research, training, health information dissemination, and other programs with respect to blinding eye diseases, visual disorders, mechanisms of visual function, preservation of sight, and the special health problems and requirements of the visually impaired. Information at the site is tailored to the needs of researchers, health professionals, the general public and patients, educators, and the media. Resources include a clinical trials database, intramural research information, funding, grants, contract information, news and events calendar, publications, visitor information, a site search engine, and an overview of the NEI offices, divisions, branches, and laboratories.

National Heart, Lung, and Blood Institute (NHLBI) ○ ○ ○
http://www.nhlbi.nih.gov

The National Heart, Lung, and Blood Institute provides leadership for a national research program in diseases of the heart, blood vessels, lungs, and blood, and in transfusion medicine through support of innovative basic, clinical, and population-based and health education research. The site provides health information, scientific resources, research funding information, news and press releases, details of committees, meetings and events, clinical guidelines, notices of studies seeking patient participation, links to laboratories at the NHLBI, and technology transfer resources. Highlights of the site include cholesterol, weight, and asthma management resources.

National Human Genome Research Institute (NHGRI) ○ ○ ○
http://www.nhgri.nih.gov

The National Human Genome Research Institute supports the NIH component of the Human Genome Project, a worldwide research effort designed to analyze the structure of human DNA and determine the location of the estimated 50,000-100,000 human genes. The NHGRI Intramural Research Program develops and implements technology for understanding, diagnosing, and treating genetic diseases. The site provides information about NHGRI, the Human Genome Project, grants, intramural research, policy and public affairs, workshops and conferences, and news items. Resources include links to the Institute's Ethical, Legal, and Social Implications Program and the Center for Inherited Disease Research, genomic and genetic resources for investigators, a glossary of genetic terms, and a site search engine.

National Institute of Allergy and Infectious Diseases (NIAID)

http://www.niaid.nih.gov

NIAID provides the major support for scientists conducting research aimed at developing better ways to diagnose, treat, and prevent the many infectious, immunologic, and allergic diseases that afflict people worldwide. This site provides NIAID news releases, contact information, calendar of events, links to related sites, a clinical trials database, grants and technology transfer information, and current research information (including meetings, publications, and research resources). Fact sheets for public use are available for different immunological disorders, allergies, asthma, and infectious diseases.

National Institute of Arthritis and Musculoskeletal and Skin Diseases (NIAMS)

http://www.nih.gov/niams

The NIAMS conducts and supports a broad spectrum of research on normal structure and function of bones, muscles, and skin, as well as the numerous and disparate diseases that affect these tissues. NIAMS also conducts research training and epidemiologic studies, and disseminates information. The site provides details of research programs at the Institute and offers personnel and employment listings, news, and an events calendar. Health information at the site is provided in the form of fact sheets, brochures, health statistics, and other resources, and contact details are available for ordering materials. Scientific resources include bibliographies of publications, consensus conference reports, grants and contracts applications, grant program announcements, and links to scientific research databases. Information on current clinical studies and transcripts of NIAMS advisory council, congressional, and conference reports are also available at the site.

National Institute of Child Health and Human Development (NICHD)

http://www.nichd.nih.gov

The NICHD conducts and supports laboratory, clinical, and epidemiological research on the reproductive, neurobiologic, developmental, and behavioral processes that determine and maintain the health of children, adults, families, and populations. Research in the areas of fertility, pregnancy, growth, development, and medical rehabilitation strives to ensure that every child is born healthy and wanted, and grows up free from disease and disability. The site provides general information about the Institute; funding and intramural research details; information about the Division of

Epidemiology, Statistics, and Prevention Research; publications bibliography; fact sheets; reports; employment and fellowship listings; and research resources.

National Institute of Dental and Craniofacial Research (NIDCR) ○ ○ ○
http://www.nidr.nih.gov

The National Institute of Dental and Craniofacial Research provides leadership for a national research program designed to understand, treat, and ultimately prevent the infectious and inherited craniofacial-oral-dental diseases and disorders that compromise millions of human lives. General information about the Institute, news and health information, details of research activities, and NIDCR employment opportunities are all found at the site. A site search engine and staff directory are also available.

National Institute of
Diabetes and Digestive and Kidney Diseases (NIDDK) ○ ○ ○
http://www.niddk.nih.gov

The National Institute of Diabetes and Digestive and Kidney Diseases conducts and supports basic and applied research, and provides leadership for a national program in diabetes, endocrinology, and metabolic diseases; digestive diseases and nutrition; and kidney, urologic, and hematologic diseases. NIDDK information at the site includes a mission statement, history, organization description, staff directory, and employment listing. Additional resources include news; a database for health information; clinical trials information, including a patient recruitment section; and information on extramural funding and intramural research at the Institute.

National Institute of Environmental Health Sciences (NIEHS) ○ ○ ○
http://www.niehs.nih.gov

The National Institute of Environmental Health Sciences reduces the burden of human illness and dysfunction from environmental causes by defining how environmental exposures, genetic susceptibility, and age interact to affect an individual's health. News and Institute events, research information, grant and contract details, fact sheets, an Institute personnel directory, employment and training notices, teacher support, and an online resource for kids are all found at this site. Library resources include a book catalog, electronic journals, database searching, NIEHS publications, and reference resources. Visitors can use search engines at the site to find environmental health information and news, publications, available grants and contracts, and library resources.

National Institute of General Medical Sciences (NIGMS) ○ ○ ○
http://www.nih.gov/nigms

The National Institute of General Medical supports basic biomedical research that is not targeted to specific diseases, but that increases the understanding of life processes, and lays the foundation for advances in disease diagnosis, treatment, and prevention. Among the most significant results of this research has been the development of recombinant DNA technology, which forms the basis for the biotechnology industry. The site provides information about NIGMS research and funding programs, information for visitors, news, publications list, reports, grant databases, a personnel and employment listing, and links to additional biomedical resources.

National Institute of Mental Health (NIMH) ◎ ◎ ◎
http://www.nimh.nih.gov

The National Institute of Mental Health provides national leadership dedicated to understanding, treating, and preventing mental illnesses through basic research on the brain and behavior, and through clinical, epidemiological, and services research. Resources available at the site include staff directories, information for visitors to the campus, employment opportunities, NIMH history, and publications from activities of the National Advisory Mental Health Council and Peer Review Committees. News, a calendar of events, information on clinical trials, funding opportunities, and intramural research are also provided. Pages tailored specifically for the public, health practitioners, or researchers contain mental disorder information, research fact sheets, statistics, science education materials, news, links to NIMH research sites, and patient education materials.

National Institute of Neurological Disorders and Stroke (NINDS) ◎ ◎ ◎
http://www.ninds.nih.gov

The National Institute of Neurological Disorders and Stroke supports and conducts research and research training on the normal structure and function of the nervous system, and on the causes, prevention, diagnosis, and treatment of more than 600 nervous system disorders including stroke, epilepsy, multiple sclerosis, Parkinson's disease, head and spinal cord injury, Alzheimer's disease, and brain tumors. The site provides visitors with an organizational diagram, e-mail directory, links to advisory groups, the mission and history of NINDS, a site search engine, employment and training opportunities, and information on research at NINDS. Information is available for patients, clinicians, and scientists, including publications, details of current clinical trials, links to other health organizations, and research funding information.

National Institute of Nursing Research (NINR) ◎ ◎ ◎
http://www.nih.gov/ninr

The National Institute of Nursing Research supports clinical and basic research to establish a scientific basis for the care of individuals across the life span, from management of patients during illness and recovery to the reduction of risks for disease and disability and the promotion of healthy lifestyles. NINR accomplishes its mission by supporting grants to universities and other research organizations as well as by conducting research intramurally at laboratories in Bethesda, Maryland. Visitors to this site can find the NINR mission statement and history, employment listings, news, conference details, publications, speech transcripts, answers to Frequently Asked Questions, information concerning legislative activities, research program and funding details, health information, highlights and outcomes of current nursing research, and links to additional Web resources.

National Institute on Aging (NIA) ○ ○ ○
http://www.nih.gov/nia

The National Institute on Aging leads a national program of research on the biomedical, social, and behavioral aspects of the aging process; the prevention of age-related diseases and disabilities; and the promotion of a better quality of life for all older Americans. The site presents recent announcements and upcoming events, employment opportunities, press releases, and media advisories of significant findings. Research resources include news from the National Advisory Council on Aging, links to extramural aging research conducted throughout the United States, and funding and training information. Health professionals and the general public can access publications on health and aging topics, or order materials online.

National Institute on Alcohol Abuse and Alcoholism (NIAAA) ○ ○ ○
http://www.niaaa.nih.gov:80

The National Institute on Alcohol Abuse and Alcoholism conducts research focused on improving the treatment and prevention of alcoholism and alcohol-related problems to reduce the enormous health, social, and economic consequences of this disease. General resources at the site include an introduction to the Institute, extramural and intramural research information, an organizational flowchart, details of legislative activities, Advisory Council roster and minutes, information on scientific review groups associated with the Institute, a staff directory, and employment announcements. Institute publications, data tables, press releases, conferences and events calendars, answers to frequently asked questions on the subject of alcohol abuse and dependence, and links to related sites are also found at the site. The ETOH Database, an online bibliographic database containing over 100,000 records on alcohol abuse and alcoholism can be accessed from the site, as well as the National Library of Medicine's MEDLINE database.

National Institute on Deafness and Other Communication Disorders (NIDCD) ○ ○ ○
http://www.nih.gov/nidcd

The National Institute on Deafness and Other Communication Disorders conducts and supports biomedical research and research training in the normal and disordered processes of hearing, balance, smell, taste, voice, speech, and language. The Institute also conducts and supports research and research training related to disease prevention and health promotion; addresses special biomedical and behavioral problems associated with people who have communication impairments or disorders; and supports efforts to create devices that substitute for lost and impaired sensory and communication function. The site provides visitors with many fact sheets and other information resources on hearing and balance; smell and taste; voice, speech, and language; hearing aids; otosclerosis; vocal abuse and misuse; and vocal cord paralysis. Other resources include a directory of organizations related to hearing, balance, smell, taste, voice, speech, and language, a glossary of terms, an online newsletter, information for kids and teachers, clinical trials details, and a site search engine. Information on research funding and intramural research activities, news and events calendar, and general information about NIDCD is also available at this site.

National Institute on Drug Abuse (NIDA) ○ ○ ○
http://www.nida.nih.gov/NIDAHome1.html
The National Institute on Drug Abuse leads the nation in bringing the power of science to bear on drug abuse and addiction through support and conduct of research across a broad range of disciplines, and rapid and effective dissemination of results of that research to improve drug abuse and addiction prevention, treatment, and policy. The site contains fact sheets on common drugs of abuse and prevention strategies, Institute announcements, media advisories, congressional testimonies, speech transcripts, online newsletters, scientific meeting dates and summaries, funding, training, legislation information, and links to related sites. Recent research reports and news related to drug addiction are highlighted at the site.

National Institutes of Health (NIH) ○ ○ ○
http://www.nih.gov
NIH is one of eight health agencies of the Public Health Service which, in turn, is part of the U.S. Department of Health and Human Services. The NIH mission is to uncover new knowledge that will lead to better health for everyone. NIH works toward that mission by conducting research in its own laboratories; supporting the research of non-federal scientists in universities, medical schools, hospitals, and research institutions throughout the country and abroad; helping in the training of research investigators; and fostering communication of biomedical information. The site provides a Director's message about the agency, e-mail and telephone directories, visitor information, employment and summer internship program information, science education program details, and a history of NIH. A site search engine and links to the home pages of all NIH Institutes and Centers are available.

National Library of Medicine (NLM) ○ ○ ○
http://www.nlm.nih.gov
The National Library of Medicine, the world's largest medical library, collects materials in all areas of biomedicine and healthcare and works on biomedical aspects of technology, the humanities, and the physical, life, and social sciences. This site contains links to government medical databases, including MEDLINE and MEDLINE plus, information on funding opportunities at the National Library of Medicine and other federal agencies, and details of services, training, and outreach programs offered by NLM. Users can access NLM's catalog of resources (LocatorPlus), as well as NLM publications, including fact sheets, published reports, and staff publications. NLM

research programs discussed at the site include topics in Computational Molecular Biology, Medical Informatics, and other related subjects.

The Web site features 15 searchable databases, covering journal searches via MEDLINE, AIDS information via AIDSLINE, AIDSDRUGS, AIDSTRIALS, bioethics via BIOETHICSLINE, and numerous other important topics. The "master search engine," nicknamed Internet Grateful Med (IGM), searches MEDLINE using the retrieval engine called PubMed. It is very user-friendly. There are 9 million citations in MEDLINE and PreMEDLINE and the other related databases. Additionally, the NLM provides sources of health statistics, serials programs, and services maintained through a system called SERHOLD.

Warren Grant Magnuson Clinical Center ◐ ◐ ◐
http://www.cc.nih.gov:80

The Warren Grant Magnuson Clinical Center is the clinical research facility of the National Institutes of Health, supporting clinical investigations conducted by the Institutes. The Clinical Center was designed to bring patient-care facilities close to research labs, allowing findings of basic and clinical scientists to move quickly from labs to the treatment of patients. The site provides visitors with news, events, details of current clinical research studies, patient recruitment resources, links to departmental Web sites, and information resources for NIH staff, patients, physicians, and scientists. Topics discussed in the Center's Medicine for the Public Lecture Series and resources in medical and scientific education offered by the Center are included at the site.

35.6 Guides to Medical Journals on the Internet

Amedeo ◐ ◐ ◐ (free registration)
http://www.amedeo.com

Amedeo is a free medical literature service, allowing users to select topics and journals of interest. The service sends a weekly e-mail with an overview of new articles reflecting the specifications indicated by the user, and creates a personal home page with abstracts of relevant articles. The site allows registered users to access a Network Center, which facilitates literature exchange among users with similar interests. This service is supported through educational grants by numerous pharmaceutical companies.

BioMedNet:
The Internet Community for Biological and Medical Researchers ◐ ◐ ◐
http://www.biomednet.com/library

Owned by publishing giant Reed Elsevier, this site contains a full text library of over 170 biomedical journals, most of which are available for a fee ranging from US$1-$20. Other features include a shopping mall for books, software, and biological supplies; an evaluated MEDLINE system; a list of biomedical site links; a job exchange; and a science news journal. Free BioMedNet membership provides access to many of the site's features. Some publications, such as the Current Biology journals, offer free access to editorials, short articles, and letters. Prices and special offers can be found on each journal's home page under "Prices/Subscriptions." All visitors to the site can search the journals library and view abstracts without incurring charges.

Blackwell Science ○ ○ ○
http://www.blackwell-science.com/uk/journals.htm

This site offers online access to information regarding well over 200 Blackwell Science Publications. Journals are sorted alphabetically by title and are available in all major fields of science and medicine. Blackwell Science provides a good general overview regarding the content and aim of each of its journals. Tables of contents are available for current and back issues of each title. Access to abstracts and articles requires a fee.

Cambridge University Press: Online Journals ○ ○ ○
http://www.journals.cup.org/journals.htm

Journal titles available online from Cambridge University Press are listed at this address. Topics encompass all subject areas, but many are devoted to medical specialties. Tables of contents and abstracts are provided once a user chooses the publication and issue of interest. Visitors can browse both current and archived issues.

Elsevier Science ○ ○ ○
http://www.elsevier.com

Covering the same Elsevier publications as Science Direct, this site's journal coverage is a bit more up-to-date, and it includes a table of contents search engine. The site also provides many links to journal-related information and subject categories for easy browsing of references in areas of interest. Information is also included on Elsevier's books, and an e-mail alerting service on subject-specific titles from Elsevier's books and journals is available free with registration.

EurekAlert ○ ○ ○
http://www.eurekalert.org

This site allows professionals and consumers to search the archives for the latest articles, news items, events, awards, and grants in science and medicine, including psychiatry. Current news from the Howard Hughes Medical Institute and the National Institutes of Health, as well as numerous links to institutions, journals, and other online resources are available.

Harcourt International: Journal Subject List ○ ○ ○
http://www.harcourt-international.com/journals/jsbrowse.cfm

Harcourt offers a directory of its publications at this address, organizaed by topic. Seventy-eight distinct topics related to medicine, biochemistry, alternative medicine, and veterinary medicine are listed. Once a specific journal is chosen, visitors are sent to a home page of the journal which typically provides a table of contents and abstracts of articles in the latest and previous issues.

Hardin Library Electronic Journal Showcase ○ ○ ○
http://www.lib.uiowa.edu/hardin/md/ej.html

The University of Iowa Hardin Library for the Health Sciences has compiled an index of free full-text journals on the Internet. Using this convenient listing, a user can go straight to a particular journal and retrieve the full text of an article, free-of-charge. Some journals are on a free-trial basis, and sample journal articles are provided for reference.

Highwire Press ○ ○ ○
http://highwire.stanford.edu

One of the largest producers of online versions of biomedical journals, Highwire Press's Web page presents an organized list (by alphabet or subject) of its biomedical journals, including detailed information regarding what is available at no charge for each title. For each journal, there is a link to its page, where tables of contents and abstracts are available. Full text of entire journals or back issues are available for a good number of titles.

Karger ○ ○ ○
http://www.karger.com

Karger provides online access to information on all of its publications. Journals are sorted by title and by subject area. Karger publishes hundreds of journals in an extensive variety of medical and related science fields. Table of contents and article abstracts are available free-of-charge. There is an extensive listing of back issues as well. A free sample issue of each publication is provided. However, a fee is assessed for access to articles.

Kluwer Academic Publishers: Journal Home Pages ○ ○
http://www.wkap.nl/jrnlsubject.htm/F+0+0+0

Journals of interest in medicine and related subjects are listed in Kluwer's directory of products. Journal titles are listed by topic, and each title links to a home page. The home page provides a list of editors, a summary of the aim and scope of the publication, information on indexing and abstracting services, instructions for authors, and contact details for the publishing editor. Visitors can also browse through the table of contents for current and archived issues, and conduct searches by keyword for returns of specific articles.

Marcel Dekker Product Catalog: Medicine ◎ ◎
http://www.dekker.com/catalog/catalog_top.htm

This online product catalog lists journals, books, and other publications offered by Marcel Dekker in the field of medicine. Publications are listed by medical specialty, and each specialty lists all journals and other publications relevant to the field. Visitors can browse these listings, click on relevant journal titles, and access free table of contents and abstract listings from the journal home page.

MDConsult ◎ ◎ ◎ (fee-based)
http://www.mdconsult.com

MDConsult is a comprehensive online medical information service specifically designed for physicians. This is service is provided for a monthly fee of US$19.95, but a 10-day free trial is available. The service includes the ability to search 35 online medical reference books for information and 48 journals for full-text articles. Searches can also be performed for full text articles through MEDLINE and other databases. Members can also search patient education handouts, drug information, and practice guidelines. Additional resources include reviews of new developments from major journals, government agencies, and medical conferences, and a section devoted to what patients are reading in the popular press.

Medical Matrix ◎ ◎ ◎ (free registration)
http://www.medmatrix.org

Following a brief free registration, this site offers a wealth of information in all major medical fields, with continuous updating, rating, and annotating provided by an editorial board and contributors' group composed of physicians and librarians. Each link also includes a description of what can be accessed free of charge at that site. Most of the journal sites covered provide free access to a table of contents and abstracts. However, some may assess a fee when accessing full-text versions of journals. Links to other Web resources in a variety of specialty areas, diseases, and clinical practice subjects are also provided, as well as a MEDLINE search engine, plus medical textbook and CME links.

MEDLINE Journal Links to Publishers ◎ ◎ ◎
http://www.ncbi.nlm.nih.gov/entrez/journals/loftext_noprov.html

Through the National Library of Medicine, the MEDLINE service provides direct access to hundreds of medical journals in all fields, listed alphabetically by name, with direct links to their respective publishers. Upon accessing an individual publication, the reader can normally view the current issue table of contents and abstracts for the articles. In certain cases, the complete article texts are available without charge, but in other cases it is necessary to pay a fee and obtain an access password. Each page explains the available information and the conditions for access, since policies vary by publisher and journal.

MedNets: Journals ○ ○ ○
http://www.mednets.com/journals.htm

MedNets offers comprehenisve directories of online journals in many medical specialties at this address. Directories are listed alphabetically by specialty. Users can also search MEDLINE for relevant articles through the site.

Mosby Publishers: Journals Arranged by Specialty ○ ○ ○
http://www1.mosby.com/scripts/om.dll/serve?action=list&listtype=spec&link=home

A directory of Mosby journals devoted to medical topics is available at this site, with journals listed by medical specialty. Visitors can access table of contents and abstracts of both current and archived issues by following the appropriate journal title link at this address.

Munksgaard
International Publishers: Alphabetical List of Journals ○ ○ ○
http://www.munksgaarddirect.dk/usr/munksgaard/tidsskrifter.nsf/Alfabetisk?OpenView

Munskgaard offers an alphabetical list of scientific publications at this address. Visitors can click on a journal of interest and access tables of contents for current and archived issues, as well as information on subscribing or accessing full-text articles online through a separate service.

National Library of Medicine (NLM):
MEDLINE Journals with Links to Publisher Web Sites ○ ○ ○
http://www.ncbi.nlm.nih.gov/PubMed/fulltextpub.html

This directory offers a comprehensive list of journals cataloged in the MEDLINE database, with links to journal home pages. Journals are listed by publisher.

PubList: Health and Medical Sciences ○ ○ ○
http://www.publist.com/indexes/health.html

This site contains an extensive list of links to medical journals, divided by subject areas. Useful information, such as frequency, publisher, and format is included for each publication, and a search engine can be used to identify titles of interest.

Science Direct ○ ○ ○
http://www.sciencedirect.com

A very useful site, Science Direct compiles an extensive list of links to online journal literature published by Elsevier Science in all major areas of scientific study, including clinical medicine. Access to full text is available by institutional subscription only; however, table of contents are provided free-of-charge for each journal. The site provides links to hundreds of journals categorized by subject and further subdivided by specialty. Journals are also listed alphabetically by title.

science.komm Internet Directory and Resource Site: Medical Journals Main Index ○ ○ ○
http://www.sciencekomm.at/journals/medicine/med-bio.html

Visitors to this address will find comprehensive listings of online journals, categorized by specialty topic. Major broad-coverage medical journals, nursing journals, and books on medical writing are also listed through the site.

Springer-Verlag's LINK ○ ○ ○ (some features fee-based)
http://link.springer.de/ol/medol/index.htm

Covering the large list of journals published by Springer-Verlag, this site mostly contains abstracts rather than full-text articles. Full text is available for those titles for which individuals or institutions maintain print subscriptions. The site covers a broad range of biomedical titles, all of which provide tables of contents from the most recent two to four years.

UnCover Web ○ ○ ○ (some features fee-based)
http://uncweb.carl.org

This enormous database of medical and nonscientific journals' tables of contents permits searching by keyword, journal title, or author. Full articles can be faxed or e-mailed for a fee. For a modest price, the "Reveal" service provides e-mailed tables of contents for specific journals as they are published and added to the database.

WebMedLit ○ ○ ○
http://webmedlit.silverplatter.com/index.html

WebMedLit provides access to the latest medical literature on the Web by indexing medical Web sites daily and presenting articles from each site organized by subject categories. All WebMedLit article links are from the original source document at the publisher's Web site, and most articles are available in full text.

Wiley Interscience ○ ○ ○
http://www3.interscience.wiley.com/index.html

This site is maintained by John Wiley and Sons, Inc. and provides links to all Wiley publications. Hundreds of titles are available online via direct link from the publisher. Journals are available in business, law, and all areas of science, including life and medical science. The Journal Finder option allows the user to search journals by title and subject. Free registration allows access to table of contents and abstracts published within the last 12 months. Full text access is available via registration to both individual and institutional subscribers of the print counterparts of the Wiley online journals.

35.7 Health and Medical Hotlines

Toll-Free Numbers for Health Information
http://nhic-nt.health.org/Scripts/Tollfree.cfm
A categorized list of toll-free health information hotlines is provided by this site. Each hotline provides educational materials for patients.

35.8 Hospital Resources

American Hospital Association
http://www.aha.org
Everything pertaining to hospitals is either available at this site or at a link from this site, including advocacy, health insurance, extensive hospital information, research and education, health statistics, and valuable links to the National Information Center for Health Services Administration as well as other organizations and resources.

HospitalDirectory.com
http://www.doctordirectory.com/hospitals/directory
This useful site provides a listing of states and territories, each of which is a hot link to a further listing of cities in the state or territory. By clicking on a city, the database provides a listing of hospitals in that area, including name, address, and telephone numbers. The site also offers other links pertaining to health plans, doctors, health news, insurance, and medical products for physicians.

HospitalWeb
http://neuro-www2.mgh.harvard.edu/hospitalwebworld.html
This site is a guide to global hospitals on the World Wide Web (not including the United States). It lists over 50 countries. Under each country, the names of a number of hospitals in that country are listed. By clicking on the hospital name, the user is taken to the hospital's Web site which provides further information.

35.9 Internet Newsgroups

General Medical Topic Newsgroups
Internet newsgroups are places where individuals can post messages on a common site for others to read. Many newsgroups are devoted to medical topics, and these groups are listed below. To access these groups you can either use a newsreader program (often part of an e-mail program), or search and browse using a popular Web site, http://www.deja.com.

Since newsgroups are mostly unmoderated, there is no editorial process or restrictions on postings. The information at these groups is therefore neither authoritative nor based on any set of standards.

sci.med	sci.med.nutrition	sci.med.vision
sci.engr.biomed	sci.med.occupational	alt.image.medical
sci.med.aids	sci.med.orthopedics	alt.med
sci.med.cardiology	sci.med.pathology	alt.med.allergy
sci.med.dentistry	sci.med.pharmacy	alt.med.cfs
sci.med.diseases.cancer	sci.med.physics	alt.med.ems
sci.med.diseases.hepatitis	sci.med.prostate.bph	alt.med.equipment
sci.med.diseases.lyme	sci.med.prostate.cancer	alt.med.fibromyalgia
sci.med.diseases.viral	sci.med.prostate.prostatitis	alt.med.outpat.clinic
sci.med.immunology	sci.med.psychobiology	alt.med.phys-assts
sci.med.informatics	sci.med.radiology	alt.med.urum-outcomes
sci.med.laboratory	sci.med.telemedicine	alt.med.veterinary
sci.med.nursing	sci.med.transcription	alt.med.vision.improve

35.10 Locating a Physician

American Medical Association (AMA): Physician Select Online Doctor Finder ○ ○ ○

http://www.ama-assn.org/aps/amahg.htm

The AMA is the primary "umbrella" professional association of physicians and medical students in the United States. The AMA Physician Select system provides information on virtually every licensed physician, including more than 650,000 physicians and doctors of osteopathy. According to the site, physician credentials have been certified for accuracy and authenticated by accrediting agencies, medical schools, residency programs, licensing and certifying boards, and other data sources. The user can search for physicians by name or by medical specialty.

HealthPages ○ ○ ○

http://www.thehealthpages.com

This search tool allows visitors to locate doctors in their area by specialty and location. Over 500,000 physicians and 120,000 dentists are listed. Doctors may update their profiles free-of-charge. Local provider choices are displayed to consumers in a comparative format. They can access charts that compare the training, office services, and fees of local physicians; the provider networks and quality measures of area managed care plans; the size, services, and fees of local hospitals; and more. Patients can post ratings and comments about their doctors.

Physicians' Practice ⊙ ⊙
http://www.physicianpractice.com

This site allows the user to search for doctors in many specialty areas. Searches are performed by specialty and zip code. Physicians must pay a fee to be listed but enjoy other benefits such as referrals, Internet presence, and a newsletter.

35.11 Medical and Health Sciences Libraries

Medical Libraries at
Universities, Hospitals, Foundations, and Research Centers ⊙ ⊙ ⊙
http://www.lib.uiowa.edu/hardin-www/hslibs.html

This site includes an up-to-date listing of libraries that can be easily accessed through links produced by staff members of the Hardin Library at the University of Iowa. Libraries are listed state by state enabling easy access to hundreds of library Web sites, and numerous foreign medical library links are also provided.

National Institutes of Health (NIH): Library Online ⊙ ⊙ ⊙
http://libwww.ncrr.nih.gov

This site presents information about the NIH Library including a staff listing, current exhibits, hours, materials available to NIH personnel and the general public, current job vacancies, maps for visitors, and answers to frequently asked questions about the Library. Users can search the Library's catalog of books, journals, and other periodicals, access public and academic medical databases, and find seminar and tutorial information, as well as links to related sites.

National Library of Medicine (NLM) ⊙ ⊙ ⊙
http://www.nlm.nih.gov

The National Library of Medicine, the world's largest medical library, collects materials in all areas of biomedicine and healthcare and works on biomedical aspects of technology, the humanities, and the physical, life, and social sciences. This site contains links to government medical databases, including MEDLINE and MEDLINE plus, information on funding opportunities at the National Library of Medicine and other federal agencies, and details of services, training, and outreach programs offered by NLM. Users can access NLM's catalog of resources (LocatorPlus), as well as NLM publications, including fact sheets, published reports, and staff publications. NLM research programs discussed at the site include topics in Computational Molecular Biology, Medical Informatics, and other related subjects.

The Web site features 15 searchable databases, covering journal searches via MEDLINE, AIDS information via AIDSLINE, AIDSDRUGS, AIDSTRIALS, bioethics via BIOETHICSLINE, and numerous other important topics. The "master search engine," nicknamed Internet Grateful Med (IGM), searches MEDLINE using the retrieval engine called PubMed. It is very user-friendly. There are 9 million citations in MEDLINE and PreMEDLINE and the other related databases.

Additionally, the NLM provides sources of health statistics, serials programs, and services maintained through a system called SERHOLD.

National Network of Libraries of Medicine (NN/LM) ◎ ◎ ◎
http://www.nnlm.nlm.nih.gov

Composed of 8 regional libraries, the NN/LM also provides access to numerous health science libraries in each region, located at universities, hospitals, and institutes. The Web site enables the user to link directly to each of the libraries in any regional of the United States. These libraries have access to the NLM's SERHOLD system database of machine-readable holdings for biomedical serial titles. There are approximately 89,000 serial titles that are accessible through SERHOLD-participating libraries.

35.12 Medical Conferences and Meetings

Doctor's Guide: Medical Conferences and Meetings ◎ ◎ ◎
http://www.pslgroup.com/medconf.htm

This address lists several hundred conferences and meetings, including continuing medical education (CME) programs worldwide, organized by date, meeting site, and subject. Location and other details are provided.

Health on the Net (HON) Foundation ◎ ◎ ◎
http://www.hon.ch/cgi-bin/conferences

This site provides a limited listing of conferences and meetings in medical specialty areas, and they are not categorized or indexed by fields. Information is chronological by month.

Medical Conferences.com ◎ ◎ ◎
http://www.medicalconferences.com

This site covers a broad range of medical conference listings, including meetings related to many different areas of healthcare including pharmaceuticals and hospital supplies, as well as the clinical medical specialties. An easy-to-use search mechanism provides access to the numerous listings, each of which links to details concerning each conference. The site claims to be updated daily, providing details on over 7,000 forthcoming conferences.

MediConf Online ○ ○ ○ (some features fee-based)
http://www.mediconf.com/online.html

This well-organized site lists conferences by medical subject, chronology, and geographic location, mostly covering meetings to be held in the next month or two. The listings include research conferences, seminars, annual meetings of professional societies, medical technology trade shows, and opportunities for CME credits. What is provided free on the Internet is only a small percentage of the complete fee-based database, which includes more than 60,000 listings of meetings to be held through 2014, and is available through the information vendors, Ovid or Dialog.

Medmeetings ○ ○ ○
http://www.medmeetings.com

The site is a service of the International Medical News Group (IMNG), which publishes six major independent newspapers for physicians. The database includes information on thousands of medical meetings and conventions. Searches can be performed by disease, specialty group, date, location, availability of CME credit, and other criteria.

Medscape: Conference Summaries and Schedules ○ ○ ○
http://www.medscape.com

This service enables members to attend important meetings, catch up on missed meetings, or review sessions later by way of "comprehensive next-day summaries by world-renowned faculty in the form of in-depth online coverage." Medscape also provides access to both free and fee-based continuing medical education courses online. Schedules for upcoming conferences in specialty areas are provided.

Physician's Guide to the Internet ○ ○ ○
http://www.physiciansguide.com/meetings.html

Dates and locations for major national medical meetings are listed alphabetically by association at this site. There are also some hyperlinks to association pages and contact persons.

Princeton Medicon: The Medical Conference Resource ○ ○ ○
http://www.medicon.com.au

This comprehensive site contains details regarding worldwide major medical conferences of interest to medical specialists and primary care professionals. It is also periodically published in printed form. Access to lists of meetings is provided through a useful search engine that permits searching by specialty, year, and geographic region.

35.13 Medical Data and Statistics

Centers for Disease Control and Prevention (CDC): Biostatistics/Statistics ⊙ ⊙ ⊙
http://www.cdc.gov/niosh/biostat.html

This address provides visitors with links to sources of national statistics. Resources include federal, county and city data, as well as statistics related to labor, current population, public health, economics, trade, and business. Sources for mathematics and software information are also found through this site.

Health Sciences Library System (HSLS): Health Statistics ⊙ ⊙ ⊙
http://www.hsls.pitt.edu/intres/guides/statcbw.html

The University of Pittsburgh's Falk Library of the Health Sciences developed this site to provide information on obtaining statistical health data from Internet and library sources. Resources include details on obtaining statistical data from United States population databases, government agencies collecting statistics, organizations and associations collecting statistics, and other Web sites providing statistical information. The site explains specific Internet and library tools for locating health statistics, and offers a glossary of terms used in statistics.

National Center for Health Statistics (NCHS) ⊙ ⊙ ⊙
http://www.cdc.gov/nchs/default.htm

The NCHS, located within the Centers for Disease Control and Prevention of the U.S. Department of Health and Human Services, provides an extensive array of health and medical statistics for the medical, research, and consumer communities. This site provides express links to numerous surveys and statistical sources at the NCHS.

University of Michigan Documents Center: Statistical Resources on the Web: Health ⊙ ⊙ ⊙
http://www.lib.umich.edu/libhome/Documents.center/sthealth.html

Online sources for health statistics are cataloged at this site, including comprehensive health statistics resources and sources for statistics by topic. Topics include abortion, accidents, births, deaths, disability, disease experimentation, hazardous substances, healthcare, health insurance, HMOs, hospitals, life tables, mental health, noise, nursing homes, nutrition, pregnancy, prescription drugs, risk behaviors, substance abuse, surgery, transplants, and vital statistics. Users can also access an alphabetical directory of sites in the database and a search engine for locating more specific resources.

World Health Organization (WHO): Statistical Information System ◉ ◉ ◉

http://www.who.int/whosis

The Statistical Information System of WHO (WHOSIS) is intended to provide access to both statistical and epidemiological data and information from this international agency in electronic form. The site provides health statistics, disease information, mortality statistics, AIDS/HIV data, immunization coverage and incidence of communicable diseases, links to statistics from other countries, as well as links to the Centers for Disease Control and Prevention in the United States. This site is the premier resource for statistics on diseases worldwide. See also the WHO main site: http://www.who.int for some additional disease-related statistics.

35.14 Medical Dictionaries, Encyclopedias, and Glossaries

BioTech's Life Science Dictionary ◉ ◉ ◉

http://biotech.icmb.utexas.edu/search/dict-search.html

This free online dictionary designed for the public and professionals contains terms that deal with biochemistry, biotechnology, botany, cell biology, and genetics. The dictionary also contains some terms relating to ecology, limnology, pharmacology, toxicology, and medicine. The search engine allows the user to search by a specific term or by a term contained within a definition.

CancerWeb Online Medical Dictionary ◉ ◉ ◉

http://www.graylab.ac.uk/omd/index.html

This site offers a comprehensive medical dictionary online for clinical, medical student, and patient audiences, although a great many of the entries are very technical. It is a convenient source for a quick definition of an unfamiliar term.

drkoop.com: Glossary of Insurance-Related Terms ◉ ◉

http://www.drkoop.com/hcr/insurance/glossary.asp

This site provides descriptions of both terms and phrases relating to health insurance. Terms are listed alphabetically.

Healthanswers.com: Disease Finder ◉ ◉ ◉

http://www.healthanswers.com/Centers/Disease/default.asp

A wide range of diseases are listed in this alphabetical directory of information for patients and consumers. Visitors can search by keyword or browse the directory for information. Details include alternative names, definitions, causes, incidences, risk factors, prevention, symptoms, signs and tests, treatment, prognosis, and complications. Any helpful diagrams or representative photographs related to the condition are also provided.

Healthanswers.com: Injury Finder ○ ○ ○

http://www.healthanswers.com/medenc/index.asp?topic=Injury

Patients can access an alphabetical directory of common injuries at this address. Information available includes a definition and important considerations about the injury, causes, symptoms, prevention, and suggested first aid.

Healthanswers.com: Test Finder ○ ○ ○

http://www.healthanswers.com/medenc/index.asp?topic=Test

Common medical tests are listed alphabetically at this address, providing patients and consumers with a definition of the test a descriptions of how the test is performed, patient preparation for the test, how the test will feel, risks, reasons the test is performed, normal values, the meaning of abnormal results, cost of the test, and special considerations.

InteliHealth: Vitamin and Nutrition Resource Center ○ ○ ○

http://www.intelihealth.com/IH/ihtIH/WSIHW000/325/20932.html

InteliHealth offers this comprehensive glossary of vitamins and minerals, listed under fat-soluble vitamins, water-soluble vitamins, and minerals. Information provided under each entry includes important facts about the vitamin or mineral, daily intake recommendations for men and women, benefits, food sources, amounts of the substance present in various food sources, and cautions in terms of health consequences of the overuse or deficiency of the substance.

List and Glossary of Medical Terms ○ ○

http://allserv.rug.ac.be/%7Ervdstich/eugloss/welcome.html

This site offers a multilingual glossary of technical and popular medical terms.

Medical Spell-Check Offered by Spellex Development ○ ○ ○

http://www.spellex.com/speller.htm

Spellex Medical and Spellex Pharmaceutical online spelling verification allows visitors to check the spelling of medical terms. The search returns possible correct spellings if the word entered was not found.

MedicineNet.com: Diseases and Conditions Index ○ ○ ○

http://www.medicinenet.com/Script/Main/AlphaIdx.asp?li=MNI&d=51&p=A_DT

Medicinenet.com offers this comprehensive, user-friendly index to common and not so common diseases and conditions for reliable consumer information. Individual entries contain related terms as well as mini forums that offer concise encyclopedic articles on each disease, related news and updates, and ask the expert sections in which physicians answer common patient inquiries. Individual entries may also contain links to fact sheets on related topics of interest.

MedicineNet.com: Medical Dictionary ○ ○ ○
http://www.medicinenet.com/Script/Main/AlphaIdx.asp?li=MNI&d=51&p=A_DICT

This valuable addition to the physician's electronic library contains all-inclusive entries that are revised on an ongoing basis for a considerable and ever-changing repertoire of classical and more modern medical terminology. The dictionary is unique in that it contains mini-encyclopedic entries for concise general information as well as definitions. With this easy to access reference tool, entries come complete with standard medical terms, related scientific terms, abbreviations, acronyms, jargon, institutions, projects, symptoms, syndromes, eponyms, and medical history.

MedicineNet.com: Procedures and Tests Index ○ ○ ○
http://www.medicinenet.com/Script/Main/AlphaIdx.asp?li=MNI&d=133&p=A_PROC

MedicineNet.com offers this comprehensive, user-friendly index to common and not so common diagnostic tests and treatment procedures. Each diagnostic and treatment mini-forum contains a main article for general information, outlining the purpose and safety of the procedure, related diseases and treatments, articles written by physicians on related topics of interest, and interesting related consumer health facts.

Merck Manual of Diagnosis and Therapy ○ ○ ○
http://www.merck.com/pubs/mmanual

This online version of the 17th edition of the *Merck Manual* (1999) contains general medical text describing disorders and diseases that affect all organ systems. The site also provides links to the *Merck Manual of Geriatrics* and the *Merck Manual of Medical Information-Home Edition*. All manuals are searchable and use of the services is free-of-charge.

National Organization for Rare Disorders (NORD) ○ ○ ○ (some features fee-based)
http://www.rarediseases.org

The National Organization for Rare Disorders, Inc. (NORD) is a federation of more than 140 nonprofit organizations serving people with rare disorders and disabilities. The site provides access to current news items, conference details, an online newsletter, a rare disease database providing useful information for patients, an organizational database providing links to support and research organizations dedicated to rare disorders, and information specific to NORD. Users must pay a fee for full access to disease information.

Phys.com Fitness Encyclopedia ○ ○
http://www.phys.com/fitness

This online encyclopedia includes exercise guides for working each part of the body. The encyclopedia also describes sports and activities, detailing the physical benefits, necessary equipment, related terms, and additional resources. It also provides tips for preparing, playing, and training for the activities.

Tests and Procedures, University of Michigan Health System ○ ○
http://www.med.umich.edu/1libr/tests/test00.htm

An alphabetical directory of medical test and procedures is found at this address. Clear, non-technical explanations of each test are offered to interested consumers. Visitors will also find discussions of health topics and other resources through this site.

Yahoo! Health: Diseases and Conditions ○ ○ ○
http://dir.yahoo.com/Health/Diseases_and_Conditions

Consumers will find an alphabetical list of health topics at this address. Each entry provides a definition or information on alternative names, causes, incidence, and risk factors, prevention, symptoms, signs and tests, treatment, and prognosis. Information is included on medical terms, diseases, medical conditions, vaccines, and other related topics.

35.15 Medical Legislation

American Medical Association (AMA): AMA in Washington ○ ○
http://www.ama-assn.org/ama/basic/category/0,1060,165,00.html

The purpose of this site is to encourage physicians around the country to get involved in the AMA's grassroots lobbying efforts. It covers information on legislation relevant to the medical profession, the AMA's Congressional agenda, and educational programs available through the AMA on political activism for physicians. The Web site is updated regularly with the latest news on medical issues in the government.

American Medical Group Association (AMGA) Public Policy and Political Affairs ○ ○
http://www.amga.org/gov/pos.htm

The AMGA Web site contains position papers concerning major issues in the medical profession currently debated in Congress, and information on ordering publications providing news, legal resources, and compliance information to healthcare professionals. One section is devoted to suggestions on communicating with Congressional representatives on policy issues.

American Medical Student Association (AMSA): Legislative Affairs ○ ○ ○
http://www.amsa.org/hp.html

The AMSA is an organization that attempts to improve healthcare and medical education. Its Legislative Affairs section of the Web site contains news of legislation that affects medical education, educational information on how to be a health policy activist, information on internship and fellowship opportunities in the field of health policy, and legislative links.

American Medical Women's Association (AMWA)
http://www.amwa-doc.org/index.html

The AMWA promotes issues related to women's health and professional development for female physicians. The site's advocacy and actions sections contain articles on news and legislation that is relevant to these issues and gives advice on how to get involved.

Public Citizen
http://www.citizen.org

Public Citizen, a group founded by Ralph Nader, is an organization dedicated to political activism in issues concerning public health and safety. Within the site, there is information on legislation and activities related to the group's purpose of "protecting health, safety, and democracy." An extensive list of links to specific subjects include medically-related topics, such as "Healthcare Legislation," "HMO Accountability," and "Medical Malpractice Reform."

Thomas-U.S. Congress on the Internet
http://thomas.loc.gov

Within Thomas, one can find information on bills, laws, reports, or any current U.S. federal legislation. The site's engine can be used to find current congressional bills by keyword or bill number.

U.S. House of Representatives Internet Office of the Law Revision Counsel
http://uscode.house.gov/fast.htm

The Office of the Law Revision Counsel of the U.S. House of Representatives prepares and publishes the United States Code. U.S. Code can be searched by keyword or other classification criteria, and titles and chapters of the Code can be downloaded from the site. Classification tables listing sections of the U.S. Code affected by recently enacted laws are also available.

35.16 Medical News

1st Headlines: Health
http://www.1sthealthnews.com/index.htm

This medical news information site offers a keyword search engine for access to nationwide health news derived from more than 70 daily publications and reputable broadcast and online networks, including *USA Today's* Health section, Reuters Health, MSNBC, and drkoop.com. News coverage includes treatment discoveries, pharmacological updates, the latest in managed care, product recalls, and hundreds of other breaking news bulletins.

CNN: Health News ○ ○ ○
http://www.cnn.com/HEALTH

Health News from CNN is produced in association with WebMD. Specific articles are available in featured topics, ethics matters, research, and home remedies, and an allergy report is also provided. National and international health news is presented, and users can access specific articles on AIDS, aging, alternative medicine, cancer, children's health, diet and fitness, men's health, and women's health. Visitors can also access patient questions and answers of doctors, chat forums, and special community resources available through WebMD. Information and articles are also offered by Mayo Clinic and AccentHealth.com.

Doctor's Guide: Medical and Other News ○ ○ ○
http://www.pslgroup.com/MEDNEWS.HTM

This site provides very current medical news and information for health professionals. Visitors can search the Doctor's Guide Medical News Database, and access medical news broadcast within the past week or the past month. News items organized by subject, firsthand conference communiqués, and journal club reviews are also available at this informative news site.

Medical Breakthroughs ○ ○ ○
http://www.ivanhoe.com/#reports

This site delivers daily News Flash Updates to your e-mail box. A fee of US$15 per quarter is required for receipt of bulletins on pending medical breakthroughs. Visitors can also search archived articles by keyword, read weekly general interest articles, find links to related sites, and watch videos related to current health issues. The site is sponsored by Ivanhoe Broadcast News, Inc., a medical news gathering organization providing stories to television stations nationwide.

Reuters Health ○ ○ (some features fee-based)
http://www.reutershealth.com

Reuters provides an excellent site for breaking medical news, updated daily, as well as a subscription-based searchable database of the News Archives of Reuters News Service. Visitors can access MEDLINE from the site. Group subscribers have access to a database of drug information.

Science News Update ○ ○
http://www.ama-assn.org/sci-pubs/sci-news/1997/pres_rel.htm

This weekly online publication provides users with *Journal of the American Medical Association* reports and a list of previous news releases. Visitors can also access site updates, search the site for specific articles, register for e-mail alerts of new issues, read classified advertisements, and find information on print subscriptions, reprints, and advertising rates.

This Week's Top Medical News Stories ⊙ ⊙ ⊙

http://www.newsfile.com/newsrx.htm

Conference coverage reports and summaries of recent research findings from weekly online publications devoted to topics such as HIV/AIDS, Alzheimer's disease, angiogenesis, blood products, cancer, gene therapy, genomics and genetics, CDC activities, hepatitis, immunotherapy, obesity, pain management, proteomics, transplants, tuberculosis and airborne diseases, vaccines, women's health, and world disease issues are available at this site.

UniSci: Daily University Science News ⊙ ⊙

http://unisci.com

This site offers current articles related to all branches of science, including medicine. Many medical articles are available, and special archives offer additional medical resources. Users can access news from the past 10 days and perform searches for archived material.

USA Today: Health ⊙ ⊙ ⊙

http://www.usatoday.com/life/health/archive.htm

USA Today's feature stories and headline archives are directly accessible at this Web site where visitors can view some of the best in nationwide medical news coverage. Articles are listed by topic, including addiction, AIDS, allergies, alternative medicine, arthritis, cancer, diabetes, genetics, hepatitis, mental health, surgery, vision, and many others. Visitors will also find the latest in groundbreaking medical and pharmacotherapeutic research.

Yahoo! Health Headlines ⊙ ⊙ ⊙

http://dailynews.yahoo.com/headlines/hl

Updated several times throughout the day, Health Headlines at Yahoo! offers full news coverage and Reuters News with top health headlines from around the globe. Earlier daily and archived stories may be accessed, and the site's powerful search engine allows viewers to browse, with full color, the latest in photographic coverage of news and events.

35.17 Medical Search Engines and Directories

Achoo Healthcare Online ⊙ ⊙ ⊙

http://www.achoo.com

This site offers a directory of Web sites in three main categories: human health and disease, business of health, and organizations and sources. The site has extensive subcategories and short descriptions for each site. Daily health news of interest to patients, the public, or medical professionals is available at the site, as well as links to journals, databases, employment directories, and discussion groups.

All The Web ⚙ ⚙ ⚙
http://www.alltheweb.com

This comprehensive site provides a variety of search engines including Fast Search. Fast Search allows users to search the Internet in 25 language catalogs and covers over 200 million high quality Web pages in very high speed. Visitors can copy the code needed to add Fast Search to their Web sites. Additionally at this site are search engines to search pictures and sounds.

Argus Clearinghouse ⚙ ⚙ ⚙
http://www.clearinghouse.net

The Argus Clearinghouse provides a central access point for value-added topical guides which identify, describe and evaluate Internet-based information resources. Its mission is to facilitate intellectual access to information resources on the Internet. Users can search for Web resources at this site using a directory or search engine. Many general categories are available including "Health & Medicine" and "Science & Mathematics." Subcategories under "Health & Medicine" include disabilities, diseases and disorders, fitness and nutrition, general health, medical specialties, medicine and medical services and sexuality and reproduction. Information about each site includes the compiler name or organization, detailed ratings, related keywords and the date the site was last checked by Argus Clearinghouse.

BigHub ⚙ ⚙ ⚙
http://www.thebighub.com

Formerly known as iSleuth.com, the BigHub allows users to search multiple engines including Yahoo, AltaVista, Infoseek, Excite, WebCrawler, Lycos, HotBot and Goto, Web directories and news databases simultaneously, and receive one summary of results. The BigHub provides advanced search options in relevant specialty topics including Health, Science and Reference resources. Users can also access news, weather, financial information, and more.

CliniWeb International ⚙ ⚙ ⚙
http://www.ohsu.edu/cliniweb

CliniWeb, a service of Oregon Health Sciences University, is a searchable index and table of contents to clinical resources available on the World Wide Web. Information found at the site is of particular interest to healthcare professional students and practitioners. Search terms can be entered in five different languages: English, German, French, Spanish, and Portuguese. The site offers links to sites for additional search resources, and is linked directly to MEDLINE.

Daily Diffs ○ ○ ○

http://www.dailydiffs.com

This site catalogs and provides updates on useful sites in many categories, including Health and Medicine. This section provides current news items related to fitness and wellness, diseases and disorders, risks, prevention, current treatments, and many specific topics covered in detail. Users can also search for resources by keyword.

Doctor's Guide ○ ○ ○

http://www.docguide.com

The Doctor's Guide to the Internet is provided by P\S\L Consulting Group, Inc. and its purpose is to provide a comfortable environment for physicians to search the Internet and World Wide Web. The site contains a professional edition for healthcare professionals and a section directed at patients. Information of medical and professional interest includes medical news and alerts, new drugs or indications, medical conferences, a Congress Resource Center, a medical bookstore, and Internet medical resources. Patient resources are organized by specific diseases or condition. Users can search the World Wide Web through Excite, InfoSeek, McKinley, and Alta Vista search engines or can search the Doctor's Guide Medical News and Conference database.

Dogpile ○ ○ ○

http://www.dogpile.com

Dogpile is a metasearch service that integrates several medium and large Web search and index guides into a single service. Visitors can complete a dogpile or geographic search (provides information about cities in the United States) or browse sites listed by categories such as "Health and Science" and their multiple subcategories. In addition this site offers yellow pages search, stock quotes, usenet articles, weather forecasts, job opportunities, shopping, and more.

drkoop.com ○ ○

http://www.drkoop.com

drkoop.com is an Internet-based consumer healthcare network. Included is a site search engine, reviews of Internet sites and multiple health-related topics and conditions to browse. In addition there are health-related news stories, a variety of resources such as information on drugs, books online, insurance, a physician locator, chat rooms, message boards, and much more.

Federal Web Locator ○ ○ ○

http://www.infoctr.edu/fwl

The Federal Web Locator is a service provided by the Center for Information Law and Policy and is intended to be the one stop shopping point for federal government information on the World Wide Web. Links to relevant sites are available in the following categories: legislative, judicial and executive branches, independent and quasi-official agencies, federal boards, commissions, committees and nongovernmental federally related sites. Additionally users can access a variety of search engines including Aliweb, Alpha Legal Directory, Alta Vista, Cyber411, EINET Galaxy, Excite, Google, Inference Find, InfoSeek, Law Crawler-Legal Search Information, Lycos, McKinley, MetaCrawler, OpenText Index, SavvySearch, Snap, WebCrawler, World Access Internet Navigator, and Yahoo.

Galaxy: Medicine ○ ○ ○

http://galaxy.einet.net/galaxy/Medicine.html

This site houses a directory of quality medical Web sites. Subcategories include diseases and disorders, health law, health occupations, history, human biology, medical informatics, operative surgery, philosophy, political issues, reference, and therapeutics. There are also several site search options available.

Galen II: The Digital Library of the University of California, San Francisco (UCSF) ○ ○ ○

http://galen.library.ucsf.edu

This online library directory includes UCSF and UC resources and services, links to the AMA Directory, Drug Info Fulltext, Harrison's Online (requires a password), the *Merck Manual*, Consumer Health, and a searchable database of additional resources and publications including electronic journals. Visitors can search the Galen II database or the World Wide Web using a variety of search engines.

Global Health Network ○ ○ ○

http://www.pitt.edu/HOME/GHNet/GHNet.html

The Global Health Network offers national and international resources with information on agencies, organizations, academic programs, workshops, and conventions. The site maintains an online newsletter and offers links to related health networks. The site is also available in Japanese, Portuguese, Spanish, German, Chinese, Turkish, and Taiwanese.

Google ○ ○ ○

http://directory.google.com

Google offers a comprehensive search tool, integrating resources from several smaller search engines. Several subject areas are available for more specific queries, including health and related subtopics. Visitors can enter a search term, view google results, and try the same query through AltaVista, Deja, Excite, HotBot, Infoseek, Lycos, and Yahoo through the site.

Hardin Meta Directory of Internet Health Services ○ ○ ○

http://www.lib.uiowa.edu/hardin/md/index.html

The purpose of the Hardin Meta Directory is to provide easy access to comprehensive resource lists in health-related subjects. It includes subject listings in large "one stop-shopping" sites such as MedWeb and Yahoo, and also independent discipline-specific lists. Sites are categorized by specific diseases and the number of links found at each site and only those that are well maintained are included. Additionally there is a list of free, full-text general medical journals available online.

Health A to Z ○ ○ ○
http://www.healthatoz.com

This site offers visitors many useful resources for locating specific health information. A site search engine locates professionally reviewed health and medical information from other Internet resources including news headlines and updates, additional general health information, and a forum for asking questions of experts. Fact pages are dedicated to many specific health topics including diseases, alternative medicine, vaccines, nutrition, and fitness.

Health on the Net (HON) Foundation: MedHunt ○ ○
http://www.hon.ch/MedHunt

Health on the Net Foundation (HON) is a nonprofit organization and international initiative with a mission to help individuals and health care providers realize the potential benefits of the World Wide Web. This site provides several widely used medical search engines including MedHunt, Honselect, and MEDLINE. Users can access databases containing information on newsgroups, LISTSERVs, medical images and movies, upcoming and past healthcare-related conferences, and daily news stories on health-related topics.

Health Sciences Information Service ○ ○ ○
http://www.lib.berkeley.edu/HSIS/other2.html

The Health Sciences Information Service at University of California, Berkeley offers links to Internet medical and health resources. Electronic journals, books, indexes, and databases on the Internet are cataloged. The Service offers links to sites providing general medical information, institutes, and organizations on the Web, current news related to health and medicine, clinical sites, and sites related to Medical Informatics.

Health Web ○ ○ ○
http://www.healthweb.org

HealthWeb provides links to specific, evaluated information resources on the World Wide Web, selected by librarians and information professionals at leading academic medical centers in the Midwest. Members, mainly universities or research centers, provide information that is sorted by alphabetical order and can be searched by keyword. Each member provides information on affiliated libraries as well as subject areas.

Indiana University: Ruth Lilly Medical Library (RLML)

http://www.medlib.iupui.edu

Although portions of this site are restricted, many Web medical resources can be accessed through links, including other libraries, government libraries and information sources, national agencies, associations, and numerous other vital resources.

Infomine

http://infomine.ucr.edu/search/bioagsearch.phtml

Provided by the University of California, Infomine provides access to all types of Internet resources in the biological, agricultural, and medical sciences. Visitors can browse sites by subject, title, or keyword, or complete a search using Infomine's search engine or a variety of Internet search and metasearch engines, virtual libraries and subject indexes, and mailing lists and newsgroups. Other features include access to BioAgMed and general references, online journals, the *Merck Manual* and educational resources.

MDchoice.com

http://www.mdchoice.com

MDchoice.com is a privately held company founded by academic physicians with the goal of making access to health and medical information on the Internet as efficient and reliable as possible. The site features an UltraWeb search with all content selected by board-certified physicians. In addition, users have access to MEDLINE, drug information, health news, and a variety of clinical calculators. Also offered are several interactive educational exercises, online journals and text books, and employment opportunities.

Med411.com: Medical Research Portal

http://www.med411.com/resources.html

This site offers access to a variety of comprehensive search tools, allowing users to search medical libraries, professional associations, online health manuals, the National Library of Medicine, peer-reviewed journals, health services, images, clinical trials, the Combined Health Information Database (CHID), CancerNet, the National Institute of Diabetes and Digestive and Kidney Diseases, HealthFinder, and WebPath directly from the site.

MedExplorer

http://www.medexplorer.com

MedExplorer is a comprehensive, searchable medical and health directory. Short descriptions of each site are provided. The site also lists related newsgroups and has information on conferences and employment.

Medical Matrix ◎ ◎ (free registration)
http://www.medmatrix.org

Medical Matrix offers peer-reviewed, annotated, updated clinical medicine resources, and assigns ranks to Internet resources based on their utility for point-of-care clinical application. Visitors can access several search engines including Medical Matrix, MEDLINE and others or access sites through categories such as medical specialties, diseases, clinical practice, literature, education, healthcare and professionals, medical computing and Internet and technology, and marketplace. Additional information available includes online journals and textbooks, news, CME, prescription assistance resources, symposia on the Web, and classifieds. Access to site requires free registration.

Medical World Search ◎ ◎ ◎
http://www.mwsearch.com

This search engine indexes Web pages from selected medical Web sites. A directory of sites is not available. Users can chose to search indexed sites, selected general search engines, or MEDLINE. The search engine utilizes a medical thesaurus to increase the amount of returns from one query.

MedicineNet.com ◎ ◎ ◎
http://medicinenet.com/Script/Main/hp.asp

MedicineNet is a network of doctors producing health information for public use. The site offers an alphabetically arranged directory that provides information about diseases, treatments, procedures, tests, and drugs. The site also provides a comprehensive medical dictionary with thousands of terms and disorders along with prefixes and association designations. Other features include news, treatment updates, and health facts.

MedMark ◎ ◎ ◎
http://www.medmark.org

This comprehensive site provides users with a searchable directory of medical resources by specialty, free MEDLINE links, and other Internet resources. A search engine is available for locating additional medical and general sites.

Medscape ◎ ◎ ◎ (free registration)
http://www.medscape.com

Medscape provides several databases from which users can search the Web. These include articles, news, information for patients, MEDLINE, AIDSline, Toxline, drug information, a dictionary, a book store, the Dow Jones Library, and medical images. There is a wealth of additional information provided including articles, case reports, conference schedules and summaries, continuing medical education resources, job listings, journals, news, patient information, practice guidelines, treatment updates, and links to medical specialty sites. Requires free online registration.

MedSurf ○ ○ ○
http://www.medsurf.com/cgi-bin/OpenPage.cgi?Home.txt;Home

MedSurf offers links and a keyword search tool to find links to health and medical resources. The "Healthy Surfing" section provides news about the latest medical technologies and breakthroughs, while "Medicine Bag" guides physicians and healthcare providers to news and in-depth information on new timesaving technologies, advanced treatment alternatives, aging research, and upcoming educational forums.

MedWeb ○ ○
http://www.medweb.emory.edu/Medweb

Offered by Emory University, this site provides a searchable database of Web sites providing medical and health information. Searching is possible by entering keywords or by browsing subject categories.

Metacrawler ○ ○
http://www.metacrawler.com

At the Metacrawler site users can search for Web resources through a directory or search engine. In addition, search engines are provided for newsgroups, audio, and shopping.

MMRL: Multimedia Medical Reference Library Medical Student Study Center ○ ○ ○
http://www.med-library.com/medlibrary

The Multimedia Medical Reference Library, developed by medical students and professionals at Tufts University School of Medicine, is a searchable database of reviewed medical Web sites. Visitors can find links to sites offering audio resources, clinical trials information, online journals, medical equipment auctions, medical reference libraries, medical services, software, products, and links to medical schools and professional organizations. Each site is listed with a short description.

NetMed.com ○ ○ ○
http://www.netmed.com/intro.html

NetMed.com provides users with links to useful sites grouped by medical condition. A relatively detailed description is given for most sites.

Online Medical Resources ○ ○
http://www.doctorbbs.com/searchall.htm

This site invites the user to search 20 different sites or online publications related to health and medicine. Links to MEDLINE and other general medical sites are also available.

Stanford MedWorld: MedBot ◎ ◎ ◎
http://www-med.stanford.edu/medworld/medbot

Offered by Stanford University, this site allows users to search medical and health resources on the Web using major general and medical search engines. More specific searches can be performed on index and reference, education and learning, news and information, and medical images, and multimedia resources topics. Users can specify engines to employ in the search.

Virtual Medical Center ◎ ◎ ◎
http://www-sci.lib.uci.edu/~martindale/Medical.html

This site, hosted by the University of California and written by Jim Martindale, provides users with links to a wealth of useful information, including travel warnings and immunization details, reference resources on a wide range of scientific subjects, and pathology and virology educational resources. Co-contributors include the UCI Science Library, the Department of Defense, the National Institutes of Health, and the National Science Foundation.

Yahoo! ◎ ◎ ◎
http://www.yahoo.com

Yahoo offers visitors the opportunity to search the Web and browse sites listed in multiple categories including health and science. Within each category are more specific subcategories that indicate the number of entries available. Most sites are suggested by users. Additionally Yahoo offers a wealth of services such as free e-mail, shopping, people search, news, travel, weather, stock reports, and more.

35.18 Pharmaceutical Information

Doctor's Guide: New Drugs and Indications ◎ ◎ ◎
http://www.pslgroup.com/NEWDRUGS.HTM

Doctor's Guide provides an ongoing source of new drug information, including FDA approvals and drug indications. Drug stories are presented in order of article datelines, with the most current stories listed first. Information for drug releases for the past 12 months is provided.

drkoop.com: Drug Interactions Search ◎ ◎
http://www.drkoop.com/drugstore/pharmacy/interactions.asp

Users can enter several drug names into a search tool, checking for drug interactions.

Drug InfoNet ⊙⊙⊙

http://www.druginfonet.com/phrminfo.htm

Information and links to areas on the Web concerning healthcare and pharmaceutical-related topics are available. The drug information is available by brand name, generic name, manufacturer, and therapeutic class. Visitors can ask questions of experts, and access disease information, pharmaceutical manufacturer information, healthcare news, and other resources.

Food and Drug Administration (FDA) ⊙⊙⊙

http://www.fda.gov

The FDA site provides extensive information on all aspects of drug research, regulations, approvals, trials, adverse reactions, enforcement, conferences, clinical alerts, reports, and drug news. The FDA Web Site Index is the first place to go to research a topic. There are several hundred subjects listed. One of these many sections covers FDA-related acronyms and abbreviations, which itself is a very useful tool in understanding much of the material at this site. For many researchers and physicians, however, information about FDA drug approvals is of central concern. A separate service, not included within the FDA, offers a concise summary of such approvals by medical specialty and condition for each year up to the present. This information can be accessed at the following Web site: www.centerwatch.com/drugs/DRUGLIST.HTM.

Food and Drug Administration (FDA): Center for Drug Evaluation and Research ⊙⊙⊙

http://www.fda.gov/cder/drug/default.htm

The Center for Drug Evaluation and Research broadcasts valuable information on prescription, consumer, and over-the-counter drugs at this address. Resources include alphabetical lists of new and generic drug approvals, new drugs approved for cancer indications, a searchable Orange Book listing all FDA approved prescription drugs, a National Drug Code directory, new over-the-counter labeling notices, patient information on over-the counter drugs, and alerts of new over-the-counter indications. Links are available to many resources related to drug safety and side effects, public health alerts and warnings, and pages offering information on major drugs. Reports and publications, special projects and programs, and cancer clinical trials information are also found through this address.

MedicineNet.com: Medications Index ⊙⊙⊙

http://www.medicinenet.com/Script/Main/AlphaIdx.asp?li=MNI&d=51&p=A_PHARM

This all-inclusive pharmacological database from Medicinenet.com includes a mini forum for each prescription and nonprescription medication, containing a brief main article pertaining to the medication, related medications, related news and updates, diseases associated with the medication, and a listing of articles pertinent to the pharmacological agent's usage.

MedWatch: The FDA Medical Products Reporting Program ○ ○ ○
http://www.fda.gov/medwatch

The FDA Medical Products Reporting Program, MedWatch, is designed to educate health professionals about the importance of being aware of, monitoring for, and reporting adverse events and problems to the FDA and/or the manufacturer. The program is also intended to disseminate new safety information rapidly within the medical community, thereby improving patient care. To these ends, the site includes an adverse event reporting form and instructions as well as safety information for health professionals, including "Dear Health Professional" letters and notifications related to drug safety. It also includes relevant full-text continuing education articles and reports regarding drug and medical device safety issues.

Pharmaceutical Information Network (PharmInfoNet) ○ ○ ○
http://pharminfo.com

PharmInfoNet is a source of information on diseases, disorders, drug treatments, and research. In addition, there are links to more than 100 pharmaceutical companies, both domestic and international. Organized by specialty areas, the site is a well-organized compilation of resources for physicians, researchers, medical students, and the public. The site is organized into information on disorders, archived articles, drugs used in the treatment of disorders, and other information sources, including newsgroups, e-mail lists, and related Web sites. An extensive medical sciences bulletin section and pharmacotherapy department provide articles on dozens of developments in research and drug therapies. Finally, the site provides a lengthy listing of drugs for treating disorders, with links to more extensive information sources. Resources are found easily at this address through the "Site Contents" link.

Pharmaceutical Research and Manufacturers of America ○ ○ ○
http://www.phrma.org

This association Web site includes a "New Medicines in Development" database; a publications section containing reports relating to the pharmaceutical industry; various links for facts and figures on pharmaceutical research and innovation; and an issues and policies section covering many current topics of interest to pharmaceutical companies, such as genetics research and healthcare liability reform.

RxList: The Internet Drug Index ○ ○ ○
http://www.rxlist.com

This site allows users to search for drug information by name, imprint code, or keyword (action, interaction, etc.) The top 200 prescribed drugs for 1998, 1997, 1996, and 1995 are listed alphabetically or by rank. Patient monographs are available for a wide range of drugs, and one section is devoted to alternative medicine information and answers to frequently asked questions. The site also provides statistics related to site visits, and a forum for drug-specific discussions.

SafeScript Limited: World Standard Drug Database ⊙ ⊙
http://209.235.64.5:8888

Information on pharmaceutical products at this address includes ingredients, dosage, routes of administration, indications, contraindications, prescribe cautions, patient cautions, toxicity, side effects, liver disease cautions, renal failure procedures, pregnancy and lactation warnings, pharmacological actions, and diagnostic procedures. Visitors can search by drug, ingredient, indications, contraindications, or side effects.

Virtual Library Pharmacy ⊙ ⊙ ⊙
http://www.pharmacy.org

This is truly a library of pharmacy information for professionals in all medical areas. The site provides information on pharmacy schools, companies, journals and books, Internet databases relating to pharmaceutical topics, conferences, hospital sites, government sites, pharmacy LISTSERVs, and news groups. Hundreds of site links are provided for the above areas.

35.19 Physician Directories

American Board of Medical Specialties (ABMS) ⊙ ⊙ ⊙
http://www.certifieddoctor.com/verify.html

This verification service contains all physicians certified by an ABMS member board. It permits the public to verify credentials and certification status of any physician, searching by name, city, state, and specialty.

Healthgrades.com ⊙ ⊙ ⊙
http://www.healthgrades.com

This resource specializes in healthcare ratings, providing hospital ratings by procedure or diagnosis, physician ratings by specialty and geographic area, and ratings of health plans. Directories of hospitals, physicians, health plans, mammography facilities, fertility clinics, assisted living facilities, dentists, and chiropractors are also available. Visitors can access tips on choosing a hospital, physician, or health plan, as well as a glossary of terms and health news articles. Online health stores offer books, videos, magazines, greeting cards, flowers and gifts, pharmaceutical products, nutritional products, and insurance quotes.

Searchpointe Physician Background Information Service ⊙ ⊙ ⊙
http://www.askmedi.com

Searchpointe provides background information on physicians licensed to practice in the United States. The physician's medical school, year of graduation, residency training record, ABMS certifications, states where certified, and records of sanctions or disciplinary actions are included. There is a fee for reports.

36. PROFESSIONAL TOPICS AND CLINICAL PRACTICE

36.1 Anatomy and Surgery

Anatomy of the Human Body ◎ ◎ ◎
http://rpisun1.mda.uth.tmc.edu/mmlearn/anatomy.html
This site offers images of the brain, elbow, arm, hand, knee, and foot. There are also sections that show slices of the ankle, foot, head, and neck in detail with nerves, muscles, and blood vessels identified.

Atlas of the Body ◎ ◎ ◎
http://www.ama-assn.org/insight/gen_hlth/atlas/atlas.htm
The Atlas of the Body is a site offered by the American Medical Association that provides detailed information and labeled illustrations of the various systems and organs of the human body. The site also provides descriptions of disorders that affect these systems and organs.

Martindale's Health Science Guide: Anatomy and Histology Center ◎ ◎
http://www-sci.lib.uci.edu/HSG/MedicalAnatomy.html
This site offers links to examinations, tutorials, and associations. It lists numerous atlases and sites with anatomical images, including some on embryology and developmental anatomy. Anatomy is just one of the many medical areas covered by the Virtual Medical Center, which also provides links to general medical dictionaries, glossaries, and encyclopedias, plus sites containing information on metabolic pathways and genetic maps.

Online Atlas Of Surgery ○ ○ ○
http://www.bgsm.edu/surg-sci/atlas/atlas.html

This site provides descriptions of specific surgical techniques, anatomy, instrumentation, positioning, room setup, and dissection. Also provided are indications leading to surgery and possible problems that may develop as a result of the surgery.

Online Surgery ○ ○ ○
http://www.onlinesurgery.com

Online Surgery gives the public an opportunity to view general and cosmetic surgical procedures online. Patients can fill out an application to finance an elective procedure and to be considered for a free procedure. Surgeries are viewed using RealPlayer.

Vesalius ○ ○ ○
http://www.vesalius.com

This site is a resource of medical illustrations with the purpose of providing educational material for surgeons and other medical professionals. Clinical Folios provide users with short educational narratives on surgical anatomy and procedures designed for online reference and study. There is an archive of images that demonstrate surgical techniques and other resources, including story boards, procedure descriptions using illustrations, photographs, x-rays, scans, animations and text, and short interactive programs or videos.

Virtual Body ○ ○ ○
http://www.medtropolis.com/vbody

This creative, informative site provides the viewer with labeled medical illustrations of various parts of the body. The human anatomy and body functions are presented in detail with interactive options that help the viewer learn the material.

Whole Brain Atlas, Harvard University ○ ○ ○
http://www.med.harvard.edu/AANLIB/home.html

This site, administered by the Harvard Medical School, shows imaging of the brain using magnetic resonance imaging (MRI), roentgen-ray computed tomography (CT), and nuclear medicine technologies. Structures within the images are labeled. Normal brain images are provided, as well as images of brains subjected to cerebrovascular disease, neoplastic disease, degenerative disease, and inflammatory or infectious disease. The entire atlas is available free-of-charge online or can be ordered on CD-ROM for a fee.

36.2 Biomedical Ethics

American Society of
Bioethics and Humanities (ASBH)
http://www.asbh.org

The American Society of Bioethics and Humanities is an organization that promotes scholarship, research, teaching, policy development, and professional development in the field of bioethics. The site offers information on the Society, the annual meeting, position papers, awards, and links.

American Society of Law, Medicine, and Ethics (ASLME)
http://www.aslme.org

This site offers information on the American Society of Law, Medicine, and Ethics; *The Journal of Law Medicine and Ethics;* and *The American Journal of Law and Medicine.* There is also information on research projects, a news section that gives information on recent developments in Law, Medicine, and Ethics, and information on future and past conferences held by the Society.

Bioethics Discussion Pages
http://www-hsc.usc.edu/~mbernste/#Welcome

This page is a forum for people to discuss and share their views on selected topics in the field of biomedical ethics. There are also polls and articles on ethical issues.

Bioethics.net
http://www.med.upenn.edu/bioethics/index.shtml

Produced by the Center for Bioethics of the University of Pennsylvania, Bioethics.net contains a host of resources relating to biomedical ethics. Included are sections on cloning and genetics, emergency room bioethics, surveys for pay, and assisted suicide. There is also a virtual library with links to Internet resources. A beginner's site (Bioethics for Beginners) contains material that is meant to educate the general public and people interested in the field about bioethics, its meaning, and its applications. At this beginner's site, there are resources for students and educators, and a list of different biomedical ethics associations.

Careers in Bioethics
http://www.ethics.ubc.ca/brynw/jobs.html

This site has information on jobs that are being offered throughout the world in the field of Bioethics. Information on postdoctorals and fellowships is also available.

Center for Medical Ethics and Mediation ○ ○ ○
http://www.wh.com/cmem

This site contains resources that help enable the Center to provide information on education, research, consultations, and mediations for healthcare professionals and organizations. These resources include information on workshops and seminars; requests for the Center to send a mediator to help with a dispute or conflict; profiles of the Center's mediators; and related links.

Health Priorities Group, Inc. ○ ○ ○
http://www.bioethics-inc.com

The Health Priorities Group is made up of professionals in the field of Ethics, Medicine, Law, Nursing, and Theology. It offers training and support of corporate and hospital ethics committees, clinical case review, and help in health policy development for private and government institutions. The Web site has sections on services, publications, and reports on ethics issues.

Human Genome Project: Ethical, Legal, and Social Issues (ELSI) ○ ○
http://www.ornl.gov/TechResources/Human_Genome/resource/elsi.html

This site attempts to disseminate information on the Human Genome Project and the ethical, legal, and social issues surrounding the availability of genetic information. Available on this site are updates, publications, description of research in progress, and basic information on the Human Genome Project.

International Bioethics Committee ○ ○
http://www.unesco.org/ibc

Includes information on various ethical issues, including a section on the Human Genome Project. The site also has information on the International Bioethics Committee and its proceedings.

Medical Ethics: Where Do You Draw the Line? ○ ○
http://www.learner.org/exhibits/medicalethics

This site deals with issues by presenting real-life scenarios and letting the viewer take part in ethical decisions. There are also links to related resources and an ethics forum.

Midwest Bioethics Center ○ ○ ○
http://www.midbio.org

This community-based Center is dedicated to the integration of ethical considerations in all health care decisions. Visitors to this address will find information about the organization, including a staff listing, membership details, and consortia information. Current events, publications, a discussion group, and advance directive pamphlets are also found at the site. Resources on community-state partnerships include policy, briefs, press releases, staff listings, a call for proposals, directories of grant seekers and recipients, and answers to questions. The Center's Compassion Sabbath program is also profiled at the site, offering information on conferences for clergy and other programs, lists of participants, answers to frequently asked questions, and links to related sites.

National Bioethics Advisory Commission (NBAC) ◉ ◉ ◉
http://bioethics.gov/cgi-bin/bioeth_counter.pl
In addition to providing information on current research trends in the biotech industry, NBAC explores the ethical implications of technological advances. The site acts a forum for the ethical concerns of the public regarding a rapidly advancing technology. NBAC's policy is outlined at the site.

National Reference Center for Bioethics Literature ◉ ◉ ◉
http://www.georgetown.edu/research/nrcbl
Linked to the Kennedy Institute of Ethics of Georgetown University, this Center holds the world's largest collections of literature on Biomedical Ethics. Serving as a resource for both the public and scholarly researchers, the library lists its resources on this Web site. The site also provides access to free searching of the world's literature in this area using BIOETHICSLINE or the Ethics and Human Genetics Database. Other relevant links are provided in the areas of Educational and Teaching Resources and other bibliographies and Internet links on bioethics.

Physicians Committee for Responsible Medicine (PCRM) ◉ ◉
http://www.pcrm.org
PCRM is dedicated to preventative medicine, higher ethical standards of research, and access to managed care. The organization provides extensive material on ethics and research as well as prevention and nutrition. The site also offers news and events about numerous PCRM activities, details on clinical research projects, and summaries of texts produced by the organization.

The Hastings Center ◉ ◉ ◉
http://www.thehastingscenter.org
The Hastings Center is a major center for the study of Biomedical Ethics. Their Web site provides information about the center as well as detailed explanations of current research activities. General listings of resources found at the Center, including an online library catalog, can also be accessed.

University of Buffalo
Center for Clinical Ethics and Humanities in Health Care ◉ ◉ ◉
http://wings.buffalo.edu/faculty/research/bioethics/nav.html
Information about the Center, news and events notices, a library of bioethics and medical humanities documents, and the Ethics Committee Core Curriculum are

available at this address. Links are presented to Internet resources on featured topics, including bioethics education, hospice and palliative care, advance directives, philosophy of mind, medical record privacy, genetics and ethics, and other relevant sites.

36.3 Biotechnology

Bio Online ○ ○ ○
http://www.bio.com
Bio Online is a comprehensive Web site for the life sciences and the biotechnology industry. This site provides general information, current news, an industry guide, academic and government links, and an extensive career center. It is an excellent resource for seeking information on the biotech industry and related sciences.

Biofind.com ○ ○ ○
http://www.biofind.com
Biofind.com provides insight into the biotechnology industry and is a resource for general information, news, and developments in emerging technologies. The site also contains a job search database, chat room, the "Biotech Rumor Mill" for anonymous public discussion of current events in the field, and links to other biotech Web sites. A subscription service is also available for a fee, which provides daily e-mail updates on jobs, candidates, business opportunities, innovations, press releases, or company "rumors" posted at the site.

Bioresearch Online ○ ○ ○
http://www.bioresearchonline.com/content/homepage
Bioresearch Online is a virtual community, forum, and marketplace for biotechnology professionals. Users have access to the latest headlines, product information, new and industry analyses, as well as career information. There are also specific pages devoted to pharmaceutical research and laboratory science.

Biotechnology: An Information Resource ○ ○ ○
http://www.nal.usda.gov/bic
Dedicated to providing current information in all areas of biotechnology, this site is a subsidiary of the National Agricultural Library and the U.S. Department of Agriculture. The site catalogs press releases and offers an exhaustive listing of links to other Web-based resources from around the world, and is an excellent source for information, especially in the area of Agricultural Biotechnology.

Biotechnology Industry Organization ○ ○ ○

http://www.bio.org/welcome.html

This industry-sponsored Web site provides weekly news updates on developing technology and world news. The site also offers general information, links to corporate Web sites, an online library, and a number of other educational resources. Although corporate sponsored, the site does not focus solely on product promotion, but has a genuine educational quality. Those seeking to learn more about this growing industry will find this site to be a valuable resources.

BioWorld Online ○ ○ ○

http://www.bioworld.com

BioWorld Online tracks the growth of the biotechnology market. In addition to providing stock and financial information, the site provides access to current industry headlines, job search resources, forums, and news worldwide.

CorpTech Database ○ ○ ○

http://www.corptech.com

This comprehensive database provides details on companies involved in high-tech industries, including biotechnology and pharmaceutical companies. Basic information such as each company's description, address, annual sales, and CEO name is available free; however, more in-depth financial and business data is only accessible to fee-paying subscribers. Searches for products or names of company officers are also available, again with some amount of information provided at no cost.

Enzyme Nomenclature Database ○ ○

http://www.expasy.ch/enzyme

Enzyme information of a very specific nature is available at this site devoted exclusively to this important medical subject. The database at this Web site provides access to enzyme information by EC (Enzyme Commission) number, enzyme class, description, chemical compound, and cofactor. There is an accompanying user manual for the enzyme database as well.

Infobiotech ○ ○ ○

http://www.cisti.nrc.ca/ibc/home.html

Infobiotech is a collaboration of government, academic, and private sector resources. This Canadian-based site provides general information, resources, and links to both Canadian and non-Canadian sites. In addition, it offers a large list of related sites providing current information on advances in the biotech industry.

International Food Information Council ◎ ◎ ◎
http://ificinfo.health.org

The International Food Information Council collects and disseminates scientific information on food safety, nutrition, and health by working with experts to help translate research findings into understandable and useful information for opinion leaders and consumers. This site provides information and news on emerging technologies in the food industry. Resources available through this site include publications, recent news articles, government guidelines and regulations, and links to other resources on the Internet.

MedWebPlus: Biotechnology ◎ ◎ ◎
http://www.medwebplus.com/subject/Biotechnology.html

MedWebPlus contains an extensive guide to online resources in biotechnology and a wide variety of other fields. The site catalogs hundreds of Internet resources containing many forms of information on the biotech industry. In addition, links are provided to journals, online publications, and recent articles of interest. Vast amounts of information are provided at this site, and links are kept current.

National Center for Biotechnology Information (NCBI) ◎ ◎ ◎
http://www.ncbi.nlm.nih.gov

A collaborative effort produced by the National Library of Medicine and the National Institutes of Health, NCBI is a national resource for molecular biology information. The Center creates public databases, conducts research in computational biology, develops software tools for analyzing genome data, and disseminates biomedical information in an effort to improve the understanding of molecular processes affecting human health and disease. In addition to conducting and cataloging its own research, NCBI tracks the progress of important research projects worldwide. The site provides access to public molecular databases containing genetic sequences, structures, and taxonomy; literature databases; catalogs of whole genomes; tools for mining genetic data; teaching resources and online tutorials; and data and software available to download. Research performed at NCBI is also discussed at the site.

Recombinant Capital ◎ ◎ ◎
http://www.recap.com

This online magazine provides analysis of the biotechnology industry. This is a good resource for those seeking to invest in companies on the forefront of the rapidly growing biotech industry. Although much of the information presented here is from a financial perspective, the site gives a good overview of the entire industry and provides daily news updates. The progress of developing technology can be closely monitored via this site.

World Wide Web Virtual Library: Biotechnology ⊙ ⊙ ⊙
http://www.cato.com/biotech

This is an excellent directory of sites in the field of Biotechnology. This site catalogs hundreds of reviewed links, including publications, educational resources, general information, and government links. There is also a rating system used by the editor of the site to point out links of specific importance.

36.4 Chronic Pain Management

American Academy of Pain Management (AAPM) ⊙ ⊙ ⊙
http://www.aapainmanage.org

The American Academy of Pain Management is the largest multidisciplinary pain society and largest physician-based pain society in the United States, providing credentials to practitioners in the area of pain management. This site provides information about AAPM and its activities, resources for finding a professional program in pain management, accreditation and continuing medical education (CME) resources, and a membership directory for locating a pain management professional. It also provides good general information on pain management and a listing of relevant links. Access to the National Pain Data Bank is available at the site, containing statistics on various pain management therapies based on an outcomes measurement system. The site is divided into two sections with information tailored to the needs of patients and healthcare professionals.

Back and Body Care ⊙ ⊙
http://www.backandbodycare.com

Produced by physical therapists, this site is a good starting point for consumers seeking an overview of the causes and treatments chronic pain. It provides general information in the areas of back, neck, arm, and wrist pain. The site lists possible causes of chronic problems, treatments and exercises, and preventive measures. A search engine for locating a local, qualified physical therapist is featured at the site.

Pain.com ⊙ ⊙ ⊙
http://www.pain.com/index.cfm

This site is an excellent resource for seeking information on pain and pain management, and contains a great deal of information for the specific needs and interests of health professionals and patients. It offers an online pain journal, articles about recent advances and news in pain management, medical forums and chat rooms, and an extensive list of other Web-based resources.

Pain Net, Inc. ○ ○
http://www.painnet.com

Pain Net, Inc. provides visitors with useful information and links on pain control and prevention. Patients can find information on new treatments as well as a listing of pain management practitioners categorized by state. Doctors can search a database of important links and organizations, and can list their practice in the public information directory.

36.5 Clinical Practice Management

Cut to the Chase ○ ○ ○ (free registration)
http://www.cuttothechase.com

Healthcare management information for physicians is available at this site, including articles about practice management issues, career development resources, publications and software sources, information about other products and services related to healthcare management, and links to sites offering additional healthcare management resources. Free site registration is required for access to these resources.

Guide to Clinical Preventive Services ○ ○ ○
http://158.72.20.10/pubs/guidecps

This guide is a comprehensive online reference source covering recommendations for clinical practice on 169 preventive interventions, including screening tests, counseling interventions, immunizations, chemoprophylactic regimens, and other preventive medical tools. Sixty (60) target conditions are discussed in the report.

Health Services/Technology Assessment Text (HSTAT) ○ ○ ○
http://text.nlm.nih.gov

This electronic resource for physicians provides access to consumer brochures, evidence reports, reference guides for clinicians, clinical practice guidelines, and other full-text documents useful in making healthcare decisions. Users can download documents from the site, access general information about the system, and browse links to additional sources for information. Searches can be comprehensive or limited to specific databases within the HSTAT system, and users can also search by keyword.

InfoMedical.com: The Medical Business Search Engine ○ ○ ○
http://www.InfoMedical.com

This engine allows users to search for companies, news, and press releases from submitted sites in the following categories: companies, distributors, products, organizations, services, and World Wide Web resources.

Martindale's Health Science Guide ○ ○ ○

http://www-sci.lib.uci.edu/~martindale/HSGuide.html

An all-encompassing site for physician resources, including clinical practice and research information, this Web service offers access to teaching files, medical cases, multimedia courses and textbooks, tutorials, and other databases. There is information on different medical disciplines including Bioscience, Chemistry, Nursing, Dental Medicine, Pharmacology, Public Health, and Biotechnology.

MDGateway ○ ○

http://www.mdgateway.com

Described as an Internet "onramp for physicians busy in clinical practice," this site offers health news articles and information on clinical, professional, and personal resources. Clinical resources include links to clinical applications, medications information, practice guidelines, and patient education literature. Professional links are available with respect to coding and billing information, resources for creating and maintaining a medical practice, medical societies, and sources for medical meetings/continuing medical education information. Personal finance information is also found at the site.

MedConnect ○ ○ ○

http://www.medconnect.com

Important medical resources at MedConnect include literature reviews, cases of the month, featured articles, journal clubs, Board reviews, free MEDLINE access, and teaching files discussing ECGs, x-rays, and CAT scans. This information is presented in separate journals of emergency medicine, pediatrics, managed care, and primary care.

MedPlanet ○ ○ ○

http://www.medplanet.com

Visitors to this site can search medical product classified advertisements, including surgical, anesthesia, monitoring, critical care, imaging, and laboratory equipment. The site also provides links to medical equipment manufacturers, dealers, and financing agencies. Users can add their own classified ads and include links to Web sites of equipment and product suppliers.

Medsite ○ ○ ○

http://www.medsite.com

This site describes itself as an e-services portal for the medical community. Services provided include books, medical software, and supplies at discounted prices; financial resources; a scheduling tool geared for medical professionals; and free e-mail accounts. The service requires free registration.

National Guideline Clearinghouse (NGC) ⊙ ⊙ ⊙

http://www.guideline.gov/index.asp

Four hundred and seventy-nine evidence-based clinical practice guidelines are offered at this indispensable site. Visitors can browse for guidelines by disease or condition or search for guidelines by keyword. Topical categories include immunologic, viral, endocrine, musculoskeletal, respiratory tract, urologic and male genital, nutritional and metabolic, otorhinolaryngologic, occupational, neonatal, eye, parasitic, nervous system, obstetric and gynecologic, skin and connective tissue, hemic and lymphatic, digestive system, and cardiovascular diseases, bacterial infections and mycoses, injuries, poisonings, and neoplasms.

Online Clinical Calculator ⊙ ⊙ ⊙

http://www.intmed.mcw.edu/clincalc.html

Directed at clinical practitioners, this site offers useful analytical tools and clinical formulas for a variety of medical purposes, including body surface calculations, heart disease risk, ingested substance blood level, pregnancy due date, weights and measures, and other subjects.

Online Directory of Medical Software ⊙ ⊙

http://www.crihealthcarepubs.com/onlindir.html

This directory provides the names, addresses, telephone numbers, and e-mail or Web site information for each of the state medical boards. Physicians can contact a board for information on licensing in that state or for other information regarding medical regulation or standards.

PDR.net ⊙ ⊙ ⊙ (some features fee-based)

http://www.PDR.net

PDR.net is a medical and healthcare Web site created by the Medical Economics Company, publisher of healthcare magazines and directories including the PDR (Physicians' Desk Reference). The site has specific areas and content for physicians, pharmacists, physician assistants, nurses, and consumers. Access to the full-text reference book is free for U.S.-based MDs, DOs and PAs in full-time practice. There is a fee for other users of this service, but most of the site's features are free.

Physician's Guide to the Internet ⊙ ⊙ ⊙

http://www.physiciansguide.com

This site contains a directory of Web sites for physicians. Features include physician lifestyle resources, such as sites offering suggestions on stress relief; news items; clinical practice resources, including access to medical databases and patient education resources; and postgraduate education and new physician resources. Other resources include links to sites selling medical books, products, and services for physicians; links to Internet search tools; and Internet tutorials.

Practice Management Information Corporation ◎ ◎
http://medicalbookstore.com/arm.htm

This site provides an opportunity for physicians to order books that offer information on topics that relate to the management of a private medical practice. Books on medical coding and reimbursement are also available.

State Medical Boards Directory ◎ ◎
http://www.fsmb.org/members.htm

This directory provides the names, addresses, telephone numbers, and e-mail or Web site information for each of the state medical boards. Physicians can contact a Board for information on licensing in that state or for other information regarding medical regulation or standards.

36.6 Genetics

Frontiers in Clinical Genetics ◎ ◎ ◎
http://www.frontiersingenetics.com/main.htm

Presented by The George Washington University Medical Center, this site offers lectures on various genetics topics presented on the Web via Real Audio. Directed at physicians requiring CME credit, the lectures assume a good deal of prior knowledge of genetics. There is also a listing of links to related sites. Lectures are archived for a period of two years to permit future study and reference.

GeneClinics ◎ ◎ ◎
http://www.geneclinics.org

GeneClinics is a knowledge base of expert-authored, up-to-date information relating genetic testing to the diagnosis, management, and counseling of individuals and families with inherited disorders. Indexed articles are of a specific and technical nature intended for use by healthcare professionals. The site also includes an extensive listing of disease profiles that is continuously updated.

Genetics Revolution at Time.com ◎ ◎
http://www.pathfinder.com/time/daily/special/genetics/index.html

This article from Time.com tracks the progress of the rapid advances in genetic technology. The site gathers a great deal of up-to-date information and offers links to a number of additional related Web-based resources.

Genetics Virtual Library ○ ○ ○

http://www.ornl.gov/TechResources/Human_Genome/genetics.html

This site contains a comprehensive listing of links to major Web sites on specific topics in genetics. Links are subdivided by organism, providing genetics information on many animals, from transgenic mice to humans. Brief descriptions are provided for many links.

Institute for Genomic Research (TIGR) ○ ○ ○

http://www.tigr.org

The Institute for Genomic Research is a not-for-profit research institute with interests in structural, functional, and comparative analysis of genomes and gene products in viruses, eubacteria, archaea, and eukaryotes. Information on recent advances in genetics and continuing research projects in the area of human genomics, an extensive searchable database of previous research, and links to other genome centers worldwide are available at this site.

Kyoto Encyclopedia of Genes and Genomes (KEGG) ○ ○ ○

http://www.genome.ad.jp/kegg

The Kyoto Encyclopedia of Genes and Genomes (KEGG) attempts to computerize current knowledge of molecular and cellular biology in terms of information pathways consisting of interacting molecules or genes, and also provides links to gene catalogs produced by genome sequencing projects. Information indexed at this site ranges from basic genetic information to extremely technical descriptions of molecular pathways. Also provided is a listing of links to other major Internet sites containing information relevant to genetic research.

Molecular Genetics Jump Station ○ ○ ○

http://www.horizonpress.com/gateway/genetics.html

This site provides a comprehensive listing of Web-based resources for geneticists. Sites indexed here are technical in nature and intended for investigators. Resources include links to molecular biology, microbiology, and genetics jump sites (containing catalogs of links); sites containing protocols on laboratory techniques; journals and other online publications, news groups, and mail lists; institutes and organizations; conferences and meetings announcements; commercial sites; and sources for ordering technical books. The site is sponsored by Beckman, Horizon Scientific Press, *Journal of Molecular Microbiology and Biotechnology,* and MWG-Biotech.

National Center for Biotechnology Information (NCBI): Online Mendelian Inheritance in Man (OMIM) ○ ○ ○

http://www.ncbi.nlm.nih.gov/Omim

Dr. Victor A. McKusick, a researcher at Johns Hopkins, and his colleagues have authored this database of human genes and genetic disorders. The database was developed for the World Wide Web by the National Center for Biotechnology Information. Reference information, texts, and images are found through the site, as well as links to the Entrez database of MEDLINE articles and sequence information. Visitors can search the OMIM Database, OMIM Gene Map, and OMIM Morbid Map (a catalog of cytogenetic map locations organized by disease) from the site. Information on the OMIM numbering system, details on creating links to OMIM, site updates, OMIM statistics, information on citing OMIM in literature, and the OMIM gene list are all found at the site. Links are available to allied resources, and the complete text of OMIM and gene maps can be downloaded from the site.

National Human Genome Research Institute (NHGRI) ⊙ ⊙ ⊙
http://www.nhgri.nih.gov
The National Human Genome Research Institute supports the NIH component of the Human Genome Project, a worldwide research effort designed to analyze the structure of human DNA and determine the location of the estimated 50,000-100,000 human genes. The NHGRI Intramural Research Program develops and implements technology for understanding, diagnosing, and treating genetic diseases. The site provides information about NHGRI, the Human Genome Project, grants, intramural research, policy and public affairs, workshops and conferences, and news items. Resources include links to the Institute's Ethical, Legal, and Social Implications Program, and the Center for Inherited Disease Research. The site also provides genetic resources for investigators, a glossary of genetic terms, and a site search engine.

Office of Genetics and Disease Prevention ⊙ ⊙ ⊙
http://www.cdc.gov/genetics
Created by the Centers for Disease Control and Prevention, this site offers access to current information on the impact of human genetic research and the Human Genome Project on public health and disease prevention. The site provides general information, indexes recent articles, lists events and training opportunities, and offers an extensive listing of links to other resources. Users can search the site by keyword and access the Human Genome Epidemiology Network (HuGENet), a global collaboration of individuals and organizations committed to the development and dissemination of population-based epidemiologic information on the human genome.

Primer on Molecular Genetics ⊙ ⊙ ⊙
http://www.ornl.gov/hgmis/publicat/primer/intro.html
The United States Department of Energy presents an excellent resource for those seeking basic background information on genetics and genetic research at this site. Discussions at the site include an introduction to genetics, DNA, genes, chromosomes, and the process of mapping the human genome. Mapping strategies, genetic linkage maps, and various physical maps are available, as well as links to mapping and sequence databases and a glossary of terms. The site also summarizes the predicted impact of the Human Genome Project on medical practice and biological research.

University of Kansas Medical Center: Genetics Education Center ⊚ ⊚ ⊚
http://www.kumc.edu/gec

Links are available at this address to Internet resources for educators interested in human genetics and the Human Genome Project. Sites are listed by topic, including the Human Genome Project, education resources, networking, genetic conditions, booklets and brochures, genetics programs and other resources, and glossaries. Lesson plans are offered both by the University of Kansas and other sources at the site. A description of different careers in genetics are also available. This site is an excellent tool for finding useful genetics Internet resources for nonprofessionals and educators.

36.7 Geriatrics

Administration on Aging: Resource Directory for Older People ⊚ ⊚ ⊚
http://www.aoa.dhhs.gov/aoa/dir/intro.html

The National Institute on Aging and the Administration on Aging has compiled this directory of resources, serving older people and their families, health and legal professionals, social service providers, librarians, researchers, and others interested in the field of aging. The directory includes names of organizations, addresses, telephone numbers (including toll-free numbers), and links to Internet sites, when available. Visitors can search the directory by keyword or view the entire table of contents from this address.

American Geriatrics Society (AGS) ⊚ ⊚ ⊚ (some features fee-based)
http://www.americangeriatrics.org

A national nonprofit association of geriatrics health professionals, research scientists, and other concerned individuals, the American Geriatrics Society is dedicated to "improving the health, independence, and quality of life for all older people." The site offers a description of the Society, adult immunization information, AGS news, conference and other events notices, legislation news, career opportunities, directories of geriatrics health care services in managed care, position statements, educational, and practice guidelines, awards information, and other professional education resources. Patient education resources, a selected bibliography in geriatrics, links to related organizations and government sites, surveys, and a site search tool are also found at this address.

36.8 Grants and Award Guides

Community of Science ◎ ◎ (free registration)
http://www.cos.com
Community of Science offers directories of current funding opportunities, profiles of researchers, career resources, professional discussion forums, information on buying laboratory equipment and supplies, news, and other valuable materials for investigators and health professionals.

Foundation Center ◎ ◎ ◎
http://fdncenter.org
The Foundation Center provides direct, hot links to thousands of grant-making organizations, including foundations, corporations, and public charities, along with a search engine to enable the user to locate sources of funding in specific fields. In addition, the site provides listings of the largest private foundations, corporate grant makers, and community foundations. There is also information on funding trends, a newsletter, and grant-seeker orientation material. More than 900 grant-making organizations are accessible through this useful site.

National Institutes of Health (NIH): Funding Opportunities ◎ ◎ ◎
http://grants.nih.gov/grants
Funding opportunities for research, scholarship, and training are extensive within the federal government. At this site for the National Institutes of Health, there is a Grants Page with information about NIH grants and fellowship programs, information on Research Contracts containing information on Requests for Proposals (RFPs), Research Training Opportunities in biomedical areas, and an NIH Guide for Grants and Contracts. The latter is the official document for announcing the availability of NIH funds for biomedical and behavioral research and research training policies. Links are provided to major divisions of NIH that have additional information on specialized grant opportunities.

National Science Foundation (NSF) Grants and Awards ◎ ◎ ◎
http://www.nsf.gov/home/grants.htm
Because approximately 20% of the federal support to academic institutions for basic research comes from the National Science Foundation, this site is an important source of information for award opportunities, programs, application procedures, and other vital information. Forms and agreements may be downloaded as well, and regulations and policy guidelines are set forth clearly.

Polaris Grants Central ○ ○

http://polarisgrantscentral.net

For the grant seeker, this site provides resources that are available from numerous organizations pertaining to grant identification and application. There are books and publications on grant sources, descriptions of grant information providers, clearinghouses for grant information, federal contacts, grant training materials, and resources on disk or CD-ROM. Within the site, useful sections provide "Tips and Hints" on writing grant proposals, "Grants News" from different government agencies and other organizations, "Scholarships or Grants to Individuals," and information on grant workshops.

Society of Research Administrators (SRA) GrantsWeb ○ ○ ○

http://www.srainternational.org/cws/sra/resource.htm

The Society of Research Administrators has created an extremely useful grant information site, with extensive links to government resources, general resources, private funding, and policy/regulation sites. The site section devoted to U.S., Canadian, and other international resources provides links to government agency funding sources, the commerce business daily, the Catalog of Federal Domestic Assistance, scientific agencies, research councils, and resources in individual fields, such as health, education, and business. Grant-application procedures, regulations, and guidelines are provided throughout the site, and extensive legal information is provided through links to patent, intellectual property, and copyright offices. Associations providing funding and grant information are also listed, with direct links.

36.9 Imaging and Pathology

Center for Biomedical Imaging Technology ○ ○ ○

http://www.cbit.uchc.edu/index.html

Current research performed by the Center for Biomedical Imaging Technology is presented at this site in the form of medical imaging examples accomplished by the Center. A short tutorial on the classification of MR images, videos, and abstracts on light microscopy of living cells, and the structure and function of the endoplasmic reticulum are available through links at the site.

Center for Human Simulation ○ ○ ○

http://www.uchsc.edu/sm/chs

This site provides a browser to view cross sections from any part of the bodies from the Visible Human Project. Also included are images, animations, videos, and 3-D polygonal models of various parts of the human anatomy that were created using new imaging technology.

CT Is Us ○ ○ ○

http://www.ctisus.org

The CT (computed tomography) site offers information on medical imaging with a specific focus on spiral CT and 3D imaging. Images of the body and various medical conditions are organized by region, and information on continuing medical education (CME) courses, teaching files, medical illustrations, and a 3D vascular atlas are all available at the site.

Digital Imaging Center ○ ○ ○

http://info.med.yale.edu/library/imaging

This Web site, provided by Cushing/Whitney Medical Library of Yale University, serves as a starting point for help on the various resources available through the Digital Imaging Center, including a digital camera, computer resource lab, color printers, scanners, and digital video editing capabilities. Resources at this site are most useful to visitors with access to the Cushing/Whitney Medical Library Digital Imaging Center.

Dr. Morimoto's Image Library of Radiology ○ ○ ○

http://www.osaka-med.ac.jp/omc-lib/noh.html

This site provides users with access to images and videos collected by Dr. Morimoto, Department of Radiology, Osaka National Hospital. Images were scanned and stored with JPEG, GIF format, and movies with QuickTime format. Visitors can download the images freely but need permission for redistribution. Ultrasonographic anatomy images related to the liver, pancreas, and bile duct include an illustration of portal anatomy, normal bile duct, tumor of liver hilum, bile duct cancer, pancreatic cancer, esophageal varix, and obstructive jaundice. Heart and major vessels images include a normal heart, major vessels of the body, and abdominal aortic aneurysm. Head images include a surface image of human head and an image of an arachnoid cyst. Images related to the kidney and urinary tract include that of a renal cell carcinoma.

Health on the Net (HON) Foundation ○ ○ ○

http://www.hon.ch/Media/anatomy.html

This site provides links to radiological and surgical images on the Internet. Images are available of the abdomen, ankle, arm, full body, brain, elbow, eye, foot, hand, head, heart, hilum, hip, kidney, knee, leg, liver, lung, muscle, neck, pancreas, pelvis, shoulder, skin, skull, teeth, thorax, trachea, blood vessels, and wrist.

Integrated Medical Curriculum: Human Anatomy ○ ○ ○ (free registration)

http://www.imc.gsm.com

An extensive database of images can be easily accessed for educational purposes. The site covers Human Anatomy, Microscopic Anatomy, Radiologic Anatomy, Cross-Sectional Anatomy, as well as essentials of Human Physiology, essentials of Immunology, and Clinical Pharmacology. A simple, free registration is required.

Medical i-Way ⊙ ⊙ ⊙

http://www.largnet.on.ca/oldlargnet

Medical i-Way demonstrates pathology through the use of medical imaging. A separate section is devoted to each anatomical group, with a list of specific pathologies available for view. Details of each image include case history, diagnosis, image findings, and descriptions of similar cases. Users can also find images through a keyword index.

Medical Images on the Web ⊙ ⊙ ⊙

http://www.unmc.edu/library/medimag.html

Eleven links are available at this address to Internet sources for medical images. All links are accompanied by short descriptions of resources at the site.

Mudi-Muse Biomedical Imaging and Processing ⊙ ⊙ ⊙

http://www.expasy.ch/LFMI

The MultiDimensional-MultiSensor/MultiModality Biomedical Imaging and Processing Web site provides examples and applications of different techniques used in biomedical imaging. Multidimensional, multimodality, and multi-sensor applications are described in detail with specific examples of medical applications, and discussions of new developments in this growing field are available.

National Library of Medicine (NLM): New Visible Human Project ⊙ ⊙ ⊙

http://www.nlm.nih.gov/research/visible/visible_human.html

The Visible Human Project, devoted to the creation of complete, anatomically detailed, three-dimensional representations of the normal male and female human bodies, is an outgrowth of the National Library of Medicine's 1986 Long Range Plan. The Project has recently completed acquisition of transverse CT, MR, and cryosection images of representative male and female cadavers. The site describes the Visible Human Data Set and how to obtain data, and provides links to primary contractors for the Project, a sampler of images and animations from the project, and links to articles and other press releases discussing the Project. Applications and tools for viewing images are discussed, and links to sources of images and animations are provided. This site is also available in Spanish.

Neurosciences on the Internet: Images ⊙ ⊙ ⊙

http://www.neuroguide.com/neuroimg.html

Internet sites are found through this address offering resources relating to human neuroanatomy and neuropathology, neuroscience images and methods, medical imaging centers, medical illustration, medical imaging indexes, and neuroanatomy atlases of animals.

Normal Radiologic Anatomy ⊙ ⊙

http://www.vh.org/Providers/TeachingFiles/NormalRadAnatomy/Text/RadM1title.html

This site provides visitors with X-Ray, CT, MR, and ultrasound images of the head and neck, thorax, abdomen, pelvis, upper extremity, and lower extremity. Images are labeled to identify normal anatomic structures.

PERLjam Online/Medical Images, Including Neuroanatomy ⊙ ⊙ ⊙

http://erl.pathology.iupui.edu

This site is an online version of the PERLjam CD-ROM of pathology, histology, and laboratory medicine resources distributed to Indiana University School of Medicine students. The Indiana University School of Medicine Pathology Educational Resources Laboratory provides general and systemic pathology, histology, laboratory medicine, and dermatology images at this site. Images are categorized by organ system.

Three-Dimensional Medical Reconstruction ⊙ ⊙ ⊙

http://www.crd.ge.com/esl/cgsp/projects/medical

Three-dimensional (3-D) reconstruction technology and medical imaging was employed to make short videos showing various sections of the human anatomy at this site. Information on the Visible Human Project and several short videos on this topic, surgical planning, and virtual endoscopy are also available.

University of Illinois College of Medicine at Urbana, Champaign: The Urbana Atlas of Pathology ⊙ ⊙ ⊙

http://www.med.uiuc.edu/PathAtlasf/framer2/path3.html

The site provides an extremely comprehensive collection of images sectioned into general, cardiovascular, endocrine, pulmonary, and renal pathology. The general pathology section includes images of the kidney, heart, spleen, thyroid, testis, cervix, small intestine, lung, artery, pancreas, liver, lymph nodes, brain, colon, skin, mesentery, joints, uterus, and peritoneal cavity.

University of Iowa: Division of Physiological Imaging Department of Radiology ⊙ ⊙ ⊙

http://everest.radiology.uiowa.edu

This site describes work done by the Division of Physiological Imaging of the University of Iowa College of Medicine. This group is dedicated to the research and advancement of medical imaging technology. Within the Web site are examples of medical imaging, selected papers on the field, descriptions of new technology and projects, and a list of links to related sites.

Visible Human Slice and Surface Server ○ ○ ○
http://visiblehuman.epfl.ch

This site provides a viewer that enables the user to see images of planar and curved surfaces from the bodies of the Visible Human Project.

36.10 Medical Informatics

American Medical Association (AMA): Coding and Medical Information Systems ○ ○ ○
http://www.ama-assn.org/med-sci/cpt/cpt.htm

This site provides information on the AMA's new current procedural terminology (CPT) information services, the resource-based relative value scale, and electronic medical systems, including systems for storing electronic medical records, telemedicine resources, and electronic data interchange. Information is also available on the National Uniform Claim Committee and Administrative Simplification Legislation.

American Medical Association (AMA): Electronic Medical Systems and Coding ○ ○ ○
http://www.ama-assn.org/med-sci/cpt/oems.htm

The American Medical Association plays a key role in the field of medical informatics. This site provides information on coding and medical information systems relative to the transmission of computerized patient and claims information. There are also links for electronic medical records, telemedicine, electronic data exchange, national uniform claim standards, and administrative simplification legislation.

American Medical Informatics Association (AMIA) ○ ○ ○
http://www.amia.org

With the proliferation of medical information, the growth of medical research, the development of medical information systems, and the creation of management systems for computerized patient data, the medical informatics field has grown substantially. This leading association provides its own organization, meeting, policy, and information access features, and also provides links to other organizations in the informatics field. Major themes of the AMIA are privacy and confidentiality of medical records, public policy development for legislation in the field, conferences of medical informatics professionals, and the issuance of papers and publications covering various aspects of the medical information field.

Health Network: Medical Informatics Resources ○ ○
http://www.healthwave.com

A dozen U.S. and international centers and medical departments dealing with Medical Informatics can be accessed from this central listing (click on Professional Medicine,

Medical Informatics), including centers at Oregon Health Sciences University, Stanford, Columbia, and at European institutions. There are also articles, directories, and discussion group links for further resources on Medical Informatics.

36.11 Patent Searches

The following sites provide easy access to patent information for medical researchers and healthcare professionals interested in learning about the latest techniques, therapies, products, and drugs.

Intellectual Property Network ○ ○ ○
http://www.patents.ibm.com

Ideal for physicians and researchers with an interest in patents, this IBM service offers a searchable database of patent information, titles and abstracts, and inventors and companies. The database brings up patents on any topic by typing in the subject, along with inventor information, dates of filing, application numbers, and an abstract of the patent.

U.S. Patent and Trademark Office ○ ○ ○
http://www.uspto.gov/patft/index.html

Access to the database of the U.S. Patent and Trademark Office is available through this site, for detailed searching of patents by number, inventor, and topic. There are both a full-text database and a bibliographic database.

37. STUDENT RESOURCES

37.1 Fellowships and Residencies

Accreditation Council for Graduate Medical Education (ACGME) ○ ○ ○
http://www.acgme.org

The ACGME reviews and accredits residency programs, establishes standards of performance, and provides a process to consider complaints and possible investigations by the Council. The site offers information about ACGME, meetings, workshops, institutional reviews, contact details, links to residency review committees, and a listing of accredited programs.

American Medical Association (AMA): Fellowship and Residency Electronic Interactive Database Access (FREIDA) Online System ○ ○ ○
http://www.ama-assn.org/physdata/datacoll/datacoll.htm

Operated as a service of the American Medical Association (AMA), the FREIDA System provides online access to a comprehensive database of information on approximately 7,500 graduate medical educational programs accredited by the Accreditation Council for Graduate Medical Education (ACGME). FREIDA enables the user to search this comprehensive database and offers other services, including label printing for mailing purposes.

Educational Commission for Foreign Medical Graduates (ECFMG) ○ ○ ○
http://www.ecfmg.org

The Educational Commission for Foreign Medical Graduates, through its certification program, "assesses the readiness of graduates of foreign medical schools to enter residency or fellowship programs in the United States that are accredited by the Accreditation Council for Graduate Medical Education (ACGME)." The site is a very useful source of information for foreign students to learn about testing and examination dates, clinical skills required, and available publications to review requirements for applications.

Electronic Residency Application Service ○ ○ ○

http://www.aamc.org

The Association of American Medical Colleges (AAMC) provides this application service for students. It transmits residency applications, recommendation letters, Dean's letters, transcripts, and other supporting credentials from medical schools to residency program directors via the Internet. At present, the service covers Obstetrics and Gynecology, Pediatrics, Surgery, and Psychiatry. The system allows tracking of an application 24 hours a day via a special document tracking system.

National Residency Matching Program (NRMP) ○ ○ ○

http://nrmp.aamc.org/nrmp/index.htm

The NRMP is a mechanism for the matching of applicants to programs according to the preferences expressed by both parties. This is an extremely useful site and service, which last year placed over 20,000 applicants for postgraduate medical training positions into 3,500 residency programs at 700 teaching hospitals in the United States. The applicants and residency programs evaluate and rank each other, producing a computerized pairing of applicants to programs, in ranked order. This process provides applicants and program directors with a uniform date of appointment to positions in March, eliminating decision pressure when options are unknown. The site offers information about the service, contact details, publications, and forms for registration. Prospective residents can register with the service for a fee and access the directory of programs.

Residency Page ○ ○ ○

http://www.Webcom.com/~wooming/residenc.html

The Residency Page Web site provides an online listing of medical residencies organized by specialty. Program directors can access resumes of residency applicants, and prospective residents can review documents related to residency matching programs and publications offering advice on obtaining a position.

37.2 Medical School Web Sites

American Universities ○ ○ ○

http://www.clas.ufl.edu/CLAS/american-universities.html

All American university home pages are listed at this site.

Gradschools.com ○ ○ ○

http://www.gradschools.com/noformsearch.html

Sponsored by several universities and other teaching institutions, Gradschools.com offers a listing of graduate programs nationwide. Programs are found by indicating a specific area of study. A directory of distance learning programs is also available.

Medical Education ◐ ◐ ◐
http://www.meducation.com/schools.html
Accredited medical schools are listed, with links, at this site.

Medical Schools ◐ ◐ ◐
http://www.scomm.net/~greg/med-ed/schools.html
This medical site provides direct links to all of the medical schools of U.S. and Canada accredited by the AAMC. These include hundreds of medical school Web sites in the United States and elsewhere.

37.3 Medical Student Resources

Amazon.com: Medical Books ◐ ◐ ◐
http://www.abcba.com/books/medical.htm
This site allows users to search by medical topic or keyword for medical textbooks. Dictionaries, encyclopedias, and Physician's Desk References on different subjects may be ordered through the site.

American Medical Association (AMA): Medical Student Section ◐ ◐ ◐
http://www.ama-assn.org/ama/pub/category/0,1120,14,FF.html
The Medical Student Section of the American Medical Association (AMA) is dedicated to representing medical students, improving medical education, developing leadership, and promoting activism for the health of America. The site offers information about the section, current issues and advocacy activities, business issues of the section, chapter information, and leadership news. Special interest groups within the section include those for residents, young physicians, organized staff, students, international medical graduates, and senior physicians.

American Medical Women's Association (AMWA) ◐ ◐ ◐
http://www.amwa-doc.org
A national association, the AMWA provides information and services to women physicians and women medical students, and promotes women's health and the professional development of women physicians. Resources include news, discussions of current issues, events, conferences, online publications, fellowship and residency information accessed through FREIDA, general information and developments from AMA staff members, advocacy activities, a listing of AMWA continuing education programs, and links to sites of interest. A variety of topics related to women's health are discussed at the site.

Association of American Medical Colleges (AAMC) ○ ○ ○

http://www.aamc.org

This nonprofit Association committed to the advancement of academic medicine consists of American and Canadian medical schools, teaching hospitals and health systems, academic and professional societies, and medical students and residents. News, membership details, publications and other information resources, meeting and conference calendars, medical education Internet resources, research findings, and discussions related to health care are all found at the site. Employment opportunities at the AAMC are also listed.

IMpact: The Internal Medicine Newsletter for Medical Students ○ ○ ○

http://www.acponline.org/journals/impact/impmenu.htm

This online newsletter focuses on different medical specialties with each issue, and includes full-text articles of interest to physicians and medical students. The newsletter is produced by the American College of Physicians—American Society of Internal Medicine (ACP-ASIM). Students can apply for free membership in the ACP-ASIM if they are currently enrolled in medical school.

Medical Student Cooperative: Medical Education Links ○ ○ ○

http://www.secondvision.com/msc/med_ed/links/index.htm

Medical education links found through this address are provided for the benefit of both medical students and patients. Specific resources are listed by organ system or medical discipline, and resources devoted to special clinical topics are also listed. Several infectious disease topics are also separately listed. All tutorials listed at the site are designated if peer-reviewed; physician oriented; providing adequate patient resources; non-commercial; multimedia enhanced; and regularly updated.

Medical Student Web Site ○ ○ ○

http://www.medicalstudent.com

This is an excellent, current site for medical students, describing itself as "a digital library of authoritative medical information for all students of medicine." It contains an extensive medical textbook section organized by discipline, patient simulations, consumer health information, access to MEDLINE and medical journals online, continuing education sources, board exam information, medical organizations, and Internet medical directories.

Stanford MedWorld ○ ○ ○

http://www-med.stanford.edu/medworld/home

MedWorld, sponsored by the Stanford Medical Alumni Association, offers information for students, patients, physicians, and the healthcare community. Resources include case reports and global rounds, links to quality medical sites and MEDLINE, doctor diaries and medical news, and newsgroups and discussion forums. Visitors can access

Stanford's medical search engine, MEDBOT, to simultaneously utilize many Internet medical search engines.

Student Doctor Network:
The Interactive Medical Student Lounge ○ ○ ○

http://www.medstudents.net

This is an excellent site for medical students with interests in all medical specialties as well as all aspects of the medical community. The site provides information on applying to medical school, financial aid, internships and residencies, medical chat rooms, databases, discussions of educational issues, links to online journals, news, updates, and broadcasts. In addition, the site provides access to discounts on medical equipment and books, the purchase and sale of used medical texts, medical software and medical CD-ROMs. Students can also access medical reference material, medical school sites, medical search engines, student groups, externships, foreign residencies, and medical missions abroad.

38. PATIENT EDUCATION AND PLANNING

38.1 Patient Resources

Patient information regarding various medical conditions and health issues can be obtained at any of the general medical search engines that are included. Below are listings of health Web sites accessible through the well-known search engines, as well as other sites that cover wide-ranging topics of interest to patients.

Allexperts.com

http://www.allexperts.com/browse.asp?Meta=24

Allexperts.com is a free online question and answer service. A message board and many frequently asked questions are present. Available medical topics are listed alphabetically, and users can choose a specific "volunteer expert" to contact after reading short biographies and descriptions of specialty areas.

allHealth.com

http://www.allhealth.com

Resources at this site include a site search engine; a drug database; information on specific conditions; weight management information; and special information centers devoted to seniors', women's, and men's health, pediatrics, mental health, sexual health, alternative medicine, asthma, headaches, smoking cessation, HIV/AIDS, heartburn, and family health. Physician directories for home and when traveling, elder care directories, interactive health calculators, an online newsletter, research information, chat forums, and news articles are also provided.

America Online (AOL) ◉ ◉
http://www.aol.com/timesavers/health.html

Sponsored by America Online, this site is a useful medical information source for the general public. The user can search for a disease; use a symptom analyzer; learn about rare illnesses; obtain advice; find support groups; and research topics on health, medicine, and wellness.

American Academy of Family Physicians Health Information Page ◉ ◉ ◉
http://familydoctor.org

This site allows visitors to search information by keyword or category, and is written and reviewed by the physicians and patient education professionals at the Academy of Family Physicians.

American Medical Association (AMA): Health Insight ◉ ◉ ◉
http://www.ama-assn.org/consumer.htm

Information for consumers at this site includes medical news; detailed information on a wide range of conditions; general health topic discussions; family health resources for children, adolescents, men, and women; interactive health calculators; healthy recipes; and general safety tips. Specific pages are devoted to comprehensive resources related to HIV/AIDS, asthma, migraines, and women's health. Patients will find this site an excellent source for accurate, useful health information. American Medical Association information at this site includes a directory of advisory board members and contact information for the Association.

BestDoctors.com ◉ ◉ (free registration)
http://www.bestdoctors.com

Best Doctors' Inc. provides information and searching services for superior medical care to major insurers, managed care companies, self-insured corporations, foreign governments, and individuals. The site provides visitors with news, feature articles from a participating doctor, drug information, general information, and suggested sites relating to over 40 health topics. Contact information, employment details, a directory of the company's medical advisory board, rating information on medical Web sites, news and events information, contact information for a physician referral service, and answers relating to recent Internet health-related rumors are all found at the site. Registered users can ask health questions, participate in chat forums, and gain access to medical newsletters.

Boston University Medical Center: Community Outreach Health Information System ◉ ◉ ◉
http://www.bu.edu/cohis

This site provides the general public with an excellent resource for health information. A wide range of health topics are discussed at the site, including AIDS/HIV, infectious diseases, sexually transmitted diseases, cancer, blood and heart diseases, nutrition, smoking cessation, domestic violence, teen pregnancy, and alcohol and substance abuse. More specific topics are also listed. Visitors can submit health questions and access a physician directory.

Columbia University: College of Physicians and Surgeons Complete Home Medical Guide ○ ○ ○

http://cpmcnet.columbia.edu/texts/guide

Patients will consider this site an excellent resource for healthcare information. Topics include receiving proper medical care, the correct use of medications, first aid and safety, preventative medicine, and good nutrition. Chapters containing more specific information on health concerns for men, women, and children; disorders; infectious diseases; mental and emotional health; and substance abuse are also available.

Combined Health Information Database (CHID) ○ ○ ○

http://chid.nih.gov

The Combined Health Information Database (CHID) is produced by several agencies of the federal government offering a searchable file of health promotion publications, education materials, and program descriptions. The site offers simple and detailed search options, and users can also indicate specific search criteria, including date and language of the publication. Availability and ordering information is provided for the resources included. Site updates are performed quarterly.

DiscoveryHealth.com ○ ○ ○

http://www.discoveryhealth.com/DH/ihtIH?t=20707&st=20707&r=WSDSC000

In association with InteliHealth, this site from the makers of the Discovery Channel offers consumer health resources. News items, feature articles and reports, a site search engine, links to health reference materials, chat forums, a forum for asking health questions, and descriptions of recent research advances are all found at this site. Visitors can learn interesting health facts and access information specific to men, women, senior citizens, children, mental health, and health in the workplace. Nutrition, fitness, and weight management tools are also available at this site.

DoctorDirectory: HealthNews Directory ○ ○

http://www.doctordirectory.com/HealthNews/Directory/Default.asp

In addition to daily news and a national directory of doctors listed by state, this site contains links to resources related to various health topics, including AIDS, allergies/asthma, alternative medicine, cancer, children's health, clinical trials, cosmetic surgery, dentistry, diabetes, women's health, geriatrics, healthcare companies, insurance, and other subjects.

drkoop.com ◉ ◉ ◉
http://www.drkoop.com

This site provides patients and the general public with an excellent source for current health information. Free registration and e-mail newsletters, site search engines, health news, chat topics, general information about clinical trials, and a drug interaction search tool are some of the most useful features. Please note that some sections of the site offering specific information are sponsored by pharmaceutical products, i.e., a company producing a smoking cessation medication sponsors a section designed to help users quit.

Family Village:
A Global Community of Disability-Related Resources ◉ ◉ ◉
http://www.familyvillage.wisc.edu/index.htmlx

This site provides the general public with cataloged information about a wide range of disorders and disabilities. Chat room links and other networking resources, support and medical resources, technology/products links, recreation programs, research programs, publications, and educational resources for children are all found at this comprehensive patient support site.

Health-Center.com ◉ ◉
http://site.health-center.com/default.htm

This site contains a variety of links to fact sheets on family issues, senior citizen related topics, general wellness topics, mental health information, and medications. There are also links to professional resources, including postings of online continuing education resources.

Healthanswers.com ◉ ◉ ◉
http://www.healthanswers.com

This site provides the general public with informational resources on a wide range of health topics, including senior health, pregnancy, alternative medicine, diseases, and healthy lifestyle tips. Partners include the American Academy of Pediatrics, the Center for Pharmacy, the National Health Council, the National Transplant Society, Reuters Health News, and other national groups and information resources.

HealthCentral ◉ ◉ ◉
http://www.healthcentral.com/home/home.cfm

News items, feature columns, quizzes and polls, a doctor's column, drug and herb information, health profiles and assessment tools, online shopping, and medical reference materials are all available at this useful site. Information centers offer specific resources on "hot topics," alternative medicine, fitness, life issues, wellness, consumer health, health improvement, such as weight loss and smoking cessation, and medical conditions.

HealthlinkUSA ○ ○ ○
http://www.healthlinkusa.com

At this site, links to many general health sites are listed in alphabetical order by topic or disorder. Interested persons can access links to specific health issues or browse for sites by medical category.

HealthWorld Online ○ ○ ○
http://www.healthy.net

A subject map appears at the beginning of this site indicating the many aspects of the health and medical world covered by numerous links. There is a topical site search engine, access to publications through MEDLINE at the National Library of Medicine, information on specific diseases and alternative therapies, a referral network, a global calendar, and information on wellness, fitness, and nutrition.

InteliHealth: Home to Harvard University Health Information ○ ○ ○
http://www.intelihealth.com/IH/ihtIH?t=408&st=408&r=WSIHW000

This comprehensive site offers consumers tips on healthy living, information, and other resources on specific conditions, a site search engine for specific information, health news by topic, special reports, an online newsletter, pharmaceutical drug information, and an online store offering health items for the home. Conditions and health topics discussed at the site include allergy, arthritis, asthma, babies, cancer, caregivers, childhood, diabetes, digestive, fitness, headache, heart, mental health, pregnancy, vitamin and nutrition, and weight management. Links are available to other sites offering consumer health resources.

Johns Hopkins Medical Institutions (InfoNet) ○ ○ ○
http://infonet.welch.jhu.edu/advocacy.html

A database of patient advocacy groups is housed at this site. Telephone contact information and links to an associated Web site is offered for most organizations. A search tool is available to find groups for specific disorders.

KidsHealth.org ○ ○ ○
http://kidshealth.org/index2.html

This site, created by the Nemours Foundation Center for Children's Health Media, provides expert health information about children from before birth through adolescence. Specific sections target kids, teens, and parents, with age-appropriate information and language.

Mayo Clinic: Health Oasis ○ ○ ○
http://www.mayohealth.org/index.htm

Visitors to this informative site will find answers to patient questions, news and articles on featured topics, registration details for e-mail alerts of site updates, and site search engines for health information and prescription drug information. Specific information centers are devoted to allergy and asthma, Alzheimer's disease, cancer, children's health, digestive health, heart health, general medicine, men's and women's health, and nutrition. A library of answers to health questions, a glossary of medical terms, and a forum for asking specific questions are also available at the site.

MDAdvice.com
http://www.mdadvice.com

In addition to containing links to informative fact sheets on a variety of health topics (arranged alphabetically), this site provides detailed information on pharmaceuticals, medicine in the news, information on health centers, expert advice, and chat rooms.

Med Help International
http://www.medhelp.org

This all-encompassing site describes itself as "the largest online consumer health information resource with tens of thousands of entries." It includes a medical search engine, library access and doctor forums, medical and health news, and support groups.

MedicineNet.com
http://www.medicinenet.com

An efficient and thorough source of information on hundreds of diseases and medical conditions, MedicineNet enables the user to click on subjects in an alphabetical list. The site's medical content is produced by Board certified physicians and allied health professionals. Topics include diseases and treatments, procedures and tests, a pharmacy section, a medical dictionary, first aid information, and a list of poison control centers.

Mediconsult.com
http://www.mediconsult.com

Mediconsult provides medical news and information on a variety of topics, including cancer, chronic pain, eating disorders, and migraines. The information at the site is drawn from journals, research centers, and other sources, and is subject to a rigorous clinical review process. Specific sections are devoted to health issues relevant to women, men, seniors, children, and caregivers. Additional resources include a medical directory of disease information, drug information, fitness and nutrition discussions, a question and answer forum, and live chat events.

MEDLINEplus
http://www.nlm.nih.gov/medlineplus

This site is a source for information on various diseases and health topics for the public, featuring a directory of links divided into categories such as health topics, dictionaries, other directories, organizations, and publications. The site links to MEDLINE, either through PubMed or the Internet Grateful Med.

National Women's Health Information Center (NWHIC) ○ ○ ○
http://www.4woman.org

This searchable site offers lists of publications and organizations for information on a wide range of women's health topics. There are also links to resources for special groups, journals, FAQs, news items and affiliated organizations, as well as information about the NWHIC itself.

NetWellness ○ ○ ○ (some features fee-based)
http://www.netwellness.org

NetWellness is a Web-based consumer health information service with one of the largest groups of medical and health experts who answer consumer questions on the Web. Developed by the University of Cincinnati Medical Center, The Ohio State University, and Case Western Reserve University, over 200 health faculty answer questions on over 40 topics. Responses are usually provided within two to three days. Users can also search archives of articles.

New York Online Access to Health (NOAH) ○ ○ ○ (some features fee-based)
http://www.noah.cuny.edu

This site is offered as a public resource by many providers, including hospitals, institutes, foundations, research centers, and city and state agencies. Users can access information concerning a wide range of health topics, including diseases, mental health, nutrition, and links to patient resources. A site-based search engine is available. A health information database containing abstracts and articles from selected health-related periodicals is only available to users accessing the site from specific institutions, including the New York Public Library branches.

OnHealth ○ ○ ○
http://www.onhealth.com/ch1/index.asp

Visitors to this site can search for health information by keyword or condition, access news and reports, ask health questions, and find many useful information resources related to specific topics, such as smoking cessation, pharmaceutical drugs, alternative medicine, vitamins and minerals, and first aid. Chat forums, information on live chat events, physician and medical center directories, online shopping opportunities, and interactive health assessment tools are all found at this site.

Prevention Magazine Online ○ ○ ○
http://www.healthyideas.com

Prevention Magazine offers resources for healthier living at this site. Health tools include a calorie calculator, exercise and weight loss information, recipes, vitamin and herb information, and tips on skin care. Online newsletters and stores, chat forums, and subscription details for the magazine are available, as well as resource centers offering specific information on health conditions, men's and women's health, and pediatrics. Links are also found to women.com for specific women's resources.

Psci-com ○ ○ ○
http://www.psci-com.org.uk

Psci-com is described as "a gateway to public understanding of science and science communication information on the Internet." The site offers a searchable catalog of Internet resources selected and cataloged by the Wellcome Trust for the benefit of the UK public.

Quackwatch ○ ○ ○
http://www.quackwatch.com

Quackwatch is a nonprofit corporation combating "health-related frauds, myths, fads, and fallacies." The group investigates questionable health claims, answers consumer inquiries, distributes publications, reports illegal marketing, generates consumer-protection lawsuits, works to improve the quality of health information on the Internet, and attacks misleading Internet advertising. Operation costs are generated solely from the sales of publications and individual donations. Sister sites, Chirobase and MLM Watch, offer a consumer's guide to chiropractors and a skeptical guide to multilevel marketing. Information for cancer patients includes alerts of questionable alternative health treatments, a discussion of how questionable practices may harm cancer patients, and other related discussions. Cancer prevention information alerts are also posted. Visitors to the site can purchase publications, read general information about questionable medical practices, and read information about specific questionable products and services. Links to government agencies and other sites providing information about health fraud are available at this important site.

ThriveOnline ○ ○ ○
http://www.thriveonline.com

ThriveOnline offers information resources in the areas of general medicine, fitness, sexuality, nutrition, serenity and mental wellness, and weight. Users can find information by choosing from a list of medical conditions, or employ search capabilities by keyword or in question form.

University of California, Davis: Medical Center Patient Care ○ ○ ○
http://www.pcs.ucdmc.ucdavis.edu

This site contains information about patient care services at UC Davis Medical Center as well as a list of health resources on the Internet. Specific resources include topics in patient care, education, and epidemiology and infection control.

Virtual Hospital:
University of Iowa Health Care ○ ○ ○ (some features fee-based)
http://www.vh.org

The Virtual Hospital is a service of the University of Iowa, providing patients and healthcare professionals with a digital library of health information. The library contains hundreds of books and brochures on health related issues, and also provides physicians with continuing medical education resources. The site provides information about the departments at the University of Iowa hospitals, a link to the Virtual Children's Hospital, continuing medical education information, and resource sections for patients and healthcare providers. Two sections are restricted to University of Iowa students, faculty, and affiliates.

Yahoo! ○ ○ ○
http://www.yahoo.com

A reliable source of information in most fields, Yahoo offers a Health Section covering diseases, medical topics, patient information, fitness, and other health topics. It is a good place to start for a patient seeking general information.

38.2 Support Groups

Ask NOAH About: Support Groups ○ ○ ○
http://www.noah.cuny.edu:8080/support1.html

This directory of Web sites and other resources includes links to other directories, general health sites, toll-free telephone numbers, face-to-face support groups, support organizations, newsgroups, mailing lists, chat forums, and other online support resources. Visitors can browse listings by type of resource or by specific medical conditions.

Support-Group.com ○ ○ ○
http://www.support-group.com

Support-Group.com allows people with health, personal, and relationship issues to share their experiences through bulletin boards and online chats, and provides plenty of links to support-related information on the Internet. The A to Z listing offers hundreds of connections to disease-related support, bereavement assistance, marriage and family issue groups, and women's/men's issues, to name a few. The Bulletin Board Tracker lists the most recent messages and provides a complete cross-reference of topics. By visiting the Support-Group.com Chat Schedule page, dates, times, and group facilitators for upcoming chat events can be viewed. Users have the option of participating in real time Chat Groups via Internet Relay Chat or JavaChat using a Java-capable Web browser. Complete instructions are available at the Web site.

38.3 Medical Planning

Blood Bank Information

America's Blood Centers ◐ ◐
http://www.americasblood.org

America's Blood Centers are found in 46 states and collect approximately 47% of the U.S. blood supply. This site provides contact information for each of this organization's centers.

American Association of Blood Banks (AABB) ◐ ◐ ◐
http://www.aabb.org

This site provides a contact list for each state on locating and arranging blood donation, including information on storing blood for an anticipated surgery or emergency (autologous blood transfusion). It also answers general questions about blood and blood transfusion.

Caregiver Resources

Caregiver Network ◐ ◐ ◐
http://www.caregiver.on.ca/content_main.html

This resource center, based in Canada, offers support, advice, seminars, and information for caregivers of the elderly and chronically ill. Text excerpts from an educational video program are available, and visitors can order the video series online. A caregiver resource guide offers telephone numbers and other contact information for government agencies, organizations, service providers, support agencies, publications, and periodicals. Suggested book and video lists and links to related Internet resources are available.

National Family Caregivers Association (NFCA) ◐ ◐
http://www.nfcacares.org

The NFCA is national organization offering education, information, support, public awareness campaigns, and advocacy to American caregivers. The address discusses caregiving and provides statistics, a survey report, news, an informational pamphlet, a reading list, caregiving tips, and contact details. Caregivers will find this site a source of support, encouragement, and information.

Chronic and Terminal Care Planning

American Association for Retired Persons (AARP): Basic Facts about Reverse Mortgages ◎ ◎ ◎
http://www.aarp.org/hecc/basicfct.html

This fact sheet within the AARP Web site describes reverse mortgages, including eligibility requirements, how reverse mortgages work, what a borrower receives from the mortgage, typical payments, and contact details for information on other programs or services not involving a loan against the home.

Chronic Pain Solutions ◎ ◎ ◎
http://www.chronicpainsolutions.com

Chronic Pain Solutions is a quarterly guide for chronic pain sufferers linking traditional and natural medical care. The site contains the online newsletter, contact and home subscription details, an online store for ordering therapeutic products, and biographies of contributing writers.

Consumer Guide to Viatical Settlements ◎ ◎
http://www.nvrnvr.com/guide.html

This online booklet, *Every Question You Need To Ask Before Selling Your Life Insurance Policy*, is provided by National Viator Representatives, a viatical settlement information source, advisor, and broker. Users can access the publication online, download the document, or order a hard copy at 1-800-932-0050.

Living Will and Values History Project ◎ ◎
http://www.euthanasia.org/lwvh.html

This site offers a Living Will package and Values History document, both available for download free-of-charge. Users can also receive hard copies for a nominal charge. The site also contains an extensive list of links to related sites.

Living Wills ◎ ◎
http://www.kepro.org/Bene_LivingWill.htm

Prepared by the Pennsylvania Medical Society, this site answers questions for the average patient regarding the development and use of a living will. It also provides a link to a free sample copy of a living will that can be completed and signed by individuals to be placed in their medical record.

National Chronic Care Consortium ◎ ◎ (some features fee-based)
http://www.nccconline.org

The National Chronic Care Consortium is dedicated to transforming the delivery of chronic care services. Members of this group strive to make the delivery of chronic care more efficient and cost effective. The site provides information on conferences, contact details, and links to related sites. Members can take part in the Alzheimer's Project Developmental Group Discussion at the site and access other services.

Organ Donation ✪ ✪ ✪
http://www.organdonor.gov

This government site answers frequently asked questions, dispels myths, and presents facts about organ donation. Visitors can download and print a donor card, and find links to related organizations on the Internet.

U.S. Living Will Registry ✪ ✪ ✪
http://www.uslivingwillregistry.com

This free service electronically stores advance directives and makes them available directly to hospitals by telephone. Registration materials are available to download online or by calling 1-800-LIV-WILL.

USAhomecare.com ✪ ✪ ✪
http://www.usahomecare.com

USAhomecare.com is a consumer-oriented home care (home health and hospice) site. The site provides answers to common questions, a bookstore, links to related sites, news, contact information, and a directory of agencies offering home care or hospice services.

Directing Healthcare Concerns and Complaints

Congress.org ✪ ✪ ✪
http://congress.org/main.html

This site offers a Capital directory, including members of Congress, the Supreme Court, state governors, and the White House. Users can also find comments on members of Congress by associations and advocacy groups, determine a bill's status through the site's search engine, send messages to Congress members, and find local congressional representatives.

Families USA ✪ ✪ ✪
http://www.familiesusa.org

Families USA is a national nonprofit, nonpartisan organization dedicated to the achievement of high-quality, affordable health, and long-term care for all Americans. The site offers a clearinghouse of information on Medicaid, Medicare, and General Managed Healthcare. Assistance and advice is provided on choosing an HMO, how to tell if a health policy or plan is good, and who to address if you have a healthcare complaint. Within the site, at www.familiesusa.org/medicaid/state.htm, a state-specific healthcare information guide is provided. This directory includes phone numbers to every state's Department of Insurance, which allows users to obtain reports on plans and information on complaint ratios.

Joint Commission of Accreditation of Healthcare Organizations (JCAHO)

http://www.jcaho.org/news/nb189.html

The JCAHO site lists a toll-free complaint hotline for patients, their families, and caregivers to express concerns about the quality of care at accredited healthcare organizations at this site. (The toll-free U.S. telephone number is 1-800-994-6610. The hotline is staffed between 8:30 a.m. and 5 p.m., central time, during weekdays.) The site also describes a mechanism for transmitting complaints via e-mail.

Medicare Rights Center (MRC)

http://www.medicarerights.org

Medicare Rights Center is a national, nonprofit organization focused to ensure that seniors and people with disabilities on Medicare have access to quality, affordable healthcare. The site offers information on specific MRC programs, news, consumer publications, information on professional membership, and details on the Initiative for the Terminally Ill on Medicare. Visitors can also subscribe for a fee to a biweekly newsletter delivered by fax.

Quality Improvement Organizations

http://www.qio.org

This site contains a directory of Peer Review Organizations (PRO) listed by state. These organizations monitor the care given to Medicare patients. Each state has a PRO that can decide whether care given to Medicare patients is reasonable, necessary, provided in the most appropriate setting, and meets standards of quality generally accepted by the medical profession. Peer Review Organizations can also be contacted to investigate beneficiary complaints.

State Insurance Commissioners

http://www.dtonline.com/insur/inlistng.htm

Deloitte and Touche Financial Counseling Services offers the addresses and phone numbers of each state's insurance commissioner at this site.

Elder and Extended Care

Administration on Aging
http://www.aoa.dhhs.gov

This site provides resources for seniors, practitioners, and caregivers, including news on aging, links to Web sites on aging, statistics about older people, consumer fact sheets, retirement and financial planning information, and help finding community assistance for seniors.

American Association for Retired Persons (AARP)
http://www.aarp.org

This nonprofit group is dedicated to the needs and rights of elderly Americans. Topics discussed at the site include caregiver support, community and volunteer organizations, Medicare, Medicaid, help with home care, finances, health and wellness, independent living, computers and the Internet, and housing options. Benefits and discounts provided to members are described, reference and research materials are available, and users can search the site by keyword.

American Association of Homes and Services for the Aging (AAHSA)
http://www.aahsa.org

This Association represents nonprofit organizations providing health care, housing, and services to the elderly. The site offers tips for consumers and family caregivers on choosing facilities and services, notices of upcoming events, press releases, fact sheets, an online bookstore, and links to sponsors, business partners, an international program, and other relevant sites.

Eldercare Locator
http://www.aoa.dhhs.gov/aoa/pages/loctrnew.html

The Eldercare Locator is a nationwide, directory assistance service designed to help older persons and caregivers locate local support resources for aging Americans. This site helps senior citizens find community assistance and Medicaid information. Interested parties can also contact the Eldercare Locator toll free at 1-800-677-1116.

Extendedcare.com (some features fee-based)
http://www.elderconnect.com/asp/default.asp

This address offers information on choosing an extended care provider, a "Geriatric Library" of information resources, a glossary of terms related to extended care, a forum for asking questions of a participating physician, and information on over 60,000 care providers. Visitors can search for care providers by type of care and zip code, subscribe to an e-mail newsletter, and read archived newsletters and press releases. A tool for assessing an individual's care needs is also available. A professional section is available to users associated with registered hospitals.

Insure.com: Answers to Seniors' Health Insurance Questions (on Medicare and Medicaid) ◉ ◉ ◉
http://www.insure.com/health/ship.html

This site provides the phone number to each state's Health Insurance Advisory Program (SHIP). SHIP is a federally funded program found in all states under different names, helping elderly and disabled Medicare and Medicaid recipients understand their rights and options for healthcare. Services include assistance with bills, advice on buying supplement policies, explanation of rights, help with payment denials or appeals, and assistance in choosing a Medicare health plan.

End of Life Decisions

American Medical Association (AMA): Education for Physicians on End-of Life Care (EPEC) ◉ ◉ ◉ (free registration)
http://www.ama-assn.org/ethic/epec/index.htm

Supported by a grant from the Robert Wood Johnson Foundation, EPEC is a two-year program designed to educate physicians nationwide on "the essential clinical competencies in end-of-life care." Visitors will find an overview of the project's purpose, design, and scope, a call for EPEC training conference applications, previous conference details, a mailing list, and an annotated list of educational resource materials. Users must complete a free registration process to view educational materials.

Before I Die ◉ ◉ ◉
http://www.pbs.org/wnet/bid

This address presents the Web companion to a public television program exploring the medical, ethical, and social issues associated with end-of-life care in the United States. Personal stories, a bulletin board, a glossary of terms, contact details for important support sources and organizations, and suggestions on forming a discussion group are available at the site. A program description, viewer's guide, outreach efforts and materials, and credits for the program are also provided.

CareOfDying.org: Supportive Care of the Dying ◉ ◉ ◉
http://www.careofdying.org

This site is presented by a coalition of 13 Catholic healthcare associations and the Catholic Health Association, advocating for an improvement in supportive care for persons with life-threatening illnesses and their caregivers. Assessment tools available at the site include patient, family caregiver, bereaved family, and professional questionnaires, and a tool assessing competency. A quarterly newsletter, research report, and hints for conducting focus groups are also available. Links are listed to related resources, including information on an upcoming PBS end-of-life series, hosted by Bill Moyers.

Choice in Dying ○ ○
http://www.choices.org

Services offered by Choice in Dying include advance directives, counseling for patients and families, professional training, advocacy, and publications. Membership details, press releases, news, information on end-of-life issues, an online newsletter, state-specific advance directive documents, and a petition for end-of-life care are all found at this site. Visitors can also order publications and videos, and access links to related sites.

Decisions Near the End of Life ○ ○
http://www.edc.org/CAE/Decisions/dnel.html

Decisions Near the End of Life is a continuing medical education program helps professional staff and patients of hospitals and nursing homes improve the way ethical decisions are made. The site describes typical program attendees, goals, format, leadership training, institutional profiles developed by the program, on-site programs, program components, and continuing medical education credit details.

End of Life: Exploring Death in America ○ ○ ○
http://www.npr.org/programs/death

National Public Radio's "All Things Considered" presents transcripts of a recent series on death and dying and other resources at this excellent site. Contact information and links to valuable organizations and other support sources, a bibliography of important publications, texts related to death, dying, and healing, and a forum for presenting personal stories are found at this address.

George Washington University:
Toolkit of Instruments to Measure End of Life ○ ○ ○
http://www.gwu.edu/~cicd/toolkit/toolkit.htm

Toolkits assessing the quality of end-of-life care are available at this address, providing healthcare institutions with information to "assess, improve, and enhance care for dying patients and their loved ones." Visitors can download a chart review instrument, surrogate questionnaires, and a patient questionnaire. Resources at the site assess quality of life, pain and other symptoms, depression and emotional symptoms, functional status, survival time and aggressiveness of care, continuity of care, spirituality, grief, caregiver and family experience, and patient and family member satisfaction with the quality of care.

Last Acts ⊙ ⊙ ⊙
http://www.lastacts.org

Designed to improve end-of-life care, Last Acts is devoted to "bring end-of-life issues out in the open and to help individuals and organizations pursue the search for better ways to care for the dying." The site presents information on Last Acts activities, a newsletter, press releases, and discussion forums. Links are available to details of recent news headlines, sites offering additional information resources, grant-making organizations, and a directory of Robert Wood Johnson Foundation end-of-life grantees.

Project on Death in America: Transforming the Culture of Dying ⊙ ⊙ ⊙
http://www.soros.org/death

The Project on Death and Dying in America supports initiatives in research, scholarship, the humanities, and the arts in transforming the American culture and experience of dying and bereavement. The Project also promotes innovations in care, public education, professional education, and public policy. Information is presented on the Project's Faculty Scholars Program, Professional Initiatives in Nursing, Social Work, and Pastoral Care, Arts and Humanities Initiative, Public Policy Initiative, Legal Initiative, and Community Initiative. Other resources described at the site include Grantmakers Concerned with Care at the End of Life, media resources, and other publications offered by the Project.

Hospice and Home Care

American Academy of Hospice and Palliative Medicine (AAHPM) ⊙ ⊙ ⊙
http://www.aahpm.org

This national nonprofit organization is comprised of physicians "dedicated to the advancement of hospice/palliative medicines, its practice, research, and education". Academy details, contact information, news, press releases, position statements, events and meetings notices, employment listings, and links to related sites are found at this address. Publications, continuing medical education opportunities, and conference tapes are also available.

Growth House, Inc. ⊙ ⊙ ⊙
http://www.growthhouse.org

Growth House, Inc. offers a comprehensive resource for hospice and home care information at this site. General information, a listing of local hospice providers, online book reviews, and an index of reviewed resources for end-of-life care are available at the site.

Hospice Association of America (HAA)

http://www.hospice-america.org

Serving the needs of the most seriously ill patients with cancer and other diseases, the HAA offers a full menu of information about the field of hospice care, as well as a directory of home care and hospice state associations. Each localized association listing offers the name of the executive director, the address, telephone, fax, and e-mail contact.

Hospice Foundation of America

http://www.hospicefoundation.org

The Hospice Foundation of America offers a range of books and training services for hospice professionals and the general public. The Web site provides general information on hospice and specific types of grief management. There is also a listing of other Web resources and useful literature for both the healthcare provider and the patient.

Hospice Net

http://www.hospicenet.org

Hospice Net is dedicated to helping patients and families facing life-threatening illnesses. The site contains a listing of useful articles, FAQ sheets, caregiver information, and a listing of well-chosen links to other major Web resources.

HospiceWeb

http://www.hospiceweb.com/index.htm

This site contains general information, a listing of frequently asked questions, discussion board, hospice locator, and an extensive list of links to valuable sites. Links to other hospice organizations are categorized by state.

National Association for Home Care (NAHC) (some features fee-based)

http://www.nahc.org

NAHC is a trade association representing more than 6,000 home care agencies, hospices, and home care aide organizations. The site offers news and Association announcements, a newsletter on pediatric home care, links to affiliates, international employment listings, legislative and regulatory information, statistics and technical papers, and directories of related state associations. Visitors can access a home care and hospice search tool for finding local service providers, and a consumer section offers information on choosing a home care provider, including descriptions of agencies providing home care, tips for finding information about agencies, and discussions of services, payment, patients' rights, accrediting agencies, and state resources. One section is restricted to members.

National Hospice Organization (NHO) ○ ○ ○
http://www.nho.org

The oldest and largest nonprofit public benefit organization devoted exclusively to hospice care, the NHO offers a comprehensive site providing information on all aspects of hospice care for the seriously and terminally ill, along with a state-by-state and city-by-city guide to hospice organizations in the United States. For each listing of a hospice facility, there is a telephone number and contact person.

Medical Insurance and Managed Care

Agency for Healthcare Research and Quality (AHRQ): Checkup On Health Insurance Choices ○ ○ ○
http://www.ahcpr.gov/consumer/insuranc.htm

This discussion of health insurance choices informs consumers on topics including why individuals need insurance, sources of health insurance, group and individual insurance, making a decision of coverage, and managed care. Types of insurance described at the site include fee-for-service and "customary" fees, health maintenance organizations, preferred provider organizations, Medicaid, Medicare, disability insurance, hospital indemnity insurance, and long-term care insurance. The site also includes a checklist and worksheet to determine features important to an individual when choosing insurance. A glossary of terms is available for reference.

American Association of Health Plans Online ○ ○ ○
http://www.aahp.org/menus/index.cfm?CFID=221345&CFTOKEN=11327695

Located in Washington, D.C., the American Association of Health Plans represents more than 1,000 HMOs, PPOs, and other network-based plans. The site offers information on government and advocacy activities, public relations materials, reports and statistics, selected bibliographies listed by subject, information on services and products, conference details, and training program information. Consumer resources include information on choosing a health plan, descriptions of different types of health plans, women's health resources, and fact sheets about health plans. Users can search each specific area of the site for information by keyword.

drkoop.com: Insurance Center ○ ○ ○
http://www.drkoop.com/hcr/insurance

This area of drkoop.com features an interactive Plan Profiler and Policy Chooser to help determine what type of plan is right for an individual consumer. An insurance library, glossary of insurance terms, and health insurance news updates are featured at the site.

Employer Quality Partnership (EQP) ○ ○
http://www.eqp.org

This site provides a guide to employees in selecting and understanding healthcare plans, provides assistance to employers in evaluating healthcare plans, and also guides employers on ways to improve the quality of their health plans. The site was developed by EQP, a volunteer coalition of employer organizations interested in promoting positive change in the healthcare marketplace and in educating employees regarding their employer-based healthcare plans.

Healthcare Financing Administration ○ ○ ○
http://www.hcfa.gov

This federal site provides a wealth of information on Medicare and Medicaid for both patients and healthcare professionals. It covers the basic features of each program and discusses laws, regulations, and statistics about federal healthcare programs. Information is also provided at the state level (state Medicaid), providing a list of sites with important state information.

Joint Commission of Accreditation of Healthcare Organizations (JCAHO) ○ ○ ○
http://www.jcaho.org

The Joint Commission of Accreditation of Healthcare Organizations evaluates and accredits nearly 18,000 healthcare organizations and programs. Quality Check, a service offered by the Commission, allows consumers to check ratings and evaluations of accredited organizations at the site. Information is available for the general public, employers, healthcare purchasers, and unions; the international community; and healthcare professionals and organizations. The site also contains information on filing complaints, career opportunities, news, and links to related sites.

Managed Care Glossary ○ ○ ○
http://mentalhelp.net/articles/glossary.htm

To be used for professional training purposes or as a general information source, this managed care glossary contains a continuously updated compilation of new terminology related to managed care with additional items in the field of information technology continuously being added. Physician and other healthcare professionals may want to bookmark this site to ensure a more complete understanding of modern health maintenance and preferred provider organization structure and service delivery.

Medical Insurance Resources ○
http://www.nerdworld.com/trees/nw1654.html

This site offers a large index of medical insurance resources on the Internet. Links are provided to major insurance companies, and other related sites. Each link is accompanied by a brief explanation of what can be found at that particular site.

Medicare ○ ○ ○
http://www.medicare.gov

The Health Care Financing Administration (HCFA) administers Medicare, the nation's largest health insurance program, which covers 39 million Americans. This site answers Medicare questions regarding eligibility, additional insurance, Medicare amounts, and enrollment. Consumer information includes answers to frequently asked questions on Medicare and helps regarding health plan options. Those interested in additional information can call 1-800-MEDICARE to receive additional help in organizing Medicare health options.

National Committee for Quality Assurance (NCQA) ○ ○ ○
http://www.ncqa.org

The National Committee for Quality Assurance (NCQA) is a private, nonprofit organization dedicated to assessing and reporting on the quality of managed healthcare plans. These activities are accomplished through accreditation and performance measurement of participating plans. Almost half the HMOs in the nation, covering three-quarters of all HMO enrollees, are involved in the NCQA accreditation process. A set of more than 50 standardized performance measures called the Health Plan Employer Data and Information Set (HEDIS), is used to evaluate and compare health plans. The NCQA Web site allows the user to search the accreditation status list. The search results will include the accreditation status designation and a summary report of the strengths and weaknesses of the plan entered. NCQA accreditation results allow users to evaluate healthcare plans in such key areas as quality of care, member satisfaction, access, and service.

Quotesmith.com ○ ○ ○
http://www.quotesmith.com

Visitors to this site can access current quotes for individual, family, and small group medical plans. Instant quotes on dental and term life insurance are also available.

U.S. News and World Report: America's Top HMOs ○ ○ ○
http://www.usnews.com/usnews/nycu/health/hetophmo.htm

This site helps consumers to rate their managed care plan by ranking HMOs by state. Other useful tools include an HMO glossary, a medical dictionary, a best hospitals finder, and a list of the 40 highest rated HMOs in the United States. Fitness tips, articles related to HMOs, and a forum for answering health professionals are all found at this site.

Yahoo! Life and Health Insurance Center ○ ○ ○
http://insurance.yahoo.com/life.html

The Yahoo insurance center is an excellent starting point for locating insurance information. Yahoo provides answers to frequently asked questions, a glossary of common terms, and quick estimates on the cost of a health insurance policy. An extensive list of links to related sites and a list of current articles of interest are available.

38.4 Nutrition and Physical Wellness

American Dietetic Association (ADA) ○ ○ ○ (fee-based)
http://www.eatright.org

The American Dietetic Association presents an ideal site for consumers, students, and dietetic professionals. This site has information on nutrition resources, government affairs, current issues and publications, job opportunities, and a public relations team to answer media questions. Users can contact other dietitians through the site. A search engine and a site map are provided to ease in the searching process. There are also links to consumer education and public policy sites; dietetic associations and networking groups; dietetic practice groups; food; food service and culinary organizations; and medical, health, and other professional organizations.

AOL Health Webcenter ○ ○ ○
http://www.aol.com/webcenters/health/diet.adp

AOL's Health Webcenter contains well-organized links to a variety of health related sites organized by topic. The site focuses on consumer needs, providing information on topics including illness and treatment; fitness and sports medicine; health and beauty; and women's, men's, children's, and seniors health. A health assessment and drug information search tool, vitamin guide, pregnancy calendar, calorie counter, and body-mass calculator are additional features of the site.

Arbor Nutrition Guide ○ ○ ○
http://www.netspace.net.au/%7Ehelmant/search.htm

The Arbor Nutrition Guide covers all areas of nutrition including applied and clinical nutrition. The site provides links to information on dietary guidelines, special diets, sports nutrition, individual vitamins and minerals, and cultural nutrition. There are also links relating to food science, such as food labeling in other countries, food regulation, food additives, science journals, phytochemistry, and other related topics.

Austin Nutritional Research ○ ○ ○
http://www.realtime.net/anr/referenc.html

This megasite provides links to various organizations and institutions worldwide regarding health and nutrition. Sites include those of professional organizations, research centers, and alternative therapy sources.

Department of Health and Human Services (HHS) ○ ○ ○
http://www.dhhs.gov

The Department of Health and Human Services (HHS) is the United States government's principal agency for protecting the health of all Americans and providing essential human services, especially for those who are least able to help themselves. HHS Operating Divisions include National Institutes of Health, Food and Drug Administration, Centers for Disease Control and Prevention, Agency for Toxic Substances and Disease Registry, Indian Health Service, Health Resources and Services Administration, Substance Abuse and Mental Health Services Administration, and the Agency for Health Care Policy and Research. This site provides news and public affairs information related to HHS, a site search engine, and notices of new site features.

Health Resource Links ○ ○ ○
http://www.rxmed.com/healthresourcelinks.html

This site provides links to many professional health-related associations and government agencies. Prescribing information, patient handouts, travel health resources, employment opportunities, medical supply resources, and investment information are all included at this comprehensive site.

International Food Information Council ○ ○ ○
http://ificinfo.health.org

The International Food Information Council presents resources at this site including current issues, up to date information for the media, food safety and nutrition facts, and extensive links to government affairs and agencies. The site also serves as a reference tool for educators, and provides users with a site search engine for locating specific information.

Nutrition and Health Linkstation ○ ○ ○
http://www.amazingstocks.com/nutrition

The Nutrition & Health Linkstation provides links to recipes, discussion groups, nutrient analysis programs, and energy calculators. The site also offers direct searches of government health organizations, associations, national health research pages, world health research pages, and pharmacy and medicine sites.

Public Health Nutritionists' Home Page ○ ○ ○
http://Weber.u.washington.edu/~phnutr/Internet/nutrlist.html

The Public Health Nutritionists' Home Page is an extensively compiled site for public health and nutrition organized by the School of Public Health and Community Medicine at the University of Washington. This site provides access to many resources, including applied nutrition, cardiovascular disease, food security, vegetarianism, growth charts, breast feeding and infant feeding. Access to the UNICEF gopher server is available to learn more about the United Nations program. Information on educational programs and newsletters are also available.

ThinkQuest Library of Entries ⊙ ⊙ ⊙
http://library.thinkquest.org/library/list.cgi?c=HEALTH_%26_SAFETY

Click on "Food and Nutrition" at this site to access in-depth information for adults, teens, and children on food and nutrition. The links provide access to information on RDA, BMI, personal caloric needs, eating out, specific sites for teens, and general information on more specific health and nutrition topics.

Tufts University Nutrition Navigator ⊙ ⊙ ⊙
http://navigator.tufts.edu

This site, presented by the Center on Nutrition Communication, School of Nutrition Science and Policy at Tufts University, is an up-to-date, rated guide to other nutrition sites. It provides information on general nutrition for parents, kids, women, health professionals, and journalists. One section is devoted to sites providing information about special dietary needs. A search engine is provided at the site for more specific resources.

U.S. Department of Agriculture (USDA) Nutrient Values ⊙ ⊙
http://www.rahul.net/cgi-bin/fatfree/usda/usda.cgi

Visitors can utilize the search engine housed at this site to find the recommended daily allowance (RDA) nutrient values of over 5,000 food items for three different serving sizes in men averaging 174 pounds, and women averaging 138 pounds, between the ages of 25 and 50.

University of Pennsylvania: Library ⊙ ⊙ ⊙
http://www.library.upenn.edu

The University of Pennsylvania Library presents an informative site containing information on health disciplines and topics. The site provides access to databases as well as lists of associations, government organizations, and other search tools. Links to alternative medicine sites are also available.

38.5 Online Drug Stores

Corner Drugstore Specialties ⊙ ⊙
http://www.cornerdrug.com

Corner Drugstore Specialties provides customers with a catalog of pharmacy products that includes nonprescription drugs, vitamins, personal care items, and other products typically found in a convenience store or pharmacy.

CVS Pharmacy ✪ ✪ ✪

http://www.cvs.com

This site offers customers a way to order prescription and nonprescription drugs along with other pharmacy items. The prescription section offers an extensive description of the purpose of the drug, side effects, precautions, drug interactions, and other prescribing information. All prescription orders are verified by the pharmacy and will be sent by either the U.S. Postal Service or UPS. Non-prescription drugs, vitamins, first aid, home care, and personal care items are also available.

Drug Emporium ✪ ✪

http://www.drugemporium.com

This Web site offers customers a wide variety of products including over-the-counter medicine, personal care items, vitamins, and electronics. Prescription medicine is also available. New patients must register by filling out an online form and provide a way to contact their doctors for prescription information. Prescriptions are processed by a registered pharmacist. Orders are shipped via UPS and shipping costs are added to the bill.

Drugstore.com ✪ ✪ ✪

http://www.drugstore.com

As one of the first online drugstores, Drugstore.com has developed an extensive and informative site that provides prescription and nonprescription medicine, personal care products, vitamins, and other products. There are also articles on solutions to some health and beauty problems, an opportunity to ask a Drugstore.com pharmacist questions, and opinions on products from customers.

Home Pharmacy ✪ ✪

http://www.homepharmacy.com

Home Pharmacy is an online drugstore that provides a variety of healthcare products at a relatively low cost. Products can be sent by standard shipping or by Federal Express.

Merck-Medco Managed Care Online ✪ ✪ ✪

http://www.merck-medco.com

An online pharmacy, the Merck-Medco site provides information on member services; a newsletter, *Optimal Health* with current health news; medication information and articles for healthy aging; client and provider services, including a list of selected FDA-approved prescription medications; a newsroom containing news releases on Merck-Medco and prescription drug-care; and important drug-related consumer announcements.

Online Drugstore.com ◎ ◎
http://www.onlinedrugstore.com

Prescription products at a low cost can be ordered from this service by phone, mail, or e-mail. Visitors can compare prices offered by competitors, access a list of products, and find a more detailed description of the service.

PlanetRx.com ◎ ◎ ◎
http://www.planetrx.com

Planet Rx, one of the first online drugstores, offers customers a variety of products and information resources. Prescription and nonprescription drugs, personal care items, beauty and spa products, and medical supplies are available. The site also offers articles on health problems and possible treatments, and opinions on products from customers.

Safeweb Medical ◎ ◎
http://drugstore.virtualave.net

The Safeweb Medical Web site provides selected popular prescription drugs and online consultations. The customer receives orders 24-48 hours after doctors approve a prescription.

Self Care ◎ ◎ ◎
http://www.selfcare.com

This Web site has sections for beauty and spa items, nonprescription drugs and medicinal supplies, alternative therapies, nutrition and fitness products, and home care merchandise. Descriptions of products are also available. Orders are sent by standard shipping, priority air delivery, or express air delivery.

Verified Internet Pharmacy Practice Sites (VIPPS) Program ◎ ◎ ◎
http://www.nabp.net/vipps/intro.asp

The Verified Internet Pharmacy Practice Sites (VIPPS) Program of the National Association of Boards of Pharmacy (NABP) was developed in 1999 out of public concern for the safety of pharmacy practices on the Internet. This site contains a menu with links providing information on the criteria for VIPPS certification; a VIPPS list (which includes the pharmacy name and Web site address); VIPPS definitions; and links to Web sites of state boards of pharmacy, state medical boards, federal agencies, and professional organizations.

39. WEB SITE AND TOPICAL INDEX

A

AACE Clinical Practice Guidelines for the Management of Thyroid Carcinoma, 139
Abbreviations and Acronyms, 425
Abetalipoproteinemia, 383
About.com
    Alcoholism
        Alcohol Metabolism, 199
    Endocrine Surgery, 123
    Hormones and Drugs Affecting the Endocrine System, 141
    Prescription Drugs for the Treatment of Obesity, 158
    Thyroid Disease and Endocrinology, 55
    Thyroid Drugs, 163
    Types of Thyroidectomy, 139
Abstract, Citation, and Full-text Search Tools, 21, 425
Accreditation Council for Continuing Medical Education (ACCME), 49
Accreditation Council for Graduate Medical Education (ACGME), 499
Achoo Healthcare Online, 463
Acid Maltase Deficiency Association (AMDA), 215, 389
Acquired Hyperlipidemia, 379
Acromegaly, 268
Acta Diabetologica, 22
ACTH Stimulation Test, 100
Acute Intermittent Porphyria, 408
Adam.com
    Hyperlipidemia, 379
    ACTH (Cortrosyn) Stimulation Test, 100

Bassen-Kornzweig Syndrome, 383
Chronic Thyroiditis (Hashimoto's Disease), 277
Dexamethasone Suppression Test, 95
Excessive Hair on Females, 308
Familial Combined Hyperlipidemia, 380
Glucagonoma, 303
Goiter, 283
Growth Hormone Stimulation Test, 94
Hereditary Fructose Intolerance, 390
Hormones, 87
Klinefelter's Syndrome, 327
McCune-Albright Syndrome, 340
Medullary Carcinoma of Thyroid, 284
Serum Calcium, 110
Addison and Cushing International Federation, 291
Addison's Disease, 293
Administration for Children and Families (ACF), 431
Administration on Aging, 431, 518
    Resource Directory for Older People, 490
Adrenal Adenoma, 299
Adrenal Glands, 78, 100, 124, 143, 291
Adrenal Hemorrhage, 294
Adrenal Hormone Overproduction, 295
Adrenal Imaging, 103
Adrenal Insufficiency, 292
Adrenal Surgery
    A Clinical Study on Incidentalomas, 124
Adrenal Tumors, 298
Adrenoleukodystrophy (ALD), 294

Adult Hormone Growth Deficiency Therapy, 157
Advanced Fertility Center of Chicago
    Hirsutism and Hyperandrogenism in Women, 308
Advanced Reproductive Care
    Hormonal Therapy, 308
Advances in Contraception, 22
Advocacy, 177
Agency for Healthcare Research and Quality (AHRQ)
    Checkup On Health Insurance Choices, 523
Agency for Toxic Substances and Disease Registry (ATSDR), 431
AIDS Knowledge Base
    Endocrine Abnormalities, 418
Aids Treatment News
    Endocrine Complications of HIV Progression, 418
Albert Einstein College of Medicine
    Division of Reproductive Endocrinology Infertility, 229
Alberta Medical Association
    Laboratory Endocrine Testing Guidelines for Investigation of Impotence and Male Androgen Insufficiency, 316
Alcaptonuria, 393
Aldosterone-Producing Adrenal Adenoma (Conn's Syndrome), 299
Alkalinizing Agents, 151
All The Web, 464
Allexperts.com, 505
allHealth.com, 505
    Early Screening for Diabetes Cost-effective, 188
    Precocious Puberty in Boys, 329
    Stein-Leventhal Syndrome, 311
Alpha and Beta Blockers, 164
AMA Health Insight
    Atlas of the Body
        Female Reproductive System, 80
        Male Reproductive System, 80
Amazon.com
    Medical Books, 501
Amedeo, 445
Amenorrhea, 307
America Online (AOL), 506
America's Blood Centers, 514

American Academy of Family Physicians
    Benefits and Risks of Controlling Blood Glucose Levels in Patients with Type 2 Diabetes Mellitus, 361
    Guidelines on the Care of Diabetic Nephropathy, 363
    Gynecomastia
        When Breasts Form in Males, 317
    Hyperparathyroidism, 344
American Academy of Family Physicians
    Health Information Page, 506
American Academy of Hospice and Palliative Medicine (AAHPM), 521
American Academy of Pain Management (AAPM), 483
American Academy of Pediatrics
    Amenorrhea in Adolescent Athletes, 307
    Causes of Growth Retardation, 348
    Endocrinology and Growth, 205
    Issues in Newborn Screening, 191
American Association for Geriatric Psychiatry
    Treating Erectile Dysfunction, 316
American Association for Retired Persons (AARP), 518
    Basic Facts about Reverse Mortgages, 515
American Association of Blood Banks (AABB), 514
American Association of Clinical Endocrinologists (AACE), 215
    Clinical Practice Guidelines, 171
    Clinical Practice Guidelines for Management of Diabetes Mellitus, 173
    Clinical Practice Guidelines for the Evaluation and Treatment of Hypogonadism in Adult Male Patients, 319
    Clinical Practice Guidelines for the Evaluation and Treatment of Male Sexual Dysfunction, 316
American Association of Diabetes Educators, 181, 216
American Association of Health Plans Online, 523
American Association of Homes and Services for the Aging (AAHSA), 518
American Association of Tissue Banks, 132, 216
American Autoimmune Related Diseases Association (AARDA), 216

Endocrine Autoimmunity, 216, 261
American Board of Medical Specialties (ABMS), 474
American College of Medical Genetics (ACMG), 200
American College of Physicians/American Society of Internal Medicine (ACP-ASIM)
 Screening for Thyroid Disease, 192
American Diabetes Association (ADA), 182, 216
 Clinical Practice Recommendations 2000, 173
 Tests of Glycemia in Diabetes, 114
 Council on Epidemiology and Statistics, 179
 Detection and Management of Lipid Disorders in Diabetes, 118
 Diabetes and Exercise, 125
 Dietary Recommendations for Persons with Diabetes, 128
 Endocrinology of Aging in the Time of Prometheus, 202
 Exercise
  Just the FAQs, 126
 In the News, 180
 Nutrition Recommendations and Principles for Diabetes Mellitus, 128
 Position Statement
  Insulin Administration, 149
 Screening for Diabetic Retinopathy, 369
 Screening for Type 2 Diabetes, 361
 Search Page, 15
 Self-Monitoring of Blood Glucose, 127
American Dietetic Association (ADA), 193, 217, 526
 Vitamin and Mineral Supplementation, 153
American Family Physician
 Abnormal Uterine Bleeding, 313
 Congenital Adrenal Hyperplasia
  Not Really a Zebra, 295
 Disorders of Puberty, 329
 Educational Guidelines for Achieving Tight Control and Minimizing Complications of Type 1 Diabetes, 360
 Oral Pharmacologic Management of Type 2 Diabetes, 361
 Type 1 Diabetes Mellitus and Use of Flexible Insulin Regimens, 360

American Foundation of Thyroid Patients, 273
 Fine Needle Aspiration Biopsy of the Thyroid, 99
American Geriatrics Society (AGS), 490
American Heart Association (AHA)
 Cholesterol-Lowering Drugs, 147
 Hyperlipidemia, 377
American Hospital Association, 451
American Journal of Clinical Nutrition, 23
American Journal of Obstetrics and Gynecology, 23
American Medical Association (AMA), 426
 AMA in Washington, 460
 CME Locator, 49
 Coding and Medical Information Systems, 496
 Education for Physicians on End-of Life Care (EPEC), 519
 Electronic Medical Systems and Coding, 496
 Fellowship and Residency Electronic Interactive Database Access (FREIDA) Online System, 499
 Health Insight, 506
 Medical Student Section, 501
 Physician Select Online Doctor Finder, 452
 The Endocrine System, 67
American Medical Group Association (AMGA) Public Policy and Political Affairs, 460
American Medical Informatics Association (AMIA), 496
American Medical Student Association (AMSA)
 Legislative Affairs, 460
American Medical Women's Association (AMWA), 461, 501
American Obesity Association (AOA), 217, 373
American Peptide Society, 217
American Porphyria Foundation, 406
American Prostate Society, 217, 321
American Society for Nutritional Sciences
 Nutrient Information, 351
American Society for Reproductive Medicine, 206, 218
American Society of Bariatric Physicians (ASBP), 218, 373

American Society of Bioethics and
    Humanities (ASBH), 477
American Society of Human Genetics
    (ASHG), 201, 218
American Society of Law, 477
American Society of Transplant Physicians
    (ASTP), 131, 218
American Society of Transplant Surgeons
    (ASTS), 131, 218
American Thyroid Association, 219, 273
    Guidelines for Detection of Thyroid
        Dysfunction, 192
    Hypothyroidism
        The Underactive Thyroid, 274
    Thyroid Disease Guidelines for Physicians,
        171
    Thyroid Hormone Treatment, 164
American Universities, 500
Amino Acid Metabolism, 84, 393
Amino Acids, 23
Amputation Prevention Global Resource
    Center, 365
Amyloidosis, 417
Amyloidosis Support Network, 417
Anabolic Steroid Abuse, 211
Anatomy and Physiology, 67
Anatomy and Surgery, 475
Anatomy of the Human Body, 475
Androgen Abnormalities, 315
Androgen Insensitivity Syndrome, 315
Androgen Insensitivity Syndrome (Male
    Pseudohermaphroditism), 331
Androgen Insensitivity Syndrome Support
    Group, 331
Androgen Therapy and Complications of
    Therapy, 159
Andrologia, 23
Andropause, 199
Andropause.com
    Impact of Low Bioavailable Testosterone,
        199
Annals of Internal Medicine
    Subclinical Thyroid Disease
        A Clinician's Perspective, 278
Annals of Nutrition and Metabolism, 23
Annual Reviews of Nutrition, 23
Anthropometric Desk Reference, 205
Antiadrenal Agent
    Aminoglutethimide, 144

Antidiuretic Hormone Testing, 92
Antigout Agents, 152
Antihypertensive Agents, 164
Antilipemic Agents, 147
Antithyroid Agents, 138, 164
Aoki Diabetes Research Institute (ADRI), 241
AOL Health Webcenter, 526
APIMALL Health Channel
    BPH Disease Management, 321
Apo E Genotype Test for Type III
    Hyperlipoproteinemia, 381
Approved and Developmental Therapeutic
    Agents, 19
Arbor Nutrition Guide, 351, 526
Archives of Andrology, 24
Argus Clearinghouse, 464
Armed Forces Institute of Pathology Lecture
    Series
    Adrenal Imaging in Adults, 103
Ask NOAH About
    Diabetes, 359
    Gastrointestinal Carcinoid Tumor, 411
    Impotence (Erectile Dysfunction), 316
    Islet Cell Carcinoma, 304
    Pregnancy
        Tay-Sachs Disease Public Health
            Education Information Sheet, 404
    Support Groups, 513
Association for the Cure of Cancer of the
    Prostate (CURE), 322
Association of American Medical Colleges
    (AAMC), 502
Association of Program Directors in
    Endocrinology and Metabolism (APDEM),
    219
Associations and Societies, 215
atEndocrine.com, 15
Atlas of the Body, 475
Austin Nutritional Research, 526
Australian Addison's Disease Association, 293
Autoimmune Polyendocrinopathy, 415

B

Back and Body Care, 483
Barbara Davis Center for Childhood Diabetes
    Exercise and Diabetes, 126
    Long-Term Complications of Diabetes, 363
Baylor

College of Medicine
  Department of Pediatrics, 229
  Grand Rounds Archive
    Primary Hyperparathyroidism, 344
  Lipid Laboratory
    Test Profiles, 118
  Metabolic Myopathies, 385
  Online Continuing Medical Education, 51
  Transplantation Primer
    Immunosuppression Medicine, 154
  Health Care System
    Diabetes Services, 244
Before I Die, 519
Benign Prostatic Hyperplasia (BPH), 321
Best Practice and Research Clinical Endocrinology and Metabolism, 24
BestDoctors.com, 506
BigHub, 464
Bio Online, 480
Biochemical Categories, 69
Biochemical Markers for Bone Turnover, 109
BioCognizance.com
  Elevated Sex Hormones are Breast Cancer Risk, 160
Bioethics, 212
Bioethics Discussion Pages, 477
Bioethics.net, 477
Biofind.com, 480
Biological Signals and Receptors, 24
Biology of Reproduction, 24
Biomedical Ethics, 477
BioMedNet
  The Internet Community for Biological and Medical Researchers, 445
Bioresearch Online, 480
BioSites, 427
Biosynthesis of Haem
  Erythropoietic Porphyria (Congenital Erythropoietic Porphyria), 408
BioTech's Life Science Dictionary, 457
Biotechnology, 480
  An Information Resource, 480
Biotechnology Industry Organization, 481
BioWorld Online, 481
Bisphosphonates, 144
Blackwell Science, 446
Blood Bank Information, 514
Blood Urea Nitrogen, 104

Blood Urea Nitrogen (BUN), 104
Bombay Hospital Journal Case Reports
  Cerebrotendinous Xanthomatosis, 399
Bone, 24
Bone and Mineral Metabolism, 81, 109, 125, 144, 335
Bone Mineral Density Testing
  Incorporating BMD into Your Practice, 111
Bone Mineralization Disorders, 338
Bone Physiology, 81
Books on Endocrinology Published in 1999/2000, 39
Boston Medical Center
  Pediatric Endocrinology Services, 229
Boston University
  Department of Medicine
    Endocrinology Section, 230
  Hereditary Fructose Intolerance and Aldolase, 390
  Medical Center
    An On-Line Adrenal Imaging Teaching Program, 103
    Community Outreach Health Information System, 506
Brain Surgery Information Center
  Pineal Region Tumors, 271
Brain Tumor Foundation of Canada
  Neuroendocrine Function, 72
Brent's Porphyria Page, 408
Brigham and Women's Hospital (BWH)
  Division of Endocrinology-Hypertension, 245
British Inherited Metabolic Diseases Group
  Homepage and U.K. Directory, 119
British Medical Journal
  Risk Factors for Coronary Artery Disease in Non-Insulin Dependent Diabetes Mellitus, 364
British Neuroendocrine Group, 72
Bromocriptine, 156
Brooke Army Medical Center
  Bone Imaging
    Metabolic Bone Disease, 112
Broomfield Hospital
  Glucose Tolerance Testing Diagnostic Criteria, 117

C

CA
- A Cancer Journal for Clinicians
  - Changing Concepts in the Pathogenesis and Management of Thyroid Carcinoma, 284

Calcitonin, 144
Calcitonin in the Prevention and Treatment of Osteoporosis, 145
Calcium, 110, 145
Calcium Metabolism Disorders, General, 335
Calcium, Phosphorus, and Vitamin D, 335
Calcium, Vitamin D, and Parathyroid Hormone, 81
Cambridge University Press
- Online Journals, 446

Canadian Diabetes Association, 182, 219
Canadian Journal of Diabetes Care, 24
Canadian Medical Association
- Journal
  - Enzyme Replacement Therapy for Gaucher's Disease, 152
    - Prevention and Management of Osteoporosis
      - Calcium Nutrition, 145
  - Vitamin D Metabolites and Analogs in the Treatment of Osteoporosis, 146

Canadian Porphyria Foundation, 406
Canadian Prostate Cancer Research Foundation (CPCRF), 322
Canadian Society for Mucopolysaccharide (MPS) and Related Diseases, 219, 391
Cancer and Genetics
- Multiple Endocrine Neoplasia, 88

Cancer Control Journal
- Gastrinoma
  - State of the Art, 302

Cancer Institute of Long Island
- Mineral and Bone Metabolism, 81

Cancer Medicine
- Adrenal Dysfunction, 419
- Corticosteroids, 143
- Endocrine Complications, 419
- Hormones and Etiology of Cancer, 161
  - Prostate Cancer, 159
- Medullary Carcinoma of the Thyroid, 284
- Multiple Endocrine Neoplasia (MEN) Syndromes, 412
- Neoplasms of the Gastroenteropancreatic Endocrine System, 302
- Neoplasms of the Neuroendocrine System
  - Medullary Thyroid Carcinoma (MTC), 412
- Vasoactive Intestinal Peptide Tumor (VIPoma), 304

CancerBACUP
- Understanding Cancer of the Pancreas Surgery, 137

Cancerlinks, 326
CancerNet
- Islet Cell Carcinoma, 304
- Thyroid Cancer, 284

CancerWeb Online Medical Dictionary, 457
Canterbury Health
- Insulin Tolerance Test (ITT), 117

Carbohydrate Metabolism, 387
Carbohydrate-Deficient Glycoprotein Syndromes, 405
Carcinoid Cancer Foundation, 411
Carcinoid Tumors and Carcinoid Syndrome, 411
Carcinoma of the Pancreas, 304
Careers in Bioethics, 477
Caregiver Network, 514
Caregiver Resources, 514
CareOfDying.org
- Supportive Care of the Dying, 519

Case Studies
- Polycystic Ovary Syndrome, 311

Case Western Reserve University
- Center for Inherited Disorders of Energy Metabolism (CIDEM), 241, 385
  - Carnitine Analysis, 121
  - General Test Information, 119
- Department of Medicine
  - Division of Endocrinology, 230
- Nuclear and Spect Teaching Files
  - Toxic Nodular Goiter, 282

CDC
- Diabetes and Public Health Resource, 359
- Division of Diabetes Translation, 62, 179
- Neuropathy, 368
- Office of Genetics and Disease Prevention, 201
- The Prevention and Treatment of Complications of Diabetes Mellitus, 364

Cell Biology Tutorials

Cell Metabolism, 84
Cellular Metabolism
    Carbohydrate, 83
    General, 82
    Lipid, 83
    Protein, 84
Center for Bioenvironmental Research of Tulane and Xavier Universities
    Environmental Estrogens and Other Hormones, 185
Center for Biomedical Imaging Technology, 492
Center for Current Research, 193
Center for Human Simulation, 492
Center for Information Technology (CIT), 436
Center for Medical Ethics and Mediation, 478
Center for Nutrition Policy and Promotion (CNPP), 431
Center for Reproductive Law and Policy (CRLP), 177
Center for Research on Reproduction and Women's Health, 241
Center for Scientific Review (CSR), 437
Centers for Disease Control and Prevention (CDC), 437
    Biostatistics/Statistics, 456
    Division of Diabetes Translation, 188
CenterWatch, 427
    Clinical Trials Listing Service, 18
    FDA Drug Approvals, 19
    National Institutes of Health (NIH) Trials Listing, 19
    Profiles of Industry Providers, 240
Central Laboratory Services
    Endocrinology, 87
    Prolactin Procedure, 93
    Urinary Free Cortisol Procedure, 104
    Urine Catecholamines Procedure, 102
Centre for Neuroendocrinology
    Cushing's Syndrome, 297
Cerebrotendinous Xanthomatosis, 399
Chicago Institute of Neurosurgery and Neuroresearch
    Pineal Tumors, 271
Children with Diabetes, 178, 194
Children's Hospital, 230
Children's Liver Alliance
    Galactosemia Links, 388

Children's Memorial Hospital in Chicago
    Department of Pediatrics
    Division of Endocrinology, 230
Children's Pompe Foundation, 390
Choice in Dying, 520
Cholesterol, 188
Cholesterol and Lipoprotein Metabolism, 84, 147
Cholesterol and Lipoproteins, 118
Cholesterol Screening in Asymptomatic Adults, 188
Chronic and Terminal Care Planning, 515
Chronic Pain Management, 483
Chronic Pain Solutions, 515
Cincinnati Children's Hospital Medical Center, 230
Cleveland Clinic
    Department of Endocrinology, 245
Clinica Diabetologica
    Insulin Types, 149
Clinical and Investigative Medicine
    Diagnosis and Management of Acromegaly, 268
Clinical Chemistry, 25
Clinical Diabetes, 25
Clinical Drug Investigations, 25
Clinical Endocrinology, 25, 39
Clinical Nutrition, 25
Clinical Pediatrics
    Diabetic Ketoacidosis Treatment Guidelines, 366
Clinical Practice and Guidelines, 171
Clinical Practice Guidelines
    Diabetes, 173
Clinical Practice Management, 484
Clinical Studies and Trials, 18
Clinical Transplantation, 25
Clinical Uses of Corticotropin-Releasing Hormone in the Evaluation of Patients with Cushing's Syndrome, 94
ClinicalTrials.com, 19
ClinicalTrials.gov, 19
CliniWeb International, 464
    Adrenal Gland Diseases, 291
    Endocrine Diseases, 57
    Search Tool, 15
CME Resources, 49
CME Unlimited, 49
CMEWeb, 50

CNN
  Health News, 462
CNN.com
  Diabetes Joins List of Heart Disease Risk Factors, 365
Collagen Disorders, 341
Colorado State University
  Adrenal Gland, 78
  Calcitonin, 81
  Endocrine Activity, 70
  Endocrine Pancreas, 85
  Gastrointestinal Hormones, 79
  Glucocorticoids, 78
  Hormone Action, 71
  Hormone Chemistry, 71
  Hormones, 71
  Hypothalamus and Pituitary Gland, 73
  Mineralocorticoids, 78
  Thyroid and Parathyroid Glands, 77
Columbia University
  Center for Continuing Education in the Health Sciences, 51
  College of Physicians and Surgeons
    Male Infertility, 318
  College of Physicians and Surgeons
    Complete Home Medical Guide, 507
  Screening for Congenital Hypothyroidism, 275
Columbia-Presbyterian Medical Center
  Department of Pediatrics
    Division of Pediatric Endocrinology, 231
  Presbyterian Hospital Department of Medicine
    Division of Endocrinology, 231
  Screening for Diabetes Mellitus, 189
  Screening for Obesity, 191
  Screening for Thyroid Disease, 192
Combined Health Information Database (CHID), 507
Common Medical Abbreviations, 425
Community of Science, 227, 491
Complete Androgen Insensitivity Syndrome, 315
Complete Guide to Medical Tests
  Abnormal Findings of Routine Urinalysis, 118
Complications, 363
Computer Retrieval of Information on Scientific Projects (CRISP), 437
Conferences, 17
Congenital Adrenal Hyperplasia, 295, 332
Congenital Adrenal Hyperplasia (CAH), 295
Congenital Adrenal Hyperplasia Support Group, 296
Congenital Erythropoietic Porphyria, 408
Congenital Hypothyroidism, 275
Congress.org, 516
Conn's Syndrome, 299
Consumer Guide to Viatical Settlements, 515
Continuing Medical Education (CME), 49
Cornell University Joan and Sanford I. Weill Medical College Office of Continuing Medical Education, 51
Corner Drugstore Specialties, 528
Coronary Complications, 364
CorpTech Database, 481
Cost-effectiveness of Screening for Type 2 Diabetes Mellitus, 189
Cosyntropin, 156
Covenant Health
  Precocious Puberty in Girls, 330
Craniopharyngiomas, 271
Creatinine, 105
CRISP
  Computer Retrieval of Information on Scientific Projects, 430
Crump Institute for Biological Imaging
  Parathyroid Embryology, 82
Cryptorchidism, 319
CT Is Us, 493
Current and Future Therapies of Diabetic Neuropathy, 128
Current Opinion in Endocrinology and Diabetes, 26
Current Problems in Obstetrics, 26
Cushing's Disease, 269
Cushing's Support and Research Foundation, 297
Cut to the Chase, 484
Cutaneous Biology Research Center, 241
CVS Pharmacy, 529
Cyberounds, 50
Cytokine and Growth Factor Reviews, 26

D

Daily Diffs, 465

Dalhousie University Cardiac Prevention
  Research Centre (CPRC)
  Diabetes and Coronary Heart Disease, 365
Databases, 209
Decisions Near the End of Life, 520
Definitive Adrenal Insufficiency Due to
  Bilateral Adrenal Hemorrhage and Primary
  Antiphospholipid Syndrome, 294
Department of Health and Human Services
  (HHS), 432, 527
Dermatologic Manifestations of Diabetes, 365
Dermatology Online Journal
  Diabetes Mellitus, 365
Detection and Management of Lipid
  Disorders in Diabetes, 377
Development and Sexual Differentiation, 327
Dexamethasone Suppression Testing, 101
Diabetes, 26, 27
  General Resources, 114
  Glucose, 115
  Glucose, Fasting, 115
  Glycated Hemoglobin, 116
  Insulin C-Peptide, 116
  Ketones, 116
  Oral Glucose Tolerance Test, 117
  Stimulation Testing, 117
  Urinalysis, 118
Diabetes Action Research and Education
  Foundation, 241
Diabetes and Endocrinology Research Center, 242
Diabetes Care, 26
  Biological Variation of Glycated
    Hemoglobin, 116
  Growth Factors and the Regulation of
    Fetal Growth, 372
  Hospital Admission Guidelines for
    Diabetes Mellitus, 174
  Insulin Administration, 149
  Optimization through Information
    Technology, 212
  Position Statement
    Gestational Diabetes Mellitus, 362
  Screening for Gestational Diabetes
    Mellitus, 189
Diabetes Caucus, 62
Diabetes Center of the Albert Einstein College
  of Medicine, 183
Diabetes Compilation Digest, 16

Diabetes Digest, 178
Diabetes Education and Research Center, 183
Diabetes Forecast, 26
Diabetes Insight
  Diabetes and Nephropathy, 367
Diabetes Insipidus, 263
Diabetes Insipidus Foundation, 220, 263
Diabetes Institutes Foundation, 184, 242
Diabetes Knowledge, 178
Diabetes Mall
  Organ Damage in Diabetes, 372
Diabetes Mellitus, 125, 147, 173, 178, 188, 359
  Understanding Laboratory Tests, 114
Diabetes Monitor
  Devices for Glucose Monitoring, 130
Diabetes News, 181
Diabetes News Home, 181
Diabetes News Library, 181
Diabetes Research and Clinical Practice, 27
Diabetes Research and Wellness Foundation,
  242
Diabetes Research Institute, 242
Diabetes Reviews, 27
Diabetes Specialist
  Treatment of Diabetes Mellitus, 147
Diabetes Spectrum, 27
  Pharmacological Properties and Clinical
    Use of Currently Available Agents, 150
Diabetes UK, 182
Diabetes Web
  Vasopressin, 155
Diabetes, General, 40
Diabetes, Nutrition, 42
Diabetes/Metabolism Reviews, 27
Diabetic Complications, 42
Diabetic Foot Disease
  An Interactive Guide, 366
Diabetic Foot Ulcers and Disease, 365
Diabetic Gourmet
  Gestational Diabetes and Exercise, 126
Diabetic Medicine, 27
Diabetic Retinopathy Foundation, 369
  Treatment of Retinopathy, 129
Diabetologia, 28
Diagnosing Diabetes, 174
Diagnostics, 42
Diagnostics and Monitoring, 87
Dietary Management of Diabetes Working
  Group, 128

Dietary Management of Individuals with
    Metabolic Disorders
    Mead Johnson Special Metabolic Diets,
        129
Differential Diagnosis of Low HDL-
    Cholesterol, 382
Digestive Diseases and Sciences, 28
DigiDoc Medical Software Endocrinology
    Cases, 167
Digital Imaging Center, 493
Directing Healthcare Concerns and
    Complaints, 516
Directories of Research Centers, 240
DiscoveryHealth.com, 507
Disease Manifestations
    Multiple Endocrine Neoplasia Type 2B,
        412
Disorders, 43
Disorders of Endocrinology and Metabolism,
    General Resources, 261
Disturbances of Acid-Base Metabolism, 356
Doctor Felix's Free MEDLINE Page, 425
Doctor's Guide, 465
    Bisphosphonates May Reduce Metastases,
        144
    Medical and Other News, 462
    Medical Conferences and Meetings, 454
        Endocrine Disorders, 17
    New Drugs and Indications, 471
    Prostate Cancer Information and
        Resources, 323
DoctorDirectory
    HealthNews Directory, 507
DoctorGeorge.com:, 278
Dogpile, 465
DotPharmacy
    Hirsute Pursuits, 311
Dr. Gale's Web Pages on Insulin Resistance,
    363
Dr. Morimoto's Image Library of Radiology,
    493
drkoop.com, 465, 508
    Drug Interactions Search, 471
    Glossary of Insurance-Related Terms, 457
    Insurance Center, 523
Drug Abuse, Endocrinologic and Metabolic
    Effects, 199
Drug Base
    Protein-Energy Malnutrition, 375

Drug Emporium, 529
Drug InfoNet, 472
Drugstore.com, 529
Duke University Medical Center
    Division of Endocrinology, 246
        Metabolism and Nutrition, 231

E

Economic Impact, 178
Ed Credits, 50
E-Doc
    Colchicine, 152
Education and Support, 178
Education Center for Prostate Cancer
    Patients, 323
Educational Commission for Foreign Medical
    Graduates (ECFMG), 499
Elder and Extended Care, 518
Eldercare Locator, 518
Electronic Residency Application Service, 500
Eli Lilly
    Managing Your Diabetes
        Patient Education Program, 179
Elsevier Science, 446
emedicine
    Addison's Disease, 293
    Adrenal Insufficiency and Adrenal Crisis,
        292
    Alcoholic Ketoacidosis, 200
    Alkaptonuria, 393
    Child Abuse and Neglect
        Psychosocial Dwarfism, 349
    Cocaine Toxicity, 200
    Diabetic Ketoacidosis, 367
    Erythropoietic Porphyria, 408
    Glucagonoma Syndrome, 303
    Hyperkalemia, 354
    Hypermagnesemia, 353
    Hypernatremia, 355
    Hyperosmolar Hyperglycemia Nonketotic
        Coma, 370
    Hyperphosphatemia, 337
    Hypocalcemia, 337
    Hypoglycemia, 370
    Hypokalemia, 354
    Hypomagnesemia, 353
    Hyponatremia, 355
    Hypophosphatemia, 337

Hypopituitarism, 265
Hypothyroidism and Myxedema Coma, 277
Infant of Diabetic Mother, 372
Klinefelter's Syndrome, 327
Maple Syrup Urine Disease, 394
Metabolic Acidosis, 356
Pituitary Apoplexy, 267
Pyruvate Carboxylase Deficiency, 392
Syndrome of Inappropriate Antidiuretic Hormone Secretion, 264
Emory University
    School of Medicine
        Department of Pediatrics
            Division of Endocrinology and Diabetes, 231
            Division of Endocrinology and Metabolism, 231
    Screening for Metabolic Disorders, 191
Employer Quality Partnership (EQP), 524
Empty Sella Syndrome, 265
End of Life
    Exploring Death in America, 520
End of Life Decisions, 519
Endocrine and Metabolic Drug Reviews, 28
Endocrine Cafe, 57
Endocrine Disorders News at Doctor's Guide, 16
Endocrine Disruptors Research Initiative, 186
Endocrine Fellows Foundation (EFF), 220
Endocrine Oncology, 44
Endocrine Research, 28
Endocrine Reviews, 28
Endocrine Rhythms, 70
Endocrine Search
    Endoscopic Thyroidectomy, 139
Endocrine Society, 220
    Comparison Between Insulin-Induced Hypoglycemia and Growth Hormone Secretion Tests for the Diagnosis of GH Deficiency in Adults, 94
    Endocrinology and Birth Defects, 201
    Endocrinology and Congenital Adrenal Hyperplasia, 296
    Endocrinology and Hormone Rhythms, 70
    Endocrinology and Premenstrual Syndrome, 312
    Endocrinology and Short Stature, 348
    Fact Sheets, 194
    News, 16
    Public Affairs, 187
    Recommendations in Response to Major Hypothyroidism Study, 287
Endocrine System Anatomy, 67
Endocrine/Estrogen Letter, 186
Endocrine-Related Cancer, 28
EndocrineWeb, 13, 55, 194
    Adrenal Disorders and Treatments, 78
    Diseases of the Adrenal Cortex
        Cushing's Syndrome, 298
    Estrogen Replacement After Menopause, 145
    Hypoparathyroidism
        Too Little Parathyroid Hormone Production, 346
    Hypothyroidism
        Too Little Thyroid Hormone, 275
    Laparoscopic Adrenalectomy, 124
    Minimally Invasive Parathyroid Surgery, 125
    Parathyroid Surgery
        The Standard Technique, 125
    Preoperative Localization of Parathyroid Tumors, 112
    Sestamibi Scanning Technical Details, 112
    Surgical Approaches to the Adrenal Gland, 124
    Tests for Parathyroid Localization, 113
    Thyroid Goiter
        Enlargement of the Thyroid, 283
    Thyroid Nodule Biopsy, 99
    Thyroid Nodules, 285
    Thyroid Operations, 139
    X-Ray Tests for Adrenal Gland Tumors, 103
    Your Parathyroid, 82
Endocrinology, 29
Endocrinology and Metabolism, 29
Endocrinology Disease Profiles, 13
Endocrinology Glossaries, 14
Endocrinology News, 16
Endocrinology of the Menstrual Cycle, 207
Endocrinology Review Articles and Commentaries, 22
Endocrinology.com, 57
Energy Metabolism, 82, 114, 373
E-note for Adult Medicine
    Hyperaldosteronism, 297

Environmed Research, 153
Environmental Endocrinology, 44
Environmental Protection Agency
  Endocrine Disruptor Screening Program, 186
Enzyme Nomenclature Database, 481
Enzyme Replacement Therapy, 152
Enzyme Replacement Therapy for Metabolic Impairment, 152
Epidemiology, 179
Epidemiology and Prevention, 44
Epidemiology Program Office, 432
Epidermoid Cyst of the Pineal Gland, 272
Erectile Dysfunction, 316
Essential Fructosuria, 387
Essential Vitamins and Minerals, 153
Estrogens, Environmental, 185
Ethics, 211
EurekAlert, 446
European Calcified Tissue Society
  Biochemical Markers of Bone Metabolism Clinical Uses in Osteoporosis, 109
European Federation of Endocrine Societies (EFES), 220
European Journal of Contraception and Reproductive Care, 29
European Journal of Endocrinology, 29
European Journal of Obstetrics and Gynecology and Reproductive Biology, 29
European Menopause Journal, 29
Evolution of Growth Hormone Therapy, 157
Exercise Regimens, 125
Extendedcare.com, 518
Extramural Research, 60

F

Fabry Disease Home Page, 399
Fabry Support and Information Group, 399
Fabry's Disease, 399
Familial Lecithin Cholesterol Acyltransferase Deficiency, 379
Families USA, 516
Family Practice Notebook.com
  Adrenal Adenoma, 300
  Aldosteronism, 297
  Allopurinol, 152
  Antithyroid Drugs, 138
  Female Pseudohermaphroditism, 332
  Gonadotropin-releasing Hormone Agonist, 156
  Hematologic, 13
  Hypogonadism, 319
  Male Pseudohermaphroditism, 331
  Precocious Puberty, 330
  Pubertal Delay, 330
  Systemic Corticosteroid, 143
  Tall Stature, 350
  Thyroid Radioiodine, 138
  Turner's Syndrome, 333
Family Village
  A Global Community of Disability Related Resources, 508
  Adrenal Hyperplasia, 296
  Diabetes Insipidus, 263
  Glycogen Storage Disease, 389
  Growth Disorders, 346
  Maple Syrup Urine Disease, 395
  McCune-Albright Syndrome, 340
  Noonan Syndrome Links, 328
  Russell-Silver Syndrome, 350
Family's Guide to Diabetes, 194
FAQs in Endocrinology
  Surgery for Pituitary Adenomas, 135
Fatty Acid Oxidation and Carnitine, 397
Federal Web Locator, 432, 465
FedStats, 17
  One Stop Shopping for Federal Statistics, 18
Feedback Control in Endocrine Systems, 70
Fellowships and Residencies, 499
Female Endocrinology, 307
Female Pseudohermaphroditism, 332
Fertilitext
  Gonadatropin-releasing Hormone GnRH, 157
  Overview of Currently Available Drugs, 207
  Prescription Medication, 207
Fertility and Sterility, 30
Fertility Drugs and Ovarian Cancer
  A Review of the Evidence Purporting a Causal Association, 309
Finch University of Health Sciences/Chicago Medical School
  Anterior Pituitary Hormones, 74
  Antibodies to Hormones and Neurotransmitters, 309

Posterior Pituitary Hormones, 74, 155
First Headlines
    Health, 461
Fluid, Electrolyte, and Acid-Base Metabolism, 353
Fogarty International Center (FIC), 438
Follicle-Stimulating Hormone, 92
Food and Drug Administration (FDA), 432, 472
    Center for Drug Evaluation and Research, 472
Food and Nutrition Service (FNS), 432
Food Safety and Inspection Service, 433
Foundation Center, 228, 491
Foundation for Osteoporosis Research and Education, 342
Foundations and Grant Support, 227
Froedtert Hospital and Medical College
    Hormones and Breast Cancer, 161
Frontiers in Bioscience
    A Tumor Atlas and Knowledge Base, 167
    Images of Thyroid Gland Neoplasms, 285
Frontiers in Clinical Genetics, 487
Frontiers in Endocrinology, 30
Frontiers in Neuroendocrinology, 30
Fructose-1,6-Bisphosphatase Deficiency, 387
Furman University
    The Endocrine System, 67

G

Galactokinase Deficiency, 388
Galactosemia, 388
Galactosylceramide Lipidosis (Krabbe's Disease), 400
Galaxy
    Medicine, 466
Galen II
    The Digital Library of the University of California, 466
Gastrinoma (Zollinger-Ellison Syndrome), 302
Gastrointestinal Tract, 79, 106, 301
Gastroparesis, 366
Gaucher Disease, 400
Gauchers Association, 220, 400
    Effect of Low-dose Enzyme Replacement Therapy on Bones, 153
    Living With Gaucher Disease, 401

Gene Therapy, 126, 133, 135
Gene Therapy Approaches for Diabetes and its Complications, 126
GeneClinics, 487
Genentech
    Familial Tall Stature and Causes of Abnormal Tall Stature, 350
    Growth Failure Caused by Hormones, 348
General and Comparative Endocrinology, 30
General Endocrinology Tests, 87
General Infirmary at Leeds
    National Guideline for the Management of Prostatitis, 325
General Medical Supersites, 426
General Medical Topic Newsgroups, 451
General Prevention Programs, 188
Generalized Gangliosidosis, 402
GeneTests, 88
Genetic Alliance, 201
Genetic Syndromes of Developmental Disorders, 327
Genetic Tests, 88
Genetics, 44, 200, 487
Genetics and In Vitro Fertilization Institute, 242
Genetics Revolution at Time.com, 487
Genetics Virtual Library, 488
GeoCities
    Med Files Case Studies in Endocrinology, 167
George Washington University
    Abnormal Prenatal Differentiation, 331
    Toolkit of Instruments to Measure End of Life, 520
Georgetown University
    Community and Family Medicine Web Server
        Diabetic Ketoacidosis, 367
    National Reference Center for Bioethics Literature, 212
    SIADH (Syndrome of Inappropriate ADH), 264
Geriatric Endocrinology, 202
Geriatrics, 44, 490
Gestational Diabetes, 362
Getting Online, 6
Gilda Radner Familial Ovarian Cancer Registry, 310
Gland Central, 273

Global Health Network, 466
Globoid Cell Leukodystrophy or Krabbe's Disease, 400
Glucagon, 148
   Insulin Antidote, 148
Glucagon.com, 85
Glucagonoma, 303
Glucocorticoid Receptor Resource (GRR), 209
Glucose Self-Monitoring, 127
Glycogen Storage Diseases
   General, 389
   Pompe Disease (Acid Maltase Deficiency), 389
Goiter, 283
Gonadal Hormone Tests, 108
Gonadotropin-Releasing Hormone and Analogs, 156
Gonadotropins, 160
Google, 466
Government Agencies and Offices, 431
Government Information Databases, 430
Government Information Locator Service, 430
Government Organizations, 431
Government Printing Office (GPO) Access, 433
Gradschools.com, 500
Grants and Award Guides, 491
Graves' Disease, 279
Great Smokies Diagnostic Laboratory
   Amino Acid Analysis, 121
   Laboratory Assessments, 87
Greenberg Center for Skeletal Dysplasias, 340
Growth and Stature, 346
Growth Hormone, 92, 157
Growth Hormone and IGF Research, 30
Growth Hormone Deficiency, 266
Growth Hormone Therapy, 45
Growth House, 521
Guide to Clinical Preventive Services, 484
Guides to Medical Journals on the Internet, 445
Gynecological Endocrinology, 30
Gynecomastia, 317

H

H. Lee Moffit Cancer Center and Research Institute

Cancer Control Journal
   Carcinoid Tumors of the Gut, 411
Harcourt International
   Journal Subject List, 447
Hardin
   Library Electronic Journal Showcase, 447
   Meta Directory of Internet Health Services, 466
      Endocrinology and Diabetes, 55
Harvard Medical School
   Department of Continuing Education, 52
   Hyperparathyroidism
      Clinical Case, 345
   Renal Osteodystrophy, 339
Harvey Mudd College
   Pineal Gland, 77
Hashimoto's Thyroiditis, 277
Hazards, Environmental, 186
Health A to Z, 467
Health and Medical Hotlines, 451
Health Aspects of Cannabis, 200
Health Education Programs, 61
Health Network
   Medical Informatics Resources, 496
Health News
   A Thyroid Dilemma, 278
Health on the Net (HON) Foundation, 427, 454, 493
   MedHunt, 467
Health Priorities Group, 478
Health Resource Links, 527
Health Resources and Services Administration (HRSA)
   Division of Transplantation, 62
   Legislative and Regulatory Activities, 187
Health Sciences Information Service, 467
Health Sciences Library System (HSLS)
   Health Statistics, 456
Health Services/Technology Assessment Text (HSTAT), 484
Health Web, 467
Healthanswers.com, 508
   Disease Finder, 457
   Injury Finder, 458
   Test Finder, 458
Healthcare Financing Administration, 433, 524
Healthcare Solutions Group On-Line CME Credits

Ultrasound of the Testis and Scrotum, 109
Health-Center.com, 508
HealthCentral, 508
   Dilutional Hyponatremia, 356
   Insulin C-Peptide, 116
   Pediatric Health Encyclopedia
      Acromegaly, 269
      Alkalosis, 357
Healthfinder, 430
HealthGate, 428
   Amylase, 107
   Bone Age, 111
   Catecholamines, 102
   Creatinine, 105
   Estrogens, 108
   Fasting Plasma Glucose, 115
   Follicle-Stimulating Hormone (FSH), 92
   Growth Hormone, 92
   Growth Hormone Suppression Test, 95
   Insulin Tolerance Test, 117
   Lipase, 107
   Lipoprotein Phenotyping, 89
   Oral Glucose Tolerance Test (OGTT), 117
   Phospholipids Test, 119
   Polycystic Ovarian Syndrome (Stein-Leventhal Syndrome), 312
   Parathyroid Hormone (Parathormone, 113
   Renal Angiography, 105
   Renal Computed Tomography, 105
   Renal Ultrasonography, 105
   Renal Venography, 106
   Retrograde Ureteropyelography, 106
   Sex Chromatin, 89
   Testosterone Testing, 108
   Thyroid Biopsy, 99
   Thyroid Ultrasonography, 97
   Total Cholesterol Test, 119
   Total Urine Estrogens, 108
   Urine Amylase, 107
   Urine Free Cortisol, 104
Healthgrades.com, 474
HealthlinkUSA, 509
   Dwarfism, 348
   Precocious Puberty, 330
HealthPages, 452
Healthtouch Online
   Endocrine, 13
HealthWeb
   Endocrinology, 58

Healthwise Knowledgebase
   Carbohydrate-Deficient Glycoprotein Syndrome Type 1, 405
   Hermaphroditism, 332
   Porphyria, Hereditary Coproporphyria, 409
   Pyruvate Dehydrogenase Deficiency, 392
HealthWorld Online, 509
Hebrew University School of Medicine Department of Endocrinology
   Pituitary Gland, 74
HeliosHealth.com
   Diabetes Type 2, 114
Hereditary Coproporphyria, 409
Hereditary Fructose Intolerance, 390
Hermaphroditism, General, 332
Highwire Press, 447
Hirsutism, 308
Histiocytosis Association Online Library
   The Facts About Diabetes Insipidus, 263
HIV, 418
Hole's Essentials of Human Anatomy and Physiology
   Growth Hormone and Growth Disorders, 266
Home Health Care Consultant
   Management of Hypoglycemia in Diabetes in the Home Care Setting, 370
Home Pharmacy, 529
Homocystinuria, 394
Hormone and Metabolic Research, 31
Hormone Foundation, 221
   Treatment Options for Menopause, 194
Hormone Replacement Therapy, 45, 145
Hormone Replacement Therapy and Complications of Therapy, 160
Hormone Research, 31
Hormones, 69, 101
Hormones and Behavior, 31
Hospice and Home Care, 521
Hospice Association of America (HAA), 522
Hospice Foundation of America, 522
Hospice Net, 522
HospiceWeb, 522
Hospital Practice
   Diagnosis and Treatment of Klinefelter Syndrome, 328
   Recognizing the Faces of Hypothyroidism, 275

Hospital Resources, 451
HospitalDirectory.com, 451
HospitalWeb, 451
Human Biological Data Interchange, 201
Human Genome Database
  Types of Dwarfism, 348
Human Genome Project
  Ethical, 478
Human Growth Foundation, 195
  Growth and Growth-Related Disorders, 347
  Growth Hormone Deficiency, 266
  Growth Hormone Treatment, 157
Human Growth Foundation (HGF), 221
Human Obesity Gene Map, 373
Human Reproduction, 31
  Menstrual Disorders and Other Common Gynecology Problems, 307
  Prolactin
    Physiologic and Pathologic Associations, 269
Hyperaldosteronism, 297
  The Facts You Need to Know, 297
Hypercalcemia, 335
Hypercalcemia Outline, 335
Hypercortisolism
  Cushing's Syndrome, 297
Hyperglycemia, Hyperosmolar, Nonketotic State, 370
Hyperkalemia, 354
Hyperlipidemia, 377
Hyperlipidemia File, 377
Hyperlipoproteinemia Classifications, 378
Hypernatremia, 355
Hyperparathyroidism
  Adenoma, 345
  Carcinoma, 345
  General, 344
Hyperphosphatemia, 337
Hyperprolactinemia and Galactorrhea, 269
Hypertension, 190
Hypertension Evaluation, Adrenal, 102
Hyperthyroidism, 287
Hypobetalipoproteinemia, 383
Hypocalcemia, 337
Hypoglycemia, 370
Hypoglycemia Association, 221, 371
Hypoglycemia Homepage Holland
  Clinical Causes of Hypoglycemia, 371

Hypokalemia, 354
Hypolipidemia, 382
Hyponatremia, 355
Hypoparathyroidism, 346
Hypophosphatemia, 337
Hypopituitarism, 265
Hypothalamic and Other Peptide Hormones, 155
Hypothalamic-Pituitary Axis Dysfunction, 263
Hypothalamic-Pituitary Hormones and Function, 73
Hypothalamic-Pituitary Testing, 91
Hypothyroidism, 287
  Causes, 275
Hypothyroidism, General, 274

I

iBionet
  Pyruvate Carboxylase Deficiency Symptoms, 392
Illinois State Academy of Science
  Andrology Databases, 209
  Endocrinology Databases, 69, 209
  Pituitary Hormone Levels in Humans, 74
  Thyroid Hormone Levels in Humans, 77
Imaging, 93, 97, 103, 105, 106, 109
  Bone Age, 111
  Bone Densitometry, 111
  Bone Scan, 112
  Parathyroid Gland, 112
Imaging and Pathology, 492
Imaginis
  Diagnosis of Osteoporosis with Bone Mineral Density Measurement, 111
Immunoassays, 98
  Thyroid Autoimmunity, 98
Immunosuppressive Drugs, 154
IMpact
  The Internal Medicine Newsletter for Medical Students, 502
Indian Health Service (IHS), 433
Indiana State University Terre Haute Center for Medical Education
  Cholesterol, 84
  Fatty Acids, 83
  Glycogen, 83
  Glycolysis, 85

Lipoproteins, 84
Medical Biochemistry Tutorial, 67
Non-Glucose Carbons in Glycolysis, 83
Peptide Hormones, 69
Steroid Hormones, 69
Indiana University
   Department of Medicine
      Endocrinology Division, 232
   Ruth Lilly Medical Library (RLML), 468
   School of Medicine
      The Endocrine System, 68
Individual Journal Web Sites, 22
Individual Research Centers, 241
Infantile Refsum's Disease, 403
Inferior Petrosal Sinus Sampling, 93
Infertility, 308, 318
Infobiotech, 481
Infomed Drug Guide
   Allopurinol, 152
   Spironolactone, 165
InfoMedical.com
   The Medical Business Search Engine, 484
Infomine, 468
   Scholarly Internet Resources, 426
Informatics and Software, 212
Institute for Genomic Research (TIGR), 488
Institute for Reproductive Medicine and Science of Saint Barnabas
   Common Questions about Human Menopausal Gonadotropins, 160
Insulin, 149
Insulin Dependent Diabetes Trust U.S. (IDDT U.S.), 177
Insulin Pumpers, 130
Insulin Resistance, 363
Insulin Resistance Information, 363
Insulin-Free World Foundation, 132, 184, 221
   Articles About Immunology, 131
   Diabetes Facts and Statistics, 184
   Facts and Statistics about Islets, 184
   General Articles, 360, 362
   Glossary of Terms, 14
   Government Relations, 177
   Pancreas Facts and Statistics, 184
   Pharmaceutical Information, 154
Insulinoma, 303
Insure.com
   Answers to Seniors' Health Insurance Questions (on Medicare and Medicaid), 519
Integrated Medical Curriculum
   Anterior Pituitary, 74
   Human Anatomy, 493
Integration and Regulation of Fuel Metabolism, 85
InteliHealth
   Home to Harvard University Health Information, 509
   Vitamin and Nutrition Resource Center, 458
Intellectual Property Network, 497
Inter Science Institute
   Growth Hormone Challenge, 95
   Hypertension, 102
   Hypothalamic-Pituitary Axis and Releasing Factor Tests, 90
   Pancreatic Tests, 107
   Pediatric and Enzyme Deficiency Tests, 120
   Reproductive Endocrinology and Gonadal Steroid Tests, 109
   Thyroid Tests, 100
International Bioethics Committee, 478
International Bone and Mineral Society, 222, 342
International Center for Fabry Disease, 399
International Diabetes Federation, 182
   Guidelines to Type 1 Diabetes Self-Monitoring of Blood Glucose, 127
International Diabetes Monitor
   Hypoglycemia
      Think Drugs, 371
International Diabetic Athletes Association (IDAA), 195, 222
International Food Information Council, 482, 527
International Islet Transplant Registry, 132
International Neuroendocrine Federation, 72, 222
International Osteoporosis Foundation, 342
International Pancreas and Islet Transplant Association (IPITA), 133, 222
International Pompe Association, 222, 390
International Society for Mannosidosis and Related Diseases, 134
International Society for Pediatric and Adolescent Diabetes, 182, 205, 223

International Society of Andrology
 Endocrinology of Aging in Males, 202
International Society of
 Psychoneuroendocrinology (ISPNE), 223
Internet Grateful Med at the National Library
 of Medicine (NLM), 426
Internet Newsgroups, 451
Internet Pathology Laboratory
 Urinalysis, 118
Internet Pathology Library
 Diabetes Mellitus, 168
 Endocrine Pathology Index, 168
Interpretation of Laboratory Test Profiles, 88
Interpreting Glycated Hemoglobin Levels, 116
Intramural Research, 60
Irish Medical Journal
 Unusual Manifestations of Type I
  Autoimmune Polyendocrinopathy, 415
Iron Disorders Institute
 Porphyria Cutanea Tarda, 409
Islet Foundation, 133
Italian Multiple Endocrine Neoplasia
 Network (MENNET), 413
IVF.com
 Male Infertility Overview
  Assessment, 318

J

Jefferson Health System
 Empty Sella Syndrome, 265
 Hypopituitarism, 265
 The Parathyroid Glands, 82
Johns Hopkins
 Bayview Medical Center
  Clinical Nutrition
   Calcium, 145
 Brain Tumor Radiosurgery
  Pituitary Tumor, 135
 Children's Center
  Syndromes of Abnormal Sex
   Differentiation, 331
 Medical Institutions
  Endocrine Surgery, 246
  Endocrine Surgery Web, 123
  Islet Cell/Endocrine Tumors of the
   Pancreas, 302
 Medical Institutions (InfoNet), 509

Office of Continuing Medical Education,
 52
School of Medicine
 Division of Endocrinology and
  Metabolism, 232
 Division of Pediatric Endocrinology, 232
Joint Commission of Accreditation of
 Healthcare Organizations (JCAHO), 517,
 524
Joslin Diabetes Center, 243
 Diabetes News, 181
Journal of Assisted Reproduction and
 Genetics, 31
Journal of Bone and Mineral Metabolism, 31
Journal of Bone and Mineral Research, 32
Journal of Cerebral Blood Flow and
 Metabolism, 32
Journal of Clinical Endocrinology and
 Metabolism, 32
Journal of Diabetes and its Complications, 32
Journal of Endocrinological Investigation, 32
Journal of Endocrinology, 32
 Thyroid Hormone Actions on Cartilage
  and Bone, 276
Journal of Gene Medicine Website, 133
Journal of Genetic Counseling, 33
Journal of Human Nutrition and Dietetics, 33
Journal of Inherited Metabolic Disease, 33
Journal of Molecular Endocrinology, 33
 Gene Therapy Strategies for the Treatment
  of Pituitary Tumors, 135
Journal of Neuroendocrinology, 33
Journal of Nutritional Biochemistry, 33
Journal of Peptide Research, 34
Journal of Pineal Research, 34
Journal of Reproductive Medicine, 34
Journal of the American Medical Association
 Cost-effectiveness of Thyroid Screening,
  193
 Women's Health Info Center
  Effects of the Menstrual Cycle on
   Medical Disorders, 309
Journal of the American Society of
 Nephrology
  Presentation and Follow-up of 30 Patients
   with Congenital Nephrogenic Diabetes
   Insipidus, 264
Journals on the Internet, 22
Journals, Articles, and Latest Books, 21

Juvenile Diabetes Foundation (JDF) International, 183, 205

K

Kansas University Medical Center
   Lipid Metabolism, 83
   Pharmacology
      Basic Pharmacology, 141
Karger, 447
Karolinska Institutet
   Endocrine Diseases, 56
Keck School of Medicine
   University of Southern California
      Department of Pediatrics
         Division of Endocrinology and Metabolism, 232
      Endocrinology Division, 233
Kelly G. Ripken Program, 195
Kennedy Krieger Institute and Academic Medical Center
   Mutation Database for X-Linked Adrenoleukodystrophy, 294
Ketoacidosis, 366
Ketone Site
   What Every Healthcare Professional Should Know, 116
Kidney, 79, 104
Kidney Pancreas Transplant Group, 195
KidsHealth.org, 509
Kimball's Biology Pages
   Adrenal Glands, 78
   Gastrointestinal Hormones, 79
   Melatonin and the Pineal Gland, 77
King Faisal Specialist Hospital and Research Centre
   Alkaptonuria
      Case Report and Review of the Literature, 393
   Wolman's Disease, 404
King's College Division of Physiology
   Pituitary and Hypothalamus, 75
Klinefelter Syndrome, 333
Klinefelter Syndrome and Associates, 333
Klinefelter's Syndrome, 327
Kluwer Academic Publishers
   Journal Home Pages, 447
Kyoto
   Encyclopedia of Genes and Genomes (KEGG), 210, 488
University Hospital
   The Pituitary
      Magnetic Resonance Imaging Protocols, 93

L

Laboratory Corporation of America
   C-Peptide, 107
Lahey Clinic Center for Sexual Dysfunction
   American Association of Clinical Endocrinologists Clinical Practice Guidelines for Male Sexual Dysfunction, 317
Last Acts, 521
Lawson Wilkins Pediatric Endocrine Society (LWPES), 206, 223
Legislation and Public Policy, 187
Leicester Royal Infirmary NHS Trust
   Thyrotoxicosis, 279
Lexi-Comp
   Clinical Reference Library
      Amino Acid Screen, 121
      Cosyntropin, 156
      Gastrin, 108
      Glucose, 115
      Glycated Hemoglobin, 116
      Ketone Bodies, 117
      Newborn Screening for Phenylketonuria and Congenital Hypothyroidism, 192
      Phenylalanine, 120
      Urea Nitrogen, 104
   Informatics Library
      Hypoglycemic Agents Comparison, 150
LifeForce Hospitals
   Amyloidosis, 417
Lipoprotein and Cholesterol Metabolism, 377
List and Glossary of Medical Terms, 458
Little People of America Dwarfism Resources
   Dwarfism Types and Definitions, 349
Living Will and Values History Project, 515
Living Wills, 515
Locating a Physician, 452
London Radiosurgical Centre
   Practice Guidelines
      Pituitary Adenomas, 136
Louisiana State University Medical Center

The Menopausal Patient and Hormone
    Replacement Therapy, 161
Loyola University
    Medical Education Network
        A Clinical Evaluation of the Thyroid in
            Health and Disease, 168
    Stritch School of Medicine, 247
Lustgarten Foundation for Pancreatic Cancer
    Research, 305
Lycos
    Health with WebMD
        Finding the Cause, 318
    Pheochromocytoma Support Site, 300
Lysosomal Disorders, 398
Lysosomal Storage Diseases, General, 398

M

Macrosomia, 372
Magnesium Metabolism Disorders, 353
Major Aspects of Growth In Children
    (MAGIC) Foundation for Children's
    Growth, 206
    Adults Who Live with Growth Hormone
        Deficiency, 267
    Russell-Silver Syndrome, 350
    Underlying Conditions of Growth
        Abnormalities, 347
Major Bone Mass Measurement Techniques,
    111
Male Endocrinology, 315
Male Gonadal Disorders, 319
Malignancy, 419
Mallinckrodt Institute of Radiology (MIR)
    and Washington University Medical Center
    MIR Nuclear Medicine Teaching File, 168
Malnutrition, 375
Managed Care Glossary, 524
Manbir Online
    Short Stature, 349
Manual of Use and Interpretation of
    Pathology Tests
    Adrenocorticotrophic Hormone (ACTH)
        Plasma, 101
    Antidiuretic Hormone (ADH) Plasma, 92
    Calcium
        Plasma or Serum, 110
    Cortisol (Plasma or Serum), 101

Dexamethasone Suppression Test
    (Overnight), 96
Gastrin, 108
Hypopituitarism, 91
Maple Syrup Urine Disease, 394
Marcel Dekker Product Catalog
    Medicine, 448
Marquette General Health System
    Organic Acids Screen, 122
Martindale's Health Science Guide, 485
    Anatomy and Histology Center, 475
Massachusetts General Hospital
    and Harvard Medical School
        Clinically Non-functioning Pituitary
            Adenomas
                Characterization and Diagnosis, 91
        Neuroendocrine Clinical Center and
            Pituitary Tumor Center, 247
        Bilateral Inferior Petrosal Sinus Sampling
            in Cushing's Syndrome, 93
        Familial Multiple Endocrine Neoplasia
            Type I, 413
        Growth Hormone Replacement in Adults,
            157
        History of Stereotactic Radiosurgery, 136
        Long-term Mortality and Morbidity after
            Transsphenoidal Surgery for Pituitary
            Adenomas, 136
    Neuroendocrine Center
        Advances in Recombinant Human
            Growth Hormone Therapy, 158
Massachusetts Prostate Cancer Research
    Institute, 323
MatWeb
    Pituitary Imaging Abnormalities, 168
    Selected Medical Images
        Adrenal Abnormalities, 169
        Thyroid Abnormalities, 169
Mayo Clinic
    Aminoglutethimide, 144
    Endocrinology, 233, 248
    Health Oasis, 509
    Primary Amyloidosis, 418
    Scottsdale Center for Reproductive
        Medicine
        Side Effects of Gonadotropins, 160
McGill University
    Gene Could Lead to New Therapy for
        Diabetes, 127

McKinley Health Center
  Pill Interactions with Other Drugs, 163
McMahon Archives
  Endoscopic Ultrasound Imaging Modality
    for a Variety of Pancreatic Diseases, 106
MDAdvice.com, 510
MDchoice.com, 468
MDConsult, 448
MDGateway, 485
MDMultimedia
  Hypercalcemia Associated with
    Malignancy, 335
  Hyperprolactinemia, 270
  Malnutrition, 375
  Osteomalacia and Rickets, 338
  Prostatic Hyperplasia, 321
  Sheehan's Syndrome, 268
Mead Johnson
  Hereditary Tyrosinemia, 396
Mechanisms of Action, 71
Med Help International, 510
Med411.com
  Medical Research Portal, 468
MedConnect, 485
MedExplorer, 468
MediCAD
  The Porphyrias, 406
Medical and Health Sciences Libraries, 453
Medical Breakthroughs, 462
Medical College of Wisconsin Health Link
  Metachromatic Leukodystrophy, 402
Medical Computing Today
  CME Sites, 50
Medical Conferences and Meetings, 454
Medical Conferences.com, 454
Medical Data and Statistics, 456
Medical Dictionaries, Encyclopedias, and
  Glossaries, 457
Medical Education, 501
Medical Ethics
  Where Do You Draw the Line?, 478
Medical Images on the Web, 494
Medical Informatics, 496
Medical Insurance and Managed Care, 523
Medical Insurance Resources, 524
Medical i-Way, 494
Medical Legislation, 460
Medical Libraries at Universities, 453
Medical Matrix, 56, 428, 448, 469

CME Courses Online, 50
Medical News, 461
Medical Pathology Course
  Graves' Disease, 279
Medical Planning, 514
Medical School Web Sites, 500
Medical Schools, 501
Medical Search Engines and Directories, 463
Medical Spell-Check Offered by Spellex
  Development, 458
Medical Student Cooperative
  Medical Education Links, 502
Medical Student Resources, 501
Medical Student Web Site, 502
Medical World Search, 469
MedicalConferences.com, 17
Medicare, 525
Medicare Rights Center (MRC), 517
MedicineNet.com, 469, 510
  Diseases and Conditions Index, 458
  Medical Dictionary, 459
  Medications Index, 472
  Procedures and Tests Index, 459
Medicines for People with Diabetes, 195
MediConf Online, 455
  Forthcoming Meetings, 17
Mediconsult.com, 510
  Random Plasma Glucose, 115
MedInfoSource
  Practical Management of Dysfunctional
    Uterine Bleeding, 313
MEDLINE Journal Links to Publishers, 448
MEDLINE/PubMed at the National Library
  of Medicine (NLM), 21, 426
MEDLINEplus, 510
MEDLINEplus Health Information, 15, 430
  Alcaptonuria, 394
  Androgens (Systemic), 159
  Bromocriptine, 156
  Calcitonin, 144
  Endocrine Overview, 196
  Genetic Testing/Counseling, 89
  Insulinoma, 303
  Toxic Nodular Goiter, 282
MEDLINEPlus Health Information
  Growth Disorders, 347
MedMark, 469
  Endocrinology, 56
Medmeetings, 17, 455

MedNets, 428
   Cushing's Disease, 298
   Journals, 449
MedPharm
   Learning Modules for Endocrinology, 172
MedPlanet, 485
Medscape, 428, 469
   Conference Summaries and Schedules, 455
   Diabetes and Endocrinology, 56
Medscout
   Diabetes Mellitus, 359
   Endocrine, 57
Medsite, 485
Medstudents
   Acromegaly and Gigantism, 269
   Endocrinology, 172
   Lysosomal Storage Diseases, 398
MedSurf, 470
Medullary Thyroid Carcinoma, 412
MedWatch
   The FDA Medical Products Reporting Program, 473
MedWeb, 470
MedWebPlus
   Biotechnology, 482
   Mitochondrial Myopathies, 385
Megasite Project
   A Metasite Comparing Health Information Megasites and Search Engines, 429
Memorial Health System
   Hyperthyroidism in Pregnancy, 287
Memorial University of Newfoundland
   The Endocrine Glands, 68
Menopause, 45, 203
Menopause and Beyond, 203
Menstrual Exacerbations of Medical Problems, 309
Merck
   Bone Physiology/Metabolism, 81
   Manual of Diagnosis and Therapy, 459
      Adrenal Cortical Hyperfunction, 295
      Adrenal Cortical Hypofunction, 292
      Benign Prostatic Hyperplasia, 322
      Calcium Metabolism, 335
      Hypolipidemia, 382
      Less Common Porphyrias, 410
      Male Hypoganadism, 320
      Nonketotic Hyperglycemic-Hyperosmolar Coma, 370
      Obesity, 374
      Secondary Hypertriglyceridemia, 379
      Type IV Hyperlipoproteinemia, 381
      Type V Hyperlipoproteinemia, 382
      Water and Sodium Metabolism, 355
   ThyroLink, 274
Merck-Medco Managed Care Online, 529
Metabolic Acidosis, 356
Metabolic Agents, 151
Metabolic Alkalosis, 357
Metabolic Disease, 133
Metabolic Disease and Stroke
   Fabry's Disease, 400
Metabolic Impairment Testing, General, 119
Metabolic Regulation, 84
Metabolic Screening and Biochemical Genetics, 120
Metabolic Testing
   Amino Acid Analysis, 121
   Carnitine Analysis, 121
   Magnetic Resonance Spectroscopy, 122
   Urine Organic Acid Analysis, 122
Metabolism, Inborn Errors, 385
Metachromatic Leukodystrophy, 402
Metacrawler, 470
Metamedix.com, 213
MetaMetrix
   Organic Compounds in Urine Metabolic Profiling to Assess Functional Nutrient Deficiencies, 122
Methodist Health Care System
   Paget's Disease of the Bone, 339
Michigan Diabetes Control Program
   Community Screening for Diabetes Recommendations, 189
Michigan Diabetes Outreach Network
   Pharmacologic Treatment of Diabetes, 148
   Quick Reference Guide to Diabetes Gestational Diabetes, 362
MidLife Passages
   Andropause or Viropause, 199
Midwest Bioethics Center, 478
Millennium Meeting on Porphyrins and Porphyrias, 407
Mineral and Electrolyte Metabolism, 34
Minerals, 154
MMRL
   Multimedia Medical Reference Library Medical Student Study Center, 470

Molecular and Cellular Endocrinology, 34
Molecular Endocrinology, 34
Molecular Genetics and Metabolism, 35
Molecular Genetics Jump Station, 488
Molecular Human Reproduction, 35
Molecular Reproduction and Development, 35
Mosby Publishers
   Journals Arranged by Specialty, 449
Mount Rogers/Mount Rainier Clinics
   Endocrinology of Aging, 203
Mount Sinai School of Medicine
   Department of Medicine
      Division of Endocrinology and Metabolism, 233
   Department of Pediatrics
      Division of Pediatric Endocrinology and Metabolism, 233
Mucopolysaccharidoses (MPS) and Related Diseases, 391
Mudi-Muse Biomedical Imaging and Processing, 494
Multiple Endocrine Neoplasia, 412
Multiple Epiphyseal Dysplasia Support Page, 341
Munksgaard International Publishers
   Alphabetical List of Journals, 449
Myxedema Coma, 277

N

Nafarelin Acetate, 157
National Adrenal Diseases Foundation, 291
National Association for Home Care (NAHC), 522
National Bioethics Advisory Commission (NBAC), 433, 479
National Cancer Institute
   Hypercalcemia, 336
   MedNews
      Pheochromocytoma, 300
National Cancer Institute (NCI), 438
   Parathyroid Cancer, 345
   Testicular Cancer, 326
National Cancer Institute MedNews
   Menopausal Hormone Replacement Therapy, 162
National Center for Biotechnology Information (NCBI), 438, 482

Genes and Disease
   Tangier Disease, 384
Online Mendelian Inheritance in Man (OMIM), 202, 210, 488
National Center for Chronic Disease Prevention and Health Promotion, 434
National Center for Complementary and Alternative Medicine (NCCAM), 438
National Center for Environmental Health (NCEH), 434
National Center for Health Statistics (NCHS), 434, 456
   Fast Stats A to Z, 18
National Center for Infectious Diseases, 434
National Center for Research Resources (NCRR), 439
National Center for Toxicological Research (NCTR), 435
National Chronic Care Consortium, 515
National Committee for Quality Assurance (NCQA), 525
National Council for Emergency Medicine Informatics (NCEMI), 425
National Diabetes Education Initiative, 183
National Diabetes Information Clearinghouse, 61
National Dysautonomia Research Foundation (NDRF)
   Tetrahydrobiopterin Deficiency, 397
National Eye Institute
   Diabetic Eye Disease, 369
National Eye Institute (NEI), 439
National Family Caregivers Association (NFCA), 514
National Gaucher Foundation, 401
   Gaucher Disease
      Clinical Course, 401
National Glycohemoglobin Standardization Program, 63
National Graves' Disease Foundation, 279
National Guideline Clearinghouse (NGC), 435, 486
   Endocrine Disease Guidelines, 172
National Heart, 374, 439
National Hospice Organization (NHO), 523
National Human Genome Research Institute (NHGRI), 439, 489
National Institute for Occupational Safety and Health (NIOSH), 435

National Institute of Allergy and Infectious
  Diseases (NIAID), 440
National Institute of Arthritis and
  Musculoskeletal and Skin Diseases
  (NIAMS), 440
National Institute of Child Health and
  Human Development (NICHD), 440
National Institute of Dental and Craniofacial
  Research (NIDCR), 441
National Institute of Diabetes and Digestive
  and Kidney Diseases (NIDDK), 58, 441
National Institute of Environmental Health
  Sciences (NIEHS), 441
National Institute of General Medical
  Sciences (NIGMS), 441
National Institute of Mental Health (NIMH),
  442
National Institute of Neurological Disorders
  and Stroke
  Cushing's Syndrome Information Page, 298
National Institute of Neurological Disorders
  and Stroke (NINDS), 442
  Adrenoleukodystrophy, 294
  Mitochondrial Myopathies Information
    Sheet, 386
  Niemann-Pick Disease, 403
National Institute of Nursing Research
  (NINR), 442
National Institute on Aging (NIA), 443
National Institute on Alcohol Abuse and
  Alcoholism (NIAAA), 443
National Institute on Deafness and Other
  Communication Disorders (NIDCD), 443
National Institute on Drug Abuse (NIDA),
  444
  Anabolic Steroid Abuse, 211
National Institute on Drug Abuse Research
  Report Series
  Anabolic Steroid Abuse, 212
National Institutes of Health (NIH), 444
  Continuing Education, 51
  Diagnosis and Management of
    Asymptomatic Primary
    Hyperparathyroidism, 344
  Fabry's Disease, 400
  Funding Opportunities, 228, 491
  Library Online, 453
  Mammary Genome Anatomy Project
    (MGAP), 210

Osteoporosis and Related Bone
  Diseases/National Resource Center, 342
Paget's Disease of Bone, 339
Screening for Hypertension, 190
National Institutes of Health News Release
  Hypothyroidism during Pregnancy Linked
    to Lower IQ for Child, 287
National Kidney and Urologic Diseases
  Information Clearinghouse, 61
National Kidney Foundation (NKF), 223
National Library of Medicine (NLM), 429,
  444, 453
  Gangliosidosis GM1, 402
  Guide to Clinical Preventive Services
    Screening for Obesity, 191
  MEDLINE Journals with Links to
    Publisher Web Sites, 449
  New Visible Human Project, 494
  Pyruvate Dehydrogenase Complex
    Deficiency, 392
  Screening for Obesity, 374
  Screening for Phenylketonuria (PKU), 395
National Mucopolysaccharidoses (MPS)
  Society, 223, 391
National Network of Libraries of Medicine
  (NN/LM), 454
National Neurofibromatosis Foundation, 413
National Niemann-Pick Disease Foundation,
  403
National Organization for Rare Disorders
  (NORD), 421, 459
National Osteoporosis Foundation, 342
  Men and Osteoporosis, 204
National Ovarian Cancer Association, 224,
  310
National Ovarian Cancer Coalition, 310
National Pancreas Foundation, 301
National PKU News, 395
National Reference Center for Bioethics
  Literature, 479
National Residency Matching Program
  (NRMP), 500
National Science Foundation, 435
National Science Foundation (NSF) Grants
  and Awards, 491
National Tay-Sachs and Allied Diseases
  Association, 224, 404
National Tay-Sachs and Allied Health
  Diseases Association, 90

National Urea Cycle Disorders Foundation, 395
National Women's Health Information Center (NWHIC), 511
Nebraska Health and Human Services System Practitioner's Manual
   Galactosemia, 388
Neoplasms of the Pancreas, 302
Neoplastic Endocrine-Like Syndromes, 303
Nephrogenic Diabetes Insipidus Foundation, 264
   Pseudohypoparathyroidism, 346
Nephropathy, 367
Netherlands Institute of Gerontology
   Endocrine System and Disorders Poster Sessions, 203
NetMed.com, 470
NetWellness, 511
Neuroendocrine Clinical Center and Pituitary Tumor Center, 243
Neuroendocrine System, 72, 135, 155, 263
Neuroendocrinology, 35, 45
Neurofibromatosis (Recklinghausen's disease), 413
Neuropathy, 128, 368
Neurosciences on the Internet
   Images, 494
Neurosurgical Focus
   Bromocriptine Therapy for Prolactin Secreting Pituitary Adenomas, 156
Neurotransmitters and Hormones, 72
New Developments in Transplantation Medicine, 154
New England Medical Center (NEMC)
   Division of Endocrinology, 248
New Scientist
   Fit For a King, 410
New York Eye and Ear Infirmary
   Diabetic Retinopathy Clinical Overview, 369
New York Hospital-Cornell Medical Center
   Division of Endocrinology, 233
New York Online Access to Health (NOAH), 511
New York Presbyterian Hospital, 249
New York Thyroid Center
   Radioactive Iodine for Testing and Treatment, 138
New York University

Insulin Receptor Signaling, 85
New York Weill Cornell Center
   Congenital Adrenal Hyperplasia, 296
New York-Presbyterian Hospital Weill Cornell Medical College, 234
News, 180
NIDDK
   Acromegaly, 269
   Clinical Trials, 59
   Devices for Taking Insulin, 130
   Diabetes in African American Populations, 179
   Diabetes in American Indians and Alaska Natives, 180
   Diabetes in Asian and Pacific Islander Americans, 180
   Diabetes in Hispanic Americans, 180
   Diabetes Prevention Program, 190
   Diabetes Research and Training Center's Demonstration and Education Divisions, 61
   Diabetes Statistics, 18, 185
   Diabetic Neuropathy, 368
   Division of Diabetes, 60
   Division of Digestive Diseases and Nutrition (DDN), 60
   Division of Nutrition Research Coordination (DNRC), 61
   Endocrine and Metabolic Diseases, 14
   Familial Multiple Endocrine Neoplasia Type I, 413
   Financial Help for Diabetes Care, 196
   Gastroparesis and Diabetes, 366
   Health Education Programs, 59
   Health Information, 59
      Endocrine and Metabolic Diseases, 262
   Hyperparathyroidism, 345
   I Have Diabetes
      What Should I Eat?, 129
   Kidney Disease of Diabetes, 367
   Laboratories, 60
   National Diabetes Clearinghouse
      Diabetes Diagnosis, 114
   Noninvasive Blood Glucose Monitors, 130
   Office of Health Research Reports
      Addison's Disease, 293
   Pancreatic Islet Transplantation, 133
   Research Funding Opportunities, 59
   Search Engine, 15

Web Site and Topical Index

Special Reports, 59
Web Site Features, 58
Welcome, 60
Niemann-Pick Disease, 403
Niemann-Pick Disease Group (UK), 403
NIH
    Autoimmunity and Endocrine Disease, 261
    Consensus Development Conference Statement
        Hyperparathyroidism, 113
    Diabetes Dictionary, 14
    Pilot Studies on Gene Therapy Vectors for Metabolic Diseases, 134
    Task Force on Genetic Testing, 89
NIH Institutes and Centers, 436
Non-Functioning Adrenal Incidentaloma, 299
Nonthyroidal Illness, 288
Noonan's Syndrome, 328
Normal Radiologic Anatomy, 495
North American Menopause Society, 203, 224
North American Society for the Study of Obesity (NASSO), 224, 374
North Carolina Baptist Hospital
    Neoplasms of the Pineal Region, 272
North Memorial Health Care Library
    Fine Needle Aspirations of Thyroid Nodules, 285
Northeastern University Pharmacology
    Catecholamines, 73
Northwestern Memorial Hospital
    Division of Endocrinology, 249
Northwestern University
    Division of Endocrinology, 234
Nuclear Imaging Tests of the Thyroid, 97
Nucmednet Featured Procedure
    Treating Thyroid Disease with Radioactive Iodine, 138
Nutrition, 35
Nutrition and Health Linkstation, 527
Nutrition and Physical Wellness, 526
Nutrition Research, 36
Nutritional Interventions, 128

O

Obesity, 191, 373
Obesity Medications, 158
Obesity Meds and Research News, 158
Office of Genetics and Disease Prevention, 489
Office of National Drug Control Policy (ONDCP), 435
Office of Naval Research
    Human Systems Department, 436
Ohio State University, 234
OncoLink
    Adrenal Cancer, 298
    Adrenal Neoplasms, 299
    Cancer of the Thyroid, 285
    Endocrine System Cancers, 262
    Hormones and Cancer, 162
    Metastatic Insulin-secreting Carcinoma of the Pancreas
        Clinical Course and the Role of Surgery, 137
    Pancreatic Cancer, 305
    Parathyroid Cancers, 345
    Pituitary Cancer, 270
    Prostate Cancer, 323
Oncology
    Pituitary Adenomas
        Current Methods of Diagnosis and Treatment, 91
OnHealth, 511
Online Atlas Of Surgery, 476
On-Line Biology Book
    The Endocrine System, 68
Online Clinical Calculator, 486
On-line Diabetes Resources, 360
    Diabetic Neuropathy, 368
    Meters, 130
    Software, 213
Online Directory of Medical Software, 486
Online Drug Stores, 528
Online Drugstore.com, 530
Online Medical Resources, 470
Online Mendelian Inheritance in Man (OMIM)
    Achondroplasia, 341
    Apolipoprotein B, 383
    Apolipoprotein E, 381
    Autoimmune Polyendocrinopathy Syndrome, 415
    Fructose Intolerance, 390
    Fructosuria, 387
    Galactokinase Deficiency, 388
    Gangliosidosis, 402

Hermaphroditism, 332
High Density Lipoprotein Deficiency, 384
Homocystinuria, 394
Hyperlipidemia, 382
Hyperlipoproteinemia, 380, 381
Kallman Syndrome, 320
Lecithin
   Cholesterol Acyltransferase Deficiency (LCAT Deficiency), 379
   Schmidt Syndrome, 415
   Wolman Disease, 404
Online Surgery, 476
Option Care Pediatric Overview
   Growth Hormone Therapy, 267
Oral Contraceptives, 163
Oral Hypoglycemic Agents, 150
Orchid Cancer Appeal, 326
Oregon Health Sciences University
   Amino Acid Metabolism, 393
   Department of Medicine
      Division of Endocrinology, 234
   Endocrine Gland Neoplasms, 262
   Hormone Antagonists, 141
   Hypolipoproteinemia, 383
   Screening for Hypertension, 190
   Studying Vitamin D as Treatment for Prostate Cancer, 146
Organ Damage, 372
Organ Donation, 516
Organic Acidemia Association
   Management of Urea Cycle Disorders, 396
Organizations, 181
Organizations and Institutions, 215
Osteogenesis Imperfecta, 341
Osteogenesis Imperfecta Foundation, 341
Osteomalacia, 338
Osteoporosis, 342
Osteoporosis in Men, 204
Osteoporosis International, 36
Osteoporosis Medical News and Alerts, 343
Osteoporosis Online
   Men and Osteoporosis
      Not Just a Woman's Disease, 204
Osteovision
   Major Biochemical Markers of Bone Turnover, 110
   Vitamin D and Analogues in the Treatment of Osteoporosis, 146

Other Government Agencies and Programs, 62
Other Topical Resources, 209
Ovarian Cancer, 309
Ovarian Cancer Alliance Canada, 310
Ovarian Cancer National Alliance, 311
Ovaries and Female Reproductive Tract, 80
Overview, 143, 147, 163
Overview of Dynamic Tests in Endocrinology, 90
Overview of Hypothalamic and Pituitary Hormones, 155
Overview of Pituitary Hormones and Analogs, 155
Overview Sites, 55
Oxford Medical Informatics
   Fructose-1, 387
   Galactokinase Deficiency, 388
   Galactose 4 Epimerase Deficiency, 391

P

Paget Foundation, 339
Paget's Disease of the Bone, 339
Pain Net, 484
Pain.com, 483
Pancreas, 137
Pancreas Cancer Home Page, 305
Pancreas.org, 301
Pancreatic Anatomy and Physiology, 85
Pancreatic Cancer Action Network, 305
Pancreatic Cancer Online, 306
Paraendocrine and Neoplastic Syndromes, 411
Parathyroid Gland, 343
Parathyroid Gland Anatomy and Physiology, 82
Parathyroid Hormone Therapy, 145
Parathyroid Scan, 113
Parathyroid Screening, 113
Parathyroid Surgery, 125
Parents' Common Sense Encyclopedia
   Bone Age, 111
Parkland Pocket Guide to HIV Care
   Endocrine Manifestations of HIV, 418
Parts and Workings of the Human Kidney, 79
Patent Searches, 497
Pathology and Case Studies, 167
Pathophysiology of the Endocrine System

Antidiuretic Hormone (Vasopressin), 92
Patient Education and Planning, 505
Patient Education and Support, 193
Patient Resources, 505
PCS Health Systems
    Hormones, 142
PDR.net, 486
PEDBASE
    Noonan Syndrome, 328
    Thyroiditis, 280
Pediatric Bulletin
    Gynecomastia, 318
Pediatric Endocrinology, 46, 205
Pediatric Screening, 191
Penn State
    Case Studies in Endocrinology, 169
    Milton S. Hershey Medical Center Endocrinology, 250
PERLjam Online/Medical Images, 495
Peroxisomal Disorders, 405
PersonalMD.com
    Male Hormones Linked to Prostate Cancer, 159
Pharmaceutical Information, 471
Pharmaceutical Information Network (PharmInfoNet), 473
Pharmaceutical Research and Manufacturers of America, 473
Pharmaceutical Research and Manufacturers of America (PhRMA)
    New Drugs under Development, 20
Pharmacology, 141
Pharmacology Central
    Peptide Hormones, 69
PharmInfoNet
    Endocrine Disease and Diabetes Center, 58, 142
    Obesity Information, 159
Phenylketonuria (PKU), 395
Pheochromocytoma, 300
Pheochromocytoma Syndromes, 413
Philipps University Marburg
    Modern Imaging Procedures in the Diagnostics of Pancreatic Disease, 106
Phys.com Fitness Encyclopedia, 459
Physician and Sportsmedicine
    Exercise for Osteoporosis, 126
Physician Directories, 474
Physician's Guide to the Internet, 455, 486

Physicians Committee for Responsible Medicine (PCRM), 479
Physicians for Social Responsibility
    Endocrine Disruptors, 186
Physicians' Practice, 453
Physiology, 46
Pineal Gland and Melatonin Physiology, 77
Pineal Gland Disorders, 271
Pittsburgh Genetics Institute
    Gaucher Disease
        A Clinical Trial of Gene Therapy, 401
Pituitary, 36
Pituitary Apoplexy, 267
Pituitary Disorders
    Conditions of Decreased Pituitary Functioning, 265
    Conditions of Hormone-secreting Pituitary Adenomas, 268
    Pituitary Tumors, 270
Pituitary Surgery, 135
Pituitary Tumor Network Association, 225, 271
    Craniopharyngiomas, 271
    Cushing's Syndrome, 269
    Empty Sella Syndrome, 265
PlanetRx.com, 530
Polaris Grants Central, 228, 492
Polycystic Ovary Syndrome, 311
    Metabolic Challenges and New Treatment Options, 150
Polyendocrine Disorders, 415
Poole Hospital
    Endocrine Dynamic Function Tests, 90
Porphyria Cutanea Tarda, 409
Porphyria Foundation of Canada
    Acute Intermittent Porphyria, 408
    Hereditary Coproporphyria (HCP), 409
    Rare Forms of Porphyria, 410
    Variegate Porphyria, 410
Porphyrias, 406
Postgraduate Medicine
    Assessment of Adrenal Glucocorticoid Function, 101
    Biochemical Markers of Bone Turnover, 110
    Coronary Artery Disease and Diabetes, 365
    How to Diagnose Hypopituitarism, 266
    Insulin Therapy, 149
    Porphyria Cutanea Tarda, 409

Sick Euthyroid Syndrome, 288
Symposium on Complications of Diabetes, 364
The Many 'Faces' of Graves' Disease, 279
Postpartum Thyroid Disease, 288
Potassium Metabolism Disorders, 354
PowerPak Pharmacy Online Continuing Education
   Androgen Replacement Therapy for Male Hypogonadism, 160
Practical Diabetes International, 36
Practice Management Information Corporation, 487
Prader-Willi Association (UK)
   Genetics of Prader-Willi Syndrome, 328
Prader-Willi Association (USA), 225, 329
Prader-Willi Syndrome, 328
Precocious Puberty and Pubertal Delay, 329
Pregnancy and Thyroid Disorders, 286
Premenstrual Syndrome, 312
Presbyterian Hospital of Dallas
   Metabolic Myopathies
      Lipid Defects, 397
   Neuromuscular Center
      Mitochondrial Myopathies, 386
Prevention Magazine Online, 511
Primary Hypogonadism
   Adult Leydig Cell Failure, 320
   General Resources, 319
Primer on Molecular Genetics, 489
Princeton Medicon
   The Medical Conference Resource, 455
Professional Topics and Clinical Practice, 475
Progesterone Advocates Network
   Ovarian, 162
Project AWARE
   Parathyroid Hormone Restores Almost Full Bone Mass to Women with Osteoporosis, 146
Project on Death in America
   Transforming the Culture of Dying, 521
Prolactin, 93
Prolonged ACTH Stimulation Test, 100
Prosite Database of Protein Families and Domains, 210
Prostaglandins, 36
Prostaglandins and Other Lipid Mediators, 36
Prostate, 37
Prostate Cancer, 322

Prostate Cancer Dot Com, 323
Prostate Cancer Research Institute, 324
Prostate Disorders, 321
Prostate Health, 321
Prostatis Foundation, 325
Prostatitis, 325
Prostatitis Foundation
   Prostatitis, 325
Psci-com, 512
Pseudohypoparathyroidism, 346
Psychoneuroendocrinology, 37
Public Citizen, 461
Public Health and Policy Topics, 177
Public Health Nutritionists' Home Page, 527
Public Health Service (PHS), 436
PubList
   Health and Medical Sciences, 449
Purine and Pyrimidine Metabolic Disorders, 398
Purine Research Society, 225, 398
Pyruvate Carboxylase Deficiency, 392
Pyruvate Dehydrogenase Complex Deficiency, 392

Q

Quackwatch, 512
Quality Improvement Organizations, 517
Quick Reference, 13
Quick Reference Guide to Diabetes for Healthcare Providers, 190
Quotesmith.com, 525

R

Radioactive Iodine, 138
Radiotherapy, 137
Radiotherapy.com, 137
Rare Disease Clinical Trials, 333
Rare Disorders, 421
Rare Genetic Diseases in Children
   Lysosomal Storage Diseases, 398
Rarer Porphyrias, 410
Ratings and Site Selection, 5
Ratings Guide, 6
Ray Williams Institute of Paediatric Endocrinology
   Age of Screening for Hypertension, 191
   Devices for Insulin Delivery, 131

Diagnostic Criteria for Diabetes in
  Childhood and Adolescence, 115
Growth and Disorders of Growth, 349
Hypoglycemia in Diabetes, 371
Normal Puberty and Pubertal Disorders,
  330
Types of Insulin Preparations, 150
Recombinant Capital, 482
Recurrent Pregnancy Loss
  Hormonal Causes, 309
Reference Information and News Sources, 425
Refsum's Disease, 403
Regional Emergency Medical Services Council
  Glucagon, 148
Reidel's Thyroiditis, 278
Renal Osteodystrophy, 339
Rensselaer Polytechnic Institute
  Adrenal Cortex, 78
Reproduction, 37
Reproductive Endocrinology, 46, 206
Reproductive Endocrinology Journals, 207
Reproductive Glands, 108
Reproductive Health Matters, 37
Reproductive Medicine Review, 37
Reproductive Organs, 80
Reproductive Science Center Network
  Glossary of Terms, 14
Reproductive System, 159
Research, 183
Research Organizations, 240
Residency Page, 500
Retinopathy, 129, 369
Reuters Health, 462
Reuters Health Information
  High Level of Estrogen Increases Breast
    Cancer Risk, 162
Reviews in Endocrine and Metabolic
  Disorders, 37
Rickets, 340
  A General Overview, 340
Ronald S. Hirshberg Memorial Foundation
  for Pancreatic Cancer Research, 306
Royal Children's Hospital
  Division of Laboratory Services
    Metabolic Disorders and Tests for Their
      Investigation, 120
  Introduction to Metabolic Testing, 120
Rush-Presbyterian-St. Luke's Medical Center
  Department of Internal Medicine, 250

RxList
  The Internet Drug Index, 473
RxMed
  Sodium Bicarbonate, 151
  Sodium Chloride, 154

S

SafeScript Limited
  World Standard Drug Database, 474
Safeweb Medical, 530
Sansum Medical Research Institute, 243
Santa Monica Thyroid Diagnostic Center, 97
Science Direct, 449
Science News Update, 462
science.komm Internet Directory and
  Resource Site
  Medical Journals Main Index, 450
ScienceDaily Magazine
  Surgical Experience Improves
    Thyroidectomy Outcome, 140
SciTalk.com
  Diabetes News Center, 16
Screening/Prevention, 188
Search the Endocrine Society Journals Online,
  21
Searchpointe Physician Background
  Information Service, 474
Secondary Hypogonadism
  Kallman Syndrome, 320
Selected Articles and Commentaries, 22
Selected Hospital Endocrinology and
  Metabolism Departments, 244
Selected Medical Images
  Metachromatic Leukodystrophy, 402
Selected Medical School CME Programs, 51
Selected Medical School Departments of
  Endocrinology and Metabolism, 229
Self Care, 530
Seoul National University College of
  Medicine
  Endocrine Pancreas, 86
Sexual Differentiation, 331
Sexual Dysfunction, 38
Sheehan's Syndrome, 268
Short Stature
  General, 348
  Psychosocial Dwarfism, 349
  Russell-Silver Syndrome, 350

Signaling Pathway Database, 211
Site Selection Criteria, 5
Skeletal Dysplasias, 340
Smith-Lemli-Opitz Syndrome, 406
Smith-Lemli-Opitz Syndrome Advocacy and Exchange, 406
Society for Behavioral Neuroendocrinology, 73, 225
Society for Endocrinology, 196, 226
   Adult Growth Hormone Replacement, 158
   Search Page, 21
Society for Neuroscience (SFN), 73
Society for the Study of Fertility (SSF), 207, 226
Society for the Study of Inborn Errors in Metabolism, 386
Society for the Study of Inborn Errors of Metabolism, 226
Society for the Study of Reproduction, 208, 226
Society of Research Administrators (SRA) GrantsWeb, 228, 492
Sodium and Water Metabolism Disorders, 355
Somatomedin C (IGF-1)
   Adult Growth Hormone Deficiency, 93
Springer-Verlag's LINK, 450
St. Thomas' Hospital
   Endocrines and Reproduction, 208
Stanford
   MedWorld, 502
      MedBot, 471
   University
      Bone Mineral Density Applet, 112
      Management of Common Lipid Disorders, 378
   University School of Medicine Department of Pediatrics
      Division of Endocrinology and Diabetes, 234
State Insurance Commissioners, 517
State Medical Boards Directory, 487
Statistics, 17, 184
Stem Cell Transplantation, 134
Stem Cell Transplantation Moves Front and Center, 135
Steroids, 38
Stimulation Testing, 94
Student Doctor Network

The Interactive Medical Student Lounge, 503
Student Resources, 499
Subacute or deQuervain's Thyroiditis, 280
Subacute Thyroiditis, 281
Subclinical Hyperthyroidism
   Just a Low Serum Thyrotropin Concentration, 281
Subclinical Hypothyroidism, 278
Subclinical Thyroid Dysfunction, 281
Subspecialty Topics, 199
Substance Abuse and Mental Health Services Administration (SAMHSA), 436
Summary of Diseases Associated with Mineral/Vitamin Deficiencies, 351
Supersites, 55
Support Groups, 513
Support-Group.com, 196, 513
Suppression Testing, 95
Surgical Experience with Pancreatic and Peripancreatic Neuroendocrine Tumors, 137
Swiss Institute of Bioinformatics (SIB) Expert Protein Analysis System (ExPASy)
   Enzyme Nomenclature Database (ENZYME), 211
Syndrome of Inappropriate ADH Secretion, 264
Synthesis, Storage, and Release, 71
Systemic Diseases
   Endocrine Manifestations, 417

T

Tall Stature, 350
Tangier Disease, 384
Tay-Sachs Disease, 404
Technological Developments in Insulin Delivery, 130
Temple University
   Hospital
      Metabolism, 251
      Principles of Endocrine Surgery, 123
   School of Medicine
      Antihyperlipidemic Agents, 147
      Hormonal Hypertension, 292
      Metabolic Acidosis, 356
      Metabolic Alkalosis, 357
Terre Haute Center for Medical Education

Abetalipoproteinemia
　Kornzweig Syndrome, 383
Defects in Fructose, 387
Glycogen Storage Diseases Database, 389
Hyperlipoproteinemias, 378
Introduction to Amino Acid Metabolism and Inborn Errors of Amino Acid Metabolism, 393
The Porphyrias, 407
Testes, 80
Testicular Cancer, 326
Testicular Cancer Resource Center, 326
Tests, 107
Tests and Procedures, 460
Tetrahydrobiopterin Home Page, 397
Texas Department of Health
　Galactosemia Handbook, 389
Texas Tech University Health Sciences Center Department of Cell Biology and Biochemistry
　Male Reproductive System, 80
The Continuing Education Network (TCEN)
　Management of the Thyroid Nodule, 286
The Endocrinologist, 38
The Hastings Center, 479
The Kidney
　Structure and Function, 79
The Peroxisome Website
　Peroxisomal Single Enzyme Disorders, 405
Therapeutics, 47
ThinkQuest Library of Entries, 528
This Week's Top Medical News Stories, 463
Thomas Jefferson University Hospital
　Division of Endocrinology, 235
Thomas-U.S. Congress on the Internet, 461
Three-Dimensional Medical Reconstruction, 495
ThriveOnline, 512
ThyCa
　Thyroid Cancer Survivors' Association, 196
Thyroid, 38
Thyroid Biopsy, 99
Thyroid Center, 274
Thyroid Disease, 192
Thyroid Disease Manager, 274
　Evaluating Thyroid Function and Anatomy, 96

Evaluation of Thyroid Function in Health and Disease, 96
Graves' Disease and the Manifestations of Thyrotoxicosis, 280
Hashimoto's Thyroiditis, 277
Hyperthyroidism Management with Antithyroid Drugs, 164
Multinodular Goiter, 283
Primary Hypothyroidism, 288
Reidel's Thyroiditis, 278
Subacute Thyroiditis, 281
Surgery of the Thyroid Gland, 140
Tests Assessing the Effects of Thyroid Hormones on Body Tissues, 97
Therapy for Toxic Nodular Goiter, 282
Thyroid Autoantibodies, 99
Thyroid Storm, 280
Thyrotoxicosis, 287
Thyrotoxicosis Factitia, 282
Thyroid Foundation of America, 197
Thyroid Foundation of Canada
　Fine Needle Aspiration Biopsy of Thyroid Nodules, 99
　Thyroid Disorders and Pregnancy, 286
　Thyroiditis, 281
Thyroid Function Tests, 100
Thyroid Gland, 77, 96, 138, 163, 273
Thyroid Hormone, 164
Thyroid Hormone Deficiency, 274
Thyroid Hormone Excess, 279
Thyroid International
　Postpartum Thyroiditis, 288
Thyroid Malignancy, 284
Thyroid Society for Education and Research, 197, 226
　Congenital Hypothyroidism, 276
Thyroid Storm, 280
Thyroid Surgery, 139
Thyroid-Cancer.net, 140, 286
Thyroiditis
　Acute, 281
Thyrotoxicosis Factitia, 282
Toll-Free Numbers for Health Information, 451
Topical Search Tools, 15
Toxic Nodular Goiter (Plummer's Disease), 282
Transplant International, 38
Transplantation, 38

Biological Specimens, 132
General Resources, 131
Pancreas and Islet Cell Transplantation, 132
TransWeb, 132
Treating Diabetes with Good Nutrition
  Dietary Guidelines, 129
Trends in Endocrinology and Metabolism, 39
Tufts University Nutrition Navigator, 528
Tulane University
  Environmental Estrogens and Other Hormones, 185
  Medical Center Department of Pathology and Laboratory Medicine
    Case Studies in Endocrine Disorders, 169
  Posterior Pituitary, 75
  Reproductive Endocrine Conference
    Delayed Puberty, 330
Turner Center
  Klinefelter's Syndrome
    An Orientation, 333
Turner's Syndrome, 333
Turner's Syndrome Society, 334
Turner's Syndrome Society of the United States, 227, 334
Tyler for Life Foundation
  Congenital Hypothyroidism, 276
  Homocystinuria, 394
Type 1 Diabetes Mellitus, 360
Type 2 Diabetes Mellitus, 361
Type I Hyperlipoproteinemia, 380
Type II Hyperlipoproteinemia, 380
Type III Hyperlipoproteinemia, 381
Type IV Hyperlipoproteinemia, 381
Type V Hyperlipoproteinemia, 382

U

U.S. Department of Agriculture (USDA)
  Nutrient Values, 528
U.S. House of Representatives Internet Office of the Law Revision Counsel, 461
U.S. Living Will Registry, 516
U.S. News and World Report
  America's Top HMOs, 525
U.S. Patent and Trademark Office, 497
UDPgalactose 4-Epimerase Deficiency, 391
UMDS Department of Endocrinology, 213
UnCover Web, 450
UniSci
  Daily University Science News, 463
United Medical and Dental Schools
  Adult Growth Hormone Deficiency, 267
United Mitochondrial Disease Foundation, 386
University Institute of Psychiatry Division of Clinical Psychopharmacology
  Steroid Hormone Metabolism, 70
University of Alabama
  Adrenal Neoplasms Clinical Resources, 299
  at Birmingham Department of Medicine
    Division of Endocrinology and Metabolism, 235
  Benign Prostatic Hyperplasia, 322
  Diabetic Nephropathy Clinical Resources, 368
  Erectile Dysfunction Clinical Resources, 317
  Health System
    Division of Endocrinology and Metabolism, 251
  Hyperlipidemia Clinical Resources, 378
  Hypofunction of the Adrenal Cortex Clinical Resources, 293
  Hypokalemia, 354
  Hyponatremia, 356
  Obesity Clinical Resources, 374
  Obesity Patient/Family Resources, 375
  Parathyroid Diseases Clinical Resources, 343
  Premenstrual Syndrome Clinical Resources, 312
  Prostatitis Clinical Resources, 325
  School of Library and Information Studies
    Endocrinology Clinical Resources, 172
  Sick Euthyroid Syndrome Clinical Resources, 289
University of Arkansas for Medical Sciences
  Hyperprolactinemia, 270
University of Buffalo Center for Clinical Ethics and Humanities in Health Care, 479
University of California
  Berkeley
    Molecular and Cell Biology
      Endocrine Pancreas, 86
  Davis
    Endocrine System Tutorial, 68
    Medical Center Patient Care, 512

Los Angeles
   Introduction to Endocrine
      Pharmacology, 142
   Medical Center
      Division of Endocrinology, 252
   Nuclear Medicine Protocols
      Parathyroid Imaging, 113
      Thyroid Uptake and Scan, 98
      Total Body Scan, 98
   Radioiodine Ablative Therapy, 139
   School of Medicine
      Hypoglycemic Agents, 151
San Francisco
   Researchers Clone Gene Vital for
      Vitamin D Metabolism, 338
   The Future of Magnetic Resonance
      Spectroscopy and Spectroscopic
      Imaging, 122
University of Chicago
   Center for Continuing Medical Education, 52
   Clinical Features of Prader-Willi
      Syndrome, 329
   Department of Pediatrics
      Section of Pediatric Endocrinology, 235
   Evaluation of New Oral Hypoglycemic
      Agents, 151
   Health Services
      Hypercalcemia Annotated Bibliography, 336
   Hospitals and Health System, 252
   Section of Endocrinology, 235
University of Cincinnati College of Medicine
   Division of Endocrinology and
      Metabolism, 236
University of Colorado Department of
   Psychology
      Hypothalamus and Its Hormonal Role, 75
University of Connecticut
   Multinodular Goiter, 283
University of Illinois
   Chicago Medical Center
      Division of Andrology, 253
   College of Medicine at Urbana, 495
   Familial Hypercholesterolemia, 380
   Primary Care Template
      Hypercalcemia, 336
University of Iowa
   Department of Physiology and Biophysics

      Mineral Metabolism, 81
   Division of Physiological Imaging
      Department of Radiology, 495
University of Iowa College of Medicine
   Department of Internal Medicine
      Division of Endocrinology and
      Metabolism, 236
   Department of Pediatrics
      Division of Endocrinology, 236
University of Kansas
   Medical Center
      Female Reproductive System, 80
      Genetics Education Center, 490
   School of Medicine Medical Pharmacology
      Learning Modules
      Adrenocorticosteroids, 143
      Diabetes, 148
      Gonadal Hormones, 76
      Hypothalamic and Pituitary Hormones, 75
      Thyroid and Antithyroid Drugs, 163
University of Louisville Pediatric Urology
   Cryptorchidism, 319
University of Manchester
   Insulin and Glucagon, 86
University of Maryland
   Center for Studies in Reproduction, 243
   Department of Medicine
      Division of Endocrinology and
      Metabolism, 236
   Endocrinology Glossary, 14
   Joslin Diabetes Center, 253
   Medical Center Department of Pediatrics
      Division of Pediatric Endocrinology, 237
University of Medicine and Dentistry of New
   Jersey (UMDNJ)
   Management of Hypernatremia, 355
University of Miami Department of Biology
   Hormones and Chemical Messages, 71
University of Michigan
   Anterior Pituitary Physiology, 76
   Comprehensive Cancer Center
      Prostate Cancer Program, 324
   Department of Internal Medicine
      Testing for Pheochromocytoma, 102
   Documents Center
      Statistical Resources on the Web
      Health, 456
   Health System

Pediatric Endocrinology Links, 206
Medical Center
    Division of Endocrinology and Metabolism, 237, 254
Ovarian Cancer and Women's Health Bibliography, 311
Review of Endocrine Surgery, 124
Turner's Syndrome
    A Case Study, 334
University of Minnesota
    Department of Medicine
        Endocrinology and Diabetes, 237
    Diabetes Institute for Immunology and Transplantation, 244
    Gene Therapy Program, 134
University of Missouri Health Sciences Center
    Thyroid Function Tests, 100
University of North Carolina, 70, 237, 254
University of Oklahoma College of Pharmacy
    A First Course in Pharmacokinetics and Biopharmaceutics, 142
University of Palermo
    Postpartum Thyroiditis, 288
University of Pennsylvania
    Adrenal Diseases, 292
    Health System
        Continuing Medical Education, 52
        Department of Medicine
            Endocrinology, 238
        Endocrinology, 255
        Institute for Human Gene Therapy, 134
    Library, 528
University of Pittsburgh
    Department of Medicine
        Screening Tests for Common Medical Management, 88
    Diabetes Health Economics Study Group, 178
    Endoscopic Transsphenoidal Pituitary Surgery, 136
    Medical Center
        Division of Endocrinology and Metabolism, 255
University of Queensland Porphyria Research Unit
    Porphyria
        A Patient's Guide, 407
University of Rochester Medical Center, 238
University of South Australia

Introductory Metabolism Module, 82
University of South Dakota
    Mechanisms of Action
        Hormone Synthesis, 71
University of Texas
    Health Science Center
        Thyroid and Parathyroid Nuclear Medicine, 98
        Thyroid Nuclear Medicine, 98
    Houston Medical School
        Acute Intermittent Porphyria, 408
        Congenital Erythropoietic Porphyria, 409
        Porphyrias, 407
    M.D. Anderson Cancer Center
        Genetic Testing for Endocrine Tumors, 90
        Management of Recurrent Persistent Hyperparathyroidism, 336
        Your Care Path, 140
    Medical Branch at Galveston (UTMB)
        Gestational Diabetes Mellitus
            An Update and Review, 362
    Southwestern Medical Center, 238
    Southwestern Medical Center Department of Pathology
        Endocrine Masses, 170
        Parathyroid, 82
        Pituitary Gland, 76
University of Utah
    Congenital Adrenal Hyperplasia, 332
    Department of Internal Medicine
        Division of Endocrinology, 238
    Gonadal Dysgenesis, 334
    Human Reproduction
        Clinical, 208
    Kallman's Syndrome, 320
    School of Medicine, 238
University of Virginia
    Pituitary Apoplexy, 268
    Variegate Porphyria Pedigree, 410
University of Virginia Health System
    Division of Endocrinology and Metabolism, 239, 256
    Posterior Pituitary Hormones, 76
University of Washington
    Bisphophonates, 144
    Diabetes Endocrinology Research Center, 244

Osteomalacia, 338
Phenylalanine Hydroxylase Deficiency, 397
School of Medicine, 239
University of Wisconsin
  Comprehensive Cancer Center
    Prostate Cancer Answers, 324
  Department of Medicine
    Section of Endocrinology, 239
Urbana Atlas of Pathology
  Endocrinology Section, 170
Urea Cycle Disorders, 395
Urine Free Cortisol, 104
Uro.com
  Undescended Testicle, 319
USA Today
  Health, 463
USAhomecare.com, 516
Uterine Bleeding Disorders, 313
UTHealth.com
  Devices to Take Insulin, 131
  Globoid Cell Leukodystrophy (GCL) A.K.A. Krabbe's Disease, 400

V

Vancouver Hospital Health Sciences Center
  Urea Cycle Defects, 396
Vanderbilt University
  Diabetes Center
    Diabetes and Research Training Center, 244
  Medical Center
    Arginine Infusion Test, 95
    Dexamethasone Suppression Tests, 101
    Division of Endocrinology, 256
    Growth Hormone Deficiency, 267
    Inferior Petrosal Sinus Sampling, 94
    Low Dose ACTH Stimulation Test, 95
    Oral Glucose Suppression Test for Growth Hormone Secretory Dynamics, 96
    Polycystic Ovary Syndrome, 312
    Secondary Amenorrhea, 308
    Traditional ACTH Stimulation Test, 101
    TRH Stimulation of TSH Test, 95
Variant Forms of Hyperphenylalaninemia, 396
Variegate Porphyria, 410

Vascular System, 164
Vasoactive Intestinal Peptide Tumor (VIPoma), 304
Verified Internet Pharmacy Practice Sites (VIPPS) Program, 530
Vesalius, 476
Vesalius Clinical Folios
  Thyroidectomy, 140
Veterans Health Administration Diabetes Program, 63
Virtual Body, 476
Virtual Children's Hospital
  Renal Osteodystrophy, 340
Virtual Drugstore
  Desmopressin, 155
Virtual Hospital
  Hematologic, 277, 280
  Pelvic Imaging, 109
  University of Iowa Health Care, 513
Virtual Library Pharmacy, 474
Virtual Medical Center, 471
Visible Human Slice and Surface Server, 496
Vitamin and Trace Mineral Deficiencies, 351
Vitamin D, 146
Vitamin D Metabolism and Rickets, 338
Vitamin D Metabolism Disorders, 338
Von Hippel Lindau Disease, 414
Von Hippel Lindau Family Alliance, 414

W

Walter Reed Army Medical Center
  Endocrine Nuclear Imaging, 170
Warren Grant Magnuson Clinical Center, 445
Washington State Department of Health
  Brief Review of Thyroid Hormone Regulation and Biological Effects of Thyroid Hormone, 164
Washington University
  Continuing Medical Education, 52
  Nutrients and Solubility, 153
  School of Medicine
    Division of Endocrinology, 239
    Division of Pediatric Endocrinology and Metabolism, 240
    Hypothalamus and Autonomic Nervous System, 76
    VIPoma Metastatic to Liver, 304
WebMD, 429

WebMedLit, 450
   Endocrinology, 22
Weight-control Information Network (WIN), 62
Weizmann Institute of Science Genome and Bioinformatics
   Molecular Biology Databases, 211
Wellman Clinic
   Hypogonadism, 320
WellnessWeb
   Prostate Cancer Center, 324
Westminster Hospital of London
   Diet Treatment of Refsum's Disease, 403
Wheeless' Textbook of Orthopedics
   Pseudohypoparathyroidism, 346
Whittier Institute for Diabetes, 244
Whole Brain Atlas, 476
Wiley Interscience, 450
Wolman's Disease, 404
Women in Endocrinology (WE), 227
Women's Health Clinical Management
   Menopause Management for the Millennium, 204
Words in a Row
   Diabetes Control and Complications Trial (DCCT), 127
World Diabetes, 39
World Health Organization (WHO)
   Diabetes, 180
   Statistical Information System, 457
World Wide Web Virtual Library
   Biotechnology, 483
World Wildlife Fund (WWF) Canada
   Endocrine Disrupting Chemicals, 187
Wound Management
   The Complexities of Wound Management in the Diabetic Foot, 366

X

XXY Information, 333

Y

Yahoo!, 471, 513
   Health
      Diseases and Conditions, 460
      Headlines, 463
   Life and Health Insurance Center, 525
   News Articles in Endocrinology, 16
Yale University
   School of Medicine
      Department of Pediatrics
         Section of Pediatric Endocrinology, 240
      Office of Postgraduate and Continuing Medical Education, 53
      Section of Endocrinology, 240
Your Parathyroid.com, 343

Z

Zollinger-Ellison Syndrome, 303

PRESCRIBING INFORMATION
AVANDIA®
brand of
rosiglitazone maleate tablets

DESCRIPTION
Avandia (rosiglitazone maleate) is an oral antidiabetic agent which acts primarily by increasing insulin sensitivity. *Avandia* is used in the management of type 2 diabetes mellitus (also known as non-insulin-dependent diabetes mellitus [NIDDM] or adult-onset diabetes). *Avandia* improves glycemic control while reducing circulating insulin levels.

Pharmacological studies in animal models indicate that rosiglitazone improves sensitivity to insulin in muscle and adipose tissue and inhibits hepatic gluconeogenesis. Rosiglitazone maleate is not chemically or functionally related to the sulfonylureas, the biguanides, or the alpha-glucosidase inhibitors.

Chemically, rosiglitazone maleate is (±)-5-[[4-[2-(methyl-2-pyridinylamino)ethoxy]-phenyl]methyl]-2,4-thiazolidinedione, (*Z*)-2-butenedioate (1:1) with a molecular weight of 473.52 (357.44 free base). The molecule has a single chiral center and is present as a racemate. Due to rapid interconversion, the enantiomers are functionally indistinguishable. The structural formula is:

rosiglitazone maleate

The molecular formula is $C_{18}H_{19}N_3O_3S \cdot C_4H_4O_4$. Rosiglitazone maleate is a white to off-white solid with a melting point range of 122° to 123°C. The pKa values of rosiglitazone maleate are 6.8 and 6.1. It is readily soluble in ethanol and a buffered aqueous solution with pH of 2.3; solubility decreases with increasing pH in the physiological range.

Each pentagonal film-coated Tiltab® tablet contains rosiglitazone maleate equivalent to rosiglitazone, 2 mg, 4 mg, or 8 mg, for oral administration. Inactive ingredients are: hydroxypropyl methylcellulose, lactose monohydrate, magnesium stearate, microcrystalline cellulose, polyethylene glycol 3000, sodium starch glycolate, titanium dioxide, triacetin, and one or more of the following: synthetic red and yellow iron oxides and talc.

CLINICAL PHARMACOLOGY
Mechanism of Action
Rosiglitazone, a member of the thiazolidinedione class of antidiabetic agents, improves glycemic control by improving insulin sensitivity. Rosiglitazone is a highly selective and potent agonist for the peroxisome proliferator-activated receptor-gamma (PPARγ). In humans, PPAR receptors are found in key target tissues for insulin action such as adipose tissue, skeletal muscle, and liver. Activation of PPARγ nuclear receptors regulates the transcription of insulin-responsive genes involved in the control of glucose production, transport, and utilization. In addition, PPARγ-responsive genes also participate in the regulation of fatty acid metabolism.

Insulin resistance is a common feature characterizing the pathogenesis of type 2 diabetes. The antidiabetic activity of rosiglitazone has been demonstrated in animal models of type 2 diabetes in which hyperglycemia and/or impaired glucose tolerance is a consequence of insulin resistance in target tissues. Rosiglitazone reduces blood glucose concentrations and reduces hyperinsulinemia in the ob/ob obese mouse, db/db diabetic mouse, and fa/fa fatty Zucker rat. Rosiglitazone also prevents the development of overt diabetes in both the db/db mouse and Zucker fa/fa Diabetic Fatty rat models.

In animal models, rosiglitazone's antidiabetic activity was shown to be mediated by increased sensitivity to insulin's action in the liver, muscle, and adipose tissues. The expression of the insulin-regulated glucose transporter GLUT-4 was increased in adipose tissue. Rosiglitazone did not induce hypoglycemia in animal models of type 2 diabetes and/or impaired glucose tolerance.

Pharmacokinetics and Drug Metabolism
Maximum plasma concentration (C_{max}) and the area under the curve (AUC) of rosiglitazone increase in a dose-proportional manner over the therapeutic dose range (Table 1). The elimination half-life is 3 to 4 hours and is independent of dose.

Table 1. Mean (SD) Pharmacokinetic Parameters for Rosiglitazone Following Single Oral Doses (N=32)

Parameter	1 mg Fasting	2 mg Fasting	8 mg Fasting	8 mg Fed
AUC_{0-inf} [ng.hr./mL]	358 (112)	733 (184)	2971 (730)	2890 (795)
C_{max} [ng/mL]	76 (13)	156 (42)	598 (117)	432 (92)
Half-life [hr.]	3.16 (0.72)	3.15 (0.39)	3.37 (0.63)	3.59 (0.70)
CL/F* [L/hr.]	3.03 (0.87)	2.89 (0.71)	2.85 (0.69)	2.97 (0.81)

* CL/F = Oral Clearance.

Absorption
The absolute bioavailability of rosiglitazone is 99%. Peak plasma concentrations are observed about 1 hour after dosing. Administration of rosiglitazone with food resulted in no change in overall exposure (AUC), but there was an approximately 28% decrease in C_{max} and a delay in T_{max} (1.75 hours). These changes are not likely to be clinically significant; therefore, Avandia (rosiglitazone maleate) may be administered with or without food.

Distribution
The mean (CV%) oral volume of distribution (Vss/F) of rosiglitazone is approximately 17.6 (30%) liters, based on a population pharmacokinetic analysis. Rosiglitazone is approximately 99.8% bound to plasma proteins, primarily albumin.

Metabolism
Rosiglitazone is extensively metabolized with no unchanged drug excreted in the urine. The major routes of metabolism were N-demethylation and hydroxylation, followed by conjugation with sulfate and glucuronic acid. All the circulating metabolites are considerably less potent than parent and, therefore, are not expected to contribute to the insulin-sensitizing activity of rosiglitazone.

In vitro data demonstrate that rosiglitazone is predominantly metabolized by Cytochrome P_{450} (CYP) isoenzyme 2C8, with CYP2C9 contributing as a minor pathway.

Excretion
Following oral or intravenous administration of [^{14}C]rosiglitazone maleate, approximately 64% and 23% of the dose was eliminated in the urine and in the feces, respectively. The plasma half-life of [^{14}C]related material ranged from 103 to 158 hours.

Population Pharmacokinetics in Patients with Type 2 Diabetes
Population pharmacokinetic analyses from three large clinical trials including 642 men and 405 women with type 2 diabetes (aged 35 to 80 years) showed that the pharmacokinetics of rosiglitazone are not influenced by age, race, smoking, or alcohol consumption. Both oral clearance (CL/F) and oral steady-state volume of distribution (Vss/F) were shown to increase with increases in body weight. Over the weight range observed in these analyses (50 to 150 kg), the range of predicted CL/F and Vss/F values varied by <1.7-fold and <2.3-fold, respectively. Additionally, rosiglitazone CL/F was shown to be influenced by both weight and gender, being lower (about 15%) in female patients.

Special Populations
Age: Results of the population pharmacokinetic analysis (n=716 <65 years; n=331 ≥65 years) showed that age does not significantly affect the pharmacokinetics of rosiglitazone.

Gender: Results of the population pharmacokinetics analysis showed that the mean oral clearance of rosiglitazone in female patients (n=405) was approximately 6% lower compared to male patients of the same body weight (n=642).

As monotherapy and in combination with metformin, *Avandia* improved glycemic control in both males and females. In metformin combination studies, efficacy was demonstrated with no gender differences in glycemic response.

In monotherapy studies, a greater therapeutic response was observed in females; however, in more obese patients, gender differences were less evident. For a given body mass index (BMI), females tend to have a greater fat mass than males. Since the molecular target PPARγ is expressed in adipose tissues, this differentiating characteristic may account, at least in part, for the greater response to *Avandia* in females. Since therapy should be individualized, no dose adjustments are necessary based on gender alone.

Hepatic Impairment: Unbound oral clearance of rosiglitazone was significantly lower in patients with moderate to severe liver disease (Child-Pugh Class B/C) compared to healthy subjects. As a result, unbound C_{max} and AUC_{0-inf} were increased 2- and 3-fold, respectively. Elimination half-life for rosiglitazone was about 2 hours longer in patients with liver disease, compared to healthy subjects.

Therapy with Avandia (rosiglitazone maleate) should not be initiated if the patient exhibits clinical evidence of active liver disease or increased serum transaminase levels (ALT >2.5X upper limit of normal) at baseline (see PRECAUTIONS, *Hepatic Effects*).

Renal Impairment: There are no clinically relevant differences in the pharmacokinetics of rosiglitazone in patients with mild to severe renal impairment or in hemodialysis-dependent patients compared to subjects with normal renal function. No dosage adjustment is therefore required in such patients receiving *Avandia*. Since metformin is contraindicated in patients with renal impairment, co-administration of metformin with *Avandia* is contraindicated in these patients.

Race: Results of a population pharmacokinetic analysis including subjects of Caucasian, black, and other ethnic origins indicate that race has no influence on the pharmacokinetics of rosiglitazone.

Pediatric Use: The safety and effectiveness of *Avandia* in pediatric patients have not been established.

Pharmacodynamics and Clinical Effects
In clinical studies, treatment with *Avandia* resulted in an improvement in glycemic control, as measured by fasting plasma glucose (FPG) and hemoglobin A1c (HbA1c), with a concurrent reduction in insulin and C-peptide. Postprandial glucose and insulin were also reduced. This is consistent with the mechanism of action of *Avandia* as an insulin sensitizer. The improvement in glycemic control was durable, with maintenance of effect for 52 weeks. The maximum recommended daily dose is 8 mg. Dose-ranging studies suggested that no additional benefit was obtained with a total daily dose of 12 mg.

The addition of *Avandia* to either metformin or a sulfonylurea resulted in significant reductions in hyperglycemia compared to any of these agents alone. These results are consistent with an additive effect on glycemic control when *Avandia* is used as combination therapy.

Reduction in hyperglycemia was associated with increases in weight. In the

Appendix A

26-week clinical trials, the mean weight gain in patients treated with *Avandia* was 1.2 kg (4 mg daily) to 3.5 kg (8 mg daily) when administered as monotherapy, 0.7 kg (4 mg daily) and 2.3 kg (8 mg daily) when administered in combination with metformin, and 1.8 kg (4 mg daily) when administered in combination with a sulfonylurea. A mean weight loss of about 1 kg was seen for both placebo and metformin alone in these studies. The mean change in weight was negligible for patients treated with a sulfonylurea alone in these studies. In the 52-week glyburide-controlled study, there was a mean weight gain of 1.75 kg and 2.95 kg for patients treated with 4 mg and 8 mg of *Avandia* daily, respectively, versus 1.9 kg in glyburide-treated patients.

Patients with lipid abnormalities were not excluded from clinical trials of *Avandia*. In all 26-week controlled trials, across the recommended dose range, *Avandia* as monotherapy was associated with increases in total cholesterol, LDL, and HDL and decreases in free fatty acids. These changes were statistically significantly different from placebo or glyburide controls (Table 2).

Increases in LDL occurred primarily during the first 1 to 2 months of therapy with *Avandia* and LDL levels remained elevated above baseline throughout the trials. In contrast, HDL continued to rise over time. As a result, the LDL/HDL ratio peaked after 2 months of therapy and then appeared to decrease over time. Because of the temporal nature of lipid changes, the 52-week glyburide-controlled study is most pertinent to assess long-term effects on lipids. At baseline, week 26, and week 52, mean LDL/HDL ratios were 3.1, 3.2, and 3.0, respectively, for *Avandia* 4 mg twice daily. The corresponding values for glyburide were 3.2, 3.1, and 2.9. The differences in change from baseline between *Avandia* and glyburide at week 52 were statistically significant.

The pattern of LDL and HDL changes following therapy with *Avandia* in combination with a sulfonylurea or metformin were generally similar to those seen with *Avandia* in monotherapy.

The changes in triglycerides during therapy with *Avandia* (rosiglitazone maleate) were variable and were generally not statistically different from placebo or glyburide controls.

Table 2. Summary of Mean Lipid Changes in 26-Week Placebo-Controlled and 52-Week Glyburide-Controlled Monotherapy Studies

	Placebo-controlled Studies Week 26			Glyburide-controlled Study Week 26 and Week 52			
		Avandia		Glyburide titration		Avandia 8 mg	
	Placebo	4 mg daily*	8 mg daily*	Wk 26	Wk 52	Wk 26	Wk 52
Free Fatty Acids							
N	207	428	436	181	168	166	145
Baseline (mean)	18.1	17.5	17.9	26.4	26.4	26.9	26.6
% Change from baseline (mean)	+0.2%	–7.8%	–14.7%	–2.4%	–4.7%	–20.8%	–21.5%
LDL							
N	190	400	374	175	160	161	133
Baseline (mean)	123.7	126.8	125.3	142.7	141.9	142.1	142.1
% Change from baseline (mean)	+4.8%	+14.1%	+18.6%	–0.9%	–0.5%	+11.9%	+12.1%
HDL							
N	208	429	436	184	170	170	145
Baseline (mean)	44.1	44.4	43.0	47.2	47.7	48.4	48.3
% Change from baseline (mean)	+8.0%	+11.4%	+14.2%	+4.3%	+8.7%	+14.0%	+18.5%

*Once daily and twice daily dosing groups were combined.

Clinical Studies
Monotherapy

A total of 2315 patients with type 2 diabetes, previously treated with diet alone or antidiabetic medication(s), were treated with *Avandia* as monotherapy in six double-blind studies, which included two 26-week placebo-controlled studies, one 52-week glyburide-controlled study, and three placebo-controlled dose-ranging studies of 8 to 12 weeks duration. Previous antidiabetic medication(s) were withdrawn and patients entered a 2 to 4 week placebo run-in period prior to randomization.

Two 26-week, double-blind, placebo-controlled trials, in patients with type 2 diabetes with inadequate glycemic control (mean baseline FPG approximately 228 mg/dL and mean baseline HbA1c 8.9%), were conducted. Treatment with *Avandia* produced statistically significant improvements in FPG and HbA1c compared to baseline and relative to placebo (Table 3).

Table 3. Glycemic Parameters in Two 26-Week Placebo-Controlled Trials

	Placebo	Avandia 2 mg twice daily	Avandia 4 mg twice daily
STUDY A			
N	158	166	169
FPG (mg/dL)			
Baseline (mean)	229	227	220
Change from baseline (mean)	19	–38	–54
Difference from placebo (adjusted mean)		–58*	–76*
Responders (≥30 mg/dL decrease from baseline)	16%	54%	64%
HbA1c (%)			
Baseline (mean)	9.0	9.0	8.8
Change from baseline (mean)	0.9	–0.3	–0.6
Difference from placebo (adjusted mean)		–1.2*	–1.5*
Responders (≥0.7% decrease from baseline)	6%	40%	42%

	Placebo	Avandia 4 mg once daily	Avandia 2 mg twice daily	Avandia 8 mg once daily	Avandia 4 mg twice daily
STUDY B					
N	173	180	186	181	187
FPG (mg/dL)					
Baseline (mean)	225	229	225	228	228
Change from baseline (mean)	8	–25	–35	–42	–55
Difference from placebo (adjusted mean)	–	–31*	–43*	–49*	–62*
Responders (≥30 mg/dL decrease from baseline)	19%	45%	54%	58%	70%
HbA1c (%)					
Baseline (mean)	8.9	8.9	8.9	8.9	9.0
Change from baseline (mean)	0.8	0.0	–0.1	–0.3	–0.7
Difference from placebo (adjusted mean)	–	–0.8*	–0.9*	–1.1*	–1.5*
Responders (≥0.7% decrease from baseline)	9%	28%	29%	39%	54%

* <0.0001 compared to placebo.

When administered at the same total daily dose, *Avandia* was generally more effective in reducing FPG and HbA1c when administered in divided doses twice daily compared to once daily doses. However, for HbA1c, the difference between the 4 mg once daily and 2 mg twice daily doses was not statistically significant.

Long-term maintenance of effect was evaluated in a 52-week, double-blind, glyburide-controlled trial in patients with type 2 diabetes. Patients were randomized to treatment with *Avandia* (rosiglitazone maleate) 2 mg twice daily (N=195) or *Avandia* 4 mg twice daily (N=189) or glyburide (N=202) for 52 weeks. Patients receiving glyburide were given an initial dosage of either 2.5 mg or 5.0 mg/day. The dosage was then titrated in 2.5 mg/day increments over the next 12 weeks, to a maximum dosage of 15.0 mg/day in order to optimize glycemic control. Thereafter the glyburide dose was kept constant.

The median titrated dose of glyburide was 7.5 mg. All treatments resulted in a statistically significant improvement in glycemic control from baseline (Figures 1 and 2). At the end of week 52, the reduction from baseline in FPG and HbA1c was –40.8 mg/dL and –0.53% with *Avandia* 4 mg twice daily; –25.4 mg/dL and –0.27% with *Avandia* 2 mg twice daily; and –30.0 mg/dL and –0.72% with glyburide. For HbA1c, the difference between *Avandia* 4 mg twice daily and glyburide was not statistically significant at week 52. The initial fall in FPG with glyburide was greater than with *Avandia*; however, this effect was less durable over time. The improvement in glycemic control seen with *Avandia* 4 mg twice daily at week 26 was maintained through week 52 of the study.

Figure 1. Mean FPG Over Time in a 52-Week Glyburide-Controlled Study

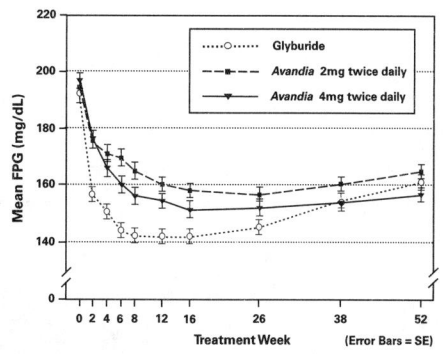

(continued)

Appendix A

Avandia® (rosiglitazone maleate) continued

Figure 2. Mean HbA1c Over Time in a 52-Week Glyburide-Controlled Study

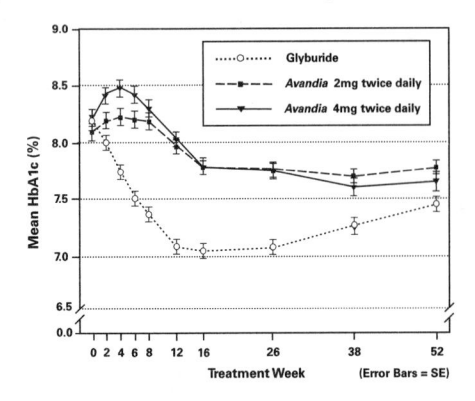

[Line graph showing Mean HbA1c (%) from 0 to 52 treatment weeks comparing Glyburide, Avandia 2mg twice daily, and Avandia 4mg twice daily. Error Bars = SE.]

Hypoglycemia was reported in 12.1% of glyburide-treated patients versus 0.5% (2 mg twice daily) and 1.6% (4 mg twice daily) of patients treated with Avandia. The improvements in glycemic control were associated with a mean weight gain of 1.75 kg and 2.95 kg for patients treated with 2 mg and 4 mg twice daily of Avandia, respectively, versus 1.9 kg in glyburide-treated patients. In patients treated with Avandia, C-peptide, insulin, pro-insulin, and pro-insulin split products were significantly reduced in a dose-ordered fashion, compared to an increase in the glyburide-treated patients.

Combination with Metformin

A total of 670 patients with type 2 diabetes participated in two 26-week, randomized, double-blind, placebo/active-controlled studies designed to assess the efficacy of Avandia (rosiglitazone maleate) in combination with metformin. Avandia, administered in either once daily or twice daily dosing regimens, was added to the therapy of patients who were inadequately controlled on a maximum dose (2.5 grams/day) of metformin.

In one study, patients inadequately controlled on 2.5 grams/day of metformin (mean baseline FPG 216 mg/dL and mean baseline HbA1c 8.8%) were randomized to receive Avandia 4 mg once daily, Avandia 8 mg once daily, or placebo in addition to metformin. A statistically significant improvement in FPG and HbA1c was observed in patients treated with the combinations of metformin and Avandia 4 mg once daily and Avandia 8 mg once daily, versus patients continued on metformin alone (Table 4).

Table 4. Glycemic Parameters in a 26-Week Combination Study

	Metformin	Avandia 4 mg once daily + metformin	Avandia 8 mg once daily + metformin
N	113	116	110
FPG (mg/dL)			
Baseline (mean)	214	215	220
Change from baseline (mean)	6	−33	−48
Difference from placebo (adjusted mean)		−40*	−53*
Responders (≥30 mg/dL decrease from baseline)	20%	45%	61%
HbA1c (%)			
Baseline (mean)	8.6	8.9	8.9
Change from baseline (mean)	0.5	−0.6	−0.8
Difference from placebo (adjusted mean)		−1.0*	−1.2*
Responders (≥0.7% decrease from baseline)	11%	45%	52%

* <0.0001 compared to metformin.

In a second 26-week study, patients with type 2 diabetes inadequately controlled on 2.5 grams/day of metformin who were randomized to receive the combination of Avandia 4 mg twice daily and metformin (N=105) showed a statistically significant improvement in glycemic control with a mean treatment effect for FPG of −56 mg/dL and a mean treatment effect for HbA1c of −0.8% over metformin alone. The combination of metformin and Avandia resulted in lower levels of FPG and HbA1c than either agent alone.

Patients who were inadequately controlled on a maximum dose (2.5 grams/day) of metformin and who were switched to monotherapy with Avandia (rosiglitazone maleate) demonstrated loss of glycemic control, as evidenced by increases in FPG and HbA1c. In this group, increases in LDL and VLDL were also seen.

Combination with a Sulfonylurea

A total of 1216 patients with type 2 diabetes participated in three 26-week randomized, double-blind, placebo/active-controlled studies designed to assess the efficacy and safety of Avandia in combination with a sulfonylurea. Avandia 2 mg or 4 mg daily, was administered either once daily or in divided doses twice daily, to patients inadequately controlled on a sulfonylurea.

In the two placebo-controlled studies, patients inadequately controlled on sulfonylureas that were randomized to single dose or divided doses of Avandia 4 mg daily plus a sulfonylurea showed significantly reduced FPG and HbA1c compared to sulfonylurea plus placebo (Table 5).

Table 5. Glycemic Parameters in Two 26-Week Combination Studies

Study C (patients on prior sulfonylurea monotherapy)	Sulfonylurea	Avandia 2 mg twice daily + sulfonylurea
N	192	183
FPG (mg/dL)		
Baseline (mean)	207	205
Change from baseline (mean)	+6	−38
Difference from placebo (adjusted mean)	−	−44*
Responders (≥30 mg/dL decrease from baseline)	21%	56%
HbA1c (%)		
Baseline (mean)	9.2	9.2
Change from baseline (mean)	+0.2	−0.9
Difference from placebo (adjusted mean)	−	−1.0*

Study D (patients on prior single or multiple therapies)	Sulfonylurea	Avandia 4 mg once daily + sulfonylurea
N	115	116
FPG (mg/dL)		
Baseline (mean)	209	214
Change from baseline (mean)	+23	−25
Difference from placebo (adjusted mean)	−	−47*
Responders (≥30 mg/dL decrease from baseline)	13%	46%
HbA1c (%)		
Baseline (mean)	8.9	9.1
Change from baseline (mean)	+0.6	−0.3
Difference from placebo (adjusted mean)	−	−0.9*

*≤0.0001 compared to sulfonylurea plus placebo.

In the third study, including patients on prior single or multiple therapies, in patients inadequately controlled on the maximal dose of glyburide (20 mg daily), Avandia 2 mg twice daily plus sulfonylurea significantly reduced FPG (n=98, mean change from baseline of −31 mg/dL) and HbA1c (mean change from baseline of −0.5%) compared to sulfonylurea plus placebo (n=99, mean change from baseline of FPG of +24 mg/dL and of HbA1c of +0.9%). The combination of sulfonylurea and Avandia resulted in lower levels of FPG and HbA1c than either agent alone. Patients who were switched from maximal dose of glyburide to 2 mg twice daily Avandia monotherapy demonstrated loss of glycemic control, as evidenced by increases in FPG and HbA1c.

INDICATIONS AND USAGE

Avandia is indicated as an adjunct to diet and exercise to improve glycemic control in patients with type 2 diabetes mellitus. Avandia is indicated as monotherapy. Avandia is also indicated for use in combination with a sulfonylurea or metformin when diet, exercise and Avandia alone or diet, exercise plus the single agent do not result in adequate glycemic control. For patients inadequately controlled with a maximum dose of a sulfonylurea or metformin, Avandia should be added to, rather than substituted for, a sulfonylurea or metformin.

Management of type 2 diabetes should include diet control. Caloric restriction, weight loss, and exercise are essential for the proper treatment of the diabetic patient because they help improve insulin sensitivity. This is important not only in the primary treatment of type 2 diabetes, but also in maintaining the efficacy of drug therapy. Prior to initiation of therapy with Avandia (rosiglitazone maleate), secondary causes of poor glycemic control, e.g., infection, should be investigated and treated.

CONTRAINDICATIONS

Avandia is contraindicated in patients with known hypersensitivity to this product or any of its components.

PRECAUTIONS

General

Due to its mechanism of action, Avandia is active only in the presence of insulin. Therefore, Avandia should not be used in patients with type 1 diabetes or for the treatment of diabetic ketoacidosis.

Patients receiving Avandia in combination with other oral hypoglycemic agents may be at risk for hypoglycemia, and a reduction in the dose of the concomitant agent may be necessary.

Ovulation: Therapy with Avandia, like other thiazolidinediones, may result in ovulation in some premenopausal anovulatory women. As a result, these patients may be at an increased risk for pregnancy while taking Avandia. (See PRECAUTIONS, Pregnancy, Pregnancy Category C.) Thus, adequate contraception in premenopausal women should be recommended. This possible effect has not been specifically investigated in clinical studies so the frequency of this occurrence is not known.

Although hormonal imbalance has been seen in preclinical studies (see Carcinogenesis, Mutagenesis, Impairment of Fertility), the clinical significance of this finding is not known. If unexpected menstrual dysfunction occurs, the benefits of continued therapy with *Avandia* should be reviewed.

Hematologic: Across all controlled clinical studies, decreases in hemoglobin and hematocrit (mean decreases in individual studies ≤1.0 gram/dL and ≤3.3%, respectively) were observed for *Avandia* alone and in combination with a sulfonylurea or metformin. The changes occurred primarily during the first 4 to 8 weeks of therapy and remained relatively constant thereafter. White blood cell counts also decreased slightly in patients treated with *Avandia*. The observed changes may be related to the increased plasma volume observed with treatment with *Avandia* and have not been associated with any significant hematologic clinical effects (see ADVERSE REACTIONS, Laboratory Abnormalities).

Edema: *Avandia* should be used with caution in patients with edema. In a clinical study in healthy volunteers who received *Avandia* 8 mg once daily for 8 weeks, there was a small, statistically significant increase in median plasma volume (1.8 mL/kg) compared to placebo.

In controlled clinical trials of patients with type 2 diabetes, mild to moderate edema was reported in patients treated with *Avandia* (See ADVERSE REACTIONS).

Since thiazolidinediones can cause fluid retention, which can exacerbate congestive heart failure, patients at risk for heart failure (particularly those on insulin) should be monitored for signs and symptoms of heart failure (See PRECAUTIONS, Use in Patients with Heart Failure).

Use in Patients with Heart Failure: In preclinical studies, thiazolidinediones, including rosiglitazone, caused plasma volume expansion and pre-load-induced cardiac hypertrophy. Two ongoing echocardiography studies in patients with type 2 diabetes (a 52-week study with *Avandia* 4 mg twice daily [n=86] and a 26-week study with 8 mg once daily [n=90]), have shown no deleterious alteration in cardiac structure or function. These studies were designed to detect a change in left ventricular mass of 10% or more.

Patients with New York Heart Association (NYHA) Class 3 and 4 cardiac status were not studied during the clinical trials. *Avandia* is not indicated in patients with NYHA Class 3 and 4 cardiac status unless the expected benefit is judged to outweigh the potential risk.

Hepatic Effects: Another drug of the thiazolidinedione class, troglitazone, has been associated with idiosyncratic hepatotoxicity, and very rare cases of liver failure, liver transplants, and death have been reported during postmarketing clinical use. In pre-approval controlled clinical trials in patients with type 2 diabetes, troglitazone was more frequently associated with clinically significant elevations in liver enzymes (ALT>3X upper limit of normal) compared to placebo, and very rare cases of reversible jaundice were reported.

In clinical studies in 4598 patients treated with *Avandia*, encompassing approximately 3600 patient years of exposure, there was no evidence of drug-induced hepatotoxicity or elevation of ALT levels.

In controlled trials, 0.2% of patients treated with *Avandia* had elevations in ALT >3X the upper limit of normal compared to 0.2% on placebo and 0.5% on active comparators. The ALT elevations in patients treated with *Avandia* were reversible and were not clearly causally related to therapy with Avandia (rosiglitazone maleate).

Although available clinical data show no evidence of *Avandia*-induced hepatotoxicity or ALT elevations, rosiglitazone is structurally related to troglitazone, which has been associated with idiosyncratic hepatotoxicity and rare cases of liver failure, liver transplants, and death. Pending the availability of the results of additional large, long-term controlled clinical trials and postmarketing safety data following wide clinical use of *Avandia* to more fully define its hepatic safety profile, it is recommended that patients treated with *Avandia* undergo periodic monitoring of liver enzymes. Liver enzymes should be checked prior to the initiation of therapy with *Avandia* in all patients. Therapy with *Avandia* should not be initiated in patients with increased baseline liver enzyme levels (ALT>2.5X upper limit of normal). In patients with normal baseline liver enzymes, following initiation of therapy with *Avandia*, it is recommended that liver enzymes be monitored every 2 months for the first 12 months, and periodically thereafter. Patients with mildly elevated liver enzymes (ALT levels one to 2.5X upper limit of normal) at baseline or during therapy with *Avandia* should be evaluated to determine the cause of the liver enzyme elevation. Initiation of, or continuation of, therapy with *Avandia* in patients with mild liver enzyme elevations should proceed with caution and include close clinical follow-up, including more frequent liver enzyme monitoring, to determine if the liver enzyme elevations resolve or worsen. If at any time ALT levels increase to >3X upper limit of normal in patients on therapy with *Avandia*, liver enzyme levels should be rechecked as soon as possible. If ALT levels remain >3X the upper limit of normal, therapy with *Avandia* should be discontinued.

There are no data available to evaluate the safety of *Avandia* in patients who experience liver abnormalities, hepatic dysfunction, or jaundice while on troglitazone. Avandia (rosiglitazone maleate) should not be used in patients who experienced jaundice while taking troglitazone. For patients with normal hepatic enzymes who are switched from troglitazone to *Avandia*, a 1-week washout is recommended before starting therapy with *Avandia*.

If any patient develops symptoms suggesting hepatic dysfunction, which may include unexplained nausea, vomiting, abdominal pain, fatigue, anorexia and/or dark urine, liver enzymes should be checked. The decision whether to continue the patient on therapy with *Avandia* should be guided by clinical judgment pending laboratory evaluations. If jaundice is observed, drug therapy should be discontinued.

Laboratory Tests
Periodic fasting blood glucose and HbA1c measurements should be performed to monitor therapeutic response.

Liver enzyme monitoring is recommended prior to initiation of therapy with *Avandia* in all patients and periodically thereafter (See PRECAUTIONS, *Hepatic Effects* and ADVERSE REACTIONS, Serum Transaminase Levels).

Information for Patients
Patients should be informed of the following:

Management of type 2 diabetes should include diet control. Caloric restriction, weight loss, and exercise are essential for the proper treatment of the diabetic patient because they help improve insulin sensitivity. This is important not only in the primary treatment of type 2 diabetes, but in maintaining the efficacy of drug therapy.

It is important to adhere to dietary instructions and to regularly have blood glucose and glycosylated hemoglobin tested. Patients should be advised that it can take 2 weeks to see a reduction in blood glucose and 2 to 3 months to see full effect. Patients should be informed that blood will be drawn to check their liver function prior to the start of therapy and every 2 months for the first 12 months, and periodically thereafter. Patients with unexplained symptoms of nausea, vomiting, abdominal pain, fatigue, anorexia, or dark urine should immediately report these symptoms to their physician.

Avandia can be taken with or without meals.

When using *Avandia* in combination with other oral hypoglycemic agents, the risk of hypoglycemia, its symptoms and treatment, and conditions that predispose to its development should be explained to patients and their family members.

Therapy with *Avandia*, like other thiazolidinediones, may result in ovulation in some premenopausal anovulatory women. As a result, these patients may be at an increased risk for pregnancy while taking *Avandia*. (See PRECAUTIONS, Pregnancy, Pregnancy Category C.) Thus, adequate contraception in premenopausal women should be recommended. This possible effect has not been specifically investigated in clinical studies so the frequency of this occurrence is not known.

Drug Interactions
Drugs Metabolized by Cytochrome P_{450}
In vitro drug metabolism studies suggest that rosiglitazone does not inhibit any of the major P_{450} enzymes at clinically relevant concentrations. *In vitro* data demonstrate that rosiglitazone is predominantly metabolized by CYP2C8, and to a lesser extent, 2C9.

Avandia (4 mg twice daily) was shown to have no clinically relevant effect on the pharmacokinetics of nifedipine and oral contraceptives (ethinylestradiol and norethindrone), which are predominantly metabolized by CYP3A4.

Glyburide: Avandia (2 mg twice daily) taken concomitantly with glyburide (3.75 to 10 mg/day) for 7 days did not alter the mean steady-state 24-hour plasma glucose concentrations in diabetic patients stabilized on glyburide therapy.

Metformin: Concurrent administration of *Avandia* (2 mg twice daily) and metformin (500 mg twice daily) in healthy volunteers for 4 days had no effect on the steady-state pharmacokinetics of either metformin or rosiglitazone.

Acarbose: Coadministration of acarbose (100 mg three times daily) for 7 days in healthy volunteers had no clinically relevant effect on the pharmacokinetics of a single oral dose of *Avandia*.

Digoxin: Repeat oral dosing of *Avandia* (8 mg once daily) for 14 days did not alter the steady-state pharmacokinetics of digoxin (0.375 mg once daily) in healthy volunteers.

Warfarin: Repeat dosing with *Avandia* had no clinically relevant effect on the steady-state pharmacokinetics of warfarin enantiomers.

Ethanol: A single administration of a moderate amount of alcohol did not increase the risk of acute hypoglycemia in type 2 diabetes mellitus patients treated with Avandia (rosiglitazone maleate).

Ranitidine: Pretreatment with ranitidine (150 mg twice daily for 4 days) did not alter the pharmacokinetics of either single oral or intravenous doses of rosiglitazone in healthy volunteers. These results suggest that the absorption of oral rosiglitazone is not altered in conditions accompanied by increases in gastrointestinal pH.

Carcinogenesis, Mutagenesis, Impairment of Fertility
Carcinogenesis: A 2-year carcinogenicity study was conducted in Charles River CD-1 mice at doses of 0.4, 1.5, and 6 mg/kg/day in the diet (highest dose equivalent to approximately 12 times human AUC at the maximum recommended human daily dose). Sprague-Dawley rats were dosed for 2 years by oral gavage at doses of 0.05, 0.3, and 2 mg/kg/day (highest dose equivalent to approximately 10 and 20 times human AUC at the maximum recommended human daily dose for male and female rats, respectively).

Rosiglitazone was not carcinogenic in the mouse. There was an increase in incidence of adipose hyperplasia in the mouse at doses ≥1.5 mg/kg/day (approximately 2 times human AUC at the maximum recommended human daily dose). In rats, there was a significant increase in the incidence of benign adipose tissue tumors (lipomas) at doses ≥0.3 mg/kg/day (approximately 2 times human AUC at the maximum recommended human daily dose). These proliferative changes in both species are considered due to the persistent pharmacological overstimulation of adipose tissue.

Mutagenesis: Rosiglitazone was not mutagenic or clastogenic in the *in vitro* bacterial assays for gene mutation, the *in vitro* chromosome aberration test in human lymphocytes, the *in vivo* mouse micronucleus test, and the *in vivo/in vitro* rat UDS assay. There was a small (about 2-fold) increase in mutation in the *in vitro* mouse lymphoma assay in the presence of metabolic activation.

Impairment of Fertility: Rosiglitazone had no effects on mating or fertility of
(continued)

Avandia® (rosiglitazone maleate) continued

male rats given up to 40 mg/kg/day (approximately 116 times human AUC at the maximum recommended human daily dose). Rosiglitazone altered estrous cyclicity (2 mg/kg/day) and reduced fertility (40 mg/kg/day) of female rats in association with lower plasma levels of progesterone and estradiol (approximately 20 and 200 times human AUC at the maximum recommended human daily dose, respectively). No such effects were noted at 0.2 mg/kg/day (approximately 3 times human AUC at the maximum recommended human daily dose). In monkeys, rosiglitazone (0.6 and 4.6 mg/kg/day; approximately 3 and 15 times human AUC at the maximum recommended human daily dose, respectively) diminished the follicular phase rise in serum estradiol with consequential reduction in the luteinizing hormone surge, lower luteal phase progesterone levels, and amenorrhea. The mechanism for these effects appears to be direct inhibition of ovarian steroidogenesis.

Animal Toxicology
Heart weights were increased in mice (3 mg/kg/day), rats (5 mg/kg/day), and dogs (2 mg/kg/day) with rosiglitazone treatments (approximately 5, 22, and 2 times human AUC at the maximum recommended human daily dose, respectively). Morphometric measurement indicated that there was hypertrophy in cardiac ventricular tissues, which may be due to increased heart work as a result of plasma volume expansion.

Pregnancy
Pregnancy Category C
There was no effect on implantation or the embryo with rosiglitazone treatment during early pregnancy in rats, but treatment during mid-late gestation was associated with fetal death and growth retardation in both rats and rabbits. Teratogenicity was not observed at doses up to 3 mg/kg in rats and 100 mg/kg in rabbits (approximately 20 and 75 times human AUC at the maximum recommended human daily dose, respectively). Rosiglitazone caused placental pathology in rats (3 mg/kg/day). Treatment of rats during gestation through lactation reduced litter size, neonatal viability, and postnatal growth, with growth retardation reversible after puberty. For effects on the placenta, embryo/fetus, and offspring, the no-effect dose was 0.2 mg/kg/day in rats and 15 mg/kg/day in rabbits. These no-effect levels are approximately 4 times human AUC at the maximum recommended human daily dose.

There are no adequate and well-controlled studies in pregnant women. Avandia (rosiglitazone maleate) should not be used during pregnancy unless the potential benefit justifies the potential risk to the fetus.

Because current information strongly suggests that abnormal blood glucose levels during pregnancy are associated with a higher incidence of congenital anomalies as well as increased neonatal morbidity and mortality, most experts recommend that insulin monotherapy be used during pregnancy to maintain blood glucose levels as close to normal as possible.

Labor and Delivery
The effect of rosiglitazone on labor and delivery in humans is not known.

Nursing Mothers
Drug related material was detected in milk from lactating rats. It is not known whether Avandia is excreted in human milk. Because many drugs are excreted in human milk, Avandia should not be administered to a nursing woman.

ADVERSE REACTIONS
In clinical trials, approximately 4600 patients with type 2 diabetes have been treated with Avandia; 3300 patients were treated for 6 months or longer and 2000 patients were treated for 12 months or longer.

Avandia Monotherapy and Oral Combination Therapy Studies
The incidence and types of adverse events reported in clinical trials of Avandia as monotherapy are shown in Table 6.

Table 6. Adverse Events (≥5% in Any Treatment Group) Reported by Patients in Double-blind Clinical Trials with Avandia as Monotherapy

Preferred Term	Avandia Monotherapy N = 2526 %	Placebo N = 601 %	Metformin N = 225 %	Sulfonylureas* N = 626 %
Upper respiratory tract infection	9.9	8.7	8.9	7.3
Injury	7.6	4.3	7.6	6.1
Headache	5.9	5.0	8.9	5.4
Back pain	4.0	3.8	4.0	5.0
Hyperglycemia	3.9	5.7	4.4	8.1
Fatigue	3.6	5.0	4.0	1.9
Sinusitis	3.2	4.5	5.3	3.0
Diarrhea	2.3	3.3	15.6	3.0
Hypoglycemia	0.6	0.2	1.3	5.9

*Includes patients receiving glyburide (N=514), gliclazide (N=91) or glipizide (N=21).

There were a small number of patients treated with Avandia who had adverse events of anemia and edema. Overall, these events were generally mild to moderate in severity and usually did not require discontinuation of treatment with Avandia.

In double-blind studies, anemia was reported in 1.9% of patients receiving Avandia compared to 0.7% on placebo, 0.6% on sulfonylureas and 2.2% on metformin. Edema was reported in 4.8% of patients receiving Avandia compared to 1.3% on placebo, 1.0% on sulfonylureas, and 2.2% on metformin. Overall, the types of adverse experiences reported when Avandia was used in combination with a sulfonylurea or metformin were similar to those during monotherapy with Avandia. Reports of anemia (7.1%) were greater in patients treated with a combination of Avandia and metformin compared to monotherapy with Avandia or in combination with a sulfonylurea.

Lower pre-treatment hemoglobin/hematocrit levels in patients enrolled in the metformin combination clinical trials may have contributed to the higher reporting rate of anemia in these studies (see Laboratory Abnormalities, Hematologic).

Laboratory Abnormalities
Hematologic: Decreases in mean hemoglobin and hematocrit occurred in a dose-related fashion in patients treated with Avandia (mean decreases in individual studies up to 1.0 gram/dL hemoglobin and up to 3.3% hematocrit). The time course and magnitude of decreases were similar in patients treated with a combination of Avandia and a sulfonylurea or metformin, or Avandia monotherapy. Pre-treatment levels of hemoglobin and hematocrit were lower in patients in metformin combination studies and may have contributed to the higher reporting rate of anemia. White blood cell counts also decreased slightly in patients treated with Avandia. Decreases in hematologic parameters may be related to increased plasma volume observed with treatment with Avandia.

Lipids: Changes in serum lipids have been observed following treatment with Avandia (see CLINICAL PHARMACOLOGY, Pharmacodynamics and Clinical Effects).

Serum Transaminase Levels: In clinical studies in 4598 patients treated with Avandia (rosiglitazone maleate) encompassing approximately 3600 patient years of exposure, there was no evidence of drug-induced hepatotoxicity or elevated ALT levels.

In controlled trials, 0.2% of patients treated with Avandia had reversible elevations in ALT >3X the upper limit of normal compared to 0.2% on placebo and 0.5% on active comparators. Hyperbilirubinemia was found in 0.3% of patients treated with Avandia compared with 0.9% treated with placebo and 1% in patients treated with active comparators.

In the clinical program including long-term, open-label experience, the rate per 100 patient years exposure of ALT increase to >3X the upper limit of normal was 0.35 for patients treated with Avandia, 0.59 for placebo-treated patients, and 0.78 for patients treated with active comparator agents.

In pre-approval clinical trials, there were no cases of idiosyncratic drug reactions leading to hepatic failure (See PRECAUTIONS, Hepatic Effects).

DOSAGE AND ADMINISTRATION
The management of antidiabetic therapy should be individualized. Avandia may be administered either at a starting dose of 4 mg as a single daily dose or divided and administered in the morning and evening. For patients who respond inadequately following 8 to 12 weeks of treatment, as determined by reduction in FPG, the dose may be increased to 8 mg daily as indicated below. Reductions in glycemic parameters by dose and regimen are described under CLINICAL PHARMACOLOGY, Clinical Studies. Avandia may be taken with or without food.

Monotherapy
The usual starting dose of Avandia is 4 mg administered either as a single dose once daily or in divided doses twice daily. In clinical trials, the 4 mg twice daily regimen resulted in the greatest reduction in FPG and HbA1c.

Combination Therapy with a Sulfonylurea or Metformin
When Avandia is added to existing therapy, the current dose of sulfonylurea or metformin can be continued upon initiation of Avandia therapy.

Sulfonylurea:
When used in combination with sulfonylurea, the recommended dose of Avandia is 4 mg administered as either a single dose once daily or in divided doses twice daily. If patients report hypoglycemia, the dose of the sulfonylurea should be decreased.

Metformin:
The usual starting dose of Avandia in combination with metformin is 4 mg administered as either a single dose once daily or in divided doses twice daily. It is unlikely that the dose of metformin will require adjustment due to hypoglycemia during combination therapy with Avandia.

Maximum Recommended Dose:
The dose of Avandia should not exceed 8 mg daily, as a single dose or divided twice daily. The 8 mg daily dose has been shown to be safe and effective in clinical studies as monotherapy and in combination with metformin. Doses of Avandia greater than 4 mg daily in combination with a sulfonylurea have not been studied in adequate and well-controlled clinical trials. In clinical trials, the 8 mg daily regimen resulted in the greatest reduction in FPG and HbA1c.

Avandia may be taken with or without food.

No dosage adjustments are required for the elderly.

No dosage adjustment is necessary when Avandia is used as monotherapy in patients with renal impairment. Since metformin is contraindicated in such patients, concomitant administration of metformin and Avandia is also contraindicated in patients with renal impairment.

Therapy with Avandia should not be initiated if the patient exhibits clinical evidence of active liver disease or increased serum transaminase levels (ALT >2.5X the upper limit of normal at start of therapy) (See PRECAUTIONS, Hepatic Effects and CLINICAL PHARMACOLOGY, Hepatic Impairment). Liver enzyme monitoring is recommended in all patients prior to initiation of therapy with Avandia and periodically thereafter (See PRECAUTIONS, Hepatic Effects).

There are no data on the use of Avandia in patients under 18 years of age; therefore, use of Avandia in pediatric patients is not recommended.

OVERDOSAGE
Limited data are available with regard to overdosage in humans. In clinical studies in volunteers, Avandia (rosiglitazone maleate) has been administered at single oral doses of up to 20 mg and was well-tolerated. In the event of an overdose, appropriate supportive treatment should be initiated as dictated by the patient's clinical status.

Appendix A

HOW SUPPLIED
Tablets: Each pentagonal film-coated Tiltab® tablet contains rosiglitazone as the maleate as follows: 2 mg–pink, debossed with SB on one side and 2 on the other; 4 mg–orange, debossed with SB on one side and 4 on the other; 8 mg–red-brown, debossed with SB on one side and 8 on the other.

2 mg bottles of 30: NDC 0029-3158-13
2 mg bottles of 60: NDC 0029-3158-18
2 mg bottles of 100: NDC 0029-3158-20
2 mg bottles of 500: NDC 0029-3158-25
2 mg SUP 100s: NDC 0029-3158-21

4 mg bottles of 30: NDC 0029-3159-13
4 mg bottles of 60: NDC 0029-3159-18
4 mg bottles of 100: NDC 0029-3159-20
4 mg bottles of 500: NDC 0029-3159-25
4 mg SUP 100s: NDC 0029-3159-21

8 mg bottles of 30: NDC 0029-3160-13
8 mg bottles of 100: NDC 0029-3160-20
8 mg bottles of 500: NDC 0029-3160-25
8 mg SUP 100s: NDC 0029-3160-21

STORAGE
Store at 25°C (77°F); excursions 15°–30°C (59°–86°F). Dispense in a tight, light-resistant container.

DATE OF ISSUANCE APR. 2000

©SmithKline Beecham, 2000

R_x only

SmithKline Beecham Pharmaceuticals
Philadelphia, PA 19101

AV:L3